NURSING DIAGNOSIS REFERENCE MANUAL

THIRD EDITION

NURSING DIAGNOSIS REFERENCE MANUAL

THIRD EDITION

Sheila M. Sparks, RN, DNSc, CS
Assistant Professor, School of Nursing
Georgetown University
Washington, D.C.

Cynthia M. Taylor, RN, MS, CS, CNAA
Independent Nurse Consultant
former Chief Operating Officer
Suburban Hospital
Bethesda, Md.

Springhouse Corporation
Springhouse, Pennsylvania

STAFF

Executive Director, Editorial
Stanley Loeb

Senior Publisher
Matthew Cahill

Art Director
John Hubbard

Senior Editor
Michael Shaw

Editors
Judd Howard, Richard Koreto

Copy Editors
Cynthia C. Breuninger (manager), Lewis Adams, Lynette High, Doris Weinstock

Designers
Stephanie Peters (associate art director), Maria Errico, Jackie B. Facciolo (cover illustration), Laurie Mirijanian

Typography
Diane Paluba (manager), Elizabeth Bergman, Joyce Rossi Biletz, Phyllis Marron, Robin Mayer, Valerie Rosenberger

Manufacturing
Deborah Meiris (director), Pat Dorshaw (manager), Anna Brindisi, T.A. Landis

Production Coordination
Patricia McCloskey

Editorial Assistants
Maree DeRosa, Beverly Lane, Mary Madden

Indexer
Janet Hodgson

The clinical procedures described and recommended in this publication are based on research and consultation with medical and nursing authorities. To the best of our knowledge, these procedures reflect currently accepted clinical practice; nevertheless, they can't be considered absolute and universal recommendations. For individual application, treatment recommendations must be considered in light of the patient's clinical condition and, before administration of new or infrequently used drugs, in light of latest package-insert information. The authors and the publisher disclaim responsibility for any adverse effects resulting directly or indirectly from the suggested procedures, from any undetected errors, or from the reader's misunderstanding of the text.

Printed in the United States of America.

DRM3-050797 ISBN 0-87434-728-9

A member of the Reed Elsevier plc group

Library of Congress Cataloging-in-Publication Data

Sparks, Sheila M.
Nursing diagnosis reference manual/Sheila M. Sparks, Cynthia M. Taylor.–3rd ed.
p. cm.
Includes bibliographical references and index.
1. Nursing–Handbooks, manuals, etc. I. Taylor, Cynthia M. II. Title
[DNLM: 1. Nursing Diagnosis–handbooks. 2. Patient Care planning–handbooks.
WY 39 S736n 1995]
RT51.S68 1995
610.73–dc20
DNLM/DLC 94-23141
ISBN 0-87434-728-9 CIP

CONTENTS

CONTRIBUTORS

SECTION EDITORS

Adult Health

Sheila M. Sparks, RN, DNSc, CS, Assistant Professor, School of Nursing, Georgetown University, Washington, D.C.

Janyce G. Dyer, RN, DNSc, CS, Assistant Professor, School of Nursing, University of Pittsburgh

Child Health

Carole Logan Kuhns, RN, MS, Assistant Professor, School of Nursing, Georgetown University, Washington, D.C.

Maternal-Neonatal Health

Lynne Hutnik Conrad, RN,C, MSN, Perinatal Clinical Nurse Specialist, Albert Einstein Medical Center, Philadelphia

Geriatric Health

Marjorie A. Maddox, RN, EdD, CANP, Associate Professor, School of Nursing, University of Louisville

CONTRIBUTORS

Rosemary G. Ambroseo, RN, BSN, Perinatal Nurse Specialist, Albert Einstein Medical Center, Philadelphia

Patricia Anasiewicz, RN, MSN, Clinical Nurse Specialist, Sacred Heart Hospital, Norristown, Pa.

Billie Dixon Barringer, RN, BSN, MA, Associate Professor, Northeast Louisiana University, Monroe, La.

Barbara Walsh Clark, RN, MSN, Professor of Nursing, Midway (Ky.) College

Christine B. Clark, RN, BSN, Head Nurse, MICU/CCU, Veterans Affairs Medical Center, Atlanta

Linda Carman Copel, RN,C, PhD, Assistant Professor, Villanova (Pa.) University

Mary Coyle-Green, RN, MSN, ARNP, Consultant, Southeastern Pain Clinic, Jacksonville, Fla.

Susan B. Dickey, RN,C, MSN, Assistant Professor, Temple University, Philadelphia

Jennifer Dooling, RN, Independent Nurse Consultant. Columbia, Mo.

Louama K. Driscoll, RN, MSN, Associate Chief, Nursing Service for Education, Veterans Affairs Medical Center, Ft. Lyon, Colo.

Teresa Eberhardt, RN, MS, Clinical Nurse Specialist, Francis Scott Key Medical Center, Baltimore

Nancy Endler, RN, MSN, Mental Health Nurse Specialist, Suburban Hospital, Bethesda, Md.

Susan Fitzgerald, RN, MBA, MS, Administrative Director, Cardiovascular Services, Suburban Hospital, Bethesda, Md.

Denise M. Fitzpatrick, RN,C, MSN, Perinatal Clinical Specialist-Educator, Holy Family College, Philadelphia

Laurel S. Garzon, RN, DNSc, PNP, Assistant Professor, School of Nursing, Old Dominion University, Norfolk, Va.

Pauline McKinney Green, RN, MSN, Assistant Professor, Howard University College of Nursing, Washington, D.C.

Kathleen J. Gutierrez, RN, PhD, CS, Associate Professor, Department of Nursing, Regis University, Denver

Betty Glenn Harris, RN, PhD, Assistant Professor, School of Nursing, University of North Carolina at Chapel Hill

Teri J. Harrison, RN, MSN, CDE, Pediatric Clinical Nurse Specialist, Methodist Hospital of Indiana, Inc., Indianapolis

Kathryn VanDyke Hayes, RN,C, MSN, Lecturer, Gwynedd-Mercy College, Gwynedd Valley, Pa.

Frances M. Johnson, RN, MSN, Assistant Chief, Community Health Nursing, Veterans Affairs Medical Center, Washington, D.C.

Darlene S. Jones, RN, BSN, Lt. Comdr., Nurse Corps, U.S. Navy, National Naval Medical Center, Bethesda, Md.

Karen Kelleher, RN, MS, Administrative Director, Mental Health Services, Suburban Hospital, Bethesda, Md.

Susan L.W. Krupnick, RN, MSN, CCRN, CS, Psychiatric Consultation Liaison Nurse, University of Pennsylvania Hospital, Philadelphia

Janice K. Lavoie, RN, MSN, Clinical Instructor, School of Nursing, Georgetown University; Staff Nurse, Surgical Intensive Care Unit, Georgetown University Medical Center, Washington, D.C.

Teresa Lien-Gieschen, RN,C, MS, GNP, Gerontology Clinical Nurse Specialist, Medical College of Virginia Hospitals, Richmond, Va.

Margaret Lunney, RN, PhD, Associate Professor, Hunter-Bellevue School of Nursing, Hunter College of the City University of New York

Maxine Maher, RN, BSN, Head Nurse, Nursing Home Care Unit, Veterans Affairs Medical Center, Atlanta

Cynthia McCormack, RN, MS, Nurse Recruiter, Department of Nursing, Veterans Affairs Medical Center, Denver

Anne McCormick, RN, MSN, Doctoral Candidate, The Catholic University of America, Washington, D.C.

Carolyn D. Moore, RN, BSN, CNOR, Clinical Instructor, Operating Room, The Arlington (Va.) Hospital

Vimala R. Philapose, RN PhD, Geriatric Nurse Consultant, Senior Health Care Services, Presbyterian-St. Luke's Medical Center, Denver

Devamma Purushotham, RN, DEd, Associate Professor, University of Windsor (Ont.), Canada

Kathleen Rhoades, RN, BSN, CCRN, Nurse Clinician IV, Critical Care Center, Suburban Hospital, Bethesda, Md.

Vanice W. Roberts, RN, DSN, Associate Professor of Nursing, Kennesaw State College, Marietta, Ga.

Patricia C. Seifert, RN, MSN, CNOR, Operating Room Coordinator, The Arlington (Va.) Hospital

Janice Ann Chaiken Sekelman, RN, DNSc, Associate Professor, Department of Nursing, College of Allied Health Sciences, Thomas Jefferson University, Philadelphia

Peggy Shedd, RN, MSN, CS, Psychiatric Liaison Clinical Nurse Specialist, Dartmouth-Hitchcock Medical Center, Hanover, N.H.

Kathleen C. Sheppard, RN, PhD, Director of Nursing, Continuity of Care, University of Texas M.D. Anderson Cancer Center, Houston

Carole J. Singer, RN, MSN, CS, Psychiatric Clinical Nurse Specialist, Private Health Care Systems Limited; Private Psychotherapy Practice, Sudbury, Mass.

Susan S. Thomason, RN, MN, CS, Clinical Nurse Specialist, Veterans Affairs Medical Center, Tampa, Fla.

Lynne Lear Tier, RN, MSN, Assistant Professor of Nursing, Manatee Community College, Bradenton, Fla.

Diane M. Wieland, RN, MSN, CS, Assistant Professor, Department of Nursing, College of Allied Health Sciences, Thomas Jefferson University, Philadelphia

Judith G. Winterhalter, RN, DNSc, Assistant Professor, Department of Nursing, College of Allied Health Sciences, Thomas Jefferson University, Philadelphia

Beryla Wolf, RN, PhD, Assistant Professor of Nursing, Department of Nursing, Regis University, Denver

Stephanie Wright, RN, PhD, Assistant Professor, School of Nursing, Georgetown University, Washington, D.C.

PREFACE

As nurses have come to realize, the nursing process is a powerful tool. It provides a framework for independent nursing action and promotes a consistent professional structure. What's more, it helps focus care on patients' actual needs. But how do you go about using the nursing process – actually applying it to patient care in a helpful, systematic, and efficient way? And how do you modify the nursing process to reflect the needs of different patients?

Well, now you have the answers to these and other questions at your fingertips with the *Nursing Diagnosis Reference Manual, Third Edition.* Incorporating all diagnoses approved by the North American Nursing Diagnosis Association (NANDA), this manual explains clearly and concisely how to apply the nursing process to patient care. It focuses on health problems that you diagnose legally and treat independently.

The manual begins with an explanation of each step of the nursing process – assessment, nursing diagnosis, outcome identification, planning, implementation, and evaluation. Included in this introductory section are clear guidelines for writing a clinically accurate diagnostic statement. This section also clarifies the distinction between a nursing diagnosis and a medical diagnosis.

After this section come the manual's five major parts: adult health, adolescent health, child health, maternal-neonatal health, and geriatric health. Together, these parts include comprehensive plans of care for 284 nursing diagnostic statements. Each plan of care has been written and reviewed by leading nursing clinicians, educators, and researchers. Each one is complete and can be used independently to avoid excessive cross-referencing.

Each plan of care uses a consistent format containing the following sections:

- *Diagnostic statement.* Each diagnostic statement includes a NANDA-approved label and, in most cases, a related etiology. This edition of the *Nursing Diagnosis Reference Manual* contains all the diagnostic labels approved by NANDA.
- *Definition.* This section offers a brief explanation of the diagnosis.
- *Assessment.* This section suggests parameters to use when collecting data to validate the diagnosis. Data may include health history, physical findings, psychosocial status, laboratory studies, patient statements, and other subjective and objective information.
- *Defining characteristics.* This section lists clinical findings that when grouped together confirm the diagnosis. For diagnoses expressing the possibility of a problem, such as "High risk for injury," this section is labeled *Risk factors.*
- *Associated medical diagnoses.* Here you'll find examples of medical problems that commonly relate to the nursing diagnosis.
- *Expected outcomes.* Here you'll find realistic goals for resolving or ameliorating the patient's health problem, written in measurable behavioral terms.

• *Interventions and rationales.* This section provides specific activities you can carry out to help attain expected outcomes. Each intervention contains a rationale, highlighted in *italic* type. Rationales receive typographic emphasis because they form the premise for every nursing action. You'll find it helpful to consider rationales before intervening. Understanding them can make repetitive or difficult interventions more interesting. And more important, it can improve critical thinking and help avoid mistakes.
• *Evaluations for expected outcomes.* Here you'll find evaluation criteria for the expected outcomes. These criteria will help you determine whether expected outcomes have been attained.
• *Documentation.* This section lists critical topics to include in your documentation—for example, patient perceptions, status, and response to treatment as well as nursing observations and interventions. Using the information provided in this section will enable you to write the careful, concise documentation required to meet professional nursing standards.

The manual includes several appendices that will help you select appropriate nursing diagnoses for virtually every clinical situation. The largest appendix lists nursing diagnoses for specific medical diagnoses. Other appendices group diagnoses by Gordon's functional health patterns, Maslow's hierarchy of needs, Orem's universal self-care demands, and Saba's home health care classification system.

As the nursing profession continues to advance, strengthening the nursing process remains an important challenge. We believe that the *Nursing Diagnosis Reference Manual, Third Edition,* will help both students and practicing nurses meet this challenge.

We would like to express our sincere appreciation to the nurses who contributed to the *Nursing Diagnosis Reference Manual, Third Edition.* Their expertise and commitment to quality patient care made this work possible. The section editors deserve special thanks for selecting excellent contributors and for writing, editing, and critiquing care plans.

We also extend special thanks to the Springhouse editorial staff—in particular, Michael Shaw, for his patience, good humor, and perseverance in helping us to complete what often seemed to be an insurmountable task. Thanks are also due to our typists, Gil Taylor and Greg Agostinelli, who proved themselves especially talented and made order out of chaos.

Finally, we dedicate this book to our nursing students and colleagues, who challenge us to think and work creatively.

Sheila M. Sparks, RN, DNSc, CS
Cynthia M. Taylor, RN, MS, CS, CNAA

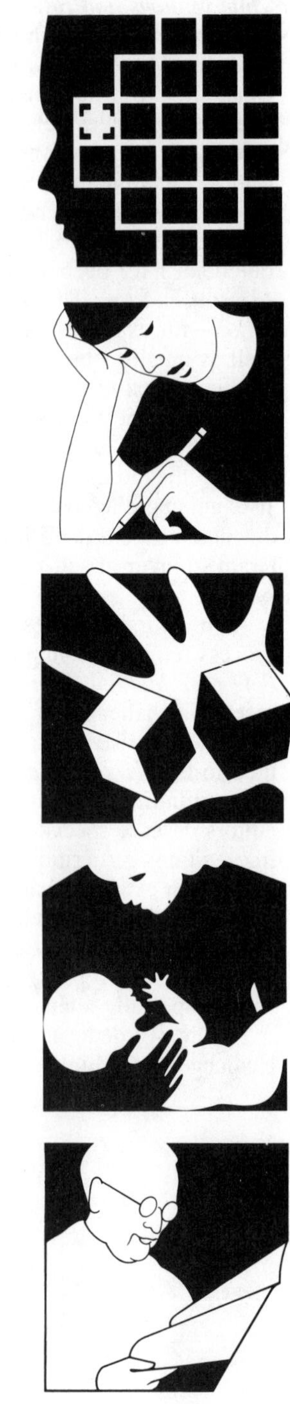

THE NURSING PROCESS

The cornerstone of clinical nursing, the nursing process is a systematic method for taking independent nursing action. Steps in the nursing process include:
- assessing the patient's problems
- forming a diagnostic statement
- identifying expected outcomes
- making a plan to achieve expected outcomes and solve the patient's problems
- implementing the plan or assigning others to implement it
- evaluating the plan's effectiveness.

The phases of the nursing process—assessment, nursing diagnosis, outcome identification, planning, implementation, and evaluation—are dynamic and flexible; they often overlap.

Becoming familiar with this process has many benefits. It will allow you to apply your knowledge and skills in an organized, goal-oriented manner. It will also enable you to communicate about professional topics with colleagues from all clinical specialties and practice settings.

The growing recognition of the nursing process is an important development in the struggle for greater professional autonomy. By clearly defining problems a nurse may treat independently, the nursing process has helped to dispel the notion that nursing practice is based solely on carrying out doctor's orders.

Despite recent advances, nursing is still in an embryonic state of professional evolution. In the years ahead, researchers and expert practitioners will continue to develop a body of knowledge specific to the field. A strong foundation in the nursing process will enable you to better assimilate emerging concepts and to incorporate these concepts into your practice (see *Nursing's approach to problem solving,* page 2).

ASSESSMENT

The vital first phase in the nursing process, assessment consists of the patient history, the physical examination, and laboratory studies. The other nursing process phases—nursing diagnosis formation, outcome identification, care planning, implementation, and evaluation—depend on the quality of the assessment data for their effectiveness.

A properly recorded initial assessment provides:
- a way to communicate patient information to other caregivers
- a method of documenting initial baseline data
- a foundation on which to build an effective plan of care.

Your initial patient assessment begins with the collection of data (patient history, physical examination findings, laboratory data) and ends with a statement of the patient's actual or potential problem—the nursing diagnosis.

Nursing's approach to problem solving

Dynamic and flexible, the phases of the nursing process resemble the steps that many other professions rely on to identify and correct problems. Here's how the nursing process phases correspond to the standard problem-solving method.

NURSING PROCESS	PROBLEM-SOLVING METHOD
Assessment • Collect and analyze subjective and objective data about the patient's health problem.	• Recognize that a problem exists. • Learn about the problem by obtaining facts.
Diagnosis • State the health problems.	• State the nature of the problem.
Outcome identification • Identify expected outcomes.	• Establish goals and a time frame for achieving them.
Planning • Write a plan of care that includes the nursing interventions designed to achieve expected outcomes.	• Think of and select ways to achieve goals and solve the problem.
Implementation • Put the plan of care into action. • Document the actions taken and their results.	• Act on ways to solve the problem.
Evaluation • Critically examine the results achieved. • Review and revise the plan of care as needed.	• Decide if the actions taken have effectively solved the problem.

Building a data base

The information you collect in taking your patient's history, performing a physical examination, and analyzing laboratory test results serves as your assessment data base. Your goal is to gather and record information that will be most helpful in assessing your patient. You can't collect or use *all* the information that exists about your patient. To limit your data base appropriately, ask yourself these questions: What data do I want to collect? How should I collect the information? How should I organize it to make care planning decisions?

Your answers will help you to be selective in collecting meaningful data during patient assessment.

The well-defined data base for a patient may begin with admission signs and symptoms, chief complaint, or medical diagnosis. It also may center on the type of patient care given in a specific nursing unit, such as the intensive care unit or the emergency department (ED). For example, you wouldn't ask a trauma victim in the ED if she has a family history of breast cancer, nor would you perform a routine breast examination on her. You would, however, do these types of assessment during a comprehensive health checkup in an ambulatory care setting.

If you work in a setting where patients with similar diagnoses are treated, choose your data base from information pertinent to this specific patient population.

Subjective and objective data

The assessment data you collect and analyze fall into two important categories, subjective and objective.

The patient's history, embodying a *personal perspective* of problems, provides **subjective data.** It's your most important assessment data source. But because it's also the most subjective source of patient information, it must be interpreted carefully.

In the *physical examination* of a patient—involving inspection, palpation, percussion, and auscultation—you collect **objective data** about your patient's health status or about the pathologic processes that may be related to his illness or injury. Besides adding to your patient data base, this information helps you interpret the patient's history more accurately by providing a basis for comparison. Use it to validate and amplify the historical data. However, don't allow the physical examination of your patient to assume undue importance.

The most objective form of assessment data, *laboratory test results* provide another source for interpreting your history and physical examination findings. The advanced technology used in laboratory tests enables you to assess anatomic, physiologic, and chemical processes that neither your senses nor your patient's are capable of measuring. For example, if your patient complains of feeling tired (history) and you observe conjunctival pallor (physical examination), check his hemoglobin and hematocrit levels (laboratory data).

You need both subjective and objective data for comprehensive patient assessment. They validate each other and together provide more data than either could provide alone.

Consider all three types of assessment information—history, physical examination, and laboratory data—in their appropriate relationships to one another. Performing an accurate physical examination requires technical skill that in itself is valuable. It becomes even more valuable, however, when you place the examination findings in perspective as one aspect of total patient assessment.

Taking a complete health history

This portion of the assessment consists of the subjective data you collect from the patient. Use your interviewing skills to help the patient describe biological, social, and psychological responses to the particular anatomic, physiologic, and chemical processes involved in his illness or injury. In addition, the patient may recall events in his own life or in relatives' lives that may indicate an increased risk for certain pathologic processes.

A complete health history provides the following information about a patient:
- biographical data
- chief complaint (or concern)
- history of present illness (or current health status)
- past history
- family history
- psychosocial history
- activities of daily living
- review of systems.

Follow this orderly format in taking your patient's history, but allow for modifications based on your patient's chief complaint or concern. For example, the health history of a patient with a localized allergic reaction will be much shorter than that of a patient who complains vaguely of mental confusion and severe headaches.

If your patient has a chief complaint, use information from your health history to decide if his problems stem from physiologic causes or psychophysiologic maladaptation and how your nursing interventions may help. The depth of such a history depends on the patient's cooperation and your skill in asking insightful questions.

A patient who requests a complete physical checkup may not even have a chief complaint. Such a patient's health history would be comprehensive, with detailed information about life-style, self-image, family and other interpersonal relationships, and degree of satisfaction with current health status.

Be sure to record health history data in an organized fashion so that the information will be meaningful to everyone involved in a patient's care. Some hospitals provide patient questionnaires or computerized checklists (see *Using an assessment checklist*). These forms make history taking easier, but they're not always available. Therefore, you must know how to take a comprehensive health history without them. This is easy to do if you develop an orderly and systematic method of interviewing. Ask the history questions in the same order every time. With experience, you'll know which types of questions to ask in specific patient situations.

Review of systems

When interviewing the patient, use this review of systems as a guide.

General: overall state of health, ability to carry out activities of daily living, weight changes, fatigue, exercise tolerance, fever, night sweats, repeated infections

Skin: changes in color, pigmentation, temperature, moisture, or hair distribution; eruptions; pruritus; scaling; bruising; bleeding; dryness; excessive oiliness; growths; moles; scars; rashes; scalp lesions; brittle, soft, or abnormally formed nails; cyanotic nail beds; pressure ulcers

Head: trauma, lumps, alopecia, headaches

Eyes: nearsightedness, farsightedness, glaucoma, cataracts, blurred vision, double vision, tearing, burning, itching, photophobia, pain, inflammation, swelling, color blindness, injuries (also ask about use of glasses or contact lenses and date of last eye examination)

Using an assessment checklist

To make sure you cover all key points during your health history interview, you may use an assessment checklist, such as the one shown below. Though the format of such guides may vary from one institution to another, all guides include the same key elements.

☐ *Reason for hospitalization or chief complaint:* As patient sees it.
☐ *Duration of this problem:* As patient recalls it. Has it affected patient's life-style?
☐ *Other illnesses and previous experience with hospitalization:* Reason? When? Results? Impressions of previous hospitalizations? Problems encountered? Effect of this hospitalization on education? Family? Child care? Employment? Finances?
☐ *Observation of patient's condition:* Level of consciousness? Well-nourished? Healthy? Color? Skin turgor? Senses? Headaches? Cough? Syncope? Nausea? Seizures? Edema? Lumps? Bruises or bleeding? Inflammation? Integrity of skin? Pressure areas? Temperature? Range of motion? Unusual sensations? Paralysis? Odors? Discharges? Pain?
☐ *Mental and emotional status:* Cooperative? Understanding? Anxious? Language? Expectations? Feelings about illness? State of consciousness? Mood? Self-image? Reaction to stress? Rapport with interviewer and staff? Compatibility with roommate?
☐ *Review of systems:* Neurologic, EENT, Pulmonary, Cardiovascular, GI, GU, Skin, Reproductive, Musculoskeletal, and so forth.
☐ *Allergies:* Food? Drugs? Type of reaction?
☐ *Medication:* Dosage? Why taken? When taken? Last dose? Does he have it with him? Any others taken occasionally? Recently? Why? Ask about over-the-counter drugs, cough preparations, and use of alcohol or illegal drugs.
☐ *Prostheses:* Pacemaker? Intermittent positive-pressure breathing unit? Tracheostomy tube? Drainage tubes? Feeding tube? Catheter? Ostomy appliance? Breast form? Hearing aid? Glasses or contacts? Dentures? Cane? Walker? Brace? False eye? Prosthetic leg? Does the patient have the device with him? Need anything?
☐ *Hygiene patterns:* Dentures? Gums? Teeth? Bath or shower? When?
☐ *Rest and sleep patterns:* Usual times? Aids? Difficulties?
☐ *Activity status:* Self-care? Ambulatory? Aids? Daily exercise?
☐ *Bladder and bowel patterns:* Continent? Frequency? Nocturia? Characteristics of stool and urine? Discharge? Pain? Ostomy? Appliances? Who cares for these? Laxatives? Medications?
☐ *Meals and diet:* Feeds self? Diet restrictions (therapeutic and cultural or preferential)? Frequency? Snacks? Allergies? Dislikes? Fad diets? Usual dietary intake?
☐ *Health practices:* Breast self-examination? Physical examination? Pap smear? Testicular self-examination? Digital rectal examination? Smoking? ECG? Annual chest X-ray? Practices related to other conditions, such as glaucoma testing, urine testing, weight control?
☐ *Life-style:* Parent? Family? Number of children? Residence? Occupation? Recreation? Diversion? Interests? Financial status? Religion? Education? Ethnic background? Living environment?
☐ *Typical day profile:* Have patient describe.
☐ *Informant:* From whom did you obtain this information? Patient? Family? Old records? Ambulance driver?

Ears: deafness, tinnitus, vertigo, discharge, pain, tenderness behind the ears, mastoiditis, otitis or other ear infections, earaches, ear surgery
Nose: sinusitis, discharge, colds, or coryza more than four times a year; rhinitis; trauma; sneezing; loss of sense of smell; obstruction; breathing problems; epistaxis
Mouth and throat: changes in color or sores on tongue, dental caries, loss of teeth, toothaches, bleeding gums, lesions, loss of taste, hoarseness, sore throats (streptococcal), tonsillitis, voice changes, dysphagia, date of last dental checkup, use of dentures, bridges, or dental appliances
Neck: pain, stiffness, swelling, limited movement
Breasts: change in development or lactation pattern, trauma, lumps, pain, discharge from nipples, gynecomastia, changes in contour or in nipples, history of breast cancer (also ask if the patient knows how to perform breast self-examination)
Cardiovascular: palpitations, tachycardia, or other rhythm irregularities; pain in chest; dyspnea on exertion; orthopnea; cyanosis; edema; ascites; intermittent claudication; cold extremities; phlebitis; postural hypotension; hypertension; rheumatic fever (also ask if an electrocardiogram has been performed recently)
Respiratory: dyspnea, shortness of breath, pain, wheezing, paroxysmal nocturnal dyspnea, orthopnea (number of pillows used), cough, sputum, hemoptysis, night sweats, emphysema, pleurisy, bronchitis, tuberculosis (contacts), pneumonia, asthma, upper respiratory tract infections (also ask about results of chest X-ray and tuberculin skin test)
Gastrointestinal: changes in appetite or weight, dysphagia, nausea, vomiting, heartburn, eructation, flatulence, abdominal pain, colic, hematemesis, jaundice (pain, fever, intensity, duration, color of urine), stools (color, frequency, consistency, odor, use of laxatives), hemorrhoids, rectal bleeding, changes in bowel habits
Renal, genitourinary: color of urine, polyuria, oliguria, nocturia (number of times per night), dysuria, frequency, urgency, problem with stream, dribbling, pyuria, retention, passage of stones or gravel, venereal disease (discharge), infections, perineal rashes and irritations (also ask if protein or sugar has ever been found in urine)
Reproductive: male—lesions, impotence, prostate problems (also ask about use of contraceptives); **female**—irregular bleeding, discharge, pruritus, pain on intercourse, protrusions, dysmenorrhea, vaginal infections (also ask about number of pregnancies; delivery dates; complications; abortions; onset, regularity, and amount of flow during menarche; last normal period; use of contraceptives; date of menopause; last Pap test)
Neurologic: headaches, seizures, fainting spells, dizziness, tremors, twitches, aphasia, loss of sensation, weakness, paralysis, numbness, tingling, balance problems
Psychiatric: changes in mood, anxiety, depression, inability to concentrate, phobias, suicidal or homicidal thoughts, hallucinations, delusions
Musculoskeletal: muscle pain, swelling, redness, pain in joints, back problems, injuries (such as broken bones, pulled tendons), gait problems, weakness, paralysis, deformities, limited motion, contractures

Hematopoietic: anemia (type, degree, treatment, response), bleeding, fatigue, bruising (also ask if patient is receiving anticoagulant therapy)
Endocrine, metabolic: polyuria, polydipsia, polyphagia, thyroid problem, heat or cold intolerance, excessive sweating, changes in hair distribution and amount, nervousness, swollen neck (goiter), moon face, buffalo hump

When documenting the health history, be sure to record negative findings as well as positive ones. Note the absence of symptoms that other history data indicate could be present. For example, if a patient reports pain and burning in his abdomen, ask him if he has experienced nausea and vomiting or noticed blood in his stools. Record the presence *or* absence of these symptoms.

Also remember that the information will be used by others who'll also care for the patient. It could even be used as a legal document in a liability case, a malpractice suit, or an insurance disability claim. With these considerations in mind, record history data thoroughly and precisely. Continue your questioning until you're satisfied that you've recorded sufficient detail. Don't be satisfied with inadequate answers, such as "a lot" or "a little." These words mean different things to different people and must be explained to be meaningful. If taking notes seems to make the patient anxious, explain the importance of keeping a written record. To facilitate accurate recording of your patient's answers, familiarize yourself with standard history data abbreviations.

Once you complete your patient's health history, it becomes part of the permanent written record. It will serve as a subjective data base with which you and other health care professionals can monitor the patient's progress. Remember that history data must be specific and precise. Avoid generalities. Instead, provide pertinent, concise, detailed information that will help determine the direction and sequence of the physical examination—the next phase in your patient assessment.

Physical examination

After taking your patient's health history, the next step in the assessment process is the *physical examination.* During this assessment phase, you obtain objective data that usually confirm or rule out suspicions raised during the health history interview.

You use four basic techniques to perform a physical examination: *inspection, palpation, percussion,* and *auscultation* (IPPA). These skills require you to use your senses of sight, hearing, touch, and smell—all necessary for an accurate appraisal of the structures and functions of body systems. If, after much careful study and practice, you learn to use IPPA skills effectively, you'll be less likely to overlook something important during the physical examination. In addition, each examination technique collects data that validate and amplify data collected through other IPPA techniques.

Accurate and complete physical assessments depend on two interrelated elements. One is the critical act of sensory perception, by which you receive and perceive external stimuli. The other element is the conceptual, or cognitive, process by which you relate these stimuli to your knowledge base. This two-step process gives meaning to your assessment data.

You need to develop a system for assessing patients that identifies their problem areas in priority order. By performing physical assessments systematically and efficiently instead of in a random or indiscriminate manner, you'll save time and identify priority problems quickly.

Choosing an examination method. The most commonly used methods for completing a total systematic physical assessment are *head to toe* and *major body systems.*

Using the head-to-toe method, you systematically assess your patient—as the name suggests—beginning at the head and working toward the toes. Examine all parts of one body region before progressing to the next region to save time and energy for yourself and your patient. Proceed from left to right within each region so that you can make symmetrical comparisons. Don't examine the patient's left side from head to toe, then his right side.

The major-body-systems method involves systematically assessing your patient by examining each body system in priority order or in a predesignated sequence.

Both the head-to-toe and the major-body-systems methods are systematic and provide a logical, organized framework for collecting physical assessment data. They also provide the same information; therefore, neither is more correct than the other. So choose the method (or a variation of it) that works well for you and is appropriate for your patient population. Follow this routine whenever you assess a patient and try not to deviate from it.

To decide which method to use, first determine whether the patient's condition is life-threatening. Identifying the *priority* problems of a patient suffering from a life-threatening illness or injury—for example, severe trauma, a heart attack, or GI hemorrhage—is essential to preserve his life and function and to prevent compounded damage.

Next, identify the *patient population* to which the patient belongs, and take the common characteristics of that population into account in choosing an examination method. For example, elderly or debilitated patients tire easily; for a patient in either category, you'd select a method that necessitates minimal position changes. Also, you'd probably defer parts of the examination to avoid tiring your patient.

Try to view your patient as an integrated whole rather than as a collection of parts, regardless of the examination method you use. Remember, the integrity of a body *region* may reflect adequate functioning of many body *systems,* both inside and outside this particular region. For example, the integrity of the chest region may provide important clues about the functioning of the cardiovascular and respiratory systems. Similarly, the integrity of a body *system* may reflect adequate functioning of many body *regions* and of the various systems within these regions.

The chief complaint. You may want to plan your physical examination around your patient's chief complaint or concern. To do this, begin by examining the body system or region that corresponds to the chief complaint. This allows you to identify priority problems promptly and reassures your patient that you are paying attention to his primary reason for seeking health care.

Consider the following example. Your patient, Sarah Clemson, is a 65-year-old, active, well-nourished woman who appears younger than her chronologic age. She complains of having difficulty breathing on exertion; she also has a dry, frequent, painful cough. Intermittent chills have persisted for 3 days. First, you'd record her vital signs: temperature, 103° F (39.4° C); pulse rate, 106 beats/minute; respiratory rate, 29 to 30 breaths/minute; blood pressure, 128/82 mm Hg.

Because Mrs. Clemson's chief complaints are difficulty breathing, a cough, and chills, your physical examination would initially focus on her *respiratory system.* You'd examine the patency of her airways, observe the color of her lips and extremities, and systematically palpate her lung fields for symmetry of expansion, crepitus, increased or decreased fremitus, and areas of tenderness. Then, after auscultating her lung fields for abnormal or adventitious sounds (such as crackles, rhonchi, or wheezing), you'd percuss her lung fields for increased or decreased resonance.

Next, you'd examine Mrs. Clemson's *cardiovascular system,* looking for further clues to the cause of her signs and symptoms. You'd inspect her neck veins for distention and her extremities for edema, venous engorgement, and pigmented areas. Then, you'd palpate her chest to see if you could feel the heart's apical impulse at the fifth intercostal space, in the midclavicular line. You'd also palpate for a precordial heave and for valvular thrills. After determining her apical pulse rate, you'd auscultate for any abnormal heart sounds.

At this point in the examination, you would probably be aware of Mrs. Clemson's level of consciousness, motor ability, and ability to use her muscles and joints. You probably wouldn't need to perform a more thorough musculoskeletal or neurologic examination. You would, however, proceed with an examination of her GI, genitourinary, and integumentary systems, modifying the examination sequence depending on your findings and Mrs. Clemson's tolerance. If her signs and symptoms worsened during the examination, you'd interrupt the procedure to report her condition to her doctor. Then you'd plan to come back and finish the examination after her condition had stabilized.

Documenting physical examination findings. Physical examination findings are crucial to arriving at a nursing diagnosis and, ultimately, to developing a sound nursing plan of care. Record your examination results thoroughly, accurately, and clearly.

Although some examiners don't like to use a printed form to record physical assessment findings, preferring to work with a blank paper, others believe that standardized data collection forms can make recording physical examination results easier. These forms simplify comprehensive data collection and documentation by providing a concise format for outlining and recording pertinent information. They also remind you to include all essential assessment data.

When documenting, describe exactly what you've inspected, palpated, percussed, or auscultated. Don't use general terms, such as *normal, abnormal, good,* or *poor.* Instead, be specific. Include positive and negative findings. Try to document as soon as possible after completing your assessment. Remember that abbreviations aid conciseness (see *Documentation tips,* page 10).

Documentation tips

Remember these rules about documenting your initial assessment.

- Always document your findings as soon as possible after you take the health history and perform the physical examination.
- Always document your assessment *away* from the patient's bedside. Jot down only key points while you're with the patient.
- Always answer every question on the assessment form if you're using one. If a question doesn't apply to your patient, write "N/A" or "not applicable" in the space.
- Always focus your questions on areas that relate to the patient's chief complaint. Record information that has significance and will help you build a plan of care.
- If you delegate the job of filling out the first section of the form to another nurse or an aide, remember—you *must* review the information gathered and validate it if you're not sure it's correct.
- Always accept accountability for your assessment by signing your name to the areas you've completed.
- Always directly quote the patient or family member who gave you the information if you fear that summarizing will make it lose some of its meaning.
- Always write or print legibly, in ink.
- Always be concise, specific, and exact when you describe your physical findings.
- Always go back to the patient's bedside to clarify or validate information that seems incomplete.

NURSING DIAGNOSIS

According to the North American Nursing Diagnosis Association (NANDA), the nursing diagnosis is a "clinical judgment about individual, family, or community responses to actual or potential health problems or to life processes. Nursing diagnoses provide the basis for selection of nursing interventions to achieve outcomes for which the nurse is accountable." The nursing diagnosis must be supported by clinical information obtained during patient assessment (see *Nursing diagnoses and the nursing process*).

Each nursing diagnosis describes a patient problem that a nurse can legally manage. Becoming familiar with nursing diagnoses will enable you to better understand how nursing practice is distinct from medical practice. Though the identification of problems commonly overlaps in nursing and medicine, the approach to treatment clearly differs. Medicine focuses on curing disease; nursing focuses on holistic care that includes cure and comfort. Nurses can independently diagnose and treat the patient's response to illness, certain health problems, and the need for patient education. Nurses comfort, counsel, and care for patients and their families until they are physically and emotionally ready to provide self-care.

Developing your diagnosis

The nursing diagnosis expresses your professional judgment of the patient's clinical status, responses to treatment, and nursing care needs. You perform this step so that you can develop your plan of care. In effect, the nursing diagnosis *defines* the practice of nursing. Translating the history, physical examination, and laboratory data about a patient into a nursing diagnosis involves organizing the data into clusters and interpreting what the clusters reveal about your patient's ability to meet basic needs. In addition to identifying the patient's needs in coping with the effects of illness, consider what assistance the patient requires to grow and develop to the fullest extent possible.

Your nursing diagnosis describes the cluster of signs and symptoms indicating an actual or potential (high risk) health problem that you can identify—and that your care can resolve.

Creating your nursing diagnosis is a logical extension of collecting assessment data. In your patient assessment, you asked each history question, performed each physical examination technique, and considered each laboratory test result because it provided evidence of how your patient could be helped by your care or because the data could affect nursing care.

To develop the nursing diagnosis, use the assessment data you've collected to develop a problem list. Less formal in structure than a fully developed nursing diagnosis, this list describes your patient's problems or needs. It's easy to generate such a list if you use a conceptual model or an accepted set of criterion norms. Examples of such norms include normal physical and psychological development, Maslow's hierarchy of needs, and Gordon's functional health patterns (see appendices, pages 591-597).

You can identify the patient's problems and needs with such simple phrases as poor circulation, high fever, or poor hydration. Next, prioritize the problems on the list and then develop the working nursing diagnosis.

Nursing diagnoses and the nursing process

When first described, the nursing process included only assessment, planning, implementation, and evaluation. However, during the past two decades, several important events have helped to establish diagnosis as a distinct part of the nursing process.

- The American Nurses' Association, in its 1973 publication *Standards of Nursing Practice,* mentioned nursing diagnosis as a separate and definable act performed by the registered nurse. In 1991, the ANA published its revised standards of clinical practice, which continued to list nursing diagnosis as a distinct step of the nursing process.
- Individual states passed nurse practice acts that listed diagnosis as part of the nurse's legal responsibility.
- In 1973, the North American Nursing Diagnosis Association (NANDA) began a formal effort to classify nursing diagnoses. NANDA continues to meet biennially to review proposed new nursing diagnoses and examine applications of nursing diagnoses in clinical practice, education, and research. Their most recent meeting was held in March 1994 in Nashville. NANDA also publishes *Taxonomy*—a classification system for nursing diagnoses based on human response patterns. Currently, members of NANDA are working in cooperation with the International Council of Nurses to develop a version of the taxonomy for inclusion in the International Classification of Diseases.
- In 1991, the Joint Commission on Accreditation of Healthcare Organizations (JCAHO) incorporated the concept of nursing diagnosis into its revised standards for nursing care. The JCAHO now requires that each patient's care be based on nursing diagnoses that have been made by a registered nurse.

Writing a nursing diagnosis

Some nurses are confused about how to document a nursing diagnosis because they think the language is too complex. But by remembering these basic guidelines, you can ensure that your diagnostic statement is correct:

- Use proper terminology that reflects the patient's *nursing* needs.
- Make your statement concise so that it's easily understood by other health team members.
- Use the most precise words possible.
- Use a problem-cause format, stating the problem and its related cause.

Whenever possible, use terminology recommended by NANDA. NANDA diagnostic headings, when combined with suspected etiology, provide a clear picture of the patient's needs. Thus, for clarity in charting, start with one of the NANDA categories as a heading for the diagnostic statement. The category can reflect an actual or potential problem. Consider this sample diagnosis:

Heading: Mobility impairment
Etiology: Related to pain and discomfort following surgery
Signs and symptoms: "I can't walk without help." Patient has not ambulated since surgery on (give date and time). Range of motion limited to 10 degrees flexion in the right hip. Patient can't walk 3′ (1 m) from the bed to the chair without the help of two nurses.

This format links the patient's problem to the etiology without stating a direct cause-and-effect relationship (which may be hard to prove). Remember to state only the patient's problems and the probable origin. Omit references to possible solutions. (Your solutions will derive from your nursing diagnosis, but they aren't part of it.)

Avoiding common errors

One major pitfall in developing a nursing diagnosis is writing one that nursing interventions can't treat. Errors can also occur when nurses take shortcuts in the nursing process, either by omitting or hurrying through assessment or by basing the diagnosis on inaccurate assessment data.

Keep in mind that a nursing diagnosis is a statement of a health problem that a nurse is licensed to treat—a problem for which you'll assume responsibility for therapeutic decisions and accountability for the outcomes. A nursing diagnosis is *not:*

- a diagnostic test ("schedule for cardiac angiography")
- a piece of equipment ("set up intermittent suction apparatus")
- a problem with equipment ("the patient has trouble using a commode")
- a nurse's problem with a patient ("Mr. Jones is a difficult patient; he's rude and won't take his medication")
- a nursing goal ("encourage fluids up to 2,000 ml per day")
- a nursing need ("I have to get through to the family that they must accept their father's dying")
- a medical diagnosis ("cervical cancer") or treatment ("catheterize after each voiding for residual urine").

At first, these distinctions may not be clear. The following examples should help clarify what a nursing diagnosis is:

- Don't state a need instead of a problem.

Incorrect: *Fluid replacement related to fever*
Correct: *Fluid volume deficit related to fever*

- Don't reverse the two parts of the statement.
  Incorrect: *Lack of understanding related to noncompliance with diabetic diet*
  Correct: *Noncompliance with diabetic diet related to lack of understanding*
- Don't identify an untreatable condition instead of the actual problem it indicates (which can be treated).
  Incorrect: *Inability to speak related to laryngectomy*
  Correct: *Social isolation related to inability to speak because of laryngectomy*
- Don't write a legally inadvisable statement.
  Incorrect: *Red sacrum related to improper positioning*
  Correct: *Skin integrity impairment related to immobility*
- Don't identify as unhealthful a response that would be appropriate, allowed for, or culturally acceptable.
  Incorrect: *Anger related to terminal illness*
  Correct: *Ineffective management of therapeutic regimen related to anger over terminal illness*
- Don't make a tautological statement (one in which both parts of the statement say the same thing).
  Incorrect: *Pain related to alteration in comfort*
  Correct: *Pain related to postoperative abdominal distention and anxiety*
- Don't identify a nursing problem instead of a patient problem.
  Incorrect: *Difficulty suctioning related to thick secretions*
  Correct: *Ineffective airway clearance related to thick tracheal secretions.*

How nursing and medical diagnoses differ

You assess your patient to obtain data for making a nursing diagnosis, just as the doctor examines a patient to establish a medical diagnosis. Learn the differences between the two, and remember that sometimes they overlap. You perform a complete patient assessment to identify patient problems that your nursing interventions can help resolve; your nursing diagnosis states these problems. (Some may occur secondary to medical treatment.) If you plan your care of a patient around only the medical aspects of his illness, you'll probably overlook significant problems.

For example, suppose your patient's medical diagnosis is a fractured femur. In your assessment, take a careful history. Include questions to determine if the patient has adequate financial resources to cope with prolonged disability. To assess the patient's capacity to adjust to the physical restrictions caused by the disability, gather data about his previous life-style.

Suppose your physical examination of this patient—in addition to uncovering signs and symptoms pertaining to the medical diagnosis—reveals actual or potential skin breakdown secondary to immobility. Your nursing diagnoses, in that case, may include home maintenance management impairment, diversional activity deficit (related to prolonged immobility), and high risk for skin integrity impairment.

The plan of care you prepare for this patient should include the nursing interventions suggested by your nursing diagnoses as well as the nursing actions necessary to fulfill the patient's medical treatment plan. When integrated into a plan of care, the nursing and medical diagnoses describe the complete nursing care your patient needs.

Study the examples below to better understand the difference between medical and nursing diagnoses:

1. Frank Smith, age 67, complains of "stubborn, old muscles." He has difficulty walking, as you can see by his shuffling gait. During the interview, Mr. Smith speaks in a monotone and seems very depressed. Physical examination shows a pill-rolling hand tremor. Laboratory tests reveal a decreased dopamine level.

Medical diagnosis

Parkinson's disease

Nursing diagnoses

- Mobility impairment related to decreased muscle control
- Body image disturbance related to physical alterations
- Knowledge deficit related to lack of information about progressive nature of illness

2. For 5 consecutive days, Judy Wilson, age 26, has had sporadic abdominal cramps of increasing intensity. Most recently, the pain has been accompanied by vomiting and a slight fever. Your examination reveals rebound tenderness and muscle guarding.

Medical diagnosis

Appendicitis

Nursing diagnoses

- Pain related to biological agents
- Fluid volume deficit related to vomiting

3. During an extensive bout with respiratory tract infections, Tom Bradley, age 7, complains of throbbing ear pain. Tom's mother notes his hearing difficulty and his fear of the pain and possible hearing loss. On inspection, his tympanic membrane appears red and bulging.

Medical diagnosis

Acute suppurative otitis media

Nursing diagnoses

- Pain related to swollen tympanic membrane
- Fear related to progressive hearing loss
- Sensory or perceptual alteration (auditory) related to obstructed middle ear.

OUTCOME IDENTIFICATION

During this phase of the nursing process, you identify expected outcomes for the patient. Expected outcomes are measurable, patient-focused goals that are derived from the patient's nursing diagnoses. These goals may be short- or long-term. Short-term goals include those of immediate concern that can be achieved quickly. Long-term goals take more time to achieve and usually involve prevention, patient teaching, and rehabilitation.

In many cases, you can identify expected outcomes by converting the nursing diagnosis into a positive statement. For instance, for the nursing diagnosis "mobility impairment related to a fracture of the right hip," the expected outcome might be "The patient will ambulate independently before discharge."

When writing the plan of care, state expected outcomes in terms of the patient's behavior—for example, "The patient correctly demonstrates turning, coughing, and deep breathing." Also identify a target time or date by which the expected outcomes should be accomplished. The expected outcomes will serve as the basis for evaluating the effectiveness of your nursing interventions.

Keep in mind that each expected outcome must be stated in measurable terms. If possible, consult with the patient and family when establishing expected outcomes. As the patient progresses, expected outcomes should be increasingly directed toward planning for discharge and follow-up care.

Tips for writing expected outcome statements

When writing expected outcomes in your plan of care, always start with a specific action verb that focuses on the patient's behavior. By telling your reader how your patient should *look, walk, eat, drink, turn, cough, speak,* or *stand,* for example, you give a clear picture by which to evaluate progress.

Avoid starting expected outcome statements with *allow, let, enable,* or similar verbs. Such words focus attention on your own and other health team members' behavior—not on the patient's.

With many documentation formats, you won't need to include the phrase "The patient will..." with each expected outcome statement. You will, however, have to specify which person the goal refers to when family, friends, or others are directly concerned.

Make sure that target dates are realistic. Be flexible enough to adjust the date if your patient needs more time to respond to your interventions.

PLANNING

The nursing plan of care refers to a written plan of action designed to help you deliver quality patient care. It includes relevant nursing diagnoses, expected outcomes, and nursing interventions. Keep in mind that the plan of care usually forms a permanent part of the patient's health record and will be used by other members of the nursing team.

Reviewing the planning stages

Planning involves the following stages:

- assigning priorities to the nursing diagnoses
- selecting appropriate nursing actions (interventions) to accomplish identified expected outcomes
- documenting the nursing diagnoses, expected outcomes, nursing interventions, and evaluations on the plan of care.

Assigning priorities. Any time you develop more than one nursing diagnosis for your patient, you must assign priorities to them and begin your plan of care with those having the highest priority. High-priority nursing diagnoses involve the patient's most urgent needs (such as emergency or immediate physical needs). Intermediate-priority diagnoses involve nonemergency needs, and low-priority diagnoses involve needs that don't directly relate to the patient's specific illness or prognosis. (To help establish priorities, you may want to refer to *Nursing diagnoses arranged by Maslow's hierarchy of needs,* pages 594 and 595.)

Selecting appropriate nursing interventions. You must develop one or more nursing interventions to achieve each of the expected outcomes identified for your patient. For example, if one expected outcome statement reads "The patient will transfer to chair with assistance," the appropriate nursing interventions include placing the wheelchair facing the foot of the bed and assisting the patient to stand and pivot into the chair. If another expected outcome statement reads "The patient will express feelings related to recent injury," appropriate interventions might include spending time with the patient each shift, conveying an open and nonjudgmental attitude, and asking open-ended questions.

Reviewing the second part of the nursing diagnosis statement (the part describing etiologic factors) may help guide your choice of nursing interventions. For example, for the nursing diagnosis "injury, high risk for, related to inadequate blood glucose levels," you'd determine the best nursing interventions for maintaining an adequate blood glucose level. Typical interventions for this goal include observing the patient for evidence of hypoglycemia and providing an appropriate diet.

Try to think creatively during this step in the nursing process. It's an opportunity to describe exactly what you and your patient would like to have happen and to establish the criteria against which you'll judge further nursing actions.

Documenting your plan. The planning phase culminates when you write the plan of care and document the nursing diagnoses, expected outcomes, nursing interventions, and evaluations for expected outcomes. Write the plan of care in concise, specific terms so that other health team members can follow it. Keep in mind that because the patient's problems and needs will change, you'll have to review your plan of care frequently and modify it when necessary.

Benefits of writing a plan of care

To provide quality care for each patient, you must plan and direct that care. Writing a plan of care lets you document the scientific method you've used throughout the nursing process. On the plan of care, you summarize the patient's problems and needs (as nursing diagnoses) and identify appropriate nursing interventions and expected outcomes. A plan of care that's well conceived and properly written helps decrease the risk of incomplete or incorrect care by:

- giving direction
- providing continuity of care
- establishing communication between you and nurses on other shifts, between you and health team members in other departments, and between you and your patient
- serving as a key for patient care assignments.

Giving direction. A written plan of care gives direction by showing colleagues the goals you've set for your patient and giving clear instructions for helping to achieve them. It also makes clear exactly what to document on the patient's progress notes. For instance, it lists what observations to make and how often, what nursing measures to take and how to implement them, and what to teach the patient and family before discharge.

Providing continuity. A written plan of care identifies the patient's needs to each hospital shift and tells what must be done to meet those needs. With this information, nurses on each shift can adjust their routines to meet the patient's care demands. A plan of care also provides each shift with specific instructions on patient care, eliminating the confusion that can exist between shifts. And if your patient is discharged from the hospital to another health care institution, the plan of care can help ease this transition.

Establishing communication. By soliciting your patient's input as you develop the plan of care, you build a rapport that lets the patient know you value his opinions and feelings. And by reviewing the plan of care with other health team members, and with other nurses during change-of-shift reports, you can regularly evaluate your patient's response or lack of response to the nursing care and medical regimen.

Guiding patient care assignments. If you're a team leader, you may want to delegate some specific routines or duties described in each nursing intervention; not all of them need your professional attention.

What your plan of care should include

Care-planning formats vary from one institution to another. For example, you may write your plan of care on a Kardex or you may use another type of form. Your institution may require you to write a traditional plan of care from scratch, or you may be allowed to customize a standardized plan of care to meet the needs of each patient. Some institutions are adopting newer documentation tools, such as protocols, which give specific sequential instructions for treating patients with particular problems. However, nearly all care-planning formats include space in which to document the nursing diagnoses, expected outcomes, and nursing interventions. In many hospitals, you may also document assessment data and discharge planning on the plan of care.

No matter which format you use, be sure to write the plan of care in ink (and sign it), even though you may have to make revisions if your nursing interventions don't work. Remember—your patient's plan of care becomes part of the permanent record and shouldn't be erased or destroyed. If you write it in pencil—so that you can erase to revise—you make it seem unimportant. The information must remain intact, enabling you and other health team members to readily refer to nursing interventions used in the past. (See *Guidelines for writing the plan of care,* page 18.)

Be specific when writing your plan of care. By discussing specific *problems,* specific *expected outcomes,* specific *nursing interventions,* and specific *evaluations for expected outcomes,* you leave no doubt as to what needs to be done by other health team members. When listing nursing interventions, for instance, be sure to include *when* the action should be implemented, *who* should be involved in each aspect of implementation, and the *method* to be used. Specify dates and times when appropriate. List target dates for each expected outcome.

If your nursing interventions have resolved the problem on which you've based the nursing diagnosis, write "discontinued" next to the diagnostic statement on the plan of care, and list the date you discontinued the interventions. If your nursing interventions haven't resolved the problem by the target date, reevaluate your plan and do one of the following:
- Extend the target date and continue the intervention until the patient responds as expected.
- Discontinue the intervention and select a new one that will achieve the expected outcome.

Keeping the plan of care current

You'll need to update and modify your patient's plan of care as problems (or their priorities) change, as problems resolve, as new assessment information becomes available, and as you evaluate the patient's responses to nursing interventions.

Guidelines for writing the plan of care

Keeping these tips in mind will help you write a plan of care that's both accurate and useful.

- Write the plan of care in ink—it's a part of the permanent record—and sign your name.
- Be specific; don't use vague terms or generalities.
- Never use abbreviations that may be confused with ones meaning something different.
- Take time to review all your assessment data *before* you select an approach for each problem. (*Note:* If you can't complete the initial assessment, immediately note "insufficient data base" on your records.)
- Write down a specific expected outcome for each problem you identify, and record a target date for its completion.
- Avoid setting an initial goal that's too high to be achieved. For example, suppose the outcome for a newly admitted patient with cerebrovascular accident says "Patient will ambulate with assistance." Several patient outcomes will need to be achieved before this goal can be addressed.
- Consider the following three phases of patient care when writing nursing interventions: what observations to make and how often; what nursing measures to implement and how to perform them; and what to teach the patient and family before discharge.
- Make each nursing intervention specific.
- Make sure nursing interventions match the resources and capabilities of the staff. Combine what is necessary to correct or modify the problem with what is reasonably possible in your setting.
- Be creative when you write your patient's plan of care; include a drawing or an innovative procedure if either will make your directions more specific.
- Don't overlook any of the patient's problems or concerns. Include them on the plan of care so that they won't be forgotten.
- Make sure your plan of care is implemented correctly.
- Evaluate the results of your plan of care and discontinue any nursing diagnoses that have been resolved. Select new approaches, if necessary, for problems that have not been resolved.

Care planning for students

Writing a plan of care helps the nursing student learn the problem-solving technique and the nursing process as well as improve written and verbal communication and organizational skills. More important, it shows how to apply classroom and textbook knowledge to practice.

Because it aims to teach the care-planning process, the student plan of care is longer than the standard plans used in the hospital. In a step-by step manner, it progresses from assessment to evaluation. However, some teaching institutions model the student plan of care on the plan used by the affiliated health care institution, adding a space for the scientific rationale for each nursing intervention selected.

IMPLEMENTATION

During this phase, you put your plan of care into action. Implementation encompasses all nursing interventions directed toward resolving the patient's nursing diagnoses and meeting health care needs. While you coordinate implementation, you also seek help from other caregivers, the patient, and the patient's family.

Implementation requires some (or all) of the following interventions:

- assessing and monitoring (for example, recording vital signs)
- performing therapeutic interventions (for example, giving medications)
- making the patient more comfortable and helping him with activities of daily living (for example, repositioning)
- supporting respiratory and elimination functions
- providing skin care
- managing the environment (for example, controlling noise to ensure a good night's sleep)
- providing food and fluids
- giving emotional support
- teaching and counseling
- referring the patient to appropriate agencies or services.

Elements of implementation

Incorporate these elements into the implementation stage:

- *Reassessment.* Although it may be brief or narrowly focused, reassessment should confirm that the planned interventions remain appropriate.
- *Reviewing and modifying the plan of care.* Never static, an appropriate plan of care changes with the patient's condition. As necessary, update the plan's assessment, nursing diagnoses, expected outcomes, implementation, and evaluation sections. (Entering the new data in different colored ink alerts other staff members to the revisions.) Date the revisions.
- *Seeking assistance.* Determine whether you need help from other staff members or additional information before you can intervene.

Documentation

Implementation isn't complete until you've documented each intervention, the time it occurred, the patient's response, and any other pertinent information. Make sure each entry relates to a nursing diagnosis. Remember that any action not documented may be overlooked during quality assurance monitoring or evaluation of care. Another good reason for thorough documentation: It offers a way for you to take rightful credit for your contribution in helping a patient achieve the highest possible level of wellness. After all, nurses use a unique and worthwhile combination of interpersonal, intellectual, and technical skills when providing care (see *Nursing interventions: Three types*).

EVALUATION

In this phase of the nursing process, you assess the effectiveness of the plan of care by answering questions like the following:

- How has the patient progressed in terms of the plan's projected outcomes?
- Does the patient have new needs?
- Does the plan of care need to be revised?

Evaluation also helps you determine whether the patient received high-quality care from the nursing staff and the hospital. Your hospital bases its own nursing quality assurance system on nursing evaluations.

Steps in the evaluation process

Include the patient, family members, and other health care professionals in the evaluation. Then follow these steps:

- *Select evaluation criteria.* The expected outcomes—the desired effects of nursing interventions—form the basis for evaluation.
- *Compare the patient's response to the evaluation criteria.* Did the patient respond as expected? If not, the plan of care may need revision.

Nursing interventions: Three types

Knowing the three types of nursing interventions will help you document implementation appropriately.

1. *Independent interventions.* These interventions fall within the purview of nursing practice and don't require a doctor's direction or supervision. Most nursing actions required by the patient's plan of care are independent interventions. Examples include patient teaching, health promotion, counseling, and helping the patient with activities of daily living.
2. *Dependent interventions.* Based on written or oral instructions from another professional—usually a doctor—dependent interventions include administering medication, inserting indwelling urinary catheters, and obtaining specimens for laboratory tests.
3. *Interdependent interventions.* Performed in collaboration with other professionals, interdependent interventions include following a protocol and carrying out standing orders.

• *Analyze your findings.* If your plan wasn't effective, determine why. You may conclude, for example, that several nursing diagnoses are inaccurate.
• *Modify the plan of care.* Make revisions (for example, change inaccurate nursing diagnoses) and implement the new plan.
• *Reevaluate.* Like all steps in the nursing process, evaluation is ongoing. Continue to assess, plan, implement, and evaluate for as long as you care for the patient.

Questions to answer

When evaluating and documenting your patient's care, collect information from all available sources—for example, the patient, his medical record, family members, and other caregivers. Also include your own observations.

During the evaluation process, ask yourself these questions:

- Has the patient's condition improved, deteriorated, or stayed the same?
- Were the nursing diagnoses accurate?
- Have the patient's nursing needs been met?
- Did the patient meet the outcome criteria documented in the plan of care?
- Which nursing interventions should I revise or discontinue?
- Why did the patient fail to achieve certain expected outcomes (if applicable)?
- Should I reorder priorities? Revise expected outcomes?

PART ONE

ADULT HEALTH

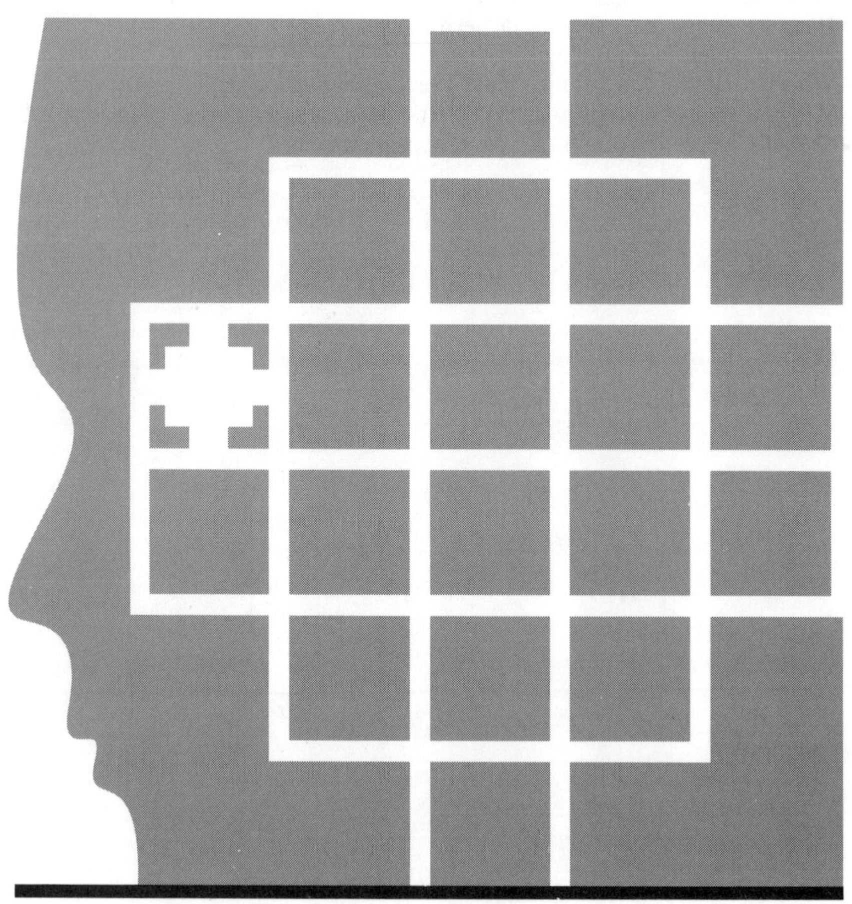

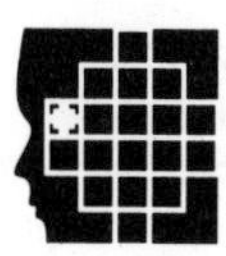

INTRODUCTION

This section includes 186 alphabetically organized diagnostic labels and associated plans of care that identify adult health problems amenable to independent nursing action. Many of them focus on meeting the patient's actual physiologic needs. For example, you'll find plans of care for ensuring the survival of a patient with decreased cardiac output, for helping an injured patient maintain joint range of motion, and for teaching an immunosuppressed patient measures to prevent infection. In addition, you'll find plans for warding off *high risk* health problems, such as infection or injury.

Other plans of care focus on the psychological and psychosocial problems of adulthood. For example, if a patient with a chronic illness experiences emotional difficulties, look up such diagnostic labels as *hopelessness, role performance alteration,* and *body image disturbance* to help pinpoint his needs. If a patient lacks adequate financial, social, or spiritual resources, appropriate plans of care provide instructions for documenting such hardships and interventions for ameliorating them.

Still other plans of care focus on more specialized patient problems. For instance, you'll find plans for patients undergoing surgery, requiring psychiatric help, or needing special attention.

In sum, the diagnostic labels and associated plans of care in this section cover the full range of nursing responsibilities. To make full use of this broad data base, you'll need to perform a complete and careful nursing assessment. When appropriate, include questions about the patient's cultural background. Ask about self-concept, stressors, daily living habits, and coping mechanisms. Discuss the patient's health goals. How well does the patient understand his condition? Will family members or friends take an active role in his care? Add information from your own observations.

Use information gathered during assessment to select an accurate diagnostic statement and an appropriate plan of care. That way, you can ensure your adult patient comprehensive, individualized, and consistent nursing care.

Activity intolerance

related to imbalance between oxygen supply and demand

Definition

Extreme fatigue or other physical symptoms caused by simple activity

Assessment

- History of circulatory disease, respiratory disease, or both
- Patient's perception of tolerance for activity
- Respiratory status, including arterial blood gases, pulmonary function studies, and respiratory rate, depth, and pattern both at rest and with activity
- Cardiovascular status, including blood pressure, complete blood count, exercise ECG results, and heart rate and rhythm both at rest and with activity
- Knowledge, including understanding of present condition, perception of need to maintain or restore an activity level consistent with capabilities, and physical, mental, and emotional readiness to learn

Defining characteristics

- Circulatory problems, respiratory problems, or both, including abnormal heart rate or blood pressure in response to activity, arrhythmia or ischemic changes on ECG, exertional discomfort, dyspnea, tachypnea, or hyperpnea
- Verbal report of fatigue or weakness

Associated medical diagnoses (selected)

Acute myocardial infarction, anemias, asthma, bronchitis, chronic obstructive pulmonary disease, congenital cardiac and valvular disorders, congestive heart failure, interstitial lung disease, peripheral vascular disorders, pulmonary edema, pulmonary embolus, respiratory failure, respiratory infections, respiratory neoplasms

Expected outcomes

- Patient states desire to increase activity level.
- Patient states understanding of the need to increase activity level gradually.
- Patient identifies controllable factors that cause fatigue.
- Blood pressure and pulse and respiratory rates remain within prescribed limits during activity.
- Patient states sense of satisfaction with each new level of activity attained.
- Patient demonstrates skill in conserving energy while carrying out daily activities to tolerance level.
- Patient explains illness and connects symptoms of activity intolerance with deficit in oxygen supply or use.

Interventions and rationales

- Discuss with patient the need for activity, *which will improve physical and psychosocial well-being.*
- Identify activities the patient considers desirable and meaningful *to enhance their positive impact.*
- Encourage patient to help plan activity progression, being sure to include activities the patient considers essential. *Participation in planning helps ensure patient compliance.*
- Instruct and help patient to alternate periods of rest and activity *to reduce the body's oxygen demand and prevent fatigue.*
- Identify and minimize factors that decrease the patient's exercise toler-

ance *to help increase the activity level.*
- Monitor physiologic responses to increased activity (including respirations, heart rate and rhythm, blood pressure), *to ensure return to normal a few minutes after exercising.*
- Teach patient how to conserve energy while performing activities of daily living—for example, sitting in a chair while dressing, wearing lightweight clothing that fastens with Velcro or a few large buttons, and wearing slip-on shoes. *These measures reduce cellular metabolism and oxygen demand.*
- Teach patient exercises for increasing strength and endurance, *which will improve breathing and gradually increase activity level.*
- Support and encourage activity to patient's level of tolerance. *This helps develop the patient's independence.*
- Before discharge, formulate a plan with the patient and caregivers that will enable the patient either to continue functioning at maximum activity tolerance or to gradually increase the tolerance. For example, teach the patient and caregivers to monitor patient's pulse during activities; to recognize need for oxygen, if prescribed; and to use oxygen equipment properly. *Participation in planning encourages patient satisfaction and compliance.*

Evaluations for expected outcomes
- Patient states a desire to increase activity level.
- Patient identifies a plan to increase activity level.
- Patient lists factors that cause fatigue.
- Patient's pulse and respiratory rates remain within normal parameters.
- Patient's blood pressure remains within normal parameters.
- Patient expresses satisfaction with increase in activity level, either verbally or through behavior.
- Patient is proficient in conserving energy while performing activities of daily living.
- Patient expresses an understanding of illness.
- Patient understands relationship between signs and symptoms of activity intolerance and deficit in oxygen supply or use.

Documentation
- Patient's perception of need for activity
- Patient's priorities in performing selected activities
- Patient's description of physical effects of various activities
- Observations made while the patient performs activities
- Skills demonstrated by patient in conserving energy during activity
- New activities patient was able to perform
- Evaluations for each expected outcome.

Activity intolerance

related to immobility

Definition
Extreme fatigue or other physical symptoms caused by simple activity

Assessment
- History of present illness
- Past experience with prolonged bed rest
- Age
- Neurologic status, including level of consciousness, orientation, motor status, and sensory status

• Respiratory status, including arterial blood gases, breath sounds, and the rate, depth, and pattern of respiration both at rest and with activity
• Cardiovascular status, including blood pressure, skin color, hemoglobin and hematocrit, and heart rate and rhythm both at rest and with activity
• Musculoskeletal status, including range of motion and muscle size, strength, and tone

Defining characteristics
• Circulatory problems, respiratory problems, or both, including exertional discomfort, arrhythmia or ischemic ECG changes, cyanosis, and abnormal heart rate, respiratory rate, or blood pressure
• Inability to move, such as from paralysis (partial or complete) or skeletal traction
• Prolonged bed rest for any reason
• Verbal report of weakness or fatigue

Associated medical diagnoses (selected)
Acute respiratory failure, cerebrovascular accident, congestive heart failure, craniocerebral trauma, encephalitis, fractures requiring skeletal traction, Guillain-Barré syndrome, meningitis, multiple sclerosis, peripheral vascular disease, rheumatoid arthritis, spinal cord injury, subacute bacterial endocarditis, vertebral fractures

Expected outcomes
• Patient regains and maintains muscle mass and strength.
• Patient maintains maximum joint range of motion.
• Patient performs isometric exercises.
• Patient helps perform self-care activities.
• Heart rate, rhythm, and blood pressure remain within expected range during periods of activity.
• Patient states understanding of and willingness to cooperate in maximizing activity level.
• Patient performs self-care activities to tolerance level.

Interventions and rationales
• Perform active or passive range-of-motion exercises to all extremities every 2 to 4 hours. *These exercises foster muscle strength and tone, maintain joint mobility, and prevent contractures.*
• Turn and reposition the patient at least every 2 hours. Establish a turning schedule for the dependent patient. Post schedule at bedside and monitor frequency. *Turning and repositioning prevents skin breakdown and improves breathing.*
• Maintain proper body alignment at all times *to avoid contractures and maintain optimal musculoskeletal balance and physiologic function.*
• Encourage active exercise:
  – Provide a trapeze or other assistive device whenever possible. *Such devices simplify moving and turning for many patients, and also allow them to strengthen some upper-body muscles.*
  – Teach isometric exercises *to allow patient to maintain or increase muscle tone and joint mobility.*
  – Have patient perform self-care activities. Begin slowly and increase daily, as tolerated. *Activities will help patient regain health.*
• Provide emotional support and encouragement *to help improve patient's self-concept and motivation to perform activities of daily living.*

• Involve patient in care-related planning and decision-making *to improve compliance.*
• Monitor physiologic responses to increased activity level, including respirations, heart rate and rhythm, and blood pressure *to ensure they return to normal within a few minutes after exercising.*
• Teach caregivers to assist patient with self-care activities in a way that maximizes patient's potential. *This enables caregivers to participate in patient's care, and also encourages them to support patient's independence.*

Evaluations for expected outcomes
• Patient regains and maintains pre-illness muscle mass and strength, as demonstrated by increased activity level.
• Patient demonstrates maximum joint range of motion.
• Patient performs isometric exercise _____ times per day.
• Patient assists caregiver in performing self-care activities.
• Patient's blood pressure, pulse rate, and rhythm remain within normal parameters.
• Patient expresses desire, either verbally or through behavior, to participate in improving his activity level.
• Patient performs self-care activities at optimal level within restrictions imposed by illness.

Documentation
• Patient's perceptions about the importance of maintaining optimal levels of activity within restrictions imposed by the illness
• Activities performed by patient
• Observations of physical findings in response to activity
• Teaching activities performed with patient or caregivers
• Evaluations for each expected outcome.

Activity intolerance, high risk for

related to immobility

Definition
Accentuated risk of extreme fatigue or other physical symptoms following simple activity

Assessment
• History of present illness
• Age
• Past experience with immobility or prescribed bed rest
• Cardiovascular status, including blood pressure, heart rate and rhythm at rest and with activity, complete blood count, skin temperature and color, edema, chest pain or discomfort.
• Respiratory status, including arterial blood gases, auscultation of breath sounds, pain or discomfort associated with respiration, and rate, rhythm, depth, and pattern of respirations at rest and with activity
• Neurologic status, including level of consciousness, orientation, mental status, sensory status, motor status
• Musculoskeletal status, including range of motion, muscle size, strength, tone, and functional mobility as follows:
0 = completely independent
1 = requires use of equipment or device
2 = requires help, supervision, or teaching from another person
3 = requires help from another person and equipment or device

4 = dependent; does not participate in activity

Risk factors
- Altered level of consciousness
- Imposed restriction of movement, including mechanical, medical protocol
- Inactivity
- Prolonged bed rest
- Severe pain

Associated medical diagnoses (selected)
Cerebrovascular accident, congestive heart failure, fractures (with traction or cast), Guillain-Barré syndrome, multiple sclerosis, severe head injury, spinal cord injury

Expected outcomes
- Patient maintains muscle strength and joint range of motion.
- Patient carries out isometric exercise regimen.
- Patient communicates understanding of rationale for maintaining activity level.
- Patient avoids risk factors that may lead to activity intolerance.
- Patient performs self-care activities to tolerance level.
- Blood pressure, pulse, and respiratory rate remain within prescribed range during periods of activity (specify).

Interventions and rationales
- Position patient to maintain proper body alignment. Use assistive devices as needed *to maintain joint function and prevent musculoskeletal deformities.*
- Turn and position the patient at least every 2 hours. Establish turning schedule for dependent patients. Post at bedside and monitor frequency. *Turning helps prevent skin breakdown by relieving pressure.*
- Assess patient's level of functioning using the functional mobility scale *to determine patient's capabilities.*
- Communicate patient's level of functioning to all staff. *Communication among staff members ensures continuity of care and enables the patient to preserve identified level of independence.*
- Unless contraindicated, perform range-of-motion exercises every 2 to 4 hours. Progress from passive to active, according to patient tolerance. *Range-of-motion exercises prevent joint contractures and muscular atrophy.*
- Encourage active movement by helping patient use trapeze or other assistive devices *to improve muscle tone and enhance self-esteem.*
- Teach patient how to perform isometric exercises *to maintain and improve muscle tone and joint mobility.*
- Assist patient in carrying out self-care activities. Increase patient's participation in self-care, as tolerated, *to foster independence and improve mobility.*
- Encourage patient to become involved in planning care and making decisions related to treatment. *Participation in planning enhances compliance.*
- Teach patient, family member, or significant other methods to maximize patient's participation in self-care. *Informed caregivers can encourage patient to become more independent.*
- Assess patient's physiologic response to increased activity (blood pressure, respirations, heart rate, and rhythm). *Monitoring vital signs helps to assess tolerance for increased exertion and activity.*
- Teach patient symptoms of over-exertion, such as dizziness, chest pain, and dyspnea, *to help patient take re-*

sponsibility for monitoring activity level.
• Explain rationale for maintaining or improving activity level. Discuss factors that increase risk of activity intolerance. *Education will help the patient avoid activity intolerance.*
• Encourage patient to carry out activities of daily living. Provide emotional support and offer positive feedback when patient displays initiative. *Offering emotional support will enhance patient's self-esteem and motivation.*

Evaluations for expected outcomes
• Functional mobility scale indicates that muscle strength and joint range of motion remain stable.
• Patient demonstrates isometric exercises.
• Patient explains rationale for maintaining activity level and states at least five risk factors for activity intolerance.
• Patient performs self-care activities in preparation for discharge.
• Patient does not exhibit evidence of cardiovascular or respiratory complications during or after activity.

Documentation
• Patient's expressions of motivation to maintain maximum activity level within restrictions imposed by illness
• Activities performed by patient
• Teaching instructions provided to patient, family, or significant other
• Patient's physiologic response to increased activity
• Evaluations for each expected outcome.

■ Adjustment impairment

related to disability

Definition
Inability to modify life-style or behavior consistent with changed health status

Assessment
• Nature of medical diagnosis
• Behavioral responses, including verbal or nonverbal, engagement or disengagement, interest or apathy, acceptance or denial, independence or dependence
• Knowledge of health condition
• Past experiences with family, friends, media
• Psychosocial factors, such as age, sex, ethnic background, religious preference and beliefs, values, occupation, family support, coping style
• Impact of medical diagnosis
• Nutritional status, including modifications in diet, weight changes

Defining characteristics
• Depression over physical changes
• Fear of rejection by staff and family
• Isolation, withdrawal, avoidance
• Poor eating habits
• Refusal to accept health status change
• Refusal to discuss treatment plans
• Refusal to participate in care activities
• Refusal to see visitors
• Somnolence or insomnia
• Unrealistic expectations

Associated medical diagnoses (selected)
Aphasia, cancer, chronic pain, deformity or disfigurement resulting from radical surgery, diabetes mellitus, hemiplegia (or paraplegia or quadri-

plegia), myocardial infarction, spinal cord injury, terminal illness, ulcerative colitis

Expected outcomes

- Patient identifies inability to cope and adjust adequately.
- Patient expresses understanding of the illness or disease.
- Patient participates in health care regimen and plans care activities.
- Patient demonstrates ability to manage health problem.
- Patient shows ability to accept and adapt to a new health status and integrate learning.
- Patient demonstrates new coping strategies.

Interventions and rationales

- Encourage patient to express feelings in a safe, nonthreatening environment. *This allows the patient to gain insight into and rationally define fears, goals, and potential problems.*
- Allow patient to grieve. *After working through denial and isolation, anger, bargaining, and depression, patient will progress toward acceptance.*
- Provide reassurance that the patient's feelings are normal *to promote coping.*
- Begin teaching patient and caregivers the skills needed to adequately manage care *to encourage compliance and adjustment to optimum wellness.*
- Spend 15 minutes per shift listening to patient's feelings. *This will help reassure patient you're interested and care.*
- Help patient identify areas where it's possible to maintain control. *This avoids feelings of powerlessness and lets patient feel part of a team effort.*
- Encourage patient to plan care activities, such as time of treatment, personal hygiene, and rest periods, *to help give patient a better sense of control.*
- Arrange for others who have suffered similar health problems to speak with patient and family. *This exposes patient to suitable role model and may allow a trusting, supportive relationship to develop.*
- Discuss health problems and implications with family *to enable them to participate in patient's care and to foster a trusting relationship.*
- Obtain a consultation with a mental health specialist if patient develops severe depression or other psychiatric problems. *Although trauma or illness commonly cause some depression, consultation with a mental health professional may help minimize it.*

Evaluations for expected outcomes

- Patient recognizes necessity of learning to live with impairment.
- Patient understands that grieving is normal response to impairment.
- Patient meets learning objectives before discharge.
- Patient identifies and contacts sources of continued psychological support, if needed.
- Patient identifies two areas in which he can maintain control despite altered health status.
- Patient meets with individual who has similar health problem and reports results of meeting.
- Patient shows ability to accept and adapt to a new health status and integrate learning.

Documentation

- Patient's nonverbal behaviors
- Patient's verbal expressions of denial, anger, or guilt due to the illness or disease process
- Patient's ability or inability to participate in care

• Evaluations for each expected outcome.

Airway clearance, ineffective

related to decreased energy or fatigue

Definition
Anatomic or physiologic obstruction of the airway that interferes with normal ventilation

Assessment
- History of present illness
- Patient's perception of ability to clear airway
- Knowledge of physical condition
- Neurologic status, including level of consciousness, orientation, sensory status, and motor status
- Respiratory status, including symmetry of chest expansion; use of accessory muscles; cough (productive or nonproductive); respiratory rate, depth, and pattern; such sputum characteristics as color, consistency, amount, odor, and changes from patient's norm; palpation for fremitus; percussion of lung fields; auscultation for breath sounds; arterial blood gases; hemoglobin and hematocrit
- Pulmonary function studies
- Psychosocial status, including interest, motivation, and knowledge

Defining characteristics
- Adventitious breath sounds, such as crackles, rhonchi, stridor, and wheezes
- Anxiety
- Apprehension
- Changes in rate, depth, or pattern of respiration
- Chest wall pain
- Choking or gasping
- Cyanosis
- Dyspnea
- Fever
- Inability to cough
- Ineffective cough
- Nasal flaring
- Noisy respirations
- Patient's report of fatigue and decreased activity tolerance
- Tachypnea

Associated medical diagnoses (selected)
Asthma, cerebrovascular accident, chronic bronchitis, congestive heart failure, emphysema, Guillain-Barré syndrome, interstitial lung disease, multiple sclerosis, myasthenia gravis, pneumonia, systemic lupus erythematosus

Expected outcomes
- Airway remains patent.
- Adventitious breath sounds are absent.
- Chest X-ray shows no abnormality.
- Oxygen level in normal range.
- Patient breathes deeply and coughs to remove secretions.
- Patient expectorates sputum.
- Patient demonstrates controlled coughing techniques.
- Ventilation is adequate.
- Patient shows no signs of pulmonary compromise.
- Patient demonstrates skill in conserving energy while attempting to clear airway.
- Patient states understanding of changes needed to diminish oxygen demands.

Interventions and rationales
- Assess respiratory status at least every 4 hours or according to established standards *to detect early signs of compromise.*
- Turn patient every 2 hours. Always position for maximal aeration of lung

fields and mobilization of secretions. *This prevents pooling and stasis of respiratory secretions.*

• When helping patient cough and deep-breathe, use whatever position best ensures cooperation and minimizes energy expenditure, such as high Fowler's position or sitting on side of bed. *Such positions promote chest expansion and ventilation of basilar lung fields.*

• Suction, as ordered, to stimulate cough and clear airways. Be alert for progression of airway compromise. *These steps prevent respiratory distress.*

• Perform postural drainage, percussion, and vibration to facilitate secretion movement. Monitor sputum, noting amount, odor, consistency. *Sputum amount and consistency may indicate hydration status and effectiveness of therapy. Foul-smelling sputum may indicate respiratory infection.*

• Teach patient an easily performed cough technique *to clear airways without fatigue.*

• Encourage sputum expectoration *to remove pathogens and prevent spread of infection.* Provide tissues and paper bag for hygienic disposal.

• Give expectorants, bronchodilators, and other drugs, as ordered, and record effectiveness. Also encourage fluids to help liquefy secretions. *These measures enhance clearance of secretions from airways.*

• Provide aerosol treatments before chest physiotherapy *to optimize results.*

• Administer oxygen, as ordered, *to help relieve respiratory distress.*

• Monitor arterial blood gases and hemoglobin *to assess oxygenation and ventilatory status;* report deviations from baseline levels.

• If conservative measures fail to maintain PaO_2 within an acceptable range, prepare for endotracheal intubation, as ordered, *to maintain artificial airway and optimize* PaO_2.

• Assess patient's learning needs and provide appropriate information *to help prevent recurrence of obstruction and promote change in daily activities to reduce oxygen demands.*

Evaluations for expected outcomes

• Patient's airway remains clear and allows for adequate ventilation.

• Auscultation of patient's lung fields does not reveal crackles, rhonchi, wheezes, or stridor.

• Patient's chest X-ray does not show any pathophysiology.

• Patient's oxygen level remains within normal range.

• Patient coughs and deep breathes to expectorate secretions.

• Patient expectorates sputum.

• Patient performs controlled coughing techniques.

• Patient does not experience dyspnea or change in respiratory pattern.

• Adventitious breath sounds are absent.

• Patient demonstrates understanding of changes needed to diminish oxygen demands.

Documentation

• Patient's perceptions of ability to cough

• Observations of physical findings

• Effectiveness of medications

• Patient's attempts to clear airway

• Maneuvers performed to clear airway

• Evaluations for each expected outcome.

Airway clearance, ineffective

related to presence of tracheobronchial obstruction or secretions

Definition

Anatomic or physiologic obstruction of the airway that interferes with normal ventilation

Assessment

- History of respiratory disorder
- Respiratory status, including rate and depth of respiration; fever; symmetry of chest expansion; use of accessory muscles; cough; sputum (color, consistency, amount, odor, and changes from patient's norm related to infection, irritation, dehydration, exposure to pollutants); palpation for fremitus; percussion of lung fields; auscultation for breath sounds; arterial blood gases; chest X-ray
- Neurologic status, including level of consciousness, orientation, and mental status
- Knowledge, including understanding of physical condition and knowledge and skill in performing maneuvers to clear airway
- Mental, physical, and emotional readiness to learn

Defining characteristics

- Adventitious breath sounds, such as crackles, rhonchi, stridor, wheezes
- Anxiety
- Apprehension
- Changes in rate or depth of respiration
- Choking or gasping
- Cough (productive or nonproductive)
- Cyanosis
- Dyspnea
- Fever
- Nasal flaring
- Noisy respirations
- Tachypnea

Associated medical diagnoses (selected)

Asthma, bronchogenic carcinoma, cerebrovascular accident, chest trauma, chronic bronchitis, chronic obstructive pulmonary disease, Guillain-Barré syndrome, interstitial lung disease, myasthenia gravis, pneumonia, spinal cord injuries, upper airway trauma

Expected outcomes

- Patient coughs effectively.
- Patient expectorates sputum.
- Adventitious breath sounds absent.
- Chest X-ray reveals no abnormality.
- Patient produces normal sputum.
- Patient drinks 3 to 4 liters of fluid daily.
- Arterial blood gas levels remain at baseline.
- Airway remains patent.
- Patient understands and can explain the need for adequate hydration, sputum monitoring, and taking medications as ordered.
- Patient demonstrates controlled coughing techniques.
- Patient performs chest physiotherapy, particularly postural drainage.
- Patient reports symptoms that indicate need for medical intervention.

Interventions and rationales

- Assess respiratory status at least every 4 hours or according to established standards *to detect early signs of compromise.*
- Place patient in Fowler's position and support upper extremities *to aid breathing and chest expansion, and to ventilate basilar lung fields.*

- Help patient turn, cough, and deep-breathe every 2 to 4 hours *to help prevent pooling of secretions and to maintain airway patency.*
- Suction as needed *to stimulate cough and clear airways.* Be alert for progression of airway compromise.
- Provide adequate humidification *to loosen secretions.*
- Encourage fluids (at least 3,000 ml daily) *to ensure adequate hydration and loosen secretions,* unless contraindicated.
- Perform postural drainage, percussion, and vibration every 4 hours or as ordered *to enhance mobilization of secretions that interfere with oxygenation.* Monitor sputum *to gauge effectiveness of therapy.*
- Mobilize patient to full capabilities *to facilitate chest expansion and ventilation.*
- Avoid supine position for extended periods. Encourage lateral, sitting, prone, and upright positions as much as possible *to enhance lung expansion and ventilation.*
- Provide tissues and paper bags for hygienic sputum disposal *to prevent spreading infection.*
- Monitor and document sputum characteristics every shift *to gauge therapy's effectiveness and detect possible respiratory infection.*
- Teach patient about:
  - maintaining adequate hydration.
  - daily monitoring of sputum and reporting changes.
  - taking prescribed drugs and avoiding over-the-counter respiratory drugs.
  - controlled coughing and postural drainage.
  - the need to remain active.

These steps involve patient in own health care.

Evaluations for expected outcomes

- Patient clears airway using controlled coughing techniques.
- Patient expectorates sputum.
- Auscultation of patient's lung fields does not reveal crackles, rhonchi, wheezes, or stridor.
- Patient's chest X-ray does not show any abnormality.
- Patient's sputum is thin, white, odorless, and moderate in quantity.
- Patient drinks 3 to 4 liters of fluid daily.
- Patient's arterial blood gas values are within normal limits.
- Patient understands necessity of adequate hydration, sputum monitoring, and taking medications as ordered.
- Patient performs chest physiotherapy, especially postural drainage.
- Patient lists symptoms that indicate a need for medical intervention.

Documentation

- Patient's statement of ability to clear airway and comfort in doing so
- Respiratory status, including cough and sputum
- Need for suctioning and its effectiveness
- Effectiveness of medications
- Teaching about airway clearance; response to interventions
- Evaluations for each expected outcome.

Altered protection

related to myelosuppression and immunosuppression

Definition

A decrease in the ability to guard the self from internal or external threats such as illness or injury

Assessment

- Vital signs
- Health maintenance, including high-risk behaviors, health-promoting activities
- Patient's knowledge of present condition, including diagnosis, treatment, prevention of complications, management of adverse effects
- Coping skills, including physical, psychosocial, and spiritual strengths
- Mobility status
- Comfort level, including symptom management
- Activities of daily living, including rest, sleep, exercise
- Cardiovascular status, including heart rate, rhythm, heart sounds, blood pressure, peripheral pulses, ECG
- Neurologic status, including sensory perception, decision-making abilities, thought processes
- Respiratory status, including gas exchange and breathing patterns
- Nutritional status, including food preferences, modifications in diet, weight changes
- Bowel and bladder elimination patterns
- Protective mechanisms, including immune, hematopoietic, integumentary, and sensorimotor systems
- Laboratory studies, including white blood cell (WBC) count, WBC differential, erythrocyte sedimentation rate, immunoelectrophoresis, enzyme-linked immunosorbent assay, and cultures of blood, body fluid, sputum, urine, wounds
- Sexuality patterns

Defining characteristics

- Altered clotting
- Anorexia
- Chills
- Cough
- Deficient immunity
- Diaphoresis
- Disorientation
- Dyspnea
- Fatigue
- Immobility
- Impaired healing
- Insomnia
- Itching
- Maladaptive stress response
- Neurosensory impairment
- Pressure ulcers
- Restlessness
- Weakness

Associated medical diagnoses (selected)

Acquired immunodeficiency syndrome, alcoholism, anemias, brain tumor, burns, coma, disseminated intravascular coagulation, graft-versus-host disease, hemophilia, idiopathic thrombocytopenia purpura, leukemia, lymphomas, malnutrition, multiple myeloma, multiple sclerosis, neutropenia, pressure sores, rheumatoid arthritis, sickle cell disease

Disorders requiring the following treatments: organ or bone marrow transplant; radiation therapy; surgery or other invasive diagnostic or therapeutic procedures; drug therapy with antineoplastics, corticosteroids, immunosuppressants, biological response modifiers, anticoagulants, thrombolytic enzymes, antibiotics

Expected outcomes
- Patient does not experience chills, fever, or other signs and symptoms of illness.
- Patient demonstrates use of protective measures, including conservation of energy, maintenance of balanced diet, and obtainment of adequate rest.
- Patient demonstrates effective coping skills.
- Patient demonstrates personal cleanliness and maintains clean environment.
- Patient maintains safe environment.
- Patient demonstrates increased strength and resistance.
- Patient's immune system response improves.

Interventions and rationales
- Spend as much time with the patient as possible *to provide comfort and support.*
- Promote personal and environmental cleanliness *to decrease threat from microorganisms.*
- Monitor vital signs. *This allows for early detection of complications.*
- Institute safety precautions *to reduce risk of falls, cuts, or other injuries and subsequent infection, bleeding, and impaired healing.*
- Teach protective measures including the need to conserve energy, obtain adequate rest, and eat a balanced diet. *Adequate sleep and nutrition enhance immune function. Energy conservation can help to decrease the weakness caused by anemia.*
- Provide relief for symptoms (fever, chills, myalgias, weakness). *Discomfort interferes with rest, disturbs nutrition intake, and places added stress on the patient.*
- Teach patient coping strategies including stress management and relaxation techniques. *Relaxation and decreased stress can increase immune function, thereby improving strength and resistance.*

Evaluations for expected outcomes
- Patient does not develop petechiae, epistaxis, melena, hematuria, fever, cough, redness, drainage, pallor, headache, weakness, or dizziness. Vital signs remain within normal limits.
- Patient demonstrates a normal pattern of rest, activity, and sleep. He consumes an adequate diet.
- Patient reports being able to cope effectively.
- Patient demonstrates personal cleanliness and maintains a clean environment.
- Patient uses safety precautions to avoid falls and other injuries.
- Patient demonstrates increased strength and resistance.
- Immune system response improves.

Documentation
- Patient's understanding of abnormal blood profiles
- Patient's description of measures to prevent or manage complications
- Observations of patient's behavior including health promoting and high-risk activities
- Signs and symptoms of decreased immune resistance in body systems assessed (cardiopulmonary, neurologic, gastrointestinal, genitourinary, integumentary)
- Observations of infection or bleeding
- Interventions to assist with coping strategies and health maintenance and promotion
- Patient's response to interventions
- Evaluations for each expected outcome.

Anxiety

related to environmental conflict (phobia)

Definition

Feeling of threat or danger to self arising from an unidentifiable source

Assessment

- History of panic symptoms (choking feeling in throat, hyperventilation, light-headedness, dizziness, other physical signs and symptoms of anxiety)
- Psychological status, including patient's explanation of problem, onset, duration, precipitating events, past coping, present coping (note excessive use of repression and denial as major psychological defenses, and note overuse of escape-avoidance behaviors), insight (note patient's understanding of irrationality of fears), motivation to change, anxiety level (+1, +2, +3, +4), secondary gains (from whom and what kinds of secondary gains are being received), current stressors, mental status examination (note escape-avoidance behavior, expression of anxiety in terms of personal fears, concentration, judgment, affect, impulse control, as well as all other aspects of mental status), personal abilities, talents, strengths
- Sociological status, including support systems, hobbies, interests, work history, family makeup, family roles (evidence of harmony or disharmony), family coping mechanisms, evidence of reinforcement of problem by family, life-style (how this reinforces irrational fears)
- Physiologic status, including medication history (response, effectiveness, side effects)

Defining characteristics

- Agoraphobia
- Behavioral measures to escape or avoid feared event (reclusiveness, avoidance)
- Depersonalization
- Feelings of weakness or failure
- High anxiety when confronting feared situation, object, or activity
- Loss of self-esteem
- Obsessive trends
- Physical symptoms
- Recognition of irrationality of behavior
- Social phobias (such as fear of public speaking, blushing, urinating in public toilet)
- Specific phobias (such as snakes, airplanes, fire)

Associated medical diagnoses (selected)

Anorexia nervosa, anxiety disorder with phobic attacks, schizophrenia

Expected outcomes

- Patient experiences reduced anxiety by identifying internal precipitating situations.
- Patient connects life events to occurrence of anxiety.
- Patient identifies current stressors.
- Patient sets limits and compromises on behavior when ready.
- Patient develops effective coping behaviors.
- Patient maintains autonomy and independence without handicapping fears and use of phobic behavior.

Interventions and rationales

- Understand own feelings toward patient, *to keep feelings from interfering with treatment.*

• Accept patient as is. *Forcing the patient to change before he or she is ready causes panic.*
• Explore factors that precipitate phobic reactions and anxiety. *This is important for understanding patient's dynamics.*
• Support patient with desensitization techniques. *Encouraging patient to expose self to fears helps patient overcome problem.*
• Give patient chance to ventilate feelings. *This reduces patient's tendency to suppress or repress; bottled-up feelings continue to affect behavior even though patient may be unaware of them.*
• Teach relaxation techniques (such as breathing exercises, progressive muscle relaxation, guided imagery, meditation). *Such measures counteract fight-or-flight response.*
• Help patient set limits and compromises on behavior when ready. Allow patient to be afraid; *fear is a feeling, neither right nor wrong.*
• Give patient facts about fear and anxiety and their consequences *to reduce anxiety and encourage patient to help in managing problem.*
• Encourage patient not to run away when afraid *to help patient learn that fear can be faced and managed.*
• Help patient develop own techniques for dealing with fears *to establish alternatives to escape or avoidance behaviors.*

Evaluations for expected outcomes
• Patient demonstrates reduced physical symptoms of anxiety, improved concentration, and reduced preoccupation with fears.
• Patient discusses possible relationship between anxiety and past and present experiences.
• Patient lists stressors.
• Patient limits phobic behavior when ready.
• Patient participates in desensitization therapy and learns to better manage stress, health, and responsibilities.
• Patient makes decisions and shows greater independence.
• Patient decreases behavior that limits spontaneous activity.

Documentation
• Nurse's observation of subjective and objective data
• Interventions to reduce anxiety and increase coping
• Patient's response to interventions
• Evaluations for each expected outcome.

■ Anxiety

related to obsessive-compulsive behavior

Definition
Feeling of threat or danger to self arising from an unidentifiable source

Assessment
• Physical status, including skin breakdown, excoriation of skin tissue, alopecia, fatigue, weight loss, sleeplessness, and other physical indications of anxiety
• Psychological status, including patient's explanation of problem; onset and duration of problem; precipitating events; past coping strategies; present coping strategies (does the patient use repression and undoing as psychological defenses?); insight; motivation to change; level of anxiety (+1, +2, +3, +4); secondary gains (what kind of secondary gains does the patient achieve? from whom?);

acting-out behavior (compulsive gambling, for example); current stressors; mental status examination (especially psychomotor behavior, thought content, concentration, judgment, affect, communication style, impulse control, presenting appearance); personal abilities, talents, strengths
• Sociologic status, including support systems, hobbies, interests, work history
• Family status, including roles of members, evidence of harmony or disharmony, family coping mechanisms, evidence of reinforcement of patient's problem by family members
• Physiologic status, including medication history (response, effectiveness, adverse reactions)

Defining characteristics
• Attempts to suppress unwanted thoughts which lead to increased anxiety
• Excessive criticism of others
• Excessive inner control, demonstrated by moralistic attitude, frequent "I should" statements, and a perception that pleasurable activity is bad
• Excessive self-restraint, demonstrated by cautiousness, deliberation, pensiveness, grave appearance, neatness, frugality, emotional distance with little affect
• Expression of hostility through ritualistic behavior
• Inability to say no to requests from others
• Indecision
• Insecurity
• Interpersonal relationships characterized by alternating periods of closeness and distance
• Recognition that behavior is irrational despite compulsion to perform rituals
• Repetitive actions or rituals, for example, obligatory hand washing, touching, counting; more elaborate ceremonies performed in an exact order
• Repetitive, unwanted thoughts
• Speech filled with facts and details
• Stubbornness

Associated medical diagnoses (selected)
Affective disorders, anorexia nervosa, bulimia, paraphilia, phobic disorders, schizophrenia, substance abuse, suicidal behavior

Expected outcomes
• Patient reduces amount of time spent each day on obsessing and ritualizing.
• Patient performs activities of daily living.
• Ritual behavior does not produce harmful effects.
• Patient expresses feelings of anxiety as they occur.
• Patient expresses anger in socially acceptable ways.
• Patient makes fewer attempts to exert control over self and environment.
• Patient copes with stress without excessive obsessive-compulsive behavior.
• Patient forms a relationship without excessive dependence or aloofness.
• Patient develops self-esteem.

Interventions and rationales
• Understand your own feelings toward patient *to prevent prejudices from interfering with treatment.*
• Understand that anxiety is the cause of the patient's problem and accept patient's need to obsess or ritualize. *An accepting attitude will nurture feelings of sympathy toward the patient and minimize feelings of disapproval.* Do not attempt to thwart ritual behavior. *Forcing pa-*

tient to change behavior can lead to panic and, possibly, psychosis.
• When possible, help the patient channel ritual behavior into constructive outlets, such as writing, painting, or physical activity, *to develop patient's self-esteem.*
• Allow patient sufficient time to engage in rituals. *Rushing the patient may increase anxiety and create hostility.*
• Avoid attempting to reason with patient regarding his obsession. *Patient already recognizes the irrationality of his symptoms. Your explanations may increase feelings of inadequacy.*
• Avoid criticizing patient's behavior, either verbally or by attitude. Only discuss ritual behavior if patient brings it up first. *Criticism will further damage patient's already low self-esteem.*
• Develop a relationship with the patient that encourages open expression of emotions *to help patient cope effectively with feelings that usually remain repressed.*
• Promote patient's self-esteem by encouraging participation in activity. Begin with simple objectives for the patient and progress to larger goals. Praise patient's efforts frequently. *Feelings of accomplishment increase patient's sense of worth and decrease anxiety, thus decreasing the need for rituals.*
• If needed, set consistent limits on self-destructive behavior *to promote the patient's physical safety. Consistent limits will help prevent the patient from vacillating.*
• Assess what secondary gain the patient achieves through ritual behavior. When possible, preempt the ritual by providing this gain when patient is not ritualizing. For example, if patient seeks attention through ritual behavior, ignore ritual behavior but pay ample attention to patient at other times. *This may help patient realize gains can be achieved without ritual behavior. Remember that, if ignored, negative behavior is less likely to be repeated.*
• If rituals interfere with nutrition, place patient on an established feeding schedule *to promote health and prevent patient from becoming indecisive about meals.*
• If patient practices washing or "picking" rituals, take steps to prevent skin breakdown. Provide hand lotion and rubber gloves, bandage hands, and keep fingernails trimmed. *These measures will prevent skin breakdown.*
• Teach relaxation techniques *to counteract anxiety.*
• Teach assertiveness skills. *Learning to say no to other people's demands can help the patient manage anger.*
• Assess patient's readiness to overcome ritual behavior. Patient can begin to change when able to manage anxiety without resorting to rituals. When patient is ready, assist in setting goals for limiting unwanted behavior *to help motivate patient to change.*

Evaluations for expected outcomes
• Patient shows less evidence of ritualizing and reports that obsessive thoughts are less frequent.
• Patient performs daily toileting activities efficiently, unhampered by distracting rituals.
• Patient eats at least 80% of meals without being distracted by obsessive thoughts or rituals.
• Patient achieves 6 to 8 hours of uninterrupted sleep each night.
• Patient's skin remains intact and supple.
• Patient expresses anxiety.

• Patient voices anger or expresses it through writing, painting, physical activity, or other healthy outlets.
• Patient participates in hobbies or other diversional activities.
• Patient uses problem-solving skills, maintains balance of work and play, and displays well-balanced use of psychological defense mechanisms.
• Patient demonstrates a less perfectionistic and moralistic outlook.
• Patient is relaxed and assertive, thinks and behaves moderately, and exhibits greater affect.

Documentation
• Observations of ritualistic behavior
• Statements indicating obsessive thoughts
• Interventions performed to reduce anxiety and to increase coping
• Patient's response to nursing interventions, including ability to relax; willingness to think flexibly, socialize, and engage in diversions; and efforts to maintain physical health
• Patient's weight, food intake, and skin condition
• Patient's ability to accept less control over self and environment
• Patient's achievement of mutually established goals
• Evaluations for each expected outcome.

Anxiety

related to situational crisis

Definition
Feeling of threat or danger to self arising from an unidentifiable source

Assessment
• Reason for hospitalization, including patient's perception of problem, onset of problem, recent stressors, life changes, other precipitants
• Mental status, including orientation to time, place, person; insight regarding current situation; judgment; abstract thinking; general information; mood; affect; recent and remote memory; thought processes; thought content
• Coping, problem-solving ability
• Ability to perform activities of daily living
• Sleep habits
• Dietary and nutritional status
• Available support systems, including family or significant other, friends, clergy, health care agencies

Defining characteristics
• Autonomic hyperactivity, including shortness of breath or smothering sensation; palpitations or tachycardia; sweating; cold, clammy hands; dry mouth; dizziness; lightheadedness; nausea, diarrhea; other abdominal distress; flushes (hot flashes) or chills; frequent urination; difficulty swallowing
• Motor tension, including trembling, twitching, shakiness, muscle tension, aches, soreness, restlessness, easily fatigued
• Vigilance and scanning (feeling keyed-up or on edge; exaggerated startle response; difficulty concentrating; insomnia; irritability)

Associated medical diagnoses (selected)
Any hospitalized patient can experience anxiety. It appears most often in patients with conditions requiring surgery, diseases that pose a threat to self-concept, diseases that require use of high-technology devices or techniques, or those who have newly diagnosed chronic or terminal diseases. High levels of anxiety can result from a situational crisis so

devastating that it requires hospitalization.

Expected outcomes

- Patient identifies factors that elicit anxious behaviors.
- Patient discusses activities that tend to decrease anxious behaviors.
- Patient practices progressive relaxation techniques ____ times a day.
- Patient copes with current medical situation (specify) without demonstrating severe signs of anxiety (specify for individual).

Interventions and rationales

- Spend 10 minutes with patient twice a shift. Convey a willingness to listen. Offer verbal reassurance; for example, "I know you're frightened. I'll stay with you." *Specific amount of uninterrupted, non-care-related time spent with anxious patient builds trust and reduces tension. Active listening helps patient ventilate feelings.*
- Give patient clear, concise explanations of anything about to occur. Avoid information overload, since the anxious patient cannot assimilate many details. *Anxiety may impair patient's cognitive abilities.*
- Listen attentively; allow patient to express feelings verbally. *This may allow patient to identify anxious behaviors and discover the source of anxiety.*
- Make no demands on patient. *Anxious patient may respond to excessive demands with hostility and abuse.*
- Identify and reduce as many environmental stressors as possible. This may apply to people as well as other stimuli. *Anxiety often results from lack of trust in the environment.*
- Have patient state what kinds of activities promote feelings of comfort, and encourage patient to perform them (specify). *This gives patient a sense of control.*
- Remain with patient during severe anxiety. *Anxiety is often related to fear of being left alone.*
- Include patient in decisions related to care when feasible. *Anxious patient may mistrust own abilities; involvement in decision making may reduce anxious behaviors.*
- Support family or significant other in coping with patient's anxious behavior. *Involving family or significant other in process of reassurance and explanation allays patient's anxiety as well as their own.*
- Allow extra visiting periods with family if this seems to allay patient's anxiety. *This allows anxious patient and family to support each other according to their abilities and at their own pace.*
- Teach patient relaxation techniques to be performed at least every 4 hours, such as guided imagery, progressive muscle relaxation, meditation. *These measures can restore psychological and physical equilibrium by decreasing autonomic response to anxiety.*
- Refer patient to community or professional mental health resources, *to provide ongoing mental health assistance.*

Evaluations for expected outcomes

- Patient describes at least two situations that increase tension.
- Patient states at least two ways to eliminate or minimize anxious behaviors.
- Patient demonstrates progressive relaxation exercises.
- Patient practices relaxation exercises a specified number of times each day.

• Patient reports being able to cope with current situation without experiencing severe anxiety.

Documentation

• Patient's statement of anxiety and feelings of relief
• Statements about observable signs of patient's anxiety
• Interventions to reduce patient's anxiety
• Effectiveness of nursing interventions that can be observed
• Evaluations for each expected outcome.

Anxiety

related to threat of death

Definition

Feeling of threat or danger to self arising from an unidentifiable source

Assessment

• History of possible stress-related symptoms, including chest pain, rapid pulse, palpitations, hyperventilation, sighing, nausea, constipation, diarrhea, anorexia, compulsive eating, sweating, hives, or rashes
• Anxiety-related behaviors, including nail biting, sleep disturbances, finger tapping, foot swinging, voice quivering, and cheek biting
• Current worries, fears, concerns
• Recent life changes
• Usual coping methods
• Mood
• Personality

Defining characteristics

• Apprehension
• Distress
• Existing problem that poses an immediate threat of death
• Extraneous movements
• Facial tension
• Fearfulness
• Feelings of inadequacy
• Focus on self
• Glancing about
• Increased helplessness
• Increased perspiration
• Increased tension
• Increased urinary frequency
• Increased wariness
• Insomnia
• Overexcitedness
• Poor eye contact
• Regretfulness
• Restlessness
• Shakiness
• Sympathetic stimulation, such as cardiovascular excitation, superficial vasoconstriction, and pupil dilation
• Trembling (hand tremors)
• Uncertainty

Associated medical diagnoses (selected)

Acute myocardial infarction, acute respiratory failure, Adams-Stokes syndrome, adult respiratory distress syndrome, malignant neoplasms, multisystem trauma, post-cardiac arrest, shock (cardiogenic, anaphylactic, hemorrhagic)

Expected outcomes

• Patient states feelings of anxiety.
• Patient identifies cause of anxiety.
• Patient uses support systems to assist with coping.
• Patient copes with threat of anxiety by being involved in decisions about care.
• Patient demonstrates abated physical symptoms of anxiety.
• Patient performs stress-reduction techniques to avoid anxiety symptoms.

Interventions and rationales

- Maintain awareness and sensitivity to threat of death experienced by patient *to recognize, respect, and cope with patient's emotions and behaviors.*
- Thoroughly attend to patient's physical needs, *thus reassuring patient and demonstrating that these needs will continue to be met.*
- Organize work to spend as much time as possible with patient *to allay fears of being neglected or forgotten.*
- Provide opportunities for patient to discuss reasons for anxiety. (Without assistance, some patients will not be able to express their fear of dying.) *By drawing patient out in conversation, you allow communication to proceed at patient's own pace.*
- Determine patient's level of knowledge about situation *so you can correct any misconceptions.*
- If patient and caregivers are coping well with their anticipatory grief, allow a family member or close friend to stay with patient *to give them time for reminiscing, sharing, and decision-making.*
- Encourage family member or friend to participate in care *to provide a more supportive environment for patient.*
- Allow patient to be involved in care-related decisions *because patient has a right to understand and participate in care.*
- Involve the family in joint planning and decision-making with patient *to foster trust between patient and family or caregivers.*
- Support patient's coping mechanisms *to increase potential for further adaptive behaviors.*
- Teach stress-reduction techniques, such as meditation, guided imagery, and progressive muscle relaxation, *to stabilize patient psychologically by diminishing sympathetic response to anxiety.*

Evaluations for expected outcomes

- Patient reports feelings of anxiety.
- Patient describes anxiety-inducing situations.
- Patient engages in conversation and activities with family, caregivers, and other support people.
- Patient makes appropriate care-related decisions.
- Patient experiences fewer physical symptoms associated with anxiety.
- Patient performs progressive relaxation techniques at least twice daily.

Documentation

- Patient's statements of anxious feelings
- Patient's perceptions of reasons for anxiety
- Observations of physical signs of anxiety
- Interventions to assist patient with coping
- Family's willingness to participate in patient's care
- Evaluations for each expected outcome.

■ Aspiration, high risk for

related to absence of protective mechanisms

Definition

State of being at risk for aspiration of gastrointestinal or oropharyngeal secretions, food, or fluids into tracheobronchial passages

Assessment

- Neurologic status, including level of consciousness, orientation, and mental status

- Gastrointestinal status, including gag and swallow reflexes, inspection of abdomen, abdominal girth, auscultation of bowel sounds, palpation for masses and tenderness, percussion of abdomen, and medications
- Nutritional status, including continuous and intermittent tube feeding
- Respiratory status, including skin color, rate and depth of respiration, cough (productive or nonproductive), auscultation of breath sounds, palpation for fremitus, sputum characteristics (color, consistency, amount, odor), arterial blood gases, chest X-ray
- Vital signs
- Laboratory studies, such as white blood cell count and sputum culture

Risk factors
- Bolus or continuous tube feedings or drug administration
- Decreased gastrointestinal motility
- Delayed gastric emptying
- Depressed cough and gag reflexes
- Feeding tubes
- Impaired swallowing
- Increased intragastric pressure
- Overinflated or underinflated tracheostomy or endotracheal tube cuff
- Reduced level of consciousness
- Situations hindering elevation of upper body
- Surgery or trauma to face, mouth, or neck
- Tracheostomy or endotracheal tube
- Wired jaws

Associated medical diagnoses (selected)
Any disease arising in adults that may require surgery with general anesthesia, tube feedings, or artificial airway; cerebrovascular accident; intestinal obstruction; decreased level of consciousness; trauma

Expected outcomes
- Patient shows no signs of aspiration.
- Patient tolerates _____ ml of tube feeding.
- Patient's temperature and white blood cell count remain normal.
- Pathogens do not appear in cultures.
- Respiratory secretions are clear and odorless.
- Auscultation reveals no adventitious breath sounds.
- Patient has normal bowel sounds.
- Patient discusses measures to prevent aspiration with caregiver.

Interventions and rationales
- Assess respiratory status at least every 4 hours *for signs of possible aspiration (increased respiratory rate, cough, sputum production, diminished breath sounds).*
- Monitor and record neurologic status *to detect altered level of consciousness, which could affect intake of food or saliva.*
- Monitor and record vital signs *to detect signs of aspiration or impaired gas exchange due to aspiration.*
- Suction as needed *to keep airway clear.*
- Assess patient for gag and swallow reflexes. *Decreased gag or swallow reflex may cause aspiration.*
- Encourage patient to cough and expectorate sputum *to mobilize secretions.* Provide tissues and paper bag.
- Auscultate bowel sounds every shift and report changes. *Delayed gastric emptying and elevated intragastric pressure may promote regurgitation of stomach contents.*
- If patient is receiving tube feedings:
  - Assess cuff inflation for patient with artificial airway and adjust appropriately *to protect lower airways from oropharyngeal secretions.*

– Add food coloring to tube feeding if patient has altered state of consciousness, diminished gag reflex, or history of aspiration, *to help monitor gastric secretions for aspiration.*
– Begin regimen with a small, diluted amount as tolerated and ordered, *to allow adjustment to formula osmolality and avoid nausea, vomiting, and diarrhea.*
– Elevate head of bed during and after feedings unless contraindicated *to prevent aspiration.*
– Check for residual tube feeding every shift and record amount. If more than 50 ml remains, withhold feeding *to prevent vomiting and aspiration.* Report findings to doctor.
– Place tube properly before feeding or giving medication *to protect airway.*
– Stop feeding immediately if you suspect aspiration. Apply suction as needed. Turn patient on side *to avoid further aspiration.*

- Assess need for antiemetic drug *to reduce nausea and vomiting.* Administer and monitor effectiveness.
- Review test results *to identify signs of infection;* report abnormalities.
- Explain treatment to patient and caregivers *to encourage compliance.*

Evaluations for expected outcomes

- Patient does not show signs of aspiration.
- Patient tolerates _____ ml of tube feeding.
- Patient's temperature remains within normal parameters.
- Patient's white blood cell count remains within normal parameters.
- No pathogens appear in patient's cultures.
- Patient's respiratory secretions remain clear and odorless.
- Auscultation of patient's lungs reveals no adventitious breath sounds.
- Auscultation of patient's abdomen reveals normal bowel sounds.
- Patient and caregiver discuss measures necessary to prevent aspiration.

Documentation

- Verification of tube placement
- Tolerance of tube feedings
- Residuals of tube feedings
- Vomiting or aspiration
- Breath sounds
- Patient's indication of situations that may lead to aspiration
- Observations of physical findings
- Interventions performed to prevent aspiration
- Evaluations for each expected outcome.

Body image disturbance

Definition

Negative perception of self that makes healthful functioning more difficult

Assessment

- Physiologic changes
- Behavioral changes
- Patient's and family's perception of the patient's present health problem
- Patient's usual pattern of coping with stress
- Marital status
- Patient's role in the family
- Patient's past experiences with health problems
- Sleep pattern
- Appetite
- Hobbies and interests
- Occupational history
- Ethnic background and cultural perceptions

Defining characteristics

- Actual change in structure or function

- Hiding or overexposing body part (intentional or unintentional)
- Missing body part
- Nonverbal response to actual or perceived change in structure or function
- Not looking at body part
- Not touching body part
- Trauma to nonfunctioning part
- Verbal response to actual or perceived change in structure or function

Associated medical diagnoses (selected)
Acromegaly; Addison's disease; bone or skin cancer; breast cancer requiring mastectomy; burns; cerebrovascular accident; colitis; conditions requiring colostomy, ileostomy, laryngectomy, limb amputation, radical neck surgery, tracheostomy or ureteroileostomy; Crohn's disease; Cushing's disease; facial trauma or tumors; Graves' disease; rheumatoid arthritis; spinal cord injury

Expected outcomes
- Patient acknowledges change in body image.
- Patient participates in decision making about his care (specify).
- Patient communicates feelings about change in body image.
- Patient expresses positive feelings about self.
- Patient talks with someone who has experienced the same problem.
- Patient demonstrates ability to practice two new coping behaviors.

Interventions and rationales
- While assisting with self-care measures, involve patient in discussions that will provide further insights into patient's coping patterns and self-esteem. *Patient's usual coping patterns and self-perception provide baseline data for assessing potential threat of current situation.*
- Accept patient's perception of self, *to validate patient's self-perception and provide reassurance that he or she can successfully overcome crisis.*
- Assess patient's readiness for decision making; then involve him in making choices and decisions related to care. *This gives patient sense of control over environment.*
- Encourage patient to participate actively in performing care. *This gives patient sense of independence.*
- Give patient opportunities to voice feelings. *This helps patient ventilate doubts and resolve concerns.*
- Show patient how bodily functions are improving or stabilizing. *Responding honestly to patient's self-doubts and describing others' successful adaptations to similar situations increases patient's confidence.*
- Provide positive reinforcement to patient's efforts to adapt, *to increase probability that healthy adaptation will continue.*
- Arrange for patient to interact with others who have similar problems. *A support group allows patient to share mutual support and caring with others who can fully understand.*
- Refer patient to a mental health professional for further counseling. *Referral to psychiatric liaison nurse is indicated when patient is adapting poorly to situation.*
- Teach patient coping strategies (specify), *to help overcome maladaptive coping behaviors.*
- Have patient provide feedback about coping behaviors that seem to work. Reinforce the practice of these behaviors. *This allows nurse to evaluate patient's adaptive abilities. Positive feedback reinforces adaptability*

and encourages similar behaviors in future.

Evaluations for expected outcomes

- Patient acknowledges change in body image.
- Patient takes an active role in planning aspects of care (specify).
- Patient expresses emotions associated with change in body image.
- Patient expresses at least one positive feeling about self daily.
- Patient participates in discussions with support group composed of individuals with a similar change in body image (specify).
- Patient uses at least two healthy coping skills to deal with change in body image.

Documentation

- Words patient uses to describe self, prostheses, adaptive equipment, limitations
- Body parts which patient focuses on or ignores
- Observations related to change in structure or function of body part
- Observed responses of patient to change in body part, such as touching or not touching
- Health education or counseling provided to help patient cope with altered body image
- Patient's response to nursing interventions
- Evaluations for each expected outcome.

Breathing pattern, ineffective

related to decreased energy or fatigue

Definition

Change in rate, depth, or pattern of breathing that alters normal gas exchange

Assessment

- History of respiratory disorder
- Respiratory status, including rate and depth of respiration, symmetry of chest expansion, use of accessory muscles, presence of cough, anterior-posterior chest diameter, palpation for fremitus, percussion of lung fields, auscultation of breath sounds, pulmonary function studies
- Neurologic and mental status, including level of consciousness and emotional level
- Knowledge, including current understanding of physical condition and physical, mental, and emotional readiness to learn

Defining characteristics

- Abnormal arterial blood gas levels
- Accessory muscle use
- Altered chest excursion
- Assumption of 3-point position
- Cough
- Cyanosis
- Dyspnea
- Exertional dyspnea
- Fremitus
- Increased anteroposterior diameter of chest wall
- Nasal flaring
- Pursed-lip breathing and prolonged expiratory phase
- Respiratory depth changes
- Tachypnea

• Verbal report of decreased energy or fatigue

Associated medical diagnoses (selected)
Anemia, chronic obstructive pulmonary disease, cirrhosis, congestive heart failure, metabolic acidosis, pulmonary edema

Expected outcomes
• Patient's respiratory rate stays within ±5 of baseline.
• Arterial blood gas levels return to baseline.
• Patient reports feeling comfortable when breathing.
• Patient reports feeling rested each day.
• Patient demonstrates diaphragmatic pursed-lip breathing.
• Patient achieves maximum lung expansion with adequate ventilation.
• Patient demonstrates skill in conserving energy while carrying out activities of daily living.

Interventions and rationales
• Assess and record respiratory rate and depth at least every 4 hours, *to detect early signs of respiratory compromise.* Assess arterial blood gas levels according to hospital policy, *to monitor oxygenation and ventilation status.*
• Auscultate breath sounds at least every 4 hours *to detect decreased or adventitious breath sounds;* report changes.
• Assist patient to a comfortable position, such as by supporting upper extremities with pillows, providing over-bed table with a pillow to lean on, or elevating head of bed. *These measures promote comfort, chest expansion, and ventilation of basilar lung fields.*
• Help patient with activities of daily living, as needed, *to conserve energy and avoid overexertion and fatigue.*
• Administer oxygen, as ordered, to help relieve respiratory distress. *Supplemental oxygen helps reduce hypoxemia and respiratory distress.*
• Suction airway, as needed, *to remove secretions.*
• Schedule necessary activities to provide periods of rest. *This prevents fatigue and reduces oxygen demands.*
• Teach patient about:
  – pursed-lip breathing
  – abdominal breathing
  – performing relaxation techniques
  – taking prescribed medications (ensuring accuracy of dosage and frequency; monitoring side effects)
  – scheduling activities to avoid fatigue and provide for rest periods.

These measures allow patient to participate in maintaining health status and improve ventilation.

Evaluations for expected outcomes
• Patient's respiratory rate remains within established limits.
• Patient's arterial blood gas levels return to and remain within established limits.
• Patient indicates feeling comfortable when breathing, either verbally or through behavior.
• Each day, patient reports that he feels rested.
• Patient performs diaphragmatic pursed-lip breathing.
• When patient carries out activities of daily living, breathing pattern remains normal.

Documentation
• Patient's expressions of comfort in breathing, emotional state, under-

standing of medical diagnosis, and readiness to learn
- Physical findings from pulmonary assessment
- Interventions carried out and patient's responses to them
- Evaluations for each expected outcome.

Breathing pattern, ineffective

related to pain

Definition

Change in the rate, depth, or pattern of breathing that alters normal gas exchange

Assessment

- History of medical or surgical problem that causes ineffective breathing
- Respiratory status, including rate and depth of respiration, symmetry of chest expansion, use of accessory muscles, presence of cough, anterior-posterior chest diameter, palpation for fremitus, percussion of lung fields, auscultation of breath sounds, and arterial blood gases
- Neurologic status, including level of consciousness and sensory and motor status
- Psychosocial status, including willingness to cooperate with treatment, coping mechanisms, and knowledge level (current understanding of physical condition)

Defining characteristics

- Accessory muscle use
- Altered chest excursion
- Altered depth of respiration
- Anxiety
- Arterial blood gas abnormalities
- Cyanosis
- Dyspnea
- Fremitus
- Inability to cough
- Nasal flaring
- Tachypnea
- Verbal report of painful respiration

Associated medical diagnoses (selected)

Chest wall injury, pericarditis, pleural effusion, pleurisy, pneumonia, pneumothorax, pulmonary embolus, rib or vertebral fractures

Expected outcomes

- Patient's respiratory rate stays within ± 5 of baseline.
- Arterial blood gas levels remain normal.
- Patient achieves comfort without depressing respirations.
- Patient demonstrates correct use of incentive spirometer.
- Auscultation reveals no adventitious breath sounds.
- Patient states understanding of importance of taking deep breaths periodically.
- Patient practices relaxation techniques _____ times a day.
- Patient reports ability to breathe comfortably.

Interventions and rationales

- Assess and record respiratory status at least every 4 hours *to detect early signs of compromise.* Also assess arterial blood gas levels according to hospital policy *to monitor oxygenation and ventilation status.*
- Assess for pain every 3 hours. *Pain reduces respiratory effort and ventilation.*
- Give pain medication, as ordered, *to allow maximal chest expansion.* Record effectiveness, and monitor respiratory depression induced by narcotic analgesic, *to guide further therapy.*

• Assist patient to a comfortable position that also allows for maximal chest expansion: Fowler's position, for example, or leaning on over-bed table with pillow *will enhance chest expansion.*
• Assist patient in using incentive spirometer or other device, as ordered, *to ensure proper use and help prevent atelectasis.*
• Teach patient how to splint chest while coughing. Keep extra pillow for patient's use. *Splinting reduces pain during coughing.*
• Perform chest physiotherapy to aid mobilization and secretion removal, if ordered. *Percussion, vibration, and postural drainage enhance airway clearance and respiratory effort.*
• Provide rest periods between breathing enhancement measures *to avoid fatigue.*
• Encourage patient to use an incentive spirometer independently. Praise patient's efforts, *to encourage compliance.*
• Provide oxygen, as ordered, *to help relieve respiratory distress caused by hypoxemia.*
• Teach relaxation techniques to help reduce anxiety. Guided imagery, progressive muscle relaxation, breathing exercises, and meditation *reduce pain and anxiety and enhance patient's sense of self-control.*
• Change patient's position frequently *to maximize comfort.*
• Encourage patient to discuss fears *to help reduce anxiety.*

Evaluations for expected outcomes
• Patient's respiratory rate remains within set limits (specify).
• Patient's arterial blood gas levels remain within set limits (specify).
• Patient does not express feelings of pain, either verbally or through behavior.
• Patient's breath sounds remain clear.
• Patient explains why periodic deep breathing is important to maintaining respiratory status.
• Patient uses incentive spirometer or other respiratory device unassisted every 2 hours, or as ordered.
• Patient practices relaxation techniques _____ times daily.
• Patient reports breathing comfortably, either verbally or through behavior.

Documentation
• Patient's reports of pain
• Patient's perception of need to take deep breaths and cough.
• Patient's expression of the effectiveness of pain medication
• Observations of physical findings
• Effectiveness of medications
• Descriptions of patient's efforts to take deep breaths and cough
• Interventions performed to enhance patient's ability to breathe effectively
• Evaluations for each expected outcome.

■ Cardiac output, decreased

related to reduced stroke volume as a result of electrophysiologic problems

Definition
Cardiovascular or respiratory symptoms resulting from insufficient blood being pumped by the heart

Assessment
• Mental status, including orientation and level of consciousness

• Cardiovascular status, including history of arrhythmias and syncope, jugular vein distention, hepatojugular reflux, heart rate and rhythm, heart sounds, blood pressure, peripheral pulses, ECG, exercise ECG, echocardiogram, phonocardiogram, serum digitalis levels, and skin color, temperature, turgor, and capillary refill
• Respiratory status, including respiratory rate and depth, breath sounds, chest X-ray, and arterial blood gases
• Renal status, including weight, intake and output, urine specific gravity, and serum electrolytes

Defining characteristics
• Arrhythmias, ECG changes
• Cold, clammy skin
• Cyanosis
• Decreased peripheral pulses
• Dizziness
• Dyspnea
• Electromechanical cardiac disorders
• Fatigue
• Jugular venous distention
• Mental status changes
• Pallor of skin and mucous membranes
• Syncope
• Variations in hemodynamic reading
• Vertigo

Associated medical diagnoses (selected)
Acute myocardial infarction, Stokes-Adams syndrome, carotid sinus syndrome, chronic heart block, congestive heart failure, digitalis toxicity, electrolyte imbalance, sick sinus syndrome

Expected outcomes
• Patient maintains hemodynamic stability: pulse not less than _____ and not greater than _____; blood pressure not less than _____ and not greater than _____.
• Skin remains warm and dry.
• Dyspneic episodes decreased or absent.
• No signs of dizziness or syncope.
• No complaint of chest pain.
• Patient practices stress-reduction techniques every 2 hours.
• Cardiac output remains adequate.
• Patient has no arrhythmias.
• Patient verbalizes reportable symptoms, diet, medication regimen, and prescribed activity level.

Interventions and rationales
• Monitor apical and radial pulse at least every 4 hours, *to better detect arrhythmias.* Immediately report abnormal pulse rates.
• Note pulse rhythm at least every 4 hours and report irregularities. *Arrhythmias may indicate cardiac arrest or other complications.*
• Assess skin temperature every 4 hours. *Cool, clammy skin may indicate decreased cardiac output.*
• Assess respiratory status at least every 4 hours. Report complaints of dyspnea or restlessness. *Adventitious breath sounds or dyspnea may indicate fluid buildup in lungs and pulmonary capillary bed (as in congestive heart failure).*
• Administer oxygen, as ordered, *to increase supply to myocardium.*
• Report complaints of dizziness or syncope promptly; *these may indicate cerebral hypoxia.*
• Tell patient to report chest pain right away, *as it may signal myocardial hypoxia or injury.*
• Plan patient's care to avoid overexertion, *which increases myocardial oxygen demand.*
• Change patient's position frequently *to promote comfort and avoid tachycardia and other sympathetic responses.*
• Teach patient how to perform stress-reduction techniques *to allay*

anxiety and avoid cardiac complications.
• Remind patient to practice stress-reduction techniques every 2 hours while awake *to help internalize learned techniques.*
• Give antiarrhythmic drugs as prescribed *to reduce or abolish arrhythmias.* Monitor for adverse effects.
• Instruct patient to avoid straining during bowel movements, *which may cause bradycardia and decreased cardiac output.*
• Administer stool softeners as prescribed *to reduce straining at stool.*
• Carry out the medical care plan as ordered. *Collaborative practice enhances care.*
• Teach patient about reportable symptoms (such as chest pain, palpitations, weakness, dizziness, syncope), prescribed diet, medications (name, dosage, frequency, therapeutic and adverse effects), and activity level. *These measures let patient and caregivers participate in patient's care and help patient make informed decisions about health status.*

Evaluations for expected outcomes
• Patient's pulse rate and blood pressure remain within set limits.
• Patient's skin remains warm and dry.
• Patient experiences fewer dyspneic episodes.
• Patient does not experience dizziness or syncope.
• Patient does not report experiencing chest pain, either verbally or through behavior.
• Patient practices stress-reduction techniques every 2 hours.
• No arrhythmias are noted during monitoring or physical examination of patient.
• Patient lists signs and symptoms of decreased cardiac output (dizziness, syncope, cool or clammy skin, fatigue, dyspnea).
• Patient expresses understanding of importance of following prescribed diet, taking medications, and maintaining activity level.

Documentation
• Patient's symptoms
• Observation of physical findings
• Incidents of chest pain, including location, character, duration, and treatment
• Patient's tolerance for activity
• Interventions to control or monitor symptoms and patient's response
• Patient teaching
• Evaluations for each expected outcome.

■ Cardiac output, decreased

related to reduced stroke volume as a result of mechanical or structural problems

Definition
Cardiovascular or respiratory symptoms resulting from insufficient blood being pumped by the heart

Assessment
• Mental status, including orientation and level of consciousness
• Cardiovascular status, including history of valvular disorder, capillary heart disease, or myopathy; skin color, temperature, turgor, and capillary refill time; jugular vein distention; hepatojugular reflux; heart rate and rhythm; heart sounds; blood pressure; peripheral pulses; ECG; exercise ECG; echocardiogram; and phonocardiogram

• Respiratory status, including respiratory rate and depth, breath sounds, chest X-ray, and arterial blood gases
• Renal status, including weight, intake and output, and urine specific gravity

Defining characteristics
• Abnormal breath sounds
• Anuria
• Arrhythmias; ECG changes
• Ascites
• Cold, clammy skin
• Cough
• Crackles
• Cyanosis
• Decreased peripheral pulses
• Dyspnea
• Fatigue
• Frothy sputum
• Jugular vein distention
• Liver engorgement and tenderness
• Mechanical or structural cardiac abnormalities
• Mental status changes
• Oliguria
• Orthopnea
• Pallor of skin and mucous membranes
• Variations in hemodynamic reading

Associated medical diagnoses (selected)
Anaphylactic shock, anemia, angina, aortic stenosis, aortic insufficiency, bacterial endocarditis, cardiogenic shock, congestive heart failure, cor pulmonale, hypovolemic shock, mitral insufficiency, mitral stenosis, myocardial infarction, neurogenic shock, Paget's disease, papillary muscle syndrome, pericarditis, pulmonary edema, pulmonary embolism, renal failure, respiratory failure, septic shock, tetralogy of Fallot, thyrotoxicosis

Expected outcomes
• Patient maintains hemodynamic stability: pulse not less than _____ and not greater than _____; blood pressure not less than _____ and not greater than _____.
• Patient exhibits no arrhythmias.
• Skin remains warm and dry.
• Patient exhibits no pedal edema.
• Patient achieves activity within limits of prescribed heart rate.
• Patient expresses sense of physical comfort after activity.
• Heart's workload diminishes.
• Patient maintains adequate cardiac output.
• Patient performs stress-reduction techniques every 4 hours while awake.
• Patient states understanding of signs and symptoms, prescribed activity level, diet, and medications.

Interventions and rationales
• Monitor and record level of consciousness, heart rate and rhythm, and blood pressure at least every 4 hours, or more often if necessary, *to detect cerebral hypoxia possibly resulting from decreased cardiac output.*
• Auscultate heart and breath sounds at least every 4 hours. Report abnormal sounds as soon as they develop. *Extra heart sounds may indicate early cardiac decompensation; adventitious breath sounds may indicate pulmonary congestion and diminished cardiac output.*
• Measure and record intake and output accurately. *Decreased urine output without lowered fluid intake may indicate decreased renal perfusion, possibly from decreased cardiac output.*
• Promptly treat life-threatening arrhythmias, as ordered, *to avoid crisis.*

- Weigh patient daily before breakfast *to detect fluid retention.*
- Inspect for pedal or sacral edema *to detect venous stasis and reduced cardiac output.*
- Provide skin care every 4 hours *to enhance skin perfusion and venous flow.*
- Gradually increase patient's activities within limits of prescribed heart rate *to allow heart to adjust to increased oxygen demand.* Monitor pulse rate before and after activity *to compare rates and gauge tolerance.*
- Plan patient's activities *to avoid fatigue and increased myocardial workload.*
- Maintain dietary restrictions, as ordered, *to reduce risk of cardiac disease.*
- Teach patient stress-reduction techniques, *to reduce patient's anxiety and provide a sense of control.*
- Explain all procedures and tests.
- Teach patient about: chest pain and other reportable symptoms; prescribed diet; medications (name, dosage, frequency, therapeutic effects, adverse effects); prescribed activity level; simple methods for lifting and bending; and stress-reduction techniques. *These measures involve patient and family in care.*
- Carry out medical care plan, as ordered. *Collaborative practice enhances overall care.*
- Administer oxygen, as ordered, *to increase supply to myocardium.*

Evaluations for expected outcomes

- Patient's pulse rate and blood pressure remain within set limits.
- Patient does not exhibit arrhythmias during monitoring or physical examination.
- Patient's skin remains warm and dry to the touch.
- Inspection and palpation of patient do not reveal pedal edema.
- Patient carries out activities of daily living without heart rate exceeding or dropping below set limits.
- Patient does not indicate, either verbally or through behavior, chest pain, dyspnea, fatigue, or other forms of discomfort after activity.
- Patient performs stress-reduction techniques every 4 hours.
- Patient describes signs and symptoms of decreased cardiac output, such as dizziness, syncope, clammy skin, fatigue, and dyspnea.
- Patient understands importance of following prescribed diet, taking medications as ordered, and maintaining activity level.

Documentation

- Patient's needs and perception of problem
- Observations of physical findings
- Patient's response to activity
- Development of skills related to diet, medication, activity, and stress management
- Evaluations for each expected outcome.

■ Caregiver role strain

related to discharge of a family member with significant home care needs

Definition

Caregiver's perceived difficulty in providing care

Assessment

- Caregiver's physical and mental status, including chronic health problems, self-care abilities, mobility limitations, level of cognitive function

• Care recipient's physical and mental status, including illness, self-care limitations, mobility limitations, level of cognitive function
• Support systems, including financial resources, family members and friends, community services, health-related services such as geriatric day-care, home health aides
• Home environment, including layout of home, structural barriers, need for equipment or assistive devices, availability of transportation
• Cultural, ethnic, and religious background
• Perceived and actual obligations of caregiver
• Caregiver's personal strengths, including coping and problem-solving abilities, participation in diversional activities or hobbies

Defining characteristics

• Caregiver reports:
  – difficulty performing specific caregiving activities, such as bathing, cleaning up after incontinence, managing behavior problems, managing pain
  – feeling a sense of loss because care recipient has changed drastically
  – feeling depressed
  – feeling that providing care interferes with other important aspects of life, including career, family, social activities
  – feeling stress or anxiety in relationship with care recipient
  – feeling that other family members aren't helping sufficiently or showing enough appreciation for caregiver's efforts
  – not having sufficient resources (time, emotional strength, physical energy, help from others) to provide care
  – worrying about such possibilities as the care recipient's deteriorating health and emotional state, institutionalization of the the care recipient, or the inability to continue to provide care

Associated medical diagnoses (selected)

Acquired immunodeficiency syndrome (AIDS); Alzheimer's disease; amyotrophic lateral sclerosis; cancer; cerebral palsy; cerebrovascular accident; chronic obstructive pulmonary disease; congestive heart failure; dementia; drug or alcohol addiction; end-stage renal, cardiac, or pulmonary disease; Huntington's disease; multiple sclerosis; muscular dystrophy; paralysis; Parkinson's disease; schizophrenia

Expected outcomes

• Caregiver describes current stressors.
• Caregiver identifies stressors that can and cannot be controlled.
• Caregiver identifies formal and informal sources of support.
• Caregiver reports increased ability to cope with stress.

Interventions and rationales

• Help the caregiver to identify current stressors *to evaluate the causes of role strain.*
• Using a nonjudgmental approach, help the caregiver evaluate which stressors are controllable and which are not *to begin to develop strategies to reduce stress.*
• Encourage the caregiver to discuss coping skills used to overcome similar stressful situations in the past *to build confidence for managing the current situation.*
• Encourage the caregiver to participate in a support group. Provide information on an organization such as

the Alzheimer's Association, Children of Aging Parents, or the referral service of the community AIDS task force *to foster mutual support and provide an opportunity for the caregiver to discuss personal feelings with empathetic listeners.*
- Help the caregiver identify informal sources of support, such as family members, friends, church groups, and community volunteers, *to provide resources for obtaining an occasional or regularly scheduled respite.*
- Help the caregiver to identify available formal support services, such as home health agencies, municipal or county social services, hospital social workers, doctors, clinics, and day-care centers, *to enhance coping by providing a reliable structure for support.*
- If the caregiver seems overly anxious or distraught, gently point out the facts about the care recipient's mental and physical condition. *Many times, especially when the care recipient is a family member, the caregiver's perspective is clouded by a long history of emotional involvement. Your input may help the caregiver view the situation more objectively.* If you believe that excessive emotional involvement is hindering the caregiver's ability to function, consider recommending Codependent's Anonymous, a support group for people whose preoccupation with a relationship leads to chronic suffering and diminished effectiveness, *to provide support.*
- Suggest ways for the caregiver to use time more efficiently. For example, the caregiver may be able to save time by filling out insurance forms while visiting and chatting with the care recipient. *Better time management may help the caregiver reduce stress.*

Evaluations for expected outcomes
- Caregiver identifies and develops a realistic appraisal of each stressful situation.
- Caregiver describes emotional response to each stressful situation.
- Caregiver utilizes appropriate coping skills for each stressful situation.
- Caregiver uses available support systems.
- Caregiver utilizes resources identified.

Documentation
- Stressors (perceived and actual) identified by caregiver
- Observations of caregiver's response to stressful situations
- Referrals provided
- Caregiver's use of informal and formal support systems
- Coping strategies identified by caregiver and nurse
- Evidence of improvement in caregiver's ability to cope
- Evaluations for each expected outcome.

■ Caregiver role strain, high risk for

Definition

Caregiver's vulnerability to experiencing difficulty in providing care

Assessment
- Caregiver's physical and mental status, including chronic health problems, self-care abilities, mobility limitations, level of cognitive function
- Care recipient's physical and mental status, including illness, self-care limitations, mobility limitations, level of cognitive function

- Support systems, including financial resources, family members and friends, community services, health-related services such as geriatric day-care, home health aids
- Home environment, including structural barriers, layout of home, need for presence of equipment or assistive devices, availability of transportation
- Cultural, ethnic, and religious background
- Perceived and actual obligations of caregiver
- Caregiver's personal strengths, including usual coping and problem-solving abilities, participation in diversional activities or hobbies

Risk factors

- Developmental
  - lack of prepararation for caregiver role – for example, a young adult who must unexpectedly care for a middle-aged parent
  - developmental delay or disability of the care recipient or caregiver
- Pathophysiologic
  - cognitive problems caused by brain dysfunction in care recipient
  - drug or alcohol addiction in caregiver or care recipient
  - severe illness
  - unpredictable illness course or instability in care recipient's health
- Psychological
  - codependency
  - deviant, bizarre behavior on the part of the care recipient
  - evidence of dysfunctional family coping patterns that existed before the caregiving situation
  - evidence of poor coping ability on the part of the caregiver
  - evidence of psychological problems in the care recipient
  - poor relationship between caregiver and care recipient
- Situational
  - competing role commitments on the part of the caregiver
  - discharge of family member with significant home care needs
  - inadequate environment or facilities for providing care
  - isolation of caregiver
  - lack of experience on the part of the caregiver
  - lack of respite or recreation for caregiver
  - long duration of caregiving anticipated
  - numerous, complex caregiving tasks
  - presence of abuse or violence
  - simultaneous occurrence of other events that cause stress for family, such as significant personal loss, natural disaster, or economic hardship

Associated medical diagnoses (selected)

Acquired immunodeficiency syndrome (AIDS); Alzheimer's disease; amyotrophic lateral sclerosis; cancer; cerebral palsy; cerebrovascular accident; chronic obstructive pulmonary disease; congestive heart failure; dementia; drug or alcohol addiction; end-stage renal, cardiac, or pulmonary disease; Huntington's disease; multiple sclerosis; muscular dystrophy; paralysis; Parkinson's disease; schizophrenia

Expected outcomes

- Caregiver identifies current stressors.
- Caregiver identifies appropriate coping strategies and states plans to

incorporate strategies into daily routine.
- Caregiver states intention to contact formal and informal sources of support.
- Caregiver states intention to incorporate recreational activities into daily routine.
- Caregiver reports satisfaction with ability to cope with stress caused by caregiving responsibilities.

Interventions and rationales
- Help the caregiver identify current stressors. Ask whether stress is likely to increase or decrease in the future *to evaluate the risk for caregiver role strain.*
- Encourage the caregiver to discuss coping skills used to overcome similar stressful situations in the past *to reinforce the caregiver's confidence in her ability to manage the current situation and explore ways to apply coping strategies before the caregiver becomes overwhelmed.*
- Help the caregiver identify informal sources of support, such as family members, friends, church groups, and community volunteers, *to plan for an occasional or regularly scheduled respite.*
- Help the caregiver to identify available formal support services, such as home health agencies, municipal or county social services, hospital social workers, doctors, clinics, and day-care centers, *to assist the caregiver and thereby lessen the risk of strain.*
- Encourage the caregiver to discuss hobbies or diversional activities. *Incorporating enjoyable activities into the daily or weekly schedule will discipline the caregiver to take needed breaks from caregiving responsibilities and thereby diminish stress.*
- Encourage the caregiver to participate in a support group. Provide information on an organization such as the Alzheimer's Association, Children of Aging Parents, or the referral service of the community AIDS task force *to foster mutual support and provide an outlet for expressing feelings before frustration becomes overwhelming.*
- If the caregiver seems overly anxious or distraught, gently point out the facts about the care recipient's mental and physical condition. *Many times, especially when the care recipient is a family member, the caregiver's perspective is clouded by a long history of emotional involvement. Your input may help the caregiver view the situation more objectively.* If you believe that excessive emotional involvement is hindering the caregiver's ability to function, consider recommending Codependent's Anonymous, a support group for people whose preoccupation with a relationship leads to chronic suffering and diminished effectiveness, *to provide support.*
- Suggest ways for the caregiver to use time efficiently; for example, the caregiver may be able to save time by filling out insurance forms while visiting and chatting with the care recipient. *Better time management may help the caregiver reduce stress.*

Evaluations for expected outcomes
- Caregiver identifies and develops a realistic appraisal of each stressful situation.
- Caregiver describes emotional response to each stressful situation.
- Caregiver utilizes appropriate coping skills for each stressful situation.
- Caregiver uses available support systems.
- Caregiver utilizes resources identified.

Documentation

- Current stressors identified by caregiver
- Risk factors (developmental, pathophysiologic, psychological, situational) for caregiver role strain identified by nurse
- Caregiver's statements indicating intention to take action to minimize stress, such as seeking help from support services, participating in a caregiver support group, and scheduling time for recreational activities
- Coping strategies identified by caregiver and nurse
- Observations of caregiver's response to stressful situations
- Referrals provided
- Evaluations for each expected outcome.

Constipation

related to gastrointestinal obstruction

Definition

Interruption of normal bowel movements resulting in infrequent or absent stools

Assessment

- History of bowel disorder or surgery
- Gastrointestinal status, including nausea and vomiting, usual bowel habits, change in bowel habits, laxative use, stool characteristics (color, amount, size, consistency), pain, inspection of abdomen, auscultation of bowel sounds, palpation for masses and tenderness, percussion for tympany and dullness, upper GI series, barium enema, sigmoidoscopy
- Nutritional status, including dietary intake, appetite, current weight, change from normal weight
- Fluid and electrolyte status, including intake and output, skin turgor, urine specific gravity, serum electrolytes
- History of ingesting nonfood items (in psychiatric patients)

Defining characteristics

- Abdominal distention
- Abdominal pain
- Amount of stool less than usual
- Clinical evidence of gastrointestinal obstruction
- Decreased appetite
- Fever
- Flatulence
- Frequency of bowel movements less than usual
- Hard, formed stools (change in stool diameter)
- Palpable abdominal mass
- Projectile vomiting
- Seizures (in controlled seizure patients)
- Straining during defecation
- Vomiting fecal material

Associated medical diagnoses (selected)

Adhesions, cancer of large bowel, diverticulitis, impaction, intussusception, mechanical intestinal obstruction, mesenteric thrombosis, neurogenic intestinal obstruction, paralytic ileus, peritonitis, spinal cord injury, strangulated hernia, vascular intestinal obstruction, volvulus

Expected outcomes

- Patient returns to usual bowel pattern.
- Patient maintains fluid balance; intake equals output.
- Patient displays normal bowel sounds.
- Patient expresses pain relief or comfort.

- Patient stops vomiting through use of antiemetics or gastrointestinal tube.
- Patient states understanding of surgical procedure.
- Patient or caregiver demonstrates use of ileostomy or colostomy equipment.
- Patient discusses fears and anxieties associated with bowel diversion.
- Patient or caregiver discusses effect of bowel diversion on life-style.

Interventions and rationales

- Carefully monitor and record frequency and characteristics of stool *to form the basis of an effective treatment plan.*
- Record intake and output accurately *to ensure correct fluid replacement therapy.* Report any imbalance.
- Auscultate bowel sounds and record every 4 hours. Report significant changes. *Absent or diminished bowel sounds may indicate peritoneal irritation or intestinal obstruction.*
- Record patient's weight daily *to detect possible fluid retention, food malabsorption, or increased adaptation requirements on body processes.*
- Administer pain medication and antiemetics, as ordered. Monitor effectiveness *to determine need for alternative treatment.*
- Promote patient comfort during vomiting episodes by providing oral care and removing vomitus promptly. Carefully record amount and characteristics of vomitus *to ensure accurate intake and output records.*
- Provide oral and nasal care every 4 hours while gastrointestinal tube is present. Keep nostrils clean and moist *to prevent irritation.*
- Prepare patient for surgery:
  - Give preoperative instruction for abdominal surgery *to reduce patient's anxiety and increase trust.*
  - Inform patient about ileostomy, colostomy, or colectomy, as indicated, *to reduce anxiety.*
- Instruct patient and caregivers in the use of ileostomy or colostomy equipment *to promote familiarity and establish therapeutic relationship.* Have patient and caregivers demonstrate use of equipment *to encourage feeling of shared responsibility.*
- Encourage patient and family to express feelings and concerns about changes in body image *to help them learn to cope.*
- Encourage visits to patient by persons from ileostomy or colostomy clubs and other support groups, *to provide patient with additional health care resources.*

Evaluations for expected outcomes

- Patient exhibits a normal bowel pattern.
- Patient drinks adequate amount of fluids, with intake equal to output.
- Patient does not exhibit weight loss or gain. Weight is consistent with body weight chart.
- Patient displays normal bowel sounds.
- Patient states that pain medication is effective and does not experience increase in severity of pain.
- Patient does not vomit. Vomitus does not appear on bed or self.
- Patient's mouth is clear and free of odor, and nostrils are clean and moist.
- Patient expresses understanding of surgical procedure, including need for ileostomy or colostomy.
- Patient or caregiver demonstrates care, changing, and irrigation of ileostomy or colostomy equipment.
- Patient states acceptance of bowel diversion.

• Patient comes to terms with effects of bowel diversion on life-style.
• Patient or caregiver identifies and contacts support group, if needed.

Documentation
• Patient's expressions of concern about vomiting, gastrointestinal tube, or surgery
• Observation of characteristics of emesis and stool, intake and output, weight, bowel sounds, and condition of oral cavity
• Patient's reaction and adaptation to ileostomy or colostomy
• Patient's and caregivers' participation in care and response to instruction
• Evaluations for each expected outcome.

Constipation

related to inadequate intake of fluid and bulk

Definition
Interruption of normal bowel movements resulting in infrequent or absent stools

Assessment
• History of bowel disorder or surgery
• Gastrointestinal status, including nausea and vomiting, usual bowel habits, change in bowel habits, laxative use, stool characteristics (color, amount, size, consistency), pain, inspection of abdomen, auscultation of bowel sounds, palpation for masses and tenderness, and percussion for tympany and dullness
• Nutritional status, including dietary intake, appetite, current weight, and change from normal weight
• Fluid status, including fluid intake, urine output, urine specific gravity, and skin turgor
• Knowledge, including ability and motivation to change current patterns, and understanding of relationship between intake, bulk, and constipation

Defining characteristics
• Amount of stool less than usual
• Decreased appetite
• Dehydration
• Fever
• Frequency less than usual pattern
• Hard, formed stools
• Straining during defecation
• Verbal report of decreased intake of fluid, food, or bulk

Associated medical diagnoses (selected)
This diagnosis may pertain to all patients undergoing periods of restricted food or fluid intake and those with anorexia nervosa or coma.

Expected outcomes
• Elimination pattern returns to normal.
• Patient experiences bowel movement every ____ day(s).
• Patient consumes high-fiber or high-bulk diet, unless contraindicated.
• Patient maintains oral fluid intake of 2,500 ml daily, unless contraindicated.
• Patient states understanding of relationship of dietary intake and bulk to constipation.
• Patient lists foods needed to prevent recurrence of problem, such as fruit, fruit juices, whole grain bread, and cereals.

Interventions and rationales

- Monitor and record frequency and characteristics of stool. *Careful monitoring forms the basis of an effective treatment plan.*
- Record intake and output accurately *to ensure correct fluid replacement therapy.*
- Unless contraindicated, encourage fluid intake of 2,500 ml daily *to ensure correct fluid replacement therapy.*
- Place patient on bedpan or commode at specific time(s) daily, as close to usual evacuation time (if known) as possible, *to aid adaptation to routine physiologic function.*
- Administer laxative or enema, as ordered, *to promote elimination of solids and gases from GI tract.* Monitor effectiveness.
- Teach patient to gently massage along the transverse and descending colon *to stimulate the bowel's spastic reflex and aid stool passage.*
- Consult with dietitian about increasing fiber and bulk in diet to maximum prescribed by doctor. *This will improve intestinal muscle tone and promote comfortable elimination.*
- Instruct patient and family in the relationship of diet, exercise, and fluid intake to constipation. Develop plan and provide for mild exercise periods. *These measures promote muscle tone and circulation and discourage departure from prescribed diet.*

Evaluations for expected outcomes

- Patient resumes regular bowel schedule.
- Without using laxatives, enemas, or suppositories, patient has bowel movement every _____ day(s).
- Patient consumes fruit, bran, and other high-fiber foods.
- Patient drinks 2,500 ml of fluid daily, unless contraindicated.
- Patient expresses understanding of the effects of diet and fluid intake on constipation.
- Patient names foods that will help prevent recurrence of constipation.

Documentation

- Patient's expressions of concern about constipation, dietary changes, laxative use, and bowel pattern
- Observations of food and fluid intake and stool characteristics
- Patient's expression of understanding of relationship between constipation and dietary intake of fluid and bulk
- Patient's response to nursing interventions
- Evaluations for each expected outcome.

■ Constipation

related to personal habits

Definition

Interruption of normal bowel movements resulting in infrequent or absent stools

Assessment

- History of bowel disorder or surgery
- Gastrointestinal status, including nausea and vomiting, usual bowel habits, change in bowel habits, stool characteristics (color, amount, size, consistency), pain, inspection of abdomen, auscultation of bowel sounds, palpation for masses and tenderness, percussion for tympany and dullness, laxative or enema use, medications (iron, narcotics)

• Nutritional status, including dietary intake, appetite, current weight, and change from normal weight
• Activity status, type and duration of exercise, and occupation (sedentary, restricted access to bathroom)
• Knowledge, including understanding of need for regular bowel habits, ability and motivation to change current patterns, and understanding of relationship between laxative and enema use, activity, and constipation

Defining characteristics
• Amount of stool less than usual
• Failure to respond to urge to defecate
• Frequency less than usual pattern
• Habitual or daily use of laxatives or enemas
• Hard, formed stools
• Interference with daily living
• Palpable abdominal mass (impaction)
• Rectal fullness or pressure
• Straining during defecation

Associated medical diagnoses (selected)
Atonic colon, depression, diverticulitis, diverticulosis, fecal impaction, hemorrhoids, spastic or irritable colon

Expected outcomes
• Elimination returns to normal.
• Patient moves bowels every _____ day(s) without laxative or enema.
• Patient states understanding of causative factors of constipation.
• Patient gets regular exercise.
• Patient describes changes in personal habits to maintain normal elimination pattern.
• Patient states plans to seek help to resolve emotional or psychological problems.

Interventions and rationales
• Monitor and record frequency and characteristics of stool. *Careful monitoring forms the basis of an effective treatment plan.*
• Administer laxatives or enemas, as ordered, *to promote elimination.* Monitor effectiveness.
• Provide privacy for elimination. Encourage establishment of daily schedule, *to aid adaptation to routine physiologic function.*
• Weigh patient weekly and record the results *to detect fluid loss or retention, food malabsorption, or increased adaptation requirement on body processes.*
• Encourage intake of high-fiber foods, such as bananas, prunes, dates, figs, and whole grain cereals and breads, *to supply bulk for normal elimination.*
• Consult with dietitian and encourage adherence to a diet modification plan *to discourage departure from prescribed diet.*
• Teach patient about:
  – effects of long-term laxative or enema use *to avoid damaging intestinal mucosa*
  – need for diet high in fiber, bulk, and fluid *to soften stool and stimulate intestinal mucosa*
  – importance of responding to defecation urge *to avoid pressure and discomfort in lower GI tract*
  – selection of regular exercise program and adherence to it.
• Make referral to psychiatric liaison nurse, community agencies, or support groups, *to provide additional health care resources to patient and family.*

Evaluations for expected outcomes
• Patient resumes regular bowel schedule.

• Without using laxatives, enemas, or suppositories, patient has bowel movement every ____ day(s).
• Patient states three ways to prevent constipation.
• Patient performs regular exercise.
• Patient states how he plans to change life-style and dietary habits to prevent constipation.
• Patient contacts at least one community resource for help with resolving psychological conflicts.

Documentation
• Patient's expressions of concern about change in diet, activity level, use of laxatives or enemas, and bowel pattern
• Observations of characteristics of stool, diet, and activity tolerance
• Patient teaching about diet, exercise, and management of constipation
• Evaluations for each expected outcome.

Constipation, colonic

Definition
Elimination pattern characterized by hard, dry stool resulting from delayed passage of food residue

Assessment
• History of neurologic or psychiatric disorder
• History of thyroid problems
• History of familial multiple polyposis
• Fluid and electrolyte status, including intake and output, skin turgor, urine specific gravity, and mucous membranes
• Age
• Gastrointestinal status, including nausea and vomiting, usual bowel pattern, bowel habits and changes in bowel habits, stool characteristics (color, amount, size, consistency), pain, auscultation of bowel sounds, palpation for masses or tenderness, percussion for tympany and dullness, laxative or enema use, medications (including iron, narcotics), rectal exam
• Nutritional status, including dietary intake, appetite, current weight and change from normal, tolerance and intolerance for foods
• Activity status, including type and duration of exercise, occupation (sedentary, restricted access to bathroom), change in activities
• Psychosocial status, including personality, stressors (finances, job, marital discord), coping mechanisms, support systems (family, significant other)
• Life-style
• Knowledge level

Defining characteristics
• Abdominal distention
• Abdominal pain
• Decreased frequency of bowel movement
• Hard, dry stool
• Headache
• Impaired appetite
• Painful defecation
• Palpable mass
• Rectal pressure
• Straining during defecation

Associated medical diagnoses (selected)
Anxiety, cerebrovascular accident, depression, hypocalcemia, hypokalemia, hypothyroidism, ulcerative colitis

Expected outcomes
• Bowel pattern returns to normal.
• Bowel movement occurs every ____ day(s) without laxatives, enemas, or suppositories.

• Patient maintains oral fluid intake of 3,000 ml daily, unless contraindicated.
• Patient states understanding of factors causing constipation.
• Patient exercises regularly.
• Patient states intention to seek additional resources, if necessary.

Interventions and rationales
• Correct dietary habits to include adequate fluids, fresh fruits, and whole-grain cereals and breads, *which supply necessary bulk for normal elimination.*
• Encourage patient to engage in active daily exercise, such as brisk walking, *to strengthen muscle tone and stimulate circulation.*
• Encourage patient to evacuate at regular times, *to encourage adaptation and routine physiologic function.*
• Urge patient to avoid taking laxatives if possible, or to gradually decrease their use, *to avoid further trauma to intestinal mucosa.*
• Inform patient not to expect to have a bowel movement every day or even every other day, *to avoid use of poor health practices to stimulate elimination.*
• Establish and implement an individualized bowel regimen based on patient's needs. *Knowledge of normal body functions will improve patient's understanding of problem.*
• Instruct patient to avoid straining during elimination, *to avoid tissue damage, bleeding, and pain.*
• If not contraindicated, raise patient's fluid intake to about 3,000 ml daily *to increase functional capacity of bowel elimination.*
• Tell patient that abdominal massage may help relieve discomfort and promote defecation. *This procedure triggers bowel's spastic reflex.*
• Obtain referral to a dietitian *for nutritional counseling.*

Evaluations for expected outcomes
• Patient resumes regular bowel schedule.
• Without using laxatives, enemas, or suppositories, patient has bowel movement every ____ day(s).
• Patient states four possible causes of constipation.
• Patient performs regular exercise.
• Patient states three ways to change personal habits to improve bowel movement pattern.
• Patient identifies community resources to help maintain dietary habits.

Documentation
• Patient's expression of concern about use of laxatives, enemas, or suppositories to establish bowel pattern
• Bowel movements
• Patient teaching about constipation management
• Evaluations for each expected outcome.

■ Constipation, perceived

Definition
State in which an individual makes a self-diagnosis of constipation and ensures daily bowel movements through use of laxatives, enemas, or suppositories

Assessment
• Family history of constipation
• History of psychiatric disorders
• Fluid and electrolyte status, including intake and output, skin turgor, urine specific gravity, mucous membranes

- Marital status
- Gastrointestinal status, including bowel habits, change in bowel habits, stool characteristics (color, amount, size, consistency), pain, auscultation of bowel sounds, laxative or enema use (time and duration), family habits concerning bowel movements, rectal examination
- Nutritional status, including dietary intake and appetite
- Activity status
- Psychosocial status, including personality, stressors (finances, job, marital discord, coping mechanisms), support systems (family, others), life-style, knowledge level

Defining characteristics
- Cultural and family health beliefs
- Daily laxative use
- Expectation of bowel movement at same time every day
- Faulty appraisal
- Impaired thought processes

Associated medical diagnoses (selected)
Acute emotional distress, chronic anxiety, laxative abuse

Expected outcomes
- Patient decreases use of laxatives, enemas, or suppositories.
- Patient states understanding of normal bowel function.
- Patient discusses feelings about elimination pattern.
- Elimination pattern returns to normal.
- Patient experiences bowel movement every _____ day(s) without laxatives, enemas, or suppositories.
- Patient states understanding of factors causing constipation.
- Patient gets regular exercise.
- Patient describes changes in personal habits to maintain normal elimination pattern.
- Patient states intent to use appropriate resources to help resolve emotional or psychological problems.

Interventions and rationales
- Correct dietary habits to include adequate fluids, fresh fruits and vegetables, and whole grain cereals and breads, *which supply necessary bulk for normal elimination.*
- Encourage patient to engage in daily exercise, such as brisk walking, *to strengthen muscle tone and stimulate circulation.*
- Encourage patient to evacuate at regular times *to aid adaptation and routine physiologic function.*
- Urge patient to avoid taking laxatives if possible, or to gradually decrease their use, *to avoid further trauma to intestinal mucosa.*
- Inform patient not to expect a bowel movement every day or even every other day, *to avoid use of poor health practices to stimulate elimination.*
- If not contraindicated, increase patient's fluid intake to about 3,000 ml daily *to increase functional capacity of bowel elimination.*
- Explain normal bowel habits *so patient can better understand normal and abnormal body functions.*
- Reassure patient that normal bowel function is possible without laxatives, enemas, or suppositories *to give patient the necessary confidence for compliance.*
- Give information about self-help groups, as appropriate, *to provide additional resources for patient and family.*
- Establish and implement an individualized bowel regimen based on patient's needs.
- Instruct patient to avoid straining during elimination *to avoid tissue damage, bleeding, and pain.*

• Instruct patient that abdominal massage may help relieve discomfort and promote defecation *because it triggers bowel's spastic reflex.*

Evaluations for expected outcomes

• Patient decreases use of laxatives, enemas, or suppositories.
• Patient describes normal bowel function and how fluid consumption, high-fiber diet, and exercise affect function.
• Patient lists factors that may cause constipation.
• Patient expresses feelings about changes in elimination pattern.
• Patient states plans to make changes in personal habits to prevent constipation, including regular exercise.
• Patient makes contact with appropriate resources to help resolve psychological conflicts.

Documentation

• Patient's expressions of concern about change in diet, activity level, laxative and enema use, and bowel pattern
• Observations of diet, stool characteristics, and activity tolerance
• Patient teaching about diet, exercise, and constipation management
• Evaluations for each expected outcome.

■ Coping, defensive

related to perceived threat to positive self-regard

Definition

Falsely positive self-evaluation based on a self-protective pattern that defends against underlying perceived threats to positive self-regard

Assessment

• Age
• Sex
• Developmental stage
• Family system, including marital status and sibling position
• Reason for hospitalization
• Past experience with illness
• Patient's perception of health problem
• Patient's perception of self, including self-worth, body image, problem-solving ability, and coping mechanisms
• Mental status, including general appearance, affect, mood, cognitive and perceptual functioning, and behavior
• Social interaction pattern
• Support systems, such as family, significant other, and friends

Defining characteristics

• Defensiveness
• Denial of obvious problems
• Difficulty establishing or maintaining relationships
• Difficulty in reality-testing perceptions
• Grandiosity
• Lack of follow-through or participation in treatment or therapy
• Projection of blame or responsibility
• Rationalization of failures

Associated medical diagnoses (selected)

Any illness or injury resulting in chronic pain, permanent disability, or disfigurement. Examples include acquired immunodeficiency syndrome, acute myocardial infarction, alcoholism, anxiety, cancer, drug addiction, end-stage disease (renal, pulmonary, or cardiac)

Expected outcomes

- Patient states reason for hospitalization.
- Patient verbally describes self, including concept, body image, successes, failures.
- Patient participates in self-care.
- Patient engages in decision-making about treatment.
- Patient accepts responsibility for own behavior.
- Patient demonstrates follow-through in decisions related to health care.
- Patient interacts with others in a socially acceptable manner.

Interventions and rationales

- Encourage patient to evaluate self, possibly by making a written list of positive and negative traits of self. *This helps patient identify aspects of self and relate changes to specific variables.*
- Have patient perform self-care to the extent possible *to provide a sense of control.*
- Provide a structured daily routine *to provide patient with alternatives to self-absorption.*
- Help patient make treatment-related decisions and encourage follow-through. *Ability to make decisions is principal component of autonomy.*
- Arrange for interaction between patient and others and observe interaction pattern. *Studying patient's verbal and nonverbal interactions with others gives clues to patient's ability to communicate effectively.*
- Provide positive feedback when patient assumes responsibility for own behavior *to reinforce effective coping behaviors.*

Evaluations for expected outcomes

- Patient states reason for hospitalization.
- Patient uses at least two positive terms to describe self.
- Patient initiates and completes at least two self-care activities daily.
- Each day, patient makes at least one decision related to activities of daily living, self-care, or treatment.
- Patient expresses responsible attitude toward own behavior.
- Patient reports specific instances of following through on decisions.
- Each day, patient socializes with others.

Documentation

- Patient's perception of self
- Behavioral responses
- Social interaction patterns
- Patient's use of defense mechanisms
- Interventions used to facilitate effective coping
- Patient's responses to nursing interventions
- Evaluations for each expected outcome.

■ Coping, family: Potential for growth

related to self-actualization needs

Definition

Inability to use adaptive behaviors in response to difficult life situations

Assessment

- Family process, including normal pattern of interaction among family members, family's understanding and knowledge of patient's present condition, support systems available (financial, social, spiritual), family's past response to crises (coping patterns), and communication patterns

used to express anger, affection, and confrontation
• Patient's illness, including progression and severity of illness, patient's perception of health problem, and problem-solving techniques used by patient to cope with life problems

Defining characteristics
• Family member attempts to describe impact of crisis on personal values, priorities, goals, or relationships.
• Family member moves in direction of health-promoting and enriching life-style that supports and monitors maturational processes and audits and negotiates treatment programs; family member generally chooses experiences that optimize wellness.

Associated medical diagnoses (selected)
Any disorder that results in long-term disability or incapacitation of family member, such as amyotrophic lateral sclerosis, cystic fibrosis, degenerative disease, genetic defects, mental retardation, multiple sclerosis, muscular dystrophy, myelomeningocele, terminal disease, and traumatic injury

Expected outcomes
• Family members discuss impact of patient's illness and feelings about it with health care professional.
• Family members participate in treatment plan.
• Family members establish a visiting routine beneficial to both patient and themselves.
• Family members demonstrate care needed to maintain patient's health status.
• Family members identify and uses available support systems.

Interventions and rationales
• Allow time for family to discuss impact of patient's illness and their feelings. Encourage expression of feelings *to allow family to realistically adjust to patient's problems.*
• Encourage family conferences; help family members identify key issues and select support services, if needed, *to develop sense of shared responsibility and feelings of safety, adequacy, and comfort.*
• Help patient and family establish a visiting routine that will not tax patient's or family's resources. Use patient's daily routine to aid in planning—for example, no visiting during treatments or during periods of uninterrupted sleep. *Involving family members reassures patient of their care and reduces family's fear and anxiety.*
• Reinforce family's efforts to care for patient, *to let them know they are doing their best and to ease adaptation and grieving process.*
• Demonstrate care procedures and encourage participation in treatment and planning decisions (such as selecting times for pulmonary toilet for patient with cystic fibrosis). *Meeting others' needs promotes self-esteem.*
• Provide family with clear, concise information about patient's condition. Be aware of what the family has already been told and help them interpret information. *This information will help alleviate their concerns.*
• Ensure privacy for patient and family visits *to foster open communication between them.*
• Help family support patient's independence. Encourage attendance at therapy sessions and allow patient to demonstrate new skills and abilities. *Independence helps patient reach maximum functional level.*

• Provide emotional support to family by being available to answer questions. *Attentive listening conveys empathy, recognition, and respect for a person.*
• Inform family of community resources and support groups available to assist in managing patient's illness and providing emotional or financial support to the caretakers, such as Easter Seals Association, Visiting Nurse Association, Meals on Wheels. *Community resources may help patient develop potential, independence, and self-reliance.*

Evaluations for expected outcomes
• Family members acknowledge their feelings about the patient's illness.
• Family members identify negative ways of responding to the patient's illness used in the past.
• Family members spend adequate time with the patient and seek to participate in care.
• Family members display competence in caring for patient through return demonstration.
• Family members establish a visiting routine beneficial to both patient and themselves.
• Family provides adequate level of care to maintain patient's health.
• Family members can name the illness and discuss its characteristics, signs and symptoms, treatment, and prognosis.
• Family members make contact with support resources available in their community.

Documentation
• Family's response to illness
• Family's current understanding of patient's illness
• Observations about family's interaction with patient and acceptance of current situation
• Evaluations for each expected outcome.

■ Coping, ineffective family: Compromised

related to inadequate or incorrect information held by primary caregiver

Definition
Behavior of family members that compromises the patient's and family's capacities to adapt

Assessment
• Family status, including normal pattern of interaction among family members, family's understanding and knowledge of patient's present condition, support systems available (financial, social, spiritual), family's response to past crises, and communication patterns used to express anger, affection, confrontation, conflict
• Patient's illness, including progression and severity of illness, patient's perception of health problem, and problem-solving techniques used by patient to cope with life problems

Defining characteristics
• Patient expresses or confirms concern about family's response to current health problem
• Family member describes or confirms and inadequate understanding or knowledge base that interferes with effective assistive or supportive behaviors.
• Family member displays protective behavior disproportionate to patient's abilities or need for autonomy

Associated medical diagnoses (selected)
Any disorder that results in long-term disability or incapacitation,

such as degenerative and terminal disorders and traumatic injuries

Expected outcomes

- Family discusses impact of patient's illness and feelings about it with health care professional.
- Family designates a spokesperson to receive information regarding the patient's illness.
- Family establishes a visiting routine beneficial to both patient and family.
- Family states understanding of patient's health status.
- Family identifies and uses available support systems.

Interventions and rationales

- Identify the spokesperson for the family *to avoid creating communication conflicts within family.*
- Facilitate family conferences; help family members identify key issues and select support services, if needed. *Involving patient and family in care planning promotes open communication throughout the illness.*
- Help patient and family establish a visiting routine that will not tax their resources. Each family member may take a day or period of time, if desired. Use patient's daily routine to aid in planning; for example, no visiting during treatments or periods of uninterrupted sleep. *This enhances family's sense of contributing to patient's overall care.*
- Encourage family to contact a community agency for continued support, if necessary. *This is an effective health-related coping skill.*
- Provide family with clear, concise information about patient's condition. Be aware of what family has already been told and help them interpret information. *This ensures clear, uncluttered communication between patient, family, and caregivers.*
- Ensure privacy for patient and family visits. *This demonstrates respect and fosters open communication between family members.*
- Help family support the patient's independence. Encourage attendance at therapy sessions and allow patient to demonstrate new skills and abilities *to help family members learn how they can help promote patient's independence and self-care.*
- Provide emotional support to family by being available to answer questions. *This demonstrates your willingness to help family seek health-related information.*

Evaluations for expected outcomes

- Family members express feelings about patient's illness and discuss its impact on family functioning.
- A family member is designated as spokesperson to receive and communicate information regarding the patient's illness.
- Family members agree to follow a consistent visiting routine.
- Family members accurately describe the patient's health status.
- Family contacts at least one support person or group.

Documentation

- Family's response to illness
- Family's current understanding of patient's illness
- Observations about family's interaction with patient and acceptance of current situation
- Evaluations for each expected outcome.

Coping, ineffective family: Compromised

related to prolonged disease

Definition

Behavior of family members that compromises the patient's and family's ability to adapt

Assessment

- Patient's illness, including course and severity, effect on family members
- Patient's health care resources, including hospital, community resources, health care providers such as therapists, case manager (outpatient)
- Family process, including involvement with patient, quality of relationships, communication patterns, coping strategies, demands posed by patient's condition, family's understanding of patient's illness, feelings regarding patient's illness, willingness of family members to commit time to patient care, family's ability to provide care

Defining characteristics

- Family interactions indicating poor coping
- Family members' expressions of concern about their ability to cope with patient's disease
- Family members experiencing prolonged and disabling feelings of anger, guilt, or sadness
- Family members' failure to support patient's decisions regarding health care
- Family's excessive or inadequate involvement with patient
- Patient's expression of concern about family's ability to cope

Associated medical diagnoses (selected)

Any disease or illness that results in long-term disability or incapacitation

Expected outcomes

- Family members express their concerns about coping with patient's illness.
- Family members identify their needs.
- Family members contact appropriate sources of support.
- Family and patient achieve better cooperation.

Interventions and rationales

- Assess effects of patient's disease on family functioning *to plan interventions that enhance the long-term well-being of the family as well as the patient.*
- Encourage family members to hold conferences. Help them identify topics appropriate for discussion. Examples of such topics include developing coping strategies for dealing with the patient's disease or resolving conflicts between meeting personal needs and meeting the patient's health care needs. *Family members may find a group problem-solving approach helpful in correcting dysfunctional behaviors.*
- Evaluate and rectify any knowledge deficit that family members have about patient's disease and treatment. *Experience does not guarantee correct knowledge. Lack of knowledge can exacerbate frustration and tension within the family.*
- Encourage family members to participate in appropriate support groups *to help them obtain social support and information and to provide an opportunity to express feelings.*
- Encourage family members to contact and use appropriate community

agencies *to help prevent burnout among family members once the patient leaves the hospital.* Families may need encouragement to use support and respite care services if past efforts to use such services proved unsuccessful.

Evaluations for expected outcomes

- Family members discuss impact of patient's prolonged disease with nurse.
- Family members communicate their needs regarding the patient's prolonged care.
- Family is aware of available sources of support and uses them appropriately.
- Family and patient negotiate meeting patient's care needs to their mutual satisfaction.

Documentation

- Assessment of family functioning (including family's level of insight into their behavior)
- Content of family conferences
- Community resources used, their effectiveness, and recommendations for future use (indicate family's level of acceptance of nurse's recommendations)
- Evaluations for each expected outcome.

Coping, ineffective family: Disabling

related to unresolved emotional conflict between patient and family members

Definition

Behavior of family members that undermines the patient's and family's ability to adapt

Assessment

- Patient's illness, including its course, severity, and effect on family members
- Patient's health care resources, including hospital, community resources, health care providers such as therapists, case manager
- Demands on family imposed by the patient's condition
- Family status, including involvement with patient, quality of relationships, communication patterns, coping strategies, family's understanding of patient's illness, feelings about patient's illness, willingness of family members to commit time to patient care, family's ability to provide care

Defining characteristics

- Family members are intolerant of the patient's physical ailments or psychological weaknesses
- Family members disregard patient's basic human needs
- Family members exhibit distorted perceptions of the patient's health problem, including extreme denial about its existence or severity
- Family members refuse to participate in care of the patient
- Patient develops helpless, dependent attitude and experiences corresponding decrease in activity level
- Patient experiences psychosomatic symptoms
- Patient expresses feelings of abandonment, agitation, depression, aggression, rejection, and hostility
- Patient reports poor relationships with family members

Associated medical diagnoses (selected)

Any disorder that results in long-term disability or incapacitation, such as degenerative and terminal disorders and traumatic injuries

Expected outcomes

- To the extent possible, family members participate in aspects of patient's care without evidence of increased conflict.
- Patient expresses confidence in his ability to make decisions, despite pressure from family members.
- Patient contacts appropriate sources of support outside the family.
- Patient takes steps to ensure that care needs are met despite family's shortcomings.
- Patient expresses greater understanding of the emotional limitations of family members.

Interventions and rationales

- Assess the effects of the patient's disease on family functioning *to plan interventions.* To the extent possible, encourage family members to participate in patient care. *Family members should have an opportunity to overcome dysfunctional behavior.*
- Maintain objectivity when dealing with family conflicts. Do not become embroiled in the dynamics of a dysfunctional family *to maintain your ability to intervene effectively.*
- If the patient and family members appear incapable of taking steps to heal their relationships, focus on being a patient advocate. Reaffirm the patient's right to make his own decisions without interference from family members. Provide necessary information to the patient to facilitate decision making. *Dysfunctional family coping patterns evolve over many years and are unlikely to change just because the patient has a serious illness. Accepting your limitations when working with family members will help you to avoid burnout and better meet the patient's needs.*
- Encourage the patient to seek the emotional support his family is unable to provide by participating in a support group. Help the patient select the support group that is best suited to his personal needs and outlook. Consider recommending Codependents Anonymous, a group for individuals who have difficulty maintaining healthy relationships as a result of being raised in a dysfunctional family. *Participation in a support group may improve the patient's ability to cope as well as provide an opportunity to form meaningful relationships.*
- Refer the patient to a home health agency, homemaker service, Meals On Wheels, or other appropriate outside agencies for assistance and follow-up. *Use of various community services may help to make up for shortcomings in the family's ability to provide care.*
- Listen openly to the patient's expressions of pain over unresolved conflicts with family members. The patient may have to grieve over the fact that he will never have an "ideal" family, capable of fully meeting his emotional needs. *Therapeutic listening helps the patient to understand himself and his family better and to understand how conflicts from the past affect his behavior.*

Evaluations for expected outcomes

- Family members demonstrate improved willingness to cooperate in the patient's care.
- Patient expresses increased confidence in his ability to make decisions.
- Patient contacts at least one support group in an effort to form meaningful relationships outside the family.
- Patient takes steps to meet his own care needs.

• Patient indicates, either verbally or through behavior, a better understanding of family members and an increased ability to accept their emotional limitations.

Documentation
• Family's response to patient's illness
• Observations of patient's interactions with family members
• Referrals made to support groups and community services
• Patient's expressions of grief, anger, and disappointment over unresolved conflicts with family members
• Evaluations for each expected outcome.

■ Coping, ineffective individual

related to personal vulnerability

Definition
Inability to use adaptive behaviors in response to difficult life situations

Assessment
• Patient's perception of present health problem or crisis
• Medical history
• Coping behaviors
• Problem-solving techniques usually employed to cope with life problems
• Presence of physical or emotional impairment
• Occupation
• Diversional activities
• Financial resources
• Support systems, including family, significant other, friends, and clergy
• Reactions of family or significant other to patient's crisis

Defining characteristics
• Chronic fatigue
• Chronic worry
• Denial of problems
• Difficulty asking for help
• Evidence of compulsive behavior
• Frequent complaints of physical symptoms not backed by organic findings
• Inability to delay gratification
• Inability to live up to age-related or gender-related role expectations
• Inability to meet basic needs or solve problems
• Low tolerance for frustration
• Obsessive thoughts
• Statements indicating inability to cope

Associated medical diagnoses (selected)
This nursing diagnosis may occur anytime an individual uses maladaptive strategies to cope with life's tasks. Associated psychiatric diagnoses include adjustment disorders, affective disorders, conversion disorder, hypochondriasis, personality disorders, schizophrenia, somatization disorder, somatoform disorder, and substance abuse.

Expected outcomes
• Patient expresses understanding of the relationship between emotional state and behavior.
• Patient becomes actively involved in planning own care.
• Patient reduces use of manipulative behavior to gratify needs.
• Patient accepts responsibility for behavior.
• Patient identifies effective and ineffective coping techniques.
• Patient uses available support systems, such as family, friends, and psychotherapist, to develop and maintain effective coping skills.

Interventions and rationales

- If possible, assign a primary nurse to patient *to provide continuity of care and promote development of a therapeutic relationship.*
- Spend consistent, uninterrupted periods of time with patient. Encourage open expression of feelings. *An open environment will help the patient ventilate intense emotion. Through discussion, you can help the patient understand the personal meaning attached to recent events and foster a realistic assessment of his situation.*
- As patient becomes able to express feelings more openly, discuss the relationship between feelings and behavior. *In order to change, patient must understand the relationship between emotions and behavior.*
- Discourage dependent behavior by assisting patient only when necessary. Provide positive reinforcement for independent behavior. *Positive reinforcement enhances self-esteem, encourages repetition of desired behavior, and promotes effective coping.*
- Encourage patient to make decisions about care *to reduce feelings of helplessness and enhance patient's sense of mastery over current situation.*
- Set limits on manipulative behavior. Provide patient with clear expectations for behavior, and describe consequences if limits are violated. *If the patient cannot curb inappropriate behavior, consistent limit-setting imposes external controls.*
- Recognize that manipulative behaviors reduce patient's sense of insecurity by increasing feelings of power. *Understanding the patient's motivation may help you deal better with manipulative behavior.*
- Help patient recognize and accept responsibility for actions. Discourage patient from unfairly placing blame on others. *Developing a sense of responsibility is necessary before change can occur.*
- Help patient recognize and feel good about positive personal qualities and accomplishments. *As self-esteem increases, patient will feel less need to manipulate others.*
- Help patient analyze current situation and evaluate the effectiveness of coping strategies *to foster an objective outlook.*
- Praise patient for identifying and using effective coping techniques *to reinforce appropriate behavior.*
- Suggest alternatives to ineffective behaviors identified by patient. Encourage patient to determine what new behaviors can be effectively incorporated into life-style. *Fostering patient participation in care promotes feelings of independence.*
- Encourage patient to use support systems, such as psychotherapist, family, friends. *Long-term support is essential to maintain effective coping skills.*

Evaluations for expected outcomes

- Patient describes emotions triggered by illness or personal crisis and usual coping behaviors.
- Patient works with primary nurses to plan care.
- Patient describes two instances where needs were met through direct communication.
- Patient describes one difficult interpersonal situation that was solved by identifying the problem, choosing alternative ways to communicate, and taking action.
- Patient describes two effective and two ineffective coping behaviors.

• Patient enlists support and assistance from family and friends.
• Patient requests a referral for psychotherapy.

Documentation
• Patient's perception of present situation
• Emotions expressed by patient
• Observations of patient's behaviors
• Interventions performed to help patient develop coping skills
• Patient's responses to nursing interventions
• Evaluations for each expected outcome.

Coping, ineffective individual

related to situational crisis

Definition
Inability to use adaptive behaviors in response to such difficult life situations as loss of health, a loved one, or job

Assessment
• Coping behaviors
• Degree of physical and emotional impairment
• Diversional activities
• Financial resources
• Occupation
• Patient's perception of present health problem or crisis
• Problem-solving techniques usually employed to cope with life problems
• Support systems, including family, companion, friends, and clergy

Defining characteristics
• Change in usual communication patterns
• Chronic fatigue
• Chronic worry
• Evidence or verification of situational crisis
• Excessive drinking
• Inability to meet role expectations, meet basic needs, or solve problems
• Inappropriate use of defense mechanisms
• Insomnia
• Irritability
• Irritable bowel
• Muscular tension
• Overeating or lack of appetite
• Verbal expression of inability to cope or ask for help
• Verbal manipulation

Associated medical diagnoses (selected)
Acute myocardial infarction, alcoholism, bipolar disease (manic or depressive phase), cancer, depression, drug addiction or overdose, drug withdrawal, end-stage disease (renal, pulmonary, or cardiac), self-inflicted injuries, trauma

Expected outcomes
• Patient communicates feelings about the present situation.
• Patient becomes involved in planning own care.
• Patient expresses feeling of having greater control over present situation.
• Patient uses available support systems, such as family and friends, to aid in coping.
• Patient identifies at least two coping behaviors.
• Patient demonstrates ability to use two healthful coping behaviors.

Interventions and rationales
• If possible, assign a primary nurse to patient *to provide continuity of care and promote development of therapeutic relationship.*
• Arrange to spend uninterrupted periods of time with patient. Encour-

age expression of feelings and accept what patient says. Try to identify factors that cause or exacerbate patient's inability to cope, such as fear of loss of health or job. *Devoting time for listening helps patient express emotions, grasp situation, and cope effectively.*

- Identify and reduce unnecessary stimuli in environment *to avoid subjecting patient to sensory or perceptual overload.*
- Initially, allow patient to depend partly on you for self-care. *Patient may regress to a lower developmental level during initial crisis phase.*
- Explain all treatments and procedures and answer patient's questions *to allay fear and allow patient to regain sense of control.*
- Encourage patient to make decisions about care *to increase sense of self-worth and mastery over current situation.*
- Have patient increase self-care performance levels gradually, *which allows progress at patient's own pace.*
- Praise patient for making decisions and performing activities *to reinforce coping behaviors.*
- Encourage patient to use support systems to assist with coping, *thereby helping restore psychological equilibrium and prevent crisis.*
- Help patient look at current situation and evaluate various coping behaviors *to encourage a realistic view of crisis.*
- Encourage patient to try coping behaviors. *A patient in crisis tends to accept interventions and develop new coping behaviors more easily than at other times.*
- Request feedback from patient about behaviors that seem to work *to encourage patient to evaluate the effect of these behaviors.*
- Refer patient for professional psychological counseling. *If patient's maladaptive behavior has high crisis potential, formal counseling helps ease nurse's frustration, increases objectivity, and fosters collaborative approach to patient's care.*

Evaluations for expected outcomes

- Patient discusses recent stressful event and describes related emotions.
- Patient cooperates with nurse to plan care.
- Patient identifies problems, makes plans, and takes action.
- Patient requests assistance from family and friends.
- Patient identifies and uses at least two healthful coping behaviors such as relaxation techniques.

Documentation

- Patient's perception of present situation and what it means
- Patient's verbal expression of feelings indicating comfort or discomfort
- Observations of patient's behaviors
- Interventions to help patient cope
- Patient's responses to interventions
- Evaluations for each expected outcome.

Decisional conflict

related to perceived threat to value system

Definition

State of uncertainty about health-related course of action when choice involves risk, loss, or challenge to personal life values

Assessment

- Perception of situation representing conflict

- Age
- Sex
- Developmental state
- Marital status
- Family system (nuclear, extended role, sibling position)
- Sociocultural factors, including educational level, occupation, socioeconomic status, ethnic group, sexual preference
- Level of functioning (cognitive, emotional, behavioral)
- Coping mechanisms
- Past experience with decision making
- Available support system

Defining characteristics
- Delayed decision making
- Physical signs of distress or tension
- Questioning personal values and beliefs while attempting to make a decision
- Vacillation between alternative choices
- Verbal report of distress related to uncertainty about choices
- Verbal report of undesired consequences of alternative actions being considered

Associated medical diagnoses (selected)
This nursing diagnosis can occur in any hospitalized patient confronted with choices related to life-sustaining or life-saving measures. Examples include any illness requiring patient's choice between palliative comfort measures, discontinuation of life-support, or cardiopulmonary resuscitation; cancers requiring radiation or chemotherapy; conditions requiring amputation of an extremity; end-stage cardiac disease requiring artificial or human heart transplant; end-stage renal disease requiring chronic hemodialysis or kidney transplant

Expected outcomes
- Patient states feelings about current situation.
- Patient discusses concerns about potential conflict between value system and treatment options.
- Patient identifies desirable and undesirable consequences of available options.
- Patient makes minor decisions related to daily activities.
- Patient accepts assistance from family, friends, clergy, and other supportive persons.
- Patient reports feeling comfortable about ability to make an appropriate, rational choice congruent with personal values.

Interventions and rationales
- Visit patient frequently, taking a nonjudgmental approach to encourage expression of feelings. *This demonstrates acceptance of patient as person of worth regardless of culture, beliefs or value system.*
- Acknowledge patient's values and beliefs; be willing to listen to patient's concerns regarding current dilemma. *Nurse must lay aside own values to enter patient's world without prejudice.*
- Help patient identify available options and their possible consequences. *This encourages thoughtful consideration of consequences of each choice and relies on patient's cognitive abilities.*
- Help patient make decisions about daily activities. *Ability to make decisions is principal component of autonomy.*
- Encourage visits with family, significant others, clergy; provide privacy during visits. *If emotional support system is less available, event will be more hazardous.*

• Demonstrate respect for patient's right to choose based on values, religious beliefs, cultural norms, or sexual preference. *Respect is demonstrated by nurse's unconditionally positive regard for patient's value system.*
• Encourage patient to continue religious practices and rituals while in the hospital; provide assistance when possible. *This demonstrates acceptance, caring, and support.*
• Support patient's right to make decisions about end-of-life care, such as writing a living will or advance directives, *to promote autonomy.*

Evaluations for expected outcomes

• Patient openly expresses feelings about current situation.
• Patient describes conflicts related to treatment.
• Patient identifies consequences of potential choices.
• Patient makes at least two care-related decisions daily.
• Patient requests assistance from family, friends, and clergy.
• Patient expresses increased comfort in dealing with conflict.

Documentation

• Assessment factors related to patient's value system
• Patient's feelings and concerns about current situation
• Cognitive, emotional, and behavioral levels of functioning
• Interventions to assist patient with conflict resolution
• Patient's response to nursing interventions
• Evaluations for each expected outcome.

■ Denial

related to fear or anxiety

Definition

Conscious or unconscious attempt to disavow the knowledge or meaning of an event to reduce anxiety or fear to the detriment of health

Assessment

• Perception of present health state, including awareness of diagnosis, perception of personal relevance or impact on life pattern, and description of symptoms
• Degree of physical and emotional functional impairment
• Mental status, including general appearance, affect, mood, memory, orientation, communication, thinking process, perception, abstract thinking, judgment, and insight
• Coping behaviors
• Problem-solving strategies
• Support systems, including family or significant other, friends, clergy, and financial resources
• Belief system, including values, norms, and religion
• Self-concept, including self-esteem and body image

Defining characteristics

• Cannot admit impact of disease on life pattern
• Delays seeking or refuses medical attention to detriment of health
• Displaces fear of condition's impact
• Displaces sources of symptoms to other organs
• Displays inappropriate affect
• Does not admit fear of death or invalidism
• Does not perceive personal relevance or danger of symptoms

• Minimizes symptoms
• Uses self-treatment to relieve symptoms

Associated medical diagnoses (selected)
Acquired immunodeficiency syndrome, acute myocardial infarction, alcoholism, anxiety, bipolar disease (manic or depressive phase), cancer, depression, end-stage disease (renal, pulmonary, or cardiac), self-destructive behaviors (anorexia nervosa, bulimia, drug addiction)

Expected outcomes
• Patient describes knowledge and perception of present health problem.
• Patient describes life pattern and reports any recent changes.
• Patient expresses knowledge of stages of grief.
• Patient demonstrates behavior associated with grief process.
• Patient discusses present health problem with physician, nurses, and family or significant other.
• Patient indicates by conversation or behavior an increased awareness of reality.

Interventions and rationales
• Provide for a specific amount of uninterrupted non-care-related time with patient each day. *This allows patient to ventilate knowledge, feelings, and concerns.*
• Encourage patient to express feelings related to present problem, its severity, and its potential impact on life pattern. *This helps patient express doubts and resolve concerns.*
• Maintain frequent communication with doctor to assess what patient has been told about illness. *This fosters consistent, collaborative approach to patient's care.*
• Listen to patient with nonjudgmental acceptance, *to demonstrate positive regard for patient as person worthy of respect.*
• Help patient learn the stages of anticipatory grieving, *to increase understanding and ability to cope.*
• Encourage patient to communicate with others, asking questions and clarifying concerns based on readiness. *Patient fixated in denial may isolate and withdraw from others.*
• Visit more frequently as patient begins to accept reality; alleviate fears when necessary. *This helps reduce patient's fear of being alone and fosters accurate reality testing.*

Evaluations for expected outcomes
• Patient describes present health problem.
• Patient describes life pattern and reports any recent changes.
• Patient communicates understanding of stages of grief.
• Patient demonstrates behavior appropriate to present phase of grieving process.
• When ready, patient discusses health problem with doctor, nurses, and family or significant other.
• Patient displays increasing awareness of reality, either verbally or through behavior.

Documentation
• Patient's perception of health problem
• Mental status (baseline and ongoing)
• Patient's knowledge of grief process
• Patient's behavioral responses
• Interventions implemented to assist patient
• Patient's response to nursing interventions
• Evaluations for each expected outcome.

Diarrhea

related to malabsorption, inflammation, or irritation of bowel

Definition

Interruption of normal elimination pattern characterized by frequent, loose stools

Assessment

- History of bowel disorder or surgery
- Gastrointestinal status, including nausea and vomiting, usual bowel habits, change in bowel habits, stool characteristics (color, amount, size, consistency), pain, inspection of abdomen, auscultation of bowel sounds, palpation for masses and tenderness, percussion for tympany and dullness, laxative and enema use, medications (especially antibiotics), stool culture, upper GI series, barium enema
- Nutritional status, including dietary intake, change from normal diet, appetite, current weight, change from normal weight, and food irritants and contaminants
- Fluid and electrolyte status, including intake and output, urine specific gravity, skin turgor, mucous membranes, serum potassium and sodium, and blood urea nitrogen
- Psychosocial status, including personality, stressors (finances, job, marital discord, disease process), coping mechanisms, support systems, life-style, and recent travel

Defining characteristics

- Abdominal pain and cramping
- Clinical evidence of malabsorption, inflammation, or irritation of bowel
- Hyperactive bowel sounds
- Increased frequency of stool
- Loose, liquid stools; possibly bloody, mucoid, fatty, or bulky
- Stool color changes
- Urgency

Associated medical diagnoses (selected)

Amebiasis, *Campylobacter* dysentery, Crohn's disease, diverticulitis, drug-induced diarrhea, irritable bowel syndrome, ischemic colitis, lactase deficiency, pseudomembranous colitis, salmonellosis, shigella, trichinosis, typhoid fever, ulcerative colitis

Expected outcomes

- Patient controls diarrhea with medication.
- Elimination pattern returns to normal.
- Patient regains and maintains fluid and electrolyte balance.
- Skin remains intact.
- Patient discusses causative factors, preventive measures, and changed body image.
- Patient practices stress-reduction techniques daily.
- Patient demonstrates skill in using ostomy devices.
- Patient seeks out persons with similar conditions or joins a support group.

Interventions and rationales

- Monitor frequency and characteristics of stool; auscultate bowel sounds and record results at least every shift *to monitor treatment effectiveness.*
- Tell patient to notify staff of each episode of diarrhea *to promote comfort and maintain communication.*
- Give antidiarrheal medications, as ordered, *to improve bodily function, promote comfort, and balance body fluids, salts, and acid-base levels.* Monitor and report efficacy.
- Monitor and record patient's intake and output, including number of

stools. Report imbalances. *Monitoring ensures correct fluid replacement therapy.*

- Check skin daily *to detect and prevent breakdown.* Report decreased skin turgor or excoriation of perianal area.
- Weigh patient daily until diarrhea is controlled *to detect fluid loss or retention.*
- Teach patient about:
  - causative and preventive factors *to promote understanding of problem.*
  - cleaning of perianal area, including use of powders and lotions, *to promote comfort and skin integrity.*
  - dietary restriction to control diarrhea, such as a lactose-free diet, *which reduces residual waste and decreases intestinal irritation and spasms.*
- Teach stress-reduction techniques and help the patient perform them daily by providing time, privacy, and needed equipment. *This temporarily relieves emotional distress.*
- Prepare patient for surgery and provide preoperative instruction for abdominal surgery *to reassure patient and maintain trust.* Provide information about ileostomy or colostomy, if indicated, *to help patient understand procedure and avoid threat to health equilibrium.*
- Demonstrate use of ostomy equipment *to encourage understanding and compliance.*
- Provide support and assistance while patient develops skill in caring for stoma, *to improve understanding and reduce anxiety.*
- Encourage expression of feelings and concerns about impact of changed body image *to allow patient to pinpoint specific fears and promote self-knowledge and growth.*
- Encourage use of support groups, such as ileostomy clubs, *to provide patient with additional support and health care resources.*

Evaluations for expected outcomes

- Patient does not experience diarrhea.
- Patient maintains weight and fluid and electrolyte balance.
- Skin breakdown does not occur.
- Patient explains cause of diarrhea and steps to prevent recurrence.
- Patient demonstrates successful use of stress reduction techniques.
- Patient demonstrates successful use of ostomy devices.
- Patient attends a support group for individuals with a similar condition.

Documentation

- Patient's expressions of concern about diarrhea, causative factors, surgery, and adaptation to changes in body image
- Observations of effects of medications, intake and output, weight, stool characteristics, skin condition, and stoma appearance
- Evaluations for each expected outcome.

■ Diarrhea

related to stress and anxiety

Definition

Interruption of normal bowel movements resulting in frequent, loose stools

Assessment

- History of bowel disorder or surgery
- Gastrointestinal status, including nausea and vomiting, usual bowel

habits, change in bowel habits, stool characteristics (color, amount, size, consistency), pain and discomfort, inspection of abdomen, auscultation of bowel sounds, palpation for masses and tenderness, percussion for tympany and dullness
• Nutritional status, including dietary intake, change from normal diet, appetite, current weight, change from normal weight
• Fluid and electrolyte status, including intake and output, urine specific gravity, skin turgor, mucous membranes, serum K^+, serum Na^+, and blood urea nitrogen
• Psychosocial status, including personality, stressors (finances, job, marital discord), coping mechanisms, support systems (family, significant other, life-style)

Defining characteristics
• Abdominal pain and cramping
• Changes in stool color
• Increased frequency of stool
• Loose, liquid stools
• Urgency
• Verbal expression of stress or anxiety

Associated medical diagnoses (selected)
Anxiety, irritable bowel syndrome (spastic colon, ulcerative colitis, mucous colitis)

Expected outcomes
• Diarrheal episodes decline or disappear.
• Usual bowel pattern resumes.
• Patient regains and maintains fluid and electrolyte balance.
• Patient keeps skin clean and free of irritation or ulcerations.
• Patient explains causative factors and preventive measures.
• Patient discusses relationship of stress and anxiety to episodes of diarrhea.
• Patient states plans to utilize stress-reduction techniques (specify).
• Patient demonstrates ability to use at least one stress-reduction technique.

Interventions and rationales
• Monitor and record frequency and characteristics of stool *to monitor treatment effectiveness.* Instruct patient to record diarrheal episodes and report them to staff *to promote comfort and maintain effective patient-staff communication.*
• Administer antidiarrheal medications, as ordered, *to improve bodily function, promote comfort, and balance body fluids, salts, and acid-base levels.* Monitor and report medications' effectiveness.
• Provide replacement fluids and electrolytes, as prescribed. Maintain accurate records *to ensure balanced fluid intake and output.*
• Monitor perianal skin for irritation and ulceration; treat according to established protocol *to promote comfort, skin integrity, and freedom from infection.*
• Identify stressors and help patient solve problems *to provide more realistic approach to care.*
• Encourage patient to ventilate stresses and anxiety; *release of pent-up emotions can temporarily relieve emotional distress.*
• Teach patient to:
  – use relaxation techniques *to reduce muscle tension and nervousness.*
  – recognize and reduce intake of diarrhea-producing foods or substances (such as dairy products, fruit), *thus reducing resid-*

ual waste matter and decreasing intestinal irritation.

- Spend at least 10 minutes with patient twice daily to discuss stress-reducing techniques; *this can help patient pinpoint specific fears.*
- Encourage and assist patient to practice relaxation techniques *to reduce tension and promote self-knowledge and growth.*

Evaluations for expected outcomes

- Episodes of diarrhea decline by at least 50%.
- Patient resumes usual bowel elimination pattern.
- Patient maintains weight and fluid and electrolyte balance.
- Patient does not experience skin breakdown, irritation, or ulcerations.
- Patient identifies cause of diarrhea and discusses steps to prevent recurrence.
- Patient explains how stress may contribute to diarrhea and steps to prevent recurrence.
- Patient describes three stress reduction techniques and successfully demonstrates one of them.

Documentation

- Patient's expressions of concern and ability to manage diarrhea produced by stress and anxiety
- Observations of effects of relaxation and stress-reduction techniques and dietary management on diarrhea
- Patient's responses and skill level in carrying out stress-reduction techniques and dietary changes
- Evaluations for each expected outcome.

■ Disuse syndrome, high risk for

related to prolonged inactivity

Definition

State of being at risk for deterioration of body systems as a result of prescribed or unavoidable inactivity

Assessment

- Condition leading to prolonged inactivity or immobility
- Age
- Neurologic status, including mental status, level of consciousness, sensory and motor ability
- Cardiovascular status, including blood pressure, heart rate, temperature, peripheral pulses, capillary refill, clotting profile, skin temperature and color, presence of edema, chest pain or discomfort
- Respiratory status, including rate and rhythm, depth of inspiration, chest symmetry, use of accessory muscles, cough and sputum, percussion of lung fields, auscultation of breath sounds, chest pain or discomfort, arterial blood gases
- Gastrointestinal status, including inspection of abdomen, auscultation of bowel sounds, palpation for tenderness and masses, percussion for areas of dullness, usual bowel habits, change in bowel habits, laxative use, pain or discomfort, characteristics of stool (color, size, amount, consistency)
- Nutritional status, including dietary intake, appetite, current weight, change from normal weight
- Fluid status, including intake and output, urine specific gravity, mucous membranes, serum electrolytes, blood urea nitrogen, creatinine

• Genitourinary status, including voiding pattern, characteristics of urine (color, odor, sediment, amount), history of urinary problems or infections, palpation of bladder, pain or discomfort, use of urinary assistive device, urinalysis and urine cultures
• Musculoskeletal status, including range of motion; muscle size, strength, and tone; coordination; and functional mobility scale:
 0 = completely independent
 1 = requires use of equipment or device
 2 = requires help, supervision, or teaching from another person
 3 = requires help from another person and equipment or device
 4 = dependent; does not participate in activity
• Integumentary status, including color, texture, turgor, temperature, elasticity, sensation, moisture, hygiene, lesions
• Psychosocial factors, including family support, coping style, current understanding of prescribed inactivity, willingness to cooperate with treatment, mood, behavior, motivation, and stressors (inactivity, finances, job, marital discord)

Risk factors
• Altered level of consciousness
• Mechanical immobilization
• Paralysis
• Prescribed immobilization
• Severe pain

Associated medical diagnoses (selected)
This diagnosis may occur in any patient subject to prescribed or unavoidable inactivity. Examples include: cerebrovascular accident, fractures (with traction or cast), neuromuscular disorders, peripheral vascular disease, rheumatoid arthritis, severe head injury, spinal cord injury, terminal cancer

Expected outcomes
• Patient displays no evidence of altered mental, sensory, or motor ability.
• Patient has no evidence of thrombus formation, venous stasis, or altered cardiovascular function.
• Patient shows no evidence of decreased chest movement, cough stimulus, or depth of ventilation; also shows no pooling of secretions or signs and symptoms of infection.
• Patient has no evidence of constipation and maintains bowel patterns.
• Patient maintains adequate dietary intake, hydration, and weight.
• Patient shows no evidence of urine retention, infection, or renal calculi.
• Patient maintains muscle strength and tone, also joint range of motion; shows no evidence of contractures.
• Patient shows no evidence of skin breakdown.
• Patient maintains normal neurologic, cardiovascular, respiratory, gastrointestinal, nutritional, genitourinary, musculoskeletal, and integumentary functioning during period of inactivity.
• Patient expresses feelings about prolonged inactivity.

Interventions and rationales
• Provide frequent contact with staff, diversionary materials (magazines, radio, TV), and orienting mechanisms (clock, calendar). *Reality orientation fosters patient awareness of environment.*
• Avoid positions that put prolonged pressure on body parts and compress blood vessels. Patient should change positions at least every 2 hours within prescribed limits. *These mea-*

sures enhance circulation and avoid tissue or skin breakdown.
• Inspect skin every shift and protect areas subject to irritation. Follow hospital policy for pressure ulcers *to prevent or mitigate skin breakdown.*
• Use pressure-reducing or -equalizing equipment as indicated or ordered (flotation pad, air pressure mattress, sheepskin pads, special bed). *This helps prevent skin breakdown by relieving pressure.*
• Apply elastic stockings; remove for 1 hour every 8 hours. *Stockings promote venous return to heart, prevent venous stasis, and decrease or prevent swelling of lower extremities.*
• Monitor clotting profile. Administer and monitor anticoagulant therapy, if ordered, and monitor for signs and symptoms of bleeding *because anticoagulant therapy may cause hemorrhage.*
• Monitor temperature, blood pressure, pulse, and respirations at least every 4 hours *to assess for signs and symptoms of infection or other complications.*
• Teach and monitor deep-breathing, coughing, and use of incentive spirometer. Maintain regimen every 2 hours. *These measures help clear airways, expand lungs, and prevent respiratory complications.*
• Encourage fluid intake of 2,500 to 3,500 ml daily, unless contraindicated, *to maintain urinary output and aid bowel elimination.* Weigh daily and monitor hydration status (serum electrolytes, blood urea nitrogen, creatinine, and intake and output every 8 hours).
• Monitor breath sounds and respiratory rate, rhythm, and depth at least every 4 hours *to rule out respiratory complications.* Monitor arterial blood gases, if indicated, *to assess oxygenation, ventilation, and metabolic status.*
• Suction airway as needed and ordered *to clear the airway and stimulate cough reflex;* note secretion characteristics.
• Establish baseline *to compare elimination patterns and habits.* Elevate head of bed and provide privacy *to allow comfortable elimination.*
• Instruct patient to avoid straining during bowel movements; administer stool softeners, suppositories, or laxatives as ordered and monitor effectiveness. *Straining at stool may be hazardous in patients with cardiovascular disorders and increased intracranial pressure.*
• Provide small, frequent meals of favorite foods *to increase dietary intake.* Increase fiber content *to enhance bowel elimination.* Increase protein and vitamin C *to promote wound healing.* Limit calcium *to reduce risk of renal and bladder calculi.*
• Monitor urine characteristics and patient's subjective complaints typical of urinary tract infection (burning, frequency, urgency). Obtain urine cultures as ordered. *These measures aid early detection of urinary tract infection.*
• Identify level of functioning *to provide baseline for future assessment* and encourage appropriate participation in care *to prevent complications of immobility and increase patient's feelings of self-esteem.*
• Perform active or passive range-of-motion exercises at least once per shift. Teach and monitor appropriate isotonic and isometric exercises. *These measures prevent joint contractures, muscular atrophy, and other complications of prolonged inactivity.*

• Provide or help with daily hygiene; keep skin dry and lubricated *to prevent cracking and possible infection.*
• Encourage patient and family to ventilate frustration. Allow open expression of all feelings associated with prolonged inactivity. *Open expression of feelings helps patient and family cope with treatment.*

Evaluations for expected outcomes
• Patient does not exhibit altered level of consciousness, mental status, sensory ability, or motor ability.
• Patient does not exhibit evidence of thrombus formation, venous stasis, or altered cardiovascular function.
• Patient's blood pressure and heart rate remain within specified ranges.
• Patient maintains clear breath sounds bilaterally and does not show evidence of fever, chills, cough, purulent sputum, pooled secretions, or rapid, shallow respirations.
• Patient shows no evidence of decreased chest movement, cough stimulus, or depth of ventilation.
• Patient's bowel elimination pattern remains normal.
• Patient's daily fluid intake remains adequate.
• Patient maintains adequate dietary intake.
• Patient does not exhibit evidence of distended bladder, fever, chills, frequent burning or painful urination, urgency, hematuria, flank pain or urine retention.
• Patient's muscle strength and tone and joint range of motion remain stable.
• Patient does not exhibit evidence of joint contractures.
• Patient does not experience skin breakdown.
• Patient maintains neurologic, cardiovascular, respiratory, gastrointestinal, nutritional, genitourinary, musculoskeletal, and integumentary functioning.
• Patient and family members openly express frustration, anger, despondency, and other feelings associated with prolonged inactivity.

Documentation
• Patient's concerns or perceptions of circumstances necessitating inactivity; willingness to accept and participate in treatment
• Assessment of body systems at risk for deterioration
• Interventions to provide preventive or supportive care and prescribed treatment
• Treatment given to patient; patient's understanding and demonstrated ability to carry out instructions
• Patient's response to nursing interventions
• Evaluations for each expected outcome.

■ Diversional activity deficit

related to lack of environmental stimulation

Definition
Restriction or decline in ability to use unoccupied time to patient's advantage or satisfaction

Assessment
• Physical status, including mobility and activity tolerance
• Cardiovascular status
• Respiratory status
• Neurologic status, including level of consciousness, orientation, mood, behavior, memory
• Psychosocial status, including family or friends, hobbies, interests, favorite music, TV, reading matter,

changes or adaptations needed to carry out activities

Defining characteristics

- Evidence of environmental deprivation
- Physical limitations affecting participation in usual activities
- Statement of boredom or wishing for something to do

Associated medical diagnoses (selected)

Any patient hospitalized for a prolonged period may be at risk. Additional diagnoses include: blindness, conditions requiring isolation or intensive care, depression, detached retina, fractures requiring skeletal traction, and hearing loss.

Expected outcomes

- Patient expresses interest in using leisure time meaningfully.
- Patent expresses interest in activities provided.
- Patient participates in chosen activity.
- Patient watches selected TV program or listens to selected music daily.
- Patient reports satisfaction with use of leisure time.
- Patient or caregiver modifies environment to provide maximum stimulation, such as with posters or cards or moving bed next to a window.

Interventions and rationales

- Encourage discussion of previously enjoyed hobbies, interests, or skills *to direct planning of new activities.* Suggest performing an activity helpful to others or otherwise productive.
- Obtain radio or TV (if desired) and allow patient to select programs. Communicate patient's desires to coworkers. Turn on TV set at _____ (time) to _____ (channel). *Selective TV or radio use can help pass time.*
- Ask volunteers (friends, family, or hospital volunteer) to read newspapers, books, or magazines to patient at specific times. *Personal contacts helps alleviate boredom.*
- Engage patient in conversation while carrying out routine care. Discuss patient's favorite topics as much as possible. *Conversation conveys caring and recognition of patient's worth.*
- Provide supplies and set time to carry out hobby; for example, give crochet hook and yarn to patient daily at _____ (time). *Specifying time for activity indicates its value.*
- Avoid scheduling procedures during patient's leisure time, *which is integral to quality of life.*
- Provide talking books or records if available. *These provide low-effort sources of enjoyment for bedridden patient.*
- Obtain an adapter for the TV *to provide captions for hearing-impaired patient.*
- Encourage patient's family or caregiver to bring in personal articles (posters, cards, pictures) to help make environment more stimulating. *Patient may respond better to objects with personal meaning.*
- Make referral to recreational, occupational, or physical therapist for consultation on adaptive equipment to carry out desired activity; arrange for therapy sessions. *Adaptive equipment allows patient to continue enjoying activities or may stimulate interest in new activities.*
- Provide plants for patient to tend. *Caring for live plants may stimulate interest.*
- Change scenery when possible; for example, place patient's bed in hall for a short period or take patient

outside in wheelchair *to help reduce boredom.*
- Identify type of music patient prefers; get help from family and hospital resources to provide selected music daily. *Music may relieve boredom.*

Evaluations for expected outcomes
- Patient expresses desire to participate in activities during leisure time.
- Patient engages in activity.
- Patient discusses content of TV or radio program.
- Patient reports reduced feelings of boredom.
- Environment is modified to increase patient stimulation.
- Patient discusses recent activity with staff, family, or significant other.

Documentation
- Patient's expression of boredom, frustration, and desire to carry out leisure activity
- Patient's interests and ability to carry out activity and necessary modifications required to accomplish activity
- Observations of patient's skill level and extent of participation in activity
- Patient's expression of satisfaction with use of unoccupied time
- Evaluations for each expected outcome.

■ Diversional activity deficit

related to long-term hospitalization or frequent, lengthy treatments

Definition
Restriction or decrease in ability to use unoccupied time to one's advantage or satisfaction

Assessment
- Physical status, including mobility and activity tolerance
- Cardiovascular status
- Respiratory status
- Neurologic status, including level of consciousness, orientation, mood, behavior, memory
- Psychosocial status, including family or significant other, hobbies, interests, favorite music, TV, reading matter, changes or adaptations needed to carry out activities

Defining characteristics
- Hospital stay beyond acute stage of illness
- Physical limitations affecting participation in usual activities
- Statement of boredom or wishing for something to do
- Treatments performed more than once a day or that require significant amounts of time

Associated medical diagnoses (selected)
Any patient hospitalized for a lengthy period of time may be at risk for this diagnosis. Examples include burns, pressure sores, isolation for contagious diseases, multiple fractures, peripheral vascular ulcers, plastic surgery involving extensive skin grafting, and spinal cord injury.

Expected outcomes
- Patient expresses interest in using leisure time meaningfully.
- Patient participates in chosen activity.
- Patient states satisfaction with use of leisure time.
- Patient expresses interest in activities provided.
- Patient makes decisions about timing and spacing of treatments.

• Patient expresses satisfaction with established schedule of treatment routines.

Interventions and rationales

• Schedule time daily to pursue leisure activities; for example, have patient sit at desk daily in wheelchair to use paint-by-number kit. *Diversional activities improve patient's quality of life; scheduling activities indicates their value.*
• Encourage family or significant other to bring in familiar objects. Provide space for favorite plants, cards, reading material, and hobby supplies. For bedridden patients, use ceiling for posters and other objects. *Maintaining personal contacts and involvement relieves boredom and stimulates interest.*
• Encourage patient to express enjoyment of past hobbies, interests, or skills. *This conveys a sense of worth and caring, and helps patient to think of new activities.*
• Work with patient and family to find ways to carry out desired activities. Use imagination and creativity; for example, a former carpenter may adapt to carving small objects rather than building large ones. *Adaptive equipment helps patient pursue previous activities within new limits.*
• Provide radio or TV at patient's request *to help relieve boredom and increase enjoyment.*
• Engage patient in conversation while carrying out procedures, if desired by patient. Discuss favorite topics. *Conversation during treatments reduces discomfort by diverting attention; it also increases patient's sense of self-worth.*
• Encourage visitors to involve patient in favorite activities through discussion, reading, and attendance at programs, if appropriate, *to reduce boredom.*
• Keep patient informed of current events through discussion; encourage patient to read newspapers or books and watch TV or listen to radio. *Keeping current helps reduce the isolation of long-term hospitalization.*
• Schedule treatments to allow adequate rest periods and pursuit of favorite activity; for example, no treatments between _____ and _____ (time), to allow time for watching TV show. *This gives patient more control over environment.*
• Streamline treatments as much as possible. Have all equipment ready before starting; thoroughly instruct new personnel in routine and plan schedule for minimal interruptions. *Efficiency conveys respect for value of patient's time.*

Evaluations for expected outcomes

• Patient expresses desire to participate in activity during leisure hours.
• Patient engages in chosen activity.
• Patient reports decrease in feelings of boredom.
• Patient makes decisions about timing and spacing of treatments.
• Patient expresses a positive attitude about the treatment schedule.

Documentation

• Patient's expressions of boredom, desire to carry out leisure activity, and frustration at being restricted
• Patient's interests, skills, and abilities to carry out activity
• Observations of patient's skill level and extent of participation in activity
• Patient's expression of satisfaction with use of non-treatment-related time
• Evaluations for each expected outcome.

Dysreflexia

related to spinal cord trauma

Definition

State in which a patient with spinal cord injury at T6 or above experiences or risks life-threatening, uninhibited sympathetic response to a noxious stimulus

Assessment

- History of spinal cord trauma, including level of injury or lesion, previous episodes of dysreflexia
- Patient's description of symptoms, including headache, nasal congestion, blurred vision, chest pain, diaphoresis and flushing above level of lesion, chilling, paresthesias, cutis anserina ("goose flesh") above level of lesion, metallic taste, nausea
- Neurologic status, including level of consciousness, orientation, pupillary response, sensory status, motor status
- Cardiovascular status, including blood pressure, heart rate and rhythm, skin temperature and color
- Genitourinary status, including urine output, palpation of bladder, signs of urinary tract infection, examination of urinary assistive devices, such as catheter
- Gastrointestinal status, including nausea and vomiting, usual bowel pattern, bowel habits, last bowel movement, inspection of abdomen, auscultation of bowel sounds, palpation for masses, percussion for areas of dullness
- Environmental conditions, including changes in temperature, for example, cold draft; objects putting pressure on skin

Defining characteristics

- Major trauma (spinal cord injury at T6 or above), including paroxysmal hypertension (sudden periodic elevated blood pressure, systolic over 140 mm Hg and diastolic over 90 mm Hg); bradycardia or tachycardia (pulse under 60 or over 100 beats/minute); diaphoresis above injury, red splotches (vasodilation) on skin above injury, pallor below injury, diffuse headache not confined to any nerve distribution area
- Minor trauma, including chilling (shivering with sensation of coldness or pallor of skin); conjunctival injection from excessive blood or tissue fluid in conjunctiva; Horner's syndrome from paralysis of cervical sympathetic nerve trunk (contracted pupils, partial ptosis, enophthalmos, sometimes loss of sweating on affected side of face); paresthesias; pilomotor reflex, blurred vision, chest pain, metallic taste, nasal congestion

Associated medical diagnoses (selected)

Spinal cord injury or tumor above T6 level

Expected outcomes

- Cause of dysreflexia is identified and corrected.
- Patient experiences cardiovascular stability as evidenced by ____ systolic range, ____ diastolic range, and ____ heart rate range.
- Patient avoids bladder distention and urinary tract infection.
- Fecal impaction is absent.
- No noxious stimuli in environment.
- Patient states relief from symptoms of dysreflexia.
- Patient encounters no or minimal complications.
- Urinary elimination remains normal.
- Fecal elimination remains normal.

- Patient, family, or caregivers demonstrate knowledge and understanding of dysreflexia and articulate care measures.
- Patient experiences few or no dysreflexic episodes.

Interventions and rationales

- Assess for signs of dysreflexia (especially severe hypertension) *in order to detect the condition promptly.*
- Place patient in sitting position or elevate head of bed *to aid venous drainage from brain, lower intracranial pressure, and temporarily reduce blood pressure.*
- Ascertain and correct probable cause of dysreflexia:
  - Check for bladder distention and patency of catheter. If necessary, irrigate catheter with small amount of solution or insert a new catheter immediately. *A blocked urinary catheter can trigger dysreflexia.*
  - Check for fecal mass in rectum. Apply dibucaine ointment (Nupercainal) or another product, as ordered, to anus and 1″ into rectum 10 to 15 minutes before removing impaction. *Failure to use ointment may aggravate autonomic response.*
  - Check environment for cold drafts and objects putting pressure on patient's skin, *which could act as dysreflexia stimuli.*
  - Send urine for culture if no other cause becomes apparent *to detect possible urinary tract infection.*
- If hypertension persists despite other measures, administer ganglionic blocking agent, vasodilator, or other medication as ordered. *Drugs may be required if hypertension persists or if noxious stimuli cannot be removed.*
- Take vital signs frequently *to monitor effectiveness of prescribed medications.*
- Instruct patient, family, or caregiver about dysreflexia, its causes, symptoms, and care measures *to prepare them to handle possible dysreflexic emergencies.*
- Implement and maintain bowel and bladder elimination programs *to avoid stimuli that could trigger dysreflexia.*

Evaluations for expected outcomes

- Cause of dysreflexia is identified and corrected.
- Patient experiences cardiovascular stability as evidenced by ____ systolic range, ____ diastolic range, and ____ heart rate range.
- Palpation does not reveal a distended bladder.
- Patient's urinary catheter is patent without kinking or blockage.
- Patient does not exhibit signs and symptoms of urinary tract infection.
- Patient's bowel elimination pattern remains normal.
- Patient's environment remains free of noxious stimuli.
- Patient expresses relief from signs and symptoms of dysreflexia.
- Patient does not experience complications of dysreflexia, including contractures, venous stasis, thrombus formation, skin breakdown, or hypostatic pneumonia.
- Patient's bladder elimination program is successfully implemented and maintained. Patient's urine output remains within specified volume.
- Patient's bowel elimination program is successfully implemented and maintained. Fecal impaction is absent.
- Patient and family or significant other express understanding of the causes, symptoms, and treatment of

autonomic dysreflexia, and demonstrate measures to implement if dysreflexia occurs.
• Because of successful maintenance of bladder and bowel elimination programs, preventive skin care measures, and patient and family teaching, patient experiences few or no dysreflexic episodes.

Documentation
• Objective assessment of dysreflexic episode
• Patient's description of dysreflexic episode
• Interventions to identify and eliminate causes of dysreflexia and patient's response to these
• Instructions given to patient, family, caregivers; patient's expressions of understanding and demonstrated ability to prevent or manage dysreflexic episode
• Implementation, alteration, or continuation of bladder and bowel programs
• Evaluations for each expected outcome.

Family process alteration

related to situational crisis

Definition
Disruption in expected role functions within the family structure because of such situational crises as protracted physical or emotional illness

Assessment
• Assumed or expected roles
• Communication patterns within family for expressing affection, anger, confrontation, despair
• Family members
• Family's financial resources
• Family's past responses to crises
• Family's spiritual practices
• Family's understanding of patient's present condition
• Normal patterns of interaction among family members
• Number and ages of children
• Perceived impact of situation on family unit or on assumed roles
• Significant others
• Support systems available to family

Defining characteristics
Family system unable or unwilling to meet the emotional or physical needs of its members

Associated medical diagnoses (selected)
Any disease or illness that results in long-term disability or incapacitation, including: cancer, cerebrovascular accident, chronic renal failure, degenerative disease, dementia, terminal disease, traumatic injury

Expected outcomes
• Family members agree on who heads the family.
• Family members develop adaptive responses by assuming duties carried out by the ill member; for example, meal preparation, transportation, shopping, laundry, cleaning, providing emotional support to other family members.
• Family members identify support systems to assist them and participate in mobilizing those systems.
• Family contacts a community agency or support group for continued assistance (depending on the type, severity, prognosis of illness); for example, American Cancer Society, American Lung Association, Arthritis Foundation, Hospice, Myasthenia Gravis Foundation, Multiple Sclerosis Society, National Kidney Foundation, Trauma Support Group.

• Family members can share feelings about illness in the family with each other.

Interventions and rationales

• Identify the individual assuming the role as head of the family *to establish family hierarchy and functional ability.*

• Provide head of family with information necessary for decision making, such as updated information on patient's condition. *This avoids potential for misinterpretation and places responsibility for communication within family unit.*

• Help head of the family decide which support systems need to be mobilized and used. *This allows opportunity to evaluate head of family's management ability and family's problem-solving ability.*

• Provide emotional support to head of family regarding altered role and additional responsibilities. *This encourages family member to ventilate feelings, ask questions, seek help, and make decisions.*

• Expedite communication within the family *to allow members to express their feelings about the present situation. This encourages supportive behavior to meet reciprocal needs in a crisis.*

• Arrange for and participate in family conferences, if appropriate.
  – Whenever possible, ensure privacy to family members for their discussions or conferences.
  – Include patient in family conferences and family interaction as often as possible.

These measures allow nurse to help family identify and work toward mutual goals and facilitate effective family coping.

• Make referrals to a psychiatric liaison nurse, social services, or community agencies, as appropriate *to provide family with access to additional coping resources.*

Evaluations for expected outcomes

• Family members identify individual to take on responsibilities of head of family.

• Family members assume responsibilities formerly carried out by ill member.

• Family members identify and contact available resources as needed.

• Family members contact community support groups and associations and attend at least two meetings.

• Family members openly share feelings about present situation.

Documentation

• Observations of family's reactions to situation

• Interventions to assist family and family's responses to those interventions

• Referrals to outside agencies

• Evaluations for each expected outcome.

■ Fatigue

Definition

Overwhelming sense of exhaustion and decreased capacity for physical and mental work, regardless of adequate sleep

Assessment

• History of underlying disease process

• Respiratory status, including dyspnea on exertion, respiratory rate and depth

• Circulatory status, including skin color, temperature, turgor, blood pressure

- Age
- Sleep pattern, including hours slept at night, amount of time awake before becoming tired
- Nutritional status, including appetite, dietary intake, current weight, change from normal weight
- Neurologic status, including headaches
- Activity status, including type and duration of exercise, occupation, use of leisure time
- Psychosocial status, including personality stressors (finances, job, marital discord), coping mechanisms, support systems (family, significant other), life-style
- Menstrual history, including length of periods, amount of menstrual flow

Defining characteristics
- Accident-prone
- Decreased libido
- Decreased performance
- Disinterest in surroundings
- Increased lability or irritability
- Introspection
- Lethargy or listlessness
- Perceived need for additional energy to accomplish routine tasks

Associated medical diagnoses (selected)
Anemia, cardiac failure, cerebrovascular accident, depression, Epstein-Barr virus, Guillain-Barré syndrome, multiple sclerosis, muscular atrophy, myasthenia gravis, poliomyelitis, rheumatoid arthritis

Expected outcomes
- Patient identifies measures to prevent or modify fatigue.
- Patient explains relationship of fatigue to disease process and activity level.
- Patient verbally expresses increased energy.
- Patient incorporates as part of daily activities those measures necessary to modify fatigue.
- Patient articulates plan to resolve fatigue problems.
- Patient employs measures to prevent and modify fatigue.

Interventions and rationales
- Prevent unnecessary fatigue; for example, avoid scheduling two energy-draining procedures on the same day. *Using energy-conserving techniques avoids overexertion and potential for exhaustion.*
- Conserve energy through rest, planning, and setting priorities *to prevent or alleviate fatigue.*
- Alternate activities with periods of rest. Encourage activities that can be completed in short periods of time or divided into several segments; for example, read one chapter of a book at a time. *Scheduling regular rest periods helps decrease fatigue and increase stamina.*
- Discuss the effect of fatigue on daily living and personal goals. Explore with patient the relationship between fatigue and the disease process *to help increase patient compliance with the schedule for activity and rest.*
- Reduce demands placed on patient; for example, ask one family member to call at specified times and relay messages to friends and other family members *to reduce physical and emotional stress.*
- Structure patient's environment; for example, set up a daily schedule based on patient's needs and desires. *This encourages compliance with treatment regimen.*
- Encourage patient to eat foods rich in iron and minerals, unless contraindicated. *This helps avoid anemia and demineralization.*

• Postpone eating when patient is fatigued *to avoid aggravating the condition.*
• Provide small, frequent feedings *to conserve patient's energy and encourage increased dietary intake.*
• Establish a regular sleeping pattern. *Eight to 10 hours of sleep nightly helps reduce fatigue.*
• Avoid highly emotional situations, *which aggravate patient's fatigue.* Encourage patient to explore feelings and emotions with a supportive counselor, clergy, or other professional *to help cope with illness.*

Evaluations for expected outcomes

• Patient describes at least three strategies to prevent or modify fatigue and incorporates at least three measures to modify fatigue into daily routine.
• Patient discusses the relationship of fatigue to disease process and activity level—for example, in heart disease, fatigue is a sign that the heart can't meet increased oxygen demands.
• Patient states that his fatigue level is reduced.
• Patient describes plan to resolve fatigue problems, including both physiologic and emotional remedies.

Documentation

• Patient's ability to describe the fatigue and its relationship to the disease process and condition
• Patient's ability to decrease fatigue by using various effective methods
• Patient's level of activity in relation to fatigue
• Patient's dietary intake
• Evaluations for each expected outcome.

Fear

related to separation from support system

Definition

Feeling of physiologic or emotional disruption related to an identifiable source

Assessment

• History of experience with illness, hospitalization, surgery
• Availability of support systems, including family, significant other, friends, clergy
• Financial resources
• History of coping with fear
• Physiologic manifestations of fear, including changes in pulse rate, respiratory rate, blood pressure, skin temperature, quality and pitch of voice
• Psychological manifestations of fear, including changes in behavior, appetite, sleep pattern

Defining characteristics

• Diaphoresis
• Feeling of loss of control (actual or perceived)
• Hospitalization may create geographic distance from family or friends
• Increased blood pressure
• Increased pulse and respiratory rate
• Increased questioning or verbalization
• Limited financial resources of family to travel
• Patient and spouse or significant other unaccustomed to separation
• Patient has no family or friends
• Voice tremors or pitch change

Associated medical diagnoses (selected)
This nursing diagnosis may occur in any hospitalized patient separated from family or friends. In elderly patients, hospitalization often disrupts routines or rituals.

Expected outcomes
- Patient identifies source(s) of fear.
- Patient communicates feelings about separation from support systems.
- Patient communicates feelings of comfort or satisfaction.
- Patient uses situational supports to reduce fear.
- Patient integrates into daily behavior at least one fear-reducing coping mechanism, such as asking questions about treatment progress, or making decisions about care.

Interventions and rationales
- Ask patient to identify source of fear; try to assess patient's understanding of situation. *Patient's perceptions may be erroneously based.*
- If patient has no visitors, spend an extra 15 minutes each shift in casual conversation; encourage other staff members to stop for brief visits *to help patient cope with separation.*
- Help patient maintain contact with family on a daily basis:
  - Arrange for telephone calls.
  - Help write letters.
  - Promptly convey messages to patient from family and vice-versa.
  - Encourage patient to have pictures of loved ones.
  - Provide privacy for visits; take patient to day room or other quiet area.

These measures help patient reestablish and maintain social relationships.
- Involve patient in planning care and setting goals *to renew confidence and give sense of control in a crisis situation.*
- Instruct patient in relaxation techniques, such as imagery and progressive muscle relaxation, *to reduce symptoms of sympathetic stimulation.*
- Administer antianxiety medications as ordered and monitor effectiveness. *Drug therapy may be needed to manage high anxiety levels or panic disorders.*
- Answer questions and help patient understand care *to reduce anxiety and correct misconceptions.*
- When feasible and where policies permit, relax visiting restrictions *to reduce patient's sense of isolation.*
- Allow a close family member or friend to participate in care *to provide an additional source of support.*
- Support family and friends in their efforts to understand patient's fear and to respond accordingly *to help them understand that patient's emotions are appropriate in context of situation.*

Evaluations for expected outcomes
- Patient states causes of fear.
- Patient expresses distress caused by separation from support systems.
- Patient reports feeling less fearful.
- Patient reaches out to others for support through phone calls, letters, or other means.
- Patient demonstrates use of at least one coping mechanism daily to reduce fear.

Documentation
- Patient's expressions of concern about illness, hospitalization, separation from support system, overt expressions of fear
- Observations of physiologic and behavioral manifestations of patient's fear

- Interventions performed to allay patient's fears and encourage healthful coping mechanisms
- Patient's response to interventions
- Evaluations for each expected outcome.

Fear

related to unfamiliarity

Definition

Feelings of threat or danger to self arising from an identifiable source

Assessment

- History of experience with illness, hospitalization, surgery, etc.
- Availability of support systems, including family, significant other, friends, clergy
- Financial resources
- History of coping with fear
- Neurologic status, including mental status, orientation, sensory status
- Physiologic manifestations of fear, including changes in pulse rate, blood pressure, respiratory rate, skin temperature
- Psychological manifestations of fear, including changes in behavior, appetite, sleep pattern
- Quality and pitch of voice

Defining characteristics

- Diaphoresis
- Expressions of feeling different from others
- Expressions indicating fear of the unknown
- Expressions of loneliness
- Inability to speak or understand English (alternatively, patient may understand English but not speak it)
- Increased blood pressure
- Increased pulse and respiratory rates
- Increased questioning or verbalization
- Lack of communication, withdrawal, poor eye contact
- Preoccupation with own thoughts
- Requests to be left alone or requests for constant bedside companionship
- Sad, dull affect
- Statements indicating that patient has no previous experience with hospitalization or illness
- Tone of voice and behavior that project hostility
- Voice tremors or pitch changes

Associated medical diagnoses (selected)

Acute renal failure with hemodialysis or peritoneal dialysis, acute respiratory failure with mechanical ventilation, bowel resection with colostomy or ileostomy, brain tumor, coronary artery bypass surgery, craniocerebral trauma, sensory loss (blindness, deafness), spinal cord injury, tracheostomy or laryngectomy

Expected outcomes

- Patient identifies source(s) of fear.
- Patient states understanding of procedures.
- Patient verbally expresses comfort with surroundings.
- Patient manifests no physical signs or symptoms of fear.
- Patient uses available support systems to assist in coping with fear.
- Patient integrates into daily behavior at least one fear-reducing coping mechanism, such as asking questions about treatment progress or making decisions about care.

Interventions and rationales

- Encourage patient to identify source(s) of fear. *Patient's perceptions may be erroneously based.*
- Explain all treatments and procedures, answering any questions patient might have. Present information at patient's level of understanding or acceptance *to reduce patient's anxiety and enhance cooperation.*
- Orient patient to surroundings. Make any adaptations to compensate for sensory deficits. *This enhances patient's ability to orient to time, place, person, and events.*
- Assign the same nurse to care for patient whenever possible *to provide consistency of care, enhance trust, and reduce threat often associated with multiple caregivers.*
- Spend time with patient each shift *to allow time for expression of feelings, provide emotional outlet, and allow feeling of acceptance.*
- Involve patient in planning and providing care *to give patient some control over the situation and restore sense of self-esteem.*
- Orient family to patient's specific needs, allowing family members to participate in giving care. *This helps them provide effective support.*
- Request that family bring pictures and other small, personal objects to patient. *This helps alleviate patient's altered mental state by familiarizing the environment.*
- Arrange for family member or friend to stay with patient *to help patient cope with fears.*
- If a language barrier is the source of fear, use family and other resources in the hospital (such as an interpreter) *to help reduce patient's fear and aid effective communication.*

Evaluations for expected outcomes

- Patient identifies causes of fear.
- Patient demonstrates comprehension of procedures.
- Patient reports feeling comfortable in hospital.
- Patient's blood pressure, pulse rate, and respirations remain within set limits.
- Patient requests assistance from support systems to diminish fears (specify).
- Patient uses at least one effective fear-reducing behavior each day.

Documentation

- Patient's verbal expressions of fear
- Behavioral and physiologic manifestations of fear
- Interventions performed to reduce patient's fear
- Patient's response to interventions
- Family's involvement in patient care
- Patient's response to family involvement
- Evaluations for each expected outcome.

Fluid volume deficit

related to active loss

Definition

Excessive loss of body fluid and electrolytes

Assessment

- History of fluid loss, such as vomiting, nasogastric tube drainage, diarrhea, hemorrhage
- Vital signs
- Fluid and electrolyte status, including weight, intake and output, urine specific gravity, skin turgor, mucous membranes
- Laboratory studies, including serum electrolytes, blood urea nitrogen, hemoglobin, hematocrit, stool cultures

Defining characteristics
- Altered electrolytes
- Clinical evidence of body fluid or blood loss
- Dry mucous membranes
- Dry or cold, clammy skin
- Fever
- Low blood pressure
- Oliguria
- Output greater than intake
- Poor skin turgor
- Rapid, shallow respirations
- Rapid, thready pulse
- Thirst
- Weakness
- Weight loss

Associated medical diagnoses (selected)
Bowel fistula, burns, dialysis, duodenal ulcer (perforated), esophageal varices (ruptured), food poisoning, fractures (femur), hemothorax, hyperosmolar nonketotic syndrome (HNKS), large amounts of diuretics, metabolic acidosis, multisystem trauma, nasogastric tubes, thoracic surgery

Expected outcomes
- Vital signs remain stable.
- Skin color and temperature are normal.
- Electrolyte levels stay within normal range.
- Fluid volume remains adequate.
- Patient produces adequate urine volume.
- Patient has normal skin turgor and moist mucous membranes.
- Urine specific gravity remains between 1.005 and 1.010.
- Fluid and blood volume return to normal.
- Patient expresses understanding of factors that caused fluid volume deficit.

Interventions and rationales
- Monitor and record vital signs every 2 hours or as often as necessary until stable. Then monitor and record vital signs every 4 hours. *Tachycardia, dyspnea, or hypotension may indicate fluid volume deficit or electrolyte imbalance.*
- Cover patient lightly. Avoid overheating *to prevent vasodilatation, blood pooling in extremities, and reduced circulating blood volume.*
- Measure intake and output every 1 to 4 hours. Record and report significant changes. Include urine, stool, vomitus, wound drainage, nasogastric drainage, chest tube drainage, and any other output. *Low urine output and high specific gravity indicate hypovolemia.*
- Administer fluids, blood or blood products, or plasma expanders, *to replace fluids and whole blood loss and facilitate fluid movement into intravascular space.* Monitor and record effectiveness and any adverse effects.
- Weigh patient at the same time daily *to give more accurate and consistent data. Weight is a good indicator of fluid status.*
- Assess skin turgor and oral mucous membranes every 8 hours *to check for dehydration.* Give meticulous mouth care every 4 hours *to avoid dehydrating mucous membranes.*
- Test urine specific gravity every 8 hours. *Elevated specific gravity may indicate dehydration.*
- Do not allow patient to sit or stand up quickly as long as circulation is compromised *to avoid orthostatic hypotension and possible syncope.*
- Measure abdominal girth every shift *to monitor for ascites and third-space shift.* Report changes.
- Administer and monitor medications *to prevent further fluid loss.*

• Explain reasons for fluid loss and teach patient how to monitor fluid volume – for example, by recording daily weight and measuring intake and output. *This encourages patient involvement in personal care.*

Evaluations for expected outcomes
• Patient's pulse rate, blood pressure, respirations, and body temperature remain within set limits.
• Patient's skin color and temperature remain normal.
• Patient's electrolyte values remain within normal range.
• Urine output remains at volume established for patient.
• Patient's skin turgor and mucous membranes remain normal.
• Patient's specific gravity remains between 1.005 and 1.010, unless specified otherwise.
• Patient's fluid volume returns to normal and remains normal, as evidenced by stable vital signs.
• Patient and caregiver demonstrate understanding of factors precipitating fluid volume deficit.

Documentation
• Patient's complaints of thirst, weakness, dizziness, palpitations
• Observations of physical findings
• Intake and output (amount and type)
• Patient's weight and abdominal girth
• Interventions performed to control fluid loss
• Patient's response to interventions
• Evaluations for each expected outcome.

Fluid volume deficit, high risk for

related to excessive loss through artificial routes (such as indwelling tubes)

Definition
Presence of risk factors that can lead to excessive fluid and electrolyte loss

Assessment
• History of problems that can cause fluid loss, such as vomiting, diarrhea, indwelling tubes, hemorrhage
• Vital signs
• Fluid and electrolyte status, including weight, intake and output, urine specific gravity, skin turgor, mucous membranes, electrolytes

Risk factors
• Altered intake
• Clinical evidence of fluid or blood loss through artificial orifices or lumens, wounds, and drainage tubes
• Increased fluid output
• Thirst
• Urinary frequency

Associated medical diagnoses (selected)
Bowel fistula, breast cancer with mastectomy, burns, esophageal fistula, esophageal varices (ruptured), intestinal obstruction, paralytic ileus

Expected outcomes
• Vital signs remain stable.
• Skin color and temperature remain normal.
• Patient maintains urine output of at least ____ ml/hour.
• Electrolyte values remain within normal range.
• Patient maintains intake at ____ ml/24 hours.

• Intake equals or exceeds output.
• Patient returns to normal, appropriate diet.

Interventions and rationales
• Monitor and record vital signs every 4 hours. *Fever, tachycardia, dyspnea, or hypotension may indicate hypovolemia.*
• Measure urine output every hour. Record and report an output of less than _____ ml/hour. *Decreased urine output may indicate reduced fluid volume.*
• Monitor serum electrolyte levels and report abnormalities. *Indwelling tube drainage may cause significant electrolyte imbalance.*
• Measure and record drainage from all tubes and catheters, *taking it into account when replacing lost fluid.*
• Obtain and record patient's weight at the same time every day *to give accurate data. Weight is good indicator of fluid status.*
• When copious drainage appears on dressings, weigh dressings every 8 hours and record with other output sources. *Excessive wound drainage causes significant fluid imbalances (1 kg dressing equals about 1 liter of fluid).*
• Cover wounds *to minimize fluid loss and prevent skin excoriation.*
• Monitor skin turgor each shift *to check for dehydration;* report any decrease.
• Maintain parenteral fluids or blood transfusions at prescribed rate *to prevent further fluid loss or overload.*
• Force oral fluids when possible and indicated *to enhance replacement of lost fluids.* (Bowel sounds should be present with patient awake before giving oral fluids.)
• Progress patient to the appropriate diet, as ordered, *to help achieve fluid and electrolyte balance.*

Evaluations for expected outcomes
• Patient's temperature, pulse rate, blood pressure, and respirations are within set limits (specify).
• Patient's skin color remains normal.
• Patient's urine output remains at specified volume.
• Patient's electrolyte values remain normal.
• Patient's daily fluid intake remains within established limits (specify).
• Patient's cumulative intake equals or exceeds cumulative output.
• Patient returns to normal, appropriate diet.

Documentation
• Observations of physical findings
• Intake and output
• Drainage from indwelling tubes and catheters, including amount, color, consistency
• Amount, color, and odor of drainage on dressings
• Patient teaching about fluid intake and diet
• Patient's response to interventions
• Evaluations for each expected outcome.

■ Fluid volume deficit, high risk for

related to excessive loss through physiologic routes

Definition
Presence of risk factors that could lead to excessive fluid and electrolyte loss

Assessment
• History of problems that can cause fluid loss, such as vomiting, diarrhea, hemorrhage
• Vital signs

• Fluid and electrolyte status, including weight, intake and output, urine specific gravity, skin turgor, mucous membranes, serum electrolytes, blood urea nitrogen

Risk factors

• Any disorder that places patient at risk for fluid volume deficit
• Hyperventilation
• Increased fluid output
• Intake alteration
• Thirst
• Urinary frequency

Associated medical diagnoses (selected)

Altered level of consciousness, diabetes insipidus, diabetes mellitus, diarrhea-producing disorders (such as salmonellosis), organic brain syndrome

Expected outcomes

• No signs of dehydration appear.
• Patient's fluid intake exceeds output (intake _____ ml/24 hours; output _____ ml/24 hours).
• Patient expresses understanding of need to maintain adequate fluid intake.
• Patient demonstrates skill in weighing self accurately and recording weight.
• Patient measures and records own intake and output.

Interventions and rationales

• Monitor skin turgor each shift and report any decrease. *Poor skin turgor is a sign of dehydration.*
• Examine oral mucous membranes each shift. *Dry mucous membranes are a sign of dehydration.*
• Test urine specific gravity each shift. Monitor laboratory values and report abnormal findings to doctor. *Increased urine specific gravity may indicate dehydration. Elevated hematocrit and hemoglobin also indicate dehydration.*
• Monitor vital signs every 4 hours. *Tachycardia, hypotension, dyspnea, or fever may indicate fluid volume deficit.*
• Weigh patient at the same time daily and record. *Daily weights help estimate body fluid status.*
• Administer and monitor parenteral fluids, as ordered, *to replace fluid losses.*
• Determine patient's fluid preferences *to enhance intake.*
• Keep oral fluids at bedside within patient's reach and encourage patient to drink. *This gives patient some control over fluid intake and supplements parenteral fluid intake.*
• Maintain accurate record of intake and output *to aid estimation of patient's fluid balance.*
• Instruct patient in maintaining appropriate fluid intake, including recording daily weight, measuring intake and output, recognizing signs of dehydration. *This encourages patient and caregiver participation in care, and enhances patient's sense of control.*
• Monitor electrolyte values and report abnormalities. *Fluid loss may cause significant electrolyte imbalance.*
• Administer and monitor medication, such as antiemetics and antidiarrheals, *to prevent fluid losses.*

Evaluations for expected outcomes

• Patient does not display signs of dehydration; skin turgor, mucous membranes, urine specific gravity, and hemoglobin and hematocrit levels are normal; hyperthermia, hypotension, tachycardia, dyspnea, and weight loss do not occur.
• Patient's cumulative intake and output remain within established limits.

• Patient demonstrates understanding of importance of maintaining fluid balance.
• Patient weighs self with same scale at same time each day and records results.
• Patient measures fluid intake and output; records are reviewed to ensure accuracy.

Documentation
• Observations of patient's fluid volume status
• Intake and output
• Patient's willingness or ability to drink enough to maintain fluid volume
• Patient's response to nursing interventions
• Evaluations for each expected outcome.

■ Fluid volume excess

related to compromised regulatory mechanisms

Definition
Excess fluid resulting from compromised regulatory mechanisms (internal physiologic controls that help the body adapt to changing needs, such as renin-angiotensin, antidiuretic hormone, aldosterone, hydrogen-bicarbonate ion exchange)

Assessment
• Neurologic status, including level of consciousness, orientation, mental status
• Cardiovascular status, including skin color, temperature, turgor, jugular venous pressure, central venous pressure and pulmonary artery pressure (if available), heart rate and rhythm, blood pressure, heart sounds, ECG, hemoglobin, and hematocrit
• Respiratory status, including rate, depth, pattern of respiration, breath sounds, chest X-ray, arterial blood gases
• Renal status, including intake and output, urine specific gravity, weight, serum electrolytes, serum and urine osmolality, blood urea nitrogen, creatinine, serum protein
• Endocrine status, including general appearance, size and body proportions, skin color and condition, distribution of body hair

Defining characteristics
• Change in cardiovascular status, including edema, jugular venous distention, central venous pressure changes and pulmonary artery changes, positive hepatojugular reflux, increased heart rate, blood pressure changes, third heart sound, ECG changes, decreased hemoglobin and hematocrit
• Change in endocrine status, including mental status changes, abnormal fat distribution, increased blood pressure
• Change in mental status, including mood and personality changes, restlessness and confusion, acute stress and anxiety
• Change in renal status, including intake greater than output, oliguria, high urine specific gravity, weight gain, anasarca, altered electrolyte levels, change in osmolality, increased blood urea nitrogen and creatinine levels, decreased serum protein levels
• Change in respiratory status, including increased respiratory rate, changes in respiration pattern, dyspnea, orthopnea, crackles, pulmonary congestion on X-ray

Associated medical diagnoses (selected)
Acute glomerulonephritis, acute renal failure, chronic renal failure, congestive heart failure, Cushing's syndrome, hypothyroidism or myxedema, Laennec's cirrhosis, malnutrition, primary aldosteronism, pyelonephritis, syndrome of inappropriate antidiuretic hormone (resulting from stress or a surgical procedure using general anesthesia, for example), systemic lupus erythematosus

Expected outcomes
- Blood pressure remains no lower than ____ and no higher than ____ .
- Patient demonstrates no signs of hyperkalemia on ECG.
- Patient maintains fluid intake of no more than ____ and output of no less than ____ .
- Urine specific gravity remains between ____ and ____ .
- Hematocrit stays above ____ .
- Blood urea nitrogen, creatinine, sodium, and potassium stay within acceptable levels for specific patient.
- Patient plans 24-hour fluid intake, as prescribed.
- Patient tolerates restricted intake with no physical or emotional discomfort.
- Patient's skin remains intact and infection-free.
- Patient assists with activities of daily living without undue fatigue.
- Patient ambulates and carries out activities of daily living safely and comfortably.
- Patient demonstrates skill in selecting permitted foods, such as those low in sodium and potassium.
- Patient describes signs and symptoms that require medical treatment.

Interventions and rationales
- Monitor blood pressure, pulse, cardiac rhythm, temperature, and breath sounds at least every 4 hours; record and report changes. *Changed parameters may indicate altered fluid or electrolyte status.*
- Carefully monitor intake, output, and urine specific gravity at least every 4 hours. *Intake greater than output and elevated specific gravity may indicate fluid retention or overload.*
- Monitor blood urea nitrogen, creatinine, electrolytes, hemoglobin, and hematocrit. *BUN and creatinine indicate renal function; electrolytes, hemoglobin and hematocrit help indicate fluid status.*
- Weigh patient daily before breakfast, as ordered, *to provide consistent readings.* Check for signs of fluid retention, such as dependent edema, sacral edema, ascites.
- Give fluids as ordered. Monitor I.V. flow rate carefully *because excess I.V. fluids can worsen patient's condition.*
- If oral fluids are allowed, help patient make a schedule for fluid intake. *Patient involvement encourages compliance.*
- Explain the reasons for fluid and dietary restrictions *to enhance patient's understanding and compliance.*
- Learn patient's food preferences and plan accordingly within prescribed dietary restrictions *to enhance compliance.*
- Provide mouth care every 4 hours. Keep mucous membranes moist with water-soluble lubricant *to prevent them from dehydrating.*
- Provide sour hard candy *to decrease thirst and improve taste.*
- Support patient with positive feedback about adherence to restrictions *to encourage compliance.*

• Give skin care every 4 hours. Change patient's position at least every 2 hours. Elevate edematous extremities. *These measures enhance venous return, reduce edema, and prevent skin breakdown.*
• Examine skin daily for signs of bruising or other discoloration. *Edema may cause decreased tissue perfusion with skin changes.*
• Encourage patient to help in performing activities of daily living. *This boosts self-image and helps mobilize fluid from edematous areas.*
• Alternate periods of rest and activity *to avoid worsening fatigue caused by electrolyte imbalance.*
• Increase patient's activity level as tolerated; for example, ambulate, increase self-care measures performed by patient. *Gradually increasing activity helps body adjust to increased tissue oxygen demand and possible increased venous return.*
• Apply antiembolism stockings or intermittent pneumatic compression stockings *to increase venous return.* Remove for 1 hour and inspect skin every 8 hours or according to hospital policy.
• Assess skin turgor *to monitor for dehydration*.
• Measure abdominal girth every shift and report changes *to monitor for ascites*.
• Have dietitian see patient *to teach or reinforce dietary restrictions.*
• Educate patient regarding:
  – environmental safety measures
  – fluid restriction and diet
  – signs and symptoms requiring immediate medical treatment
  – medications (name, dosage, frequency, therapeutic effects, and adverse effects)
  – activity level
  – ways to prevent infection.

These measures encourage patient and significant others to participate more fully in care.

Evaluations for expected outcomes
• Patient's blood pressure remains within established limits.
• Signs of hyperkalemia (peaked or elevated T waves, prolonged P-R intervals, widened QRS complexes, or depressed ST segments) do not appear on ECG.
• Patient's fluid intake and output remain within established limits.
• Patient's urine specific gravity remains within established limits.
• Patient's hematocrit remains above specified level.
• Patient's electrolyte levels remain within established limits.
• Patient plans 24-hour fluid intake.
• Patient does not indicate discomfort with restricted fluid intake, either verbally or through behavior.
• Patient's skin remains intact and free of infection.
• Patient assists caregiver with activities of daily living without undue fatigue.
• Patient ambulates and carries out activities of daily living comfortably and safely.
• Patient plans own menu and selects foods low in sodium and potassium. Patient follows other dietary restrictions (specify).
• Patient and caregiver list signs and symptoms that require medical attention.

Documentation
• Expression of patient's needs, desires, or perceptions of the situation
• Specific changes in patient's physical status
• Observations about patient's response to treatment

• Observations about how patient appears to be coping with fluid and dietary restrictions
• Condition of skin and mucous membranes
• Interventions performed to alleviate or resolve diagnosis
• Evaluations for each expected outcome.

Fluid volume excess

related to excess fluid intake or retention, or excess sodium intake or retention

Definition

Imbalance of water or sodium causing increased total body fluid or fluid volume shift from one compartment to another

Assessment

• Neurologic status, including level of consciousness, orientation, mental status
• Cardiovascular status, including skin color, temperature, and turgor; jugular venous pressure; central venous pressure and pulmonary artery pressure (if available); heart rate and rhythm; blood pressure; heart sounds; ECG; hemoglobin; and hematocrit
• Respiratory status, including breath sounds, chest X-ray, arterial blood gases, and rate, depth, and pattern of respiration
• Renal status, including intake and output, urine specific gravity, weight, serum electrolytes, serum and urine osmolality, blood urea nitrogen, urine and serum creatinine, serum protein

Defining characteristics

• Altered electrolytes
• Anasarca
• Azotemia
• Central venous pressure changes
• Clinical evidence of increased fluids or salt intake or retention
• Edema
• Effusion
• Hepatojugular reflux
• Intake greater than output
• Mental status changes
• Oliguria
• Pulmonary congestion
• Restlessness and anxiety
• Shortness of breath, orthopnea
• Specific gravity changes
• Third heart sound
• Weight gain

Associated medical diagnoses (selected)

Cirrhosis, congestive heart failure, hypertension, hypoalbuminemia, portal vein thrombosis, psychogenic polydipsia, renal disease, small-bowel obstruction, severe burns

Expected outcomes

• Patient states ability to breathe comfortably.
• Patient maintains fluid intake at _____ ml/day.
• Patient returns to baseline weight.
• Patient maintains vital signs within normal limits (specify).
• Patient exhibits urine specific gravity of 1.005 to 1.010.
• Patient has normal skin turgor.
• Patient shows electrolytes within normal range (specify).
• Patient avoids complications of excess fluid.
• Patient states understanding of health problem.
• Patient demonstrates skill in health-related behaviors.

Interventions and rationales

• Help patient into a position that aids breathing, such as Fowler's or semi-Fowler's, *to increase chest expansion and improve ventilation.*

• Administer oxygen, as ordered, *to enhance arterial blood oxygenation.*

• Restrict fluids to _____ ml per shift. *Excessive fluids will worsen patient's condition.*

• Monitor and record vital signs at least every 4 hours. *Changes may indicate fluid or electrolyte imbalances.*

• Measure and record intake and output. *Intake greater than output may indicate fluid retention and possible overload.*

• Weigh patient at same time each day *to obtain consistent readings.*

• Administer diuretics *to promote fluid excretion.* Record effects.

• Test urine specific gravity every 8 hours and record results. Monitor laboratory values and report significant changes to doctor. *High specific gravity indicates fluid retention. Fluid overload may alter electrolyte levels.*

• Assess patient daily for edema, including ascites and dependent or sacral edema. *Fluid overload or decreased osmotic pressure may result in edema, especially in dependent areas.*

• Maintain patient on sodium-restricted diet, as ordered, *to reduce excess fluid and prevent reaccumulation.*

• Reposition patient every 2 hours, inspect skin for redness with each turn, and institute measures as needed *to prevent skin breakdown.*

• Apply antiembolism stockings or intermittent pneumatic compression stockings *to increase venous return.* Remove for 1 hour every 8 hours or according to institutional policy.

• Encourage patient to cough and deep-breathe every 2 to 4 hours *to prevent pulmonary complications.*

• Educate patient regarding:
  – maintenance of daily weight record
  – daily measuring and recording of intake and output
  – diuretic therapy
  – dietary restrictions, especially sodium.

These measures encourage patient and caregivers to participate more fully.

Evaluations for expected outcomes

• Patient indicates, verbally and through behavior, ability to breathe comfortably.

• Patient's fluid intake remains at established daily limit (specify).

• Patient's weight returns to baseline and remains stable.

• Patient's pulse and respiratory rates, blood pressure, and temperature remain within established limits.

• Patient's urine specific gravity remains between 1.005 and 1.010.

• Patient's skin turgor remains normal.

• Patient's electrolyte levels remain within established range.

• Complications of excess fluid do not occur.

• Patient expresses understanding of health problem.

• Patient demonstrates skill in health-related behaviors, such as maintaining weight and monitoring intake and output.

Documentation

• Patient's perceptions of the situation

• Observations of physical findings

• Interventions to correct fluid volume excess

• Patient's responses to fluid and dietary restrictions

- Patient's demonstration of skills
- Evaluations for each expected outcome.

Gas exchange impairment

related to altered oxygen-carrying capacity of the blood

Definition

Interference in cellular respiration resulting from inadequate exchange or transport of oxygen and carbon dioxide

Assessment

- Neurologic status, including level of consciousness, orientation, mental status
- Respiratory status, including respiratory rate and depth, symmetry of chest expansion, accessory muscle use, cough, sputum, palpation for fremitus, percussion of lung fields, auscultation of breath sounds, arterial blood gases, pulmonary function studies
- Cardiovascular status, including skin color and temperature, heart rate and rhythm, blood pressure, hemoglobin and hematocrit, red blood cell (RBC) count, white blood cell count, platelet count, prothrombin time, partial thromboplastin time, serum iron
- Activity status, including such functional capabilities as range of motion and muscle strength, activities of daily living, occupation

Defining characteristics

- Anxiety
- Bleeding tendency
- Confusion
- Cyanosis
- Decreased mental acuity
- Dizziness
- Dyspnea
- Fatigue
- Hypoxia
- Irritability
- Lethargy
- RBC abnormalities
- Restlessness

Associated medical diagnoses (selected)

Carbon monoxide poisoning, chronic obstructive pulmonary disease, folic acid deficiency, hemophilia, hypoplastic anemia, iron-deficiency anemia, leukemia, pernicious anemia, polycythemia vera, sickle-cell anemia, thalassemia, thrombocytopenic purpura

Expected outcomes

- Patient carries out activities of daily living without weakness or fatigue.
- No signs of active bleeding appear.
- Hemoglobin and hematocrit return to normal level (specify).
- Clotting profile remains within normal limits (specify).
- Patient maintains adequate ventilation.
- Patient communicates understanding of precautions needed to prevent bleeding.

Interventions and rationales

- Encourage patient to alternate periods of rest and activity. *Activity increases tissue oxygen demand; rest enhances tissue oxygen perfusion.*
- If patient is on bed rest, help him into a comfortable position and raise the side rails *to prevent falls.* Have patient turn, cough, and deep-breathe every 4 hours *to prevent atelectasis or fluid buildup in lungs, and enhance blood oxygen level.*
- Move patient slowly *to avoid orthostatic hypotension.* Assist patient

when out of bed *in case of dizziness.* Avoid bumps and scratches, *which may cause trauma and tissue bleeding.*
• Plan patient's activities within level of tolerance, *to avoid fatigue.*
• Provide gentle oral hygiene, *to avoid injuring oral mucosa.*
• Check all urine and stools for blood *to detect internal bleeding.* Check for evidence of bleeding at least once every 8 hours. *Hemorrhage or bleeding may cause anemia.*
• Administer blood or blood products and monitor for adverse reactions.
• Consolidate laboratory work *to avoid multiple needle-sticks and reduce chance of hematoma or hemorrhage in patients with altered clotting mechanisms.* Apply pressure for at least 1 minute after puncture *to promote clotting.*
• Auscultate lungs every 4 hours and report abnormalities.
• Monitor vital signs, cardiac rhythm, and arterial blood gas and hemoglobin levels. Report abnormalities.
• Teach patient about safety at home and work, including:
  – use of soft toothbrush
  – use of an electric razor for shaving
  – careful use of sharp objects, such as knives, tweezers, scissors
  – monitoring of urine, stools, and sputum for blood and reporting results immediately if blood is present
  – disadvantages and risks of smoking
  – using medications (name, dosage, therapeutic effect, adverse effects, precautions).

These measures encourage patient and caregivers to participate in care.

Evaluations for expected outcomes

• Patient carries out activities of daily living without fatigue or weakness.
• Patient does not exhibit signs of active bleeding, including oozing from wounds or puncture site, bruising, petechiae, or occult blood in stool or urine.
• Patient's hemoglobin and hematocrit remain within established limits.
• Patient's clotting profile, including platelet count, partial thromboplastin time, prothrombin time, fibrinogen, and fibrin split products, remains within normal limits.
• Patient maintains adequate ventilation.
• Patient communicates understanding of precautions needed to prevent bleeding episodes.

Documentation

• Patient's expression of personal feelings
• Observations about physical findings
• Results of laboratory studies that significantly affect nursing care
• Patient's response to interventions
• Evaluations for each expected outcome.

■ Gas exchange impairment

related to altered oxygen supply

Definition

Interference in cellular respiration resulting from inadequate exchange or transport of oxygen and carbon dioxide

Assessment

- Neurologic status, including level of consciousness, orientation, mental status
- Respiratory status, including respiratory rate and depth, symmetry of chest expansion, use of accessory muscles, cough, sputum, palpation for fremitus, percussion of lung fields, auscultation of breath sounds, arterial blood gas (ABG) levels, pulmonary function studies
- Cardiovascular status, including skin color and temperature, heart rate and rhythm, blood pressure, complete blood count
- Activity status, including such functional capabilities as range of motion and muscle strength, activities of daily living, occupation

Defining characteristics

- Abnormal ABG levels
- Anxiety
- Confusion
- Cyanosis
- Dyspnea
- Hypercapnia
- Hypoxia
- Inability to move secretions
- Irritability
- Mental acuity decrease
- Restlessness
- Somnolence
- Tachycardia, arrhythmias

Associated medical diagnoses (selected)

Acute pulmonary edema, acute respiratory failure, adult respiratory distress syndrome, altitude sickness, carbon monoxide poisoning, cerebrovascular accident, gallbladder disorders requiring cholecystectomy, drug overdose (narcotics, barbiturates, tranquilizers), Guillain-Barré syndrome, head injury, myasthenia gravis, pneumonia, pulmonary embolism, spinal cord injury, conditions requiring thoracotomy

Expected outcomes

- Patient maintains respiratory rate within ± 5 of baseline.
- Patient expresses feeling of comfort in maintaining air exchange.
- Patient coughs effectively.
- Patient expectorates sputum.
- Patient sustains sufficient fluid intake to prevent dehydration: _____ ml/24 hours.
- Patient performs activities of daily living to level of tolerance.
- Patient has normal breath sounds.
- Patient's ABG levels return to baselines: _____ pH; _____ PaO_2; _____ $PaCO_2$.
- Patient performs relaxation techniques every 4 hours.

Interventions and rationales

- Assess and record pulmonary status every 4 hours or more frequently if patient's condition is unstable. *Poor pulmonary status may result in hypoxemia.*
- Monitor vital signs and cardiac rhythm at least every 4 hours *to detect tachycardia and tachypnea, which could indicate hypoxemia.*
- Place patient in position that best facilitates chest expansion *to enhance gas exchange.*
- Change patient's position at least every 2 hours *to mobilize secretions and allow aeration of all lung fields.*
- Perform bronchial hygiene as ordered, including coughing, percussion, postural drainage, suctioning. *These measures promote drainage and keep airways clear.*
- Give medications, as ordered, *to improve oxygenation.* Monitor and re-

cord efficacy and adverse reactions, *to guide treatment.*
- Monitor oxygen therapy, *which increases alveolar oxygen concentration and enhances arterial blood oxygenation.*
- Record intake and output, *to monitor patient's fluid status.*
- Report signs of dehydration or fluid overload immediately. *Dehydration may hinder tissue perfusion and secretion mobilization; fluid overload may cause pulmonary edema.*
- Assist patient with activities of daily living, *to decrease tissue oxygen demand.*
- Include periods of rest in care plan *to reduce patient's tissue oxygen demand.*
- Monitor ABG levels and notify doctor immediately if PaO_2 or SaO_2 drops or $PaCO_2$ rises. Administer endotracheal intubation and mechanical ventilation if needed. *This helps increase ventilation and gas exchange.*
- Teach patient relaxation techniques, *to reduce tissue oxygen demand.*
- Have patient perform relaxation techniques every 4 hours *to establish the routine and reduce oxygen demand.*

Evaluations for expected outcomes
- Patient's respiratory rate remains within established limits.
- Patient does not experience dyspnea.
- Patient demonstrates ability to cough and produce sputum.
- Patient expectorates sputum produced by coughing and deep breathing.
- Patient's PaO_2 and SaO_2 remain within established limits.
- Patient's fluid intake remains sufficient to prevent dehydration.
- Patient performs activities of daily living without exhibiting dyspnea or other signs of abnormal ABG levels.
- Patient has normal breath sounds.

Documentation
- Patient's complaints of dyspnea, headache, restlessness
- Patient's expression of well-being
- Observations of physical findings
- Effectiveness of medications
- Other treatments performed by the nurse
- Evaluations for each expected outcome.

Grieving, anticipatory

related to perceived potential loss of significant object (such as person, job, possessions)

Definition
Grief response in anticipation of perceived personal loss

Assessment
- Type of loss expected
- Feelings about control of situation
- Usual patterns of coping with loss
- Ability of patient and family to grieve over loss
- Greatest fear about the loss
- Behavioral manifestations of grieving
- Somatic problems associated with grieving process, including appetite, sleep patterns, activity, libido
- Support systems, including family or significant other, friends, clergy

Defining characteristics
- Altered activity level
- Altered communication pattern
- Altered libido
- Anger

- Changes in eating habits
- Changes in sleep patterns
- Choked feelings
- Denial of potential loss
- Expression of distress at potential loss
- Guilt
- Potential loss of significant object
- Sorrow

Associated medical diagnoses (selected)

Diagnoses may include recently diagnosed chronic or terminal diseases, such as acquired immunodeficiency syndrome, amyotrophic lateral sclerosis, cancer, chronic obstructive pulmonary disease, diabetes mellitus, leukemia, lupus erythematosus, multiple sclerosis, and rheumatoid arthritis. Also conditions that require radical surgery, such as amputation of a limb, mastectomy, permanent tracheostomy or laryngectomy, radical neck surgery

Expected outcomes

- Patient identifies the perceived potential loss.
- Patient expresses feelings about the potential loss.
- Patient communicates understanding of grieving process and willingness to experience the process.
- Patient exercises control by making decisions about care.
- Patient uses healthful coping mechanisms to deal with potential loss.
- Patient seeks support groups.
- Patient makes plans for future.

Interventions and rationales

- Help patient identify the potential loss *because patient may be unable to pinpoint cause of anxiety.*
- Plan time each shift to sit and listen to patient. If patient isn't ready to talk, spend the time in silence. *This demonstrates concern, understanding, and support for the patient.*
- Encourage patient to express feelings about the potential loss and its impact on well-being and life-style. *This reinforces reality and helps alleviate guilt through self-assurance that effort was made to prevent loss.*
- Help patient understand grieving process and accept feelings being experienced as normal under the present circumstances. *This enhances patient's understanding and ability to cope.*
- Encourage patient to make simple decisions related to care issues *to give patient a sense of functional ability and control.*
- Emphasize patient's identified strengths. Provide positive reinforcement as patient demonstrates effective coping behavior. *This helps patient reestablish positive self-image and gain confidence.*
- Encourage patient to use family, friends, or other support systems *to bolster coping ability.*
- Inform patient about existing support groups in the facility and the community *to encourage patient to seek help from available resources.*
- Help make a specific plan for coping after discharge *to enable patient to integrate the loss and adjust to life-style.*

Evaluations for expected outcomes

- Patient identifies potential loss.
- Patient expresses feelings about potential loss.
- Patient communicates understanding of stages of grief.
- Patient accepts feelings and behavior brought on by potential loss.
- Patient plans own daily plan of care, such as deciding best time for bathing, resting, and receiving visitors.

- Patient uses healthful coping mechanisms to deal with potential loss.
- Patient contacts support groups for help in coping with potential loss.
- Patient discusses future plans for coping with potential loss.

Documentation
- Patient's verbal expressions
- Patient's eating, sleeping, activity patterns
- Observation of emotional responses, such as crying, anger, withdrawal
- Patient's attempt to gain control, such as making decisions, use of support systems
- Interventions performed to assist patient
- Patient's response to intervention
- Evaluations for each expected outcome.

Grieving, dysfunctional

related to actual object loss

Definition
Prolongation of the normal grief response beyond the time one would expect resolution to have occurred

Assessment
- History of recent loss
- Patient's usual patterns of coping with loss, including cultural, intellectual, emotional
- Verbal expressions of feelings of control over the situation
- Behavioral manifestations of grieving, including presence and intensity of specific behaviors
- Somatic problems associated with grieving process, including appetite, sleep patterns, activity level, libido
- Support systems, including family or significant other, friends, clergy

Defining characteristics
- Alterations in concentration or pursuit of tasks
- Alterations in eating habits, sleep patterns, dream patterns, activity level, libido
- Anger
- Crying
- Denial of loss
- Developmental regression
- Difficulty in expressing loss
- Expressions of guilt
- Expressions of unresolved issues
- Idealization of lost object
- Interference with life functioning
- Labile affect
- Loss of health, significant other, job, or anything of importance to patient
- Reliving of past experiences
- Sadness
- Verbal expression of distress at loss

Associated medical diagnoses (selected)
The presence and degree of dysfunctional grieving depends greatly on the inner personal strength and support systems of the patient. Examples of medical diagnoses in which dysfunctional grieving may occur include abruptio placentae or placenta previa resulting in fetal death; end-stage diseases of any kind; hysterectomy, mastectomy, orchiectomy, severe burns, spinal cord injury (partial or total paralysis), spontaneous or therapeutic abortion, surgical or traumatic limb amputation.

Expected outcomes
- Patient identifies the loss.
- Patient expresses feelings about the loss.
- Patient allows others to help in coping.
- Patient begins using healthful coping mechanisms.

- Patient communicates understanding that it's normal to grieve.
- Patient seeks out healthful support systems.
- Patient allows self to experience grieving process alone and with family.
- Patient uses appropriate support systems.
- Patient begins planning for future.

Interventions and rationales

- Encourage patient to use expressions of feeling that are most comfortable; for example, crying, talking, writing, drawing. *Dysfunctional grieving may result from inability to express feelings freely.*
- Spend at least 15 minutes each shift with patient. Allow this time for expression of feelings. Place limits on behaviors that are destructive or exaggerated. *Inability to identify anger as normal response to loss may cause patient to behave aggressively toward self or others.*
- Help patient focus realistically on changes the loss has brought about. *This is an initial step in planning for future, and helps patient find new patterns of rewarding interactions.*
- Encourage patient's help in self-care activities, *to reduce intensity of patient's mourning and enhance sense of functional ability.*
- Encourage patient to use available support systems, *to provide emotional strength.*
- Encourage patient and family to reminisce. *Helping them engage in "life-review" often creates peaceful atmosphere in which loss acquires purpose and meaning.*
- Inform patient and family about existing support groups in the agency and in the community, *to help prevent or reduce maladaptive emotional responses to loss.*
- Help patient formulate goals for discharge and the future. *This helps patient to place loss in perspective and to move on to new situations and relationships.*
- Refer patient to an appropriate mental health professional. *Delayed grief reaction may indicate depression, which requires psychiatric intervention.*

Evaluations for expected outcomes

- Patient identifies recent loss.
- Patient discusses feelings about recent loss.
- Patient allows others to help cope with loss.
- Patient uses coping mechanisms, including discussing loss with others.
- Patient communicates understanding that grieving is an appropriate response to loss and comes to terms with own grief response.
- Patient actively participates in discussions about loss with support groups or seeks help from mental health professional.
- Patient shares grief with family members.
- Patient describes future plans for coping with loss and getting on with life.

Documentation

- Patient's verbal expressions of grieving.
- Patient's observable behaviors, such as attempts at coping, interactions with family and staff.
- Description of nursing interventions and patient's responses.
- Evaluations for each expected outcome.

Growth and development alteration

related to effects of physical disability

Definition
State in which an individual deviates from norms for age

Assessment
- Age (chronological, developmental stage)
- Sex
- Nature of physical disability
- Past experience with hospitalization
- Family system (nuclear, extended, sibling position)
- Communication skills (verbal, nonverbal)
- Motor skills
- Socialization pattern
- Knowledge, including educational background, understanding of physical disability
- Mental status, including orientation, cognitive and perceptual ability, memory, affect, and mood behavior

Defining characteristics
- Delay or difficulty in performing skills typical of age group (motor, social, expressive)
- Flat affect, listlessness, decreased verbal or nonverbal response
- Inability to perform self-care or self-control activities appropriate for age

Associated medical diagnoses (selected)
This nursing diagnosis may apply to patients of all ages but will be limited here to include only those age 12 or older. Diagnoses include cerebrovascular accident, conditions requiring amputation, head trauma, metastatic illness, orthopedic injuries, spinal cord injuries.

Expected outcomes
- Patient expresses concerns about physical disability.
- Patient identifies changes in usual communication, motor, and socialization skills.
- Patient states a desire to regain age-appropriate skills and behaviors to the extent possible.
- Patient demonstrates age-appropriate skills and behaviors to the extent possible.
- Patient, family, or significant other agrees to seek help from peer support groups or professional counselors to increase adaptive coping behaviors.

Interventions and rationales
- Spend specified amount of uninterrupted non–care-related time, perhaps 20 minutes twice daily, using active listening to encourage patient to express concerns. *Active listening, which includes attentive involvement and openness to patient's concerns without interpretation, allows patient to reveal concerns at own pace.*
- Urge patient to identify normal skills and behaviors and then describe how they could be altered in light of current disability. *Self-monitoring helps patient identify normal behaviors and relate behavioral changes to specific variables.*
- Instruct patient on age-appropriate skills and behaviors (chronological and developmental) and request feedback on possible ways for patient to regain as many as possible. *This helps patient to recognize regressive behavior and noncompliance and to adjust accordingly.*
- Give patient positive reinforcement for demonstrating appropriate skills

and behaviors *to promote similar behavior in future.*
- Tell patient, family, or significant other about social and professional support available and advise about the benefits of using services after discharge. *This encourages patient to seek help from available resources.*

Evaluations for expected outcomes
- Patient expresses concerns about physical disability.
- Patient provides information about usual abilities and behaviors and reports changes seen as result of current situation (specify).
- Patient expresses a desire to regain appropriate skills and behaviors (specify).
- As much as possible, patient demonstrates age-appropriate skills and behavior.
- Patient and caregiver describe plans for participating in support groups after discharge.

Documentation
- Assessment of observed deviations from norm for patient's age group
- Patient's report of concern about disability
- Interventions performed to assist patient in regaining age-appropriate skills and behaviors
- Patient's response to nursing interventions
- Evaluations for each expected outcome.

Health maintenance alteration

related to lack of motor skills

Definition
Inability to maintain a healthy state

Assessment
- Neuromuscular status, including muscle strength and mass, gross and fine motor skills, joint mobility, electromyelogram and electroencephalogram
- Abilities and limitations, including turning, transferring, ambulation, wheelchair use, driving, activities of daily living
- Knowledge of health practices, including body maintenance, preventive health needs, health team follow-up, safety measures
- Psychosocial support, including life-style, communication status (verbal, nonverbal, phone, written); family or significant other, finances

Defining characteristics
- Clinical evidence of deficiency in motor skills or ability
- Demonstrated lack of adaptive behaviors to internal or external environmental changes
- Demonstrated lack of knowledge regarding basic health practices
- Reported or observed inability to take responsibility for meeting basic health needs in any or all functional pattern areas

Associated medical diagnoses (selected)
Amyotrophic lateral sclerosis, brain tumor, cerebral palsy, cerebrovascular accident, head trauma, mental retardation, multiple sclerosis, muscular dystrophy, poliomyelitis, rheumatoid arthritis, spinal cord injury (quadriplegia, paraplegia), trauma

Expected outcomes
- Patient identifies necessary health maintenance activities.
- Patient makes decisions about daily schedule.

• Patient performs health maintenance activities according to level of ability (specify).
• Patient communicates understanding of necessity for continuous self-monitoring of body functions.
• Patient maintains muscle strength and joint mobility.
• Patient demonstrates specific motor skills, such as brushing teeth.
• Family or significant other demonstrates skill in carrying out activities patient cannot perform.
• Patient identifies community and social resources available to help with health maintenance.

Interventions and rationales

• Discuss health maintenance needs with patient while carrying out routine activities *to reinforce their importance.*
• Involve patient in decision making by allowing choices in determining where, when, and how activities are to be carried out. Ask, for example, "Would you like a bath or shower in the morning or evening?" *Participation in decision making increases feelings of independence.*
• Help patient perform health maintenance activities, such as daily skin inspection and weekly catheterization for residual urine. *Skill development should be encouraged to promote continuation after discharge.*
• Instruct patient in specific skills needed in monitoring health status *to prompt participation in self-care.* Allow patient to carry out skills *to encourage independence.*
• Perform or help patient perform passive and active range-of-motion exercises *to help maintain joint mobility and muscle strength.*
• Identify level of mobility (independent in feeding, bathing; needs assistance to brush teeth; dependent in use of wheelchair) and communicate skill level to all personnel *to provide continuity and preserve level of independence.*
• Educate family or significant other in skills that patient cannot perform unassisted, such as bathing, maintaining hygiene, driving to appointments, transferring, or using walker. *This allows patient, family, or significant other to take active role in care.*
• Consult with social service or other health team members to identify health resources (for example, Meals On Wheels or homemaker services), and help patient contact and arrange for follow-up. *These resources can help patient maintain independence after discharge.*

Evaluations for expected outcomes

• Patient identifies health maintenance activities.
• Patient plans daily schedule.
• Patient's functional level is appropriate to capability level.
• Patient communicates understanding of importance of monitoring body functions, such as blood glucose levels, blood pressure, and pulse rate.
• Patient maintains muscle strength and joint mobility.
• Patient demonstrates motor skills correctly without prompting.
• Family or significant other demonstrates skill in carrying out activities patient cannot perform.
• Patient identifies and contacts community resources to assist with health maintenance, if needed.

Documentation

• Patient's identified health needs and perceptions and limitations in achieving them
• Patient's willingness to make decisions and participate in health maintenance activities

• Observations of motor abilities, level of skill performance, and health status
• Patient's response to nursing interventions
• Evaluations for each expected outcome.

Health maintenance alteration

related to perceptual or cognitive impairment

Definition

Inability to maintain a healthy state

Assessment

• Age
• Current health status
• History of neurologic, sensory, or psychological impairment
• Neurologic status, including level of consciousness, orientation, cognition (memory, insight, or judgment), sensory ability, motor ability
• Personal habits, such as smoking or alcohol consumption
• Psychosocial status, including support systems, personality, coping mechanisms, drug use, and communication status (verbal, nonverbal, phone, written)

Defining characteristics

• Impaired perceptual or cognitive functioning
• Impaired short-term or long-term memory
• Inability to concentrate or to follow instructions
• Lack of adaptive behaviors to internal or external environmental changes
• Lack of interest in health maintenance
• Reported or observed inability to take responsibility for meeting basic health needs in any or all functional pattern areas

Associated medical diagnoses (selected)

Alcoholic psychosis, Alzheimer's disease, anoxic encephalopathy, autism, bipolar disease (manic or depressive phase), brain tumor, cerebrovascular accident, drug dependence, head injury, Huntington's disease, Laennec's cirrhosis, mental retardation, organic brain syndrome

Expected outcomes

• Patient maintains current health status.
• Patient sustains no harm or injury.
• Patient, family member, or significant other verbalizes feelings and concerns.
• Patient, family member, or significant other explains health maintenance program.
• Patient, family member, or significant other demonstrates health maintenance program.
• Patient, family member, or significant other identifies health resources available.
• Patient, family member, or significant other demonstrates appropriate coping skills.

Interventions and rationales

• Determine patient's capability to maintain health, degree of support available from family or significant other, degree of motivation, and level of dependence. Report any changes. *Comprehensive assessment provides a basis for evaluating future functional changes.*
• Perform prescribed treatment for condition causing perceptual or cognitive impairment. Monitor progress and report favorable and adverse re-

sponses. *Evaluating patient's responses to treatment and collaborating with doctor fosters appropriate care planning.*

• Help the patient and family or significant other identify strengths and weaknesses in maintaining health (such as self-care deficits) *to provide focus for interventions.* Also help family or significant other communicate with patient and understand what patient's behaviors mean. *This reduces patient's feelings of helplessness and gives a sense of control over the situation.*

• Plan a health maintenance program with the patient and family or significant other, addressing current disabilities.
  – Reorient patient as often as necessary, *to enhance reality testing and mental status.* Adapt environment to appear somewhat familiar to patient. Display such personal objects as pictures and clocks from patient's home.
  – Provide a structured care program in writing *to give patient sense of security.*
  – Have the same person provide care on an ongoing basis *to provide stability.*
  – Fully describe all aspects of care *to elicit patient's cooperation.*
  – When discussing care, give short, simple explanations geared to patient's level of understanding. *This also enhances cooperation.*
  – If possible, prepare patient for any unexpected change *to minimize disruption.*
  – Provide ample time for patient to perform health maintenance tasks *to reduce frustration and encourage success.*

• Urge family or significant other to carry out health maintenance practices. Demonstrate such necessary skills as bathing, feeding, and reality orientation; then have family member or significant other perform them under supervision. *Involving family or significant other allows them to solve problems with supervision and support.*

• Instruct family member or significant other on how to maintain a safe environment *to reduce risk of patient injury.*

• Encourage patient and family or significant other to verbalize feelings and concerns related to health maintenance *to help them develop greater understanding and better manage their health.*

• Help family or significant other develop coping skills necessary to deal with patient. *If patient's illness is prolonged, family members or significant other could develop maladaptive coping strategies.*

• Help family or significant other identify available social and community resources, such as a stroke support group or an Alzheimer's family support group. *This helps them gain social support and factual information, and allows them to express feelings associated with patient's disorder.*

• Make referrals, as appropriate, to psychiatric liaison nurse, social services, etc., *to help prevent burnout among family members.*

Evaluations for expected outcomes

• Patient maintains health.

• Patient does not show signs of injury.

• Patient discusses impact of illness and self-care needs on others' lives. Family member or significant other voices feelings about patient's illness.

• Patient, family member, or significant other states at least three health maintenance strategies.
• Patient performs health maintenance practices to extent possible. Family member or significant other assists patient as needed.
• Patient, family member, or significant other identifies and contacts sources of support.
• Patient copes with current situation without experiencing severe emotional upset. Family member or significant other also displays effective coping.

Documentation
• Expressions of concern by patient and family or significant other about patient's inability to maintain health
• Observations of patient's impaired ability to perform self-care and response to treatment
• Patient's response to nursing interventions
• Instructions given to patient and family or significant other, their level of understanding, and demonstrated skill in carrying out the health maintenance program
• Referrals made for patient and family or significant other
• Evaluations for each expected outcome.

■ Health-seeking behaviors

related to absence of aerobic exercise as a risk factor for coronary artery disease

Definition
State in which a patient in stable health actively seeks ways to alter personal health habits or the environment in order to move toward optimal health

Assessment
• Risk factor analysis, including age, diabetes, elevated cholesterol level, family history, lack of exercise, obesity, sex, smoking, stress
• Current health status
• Psychosocial status, including lifestyle and motivation
• Recognition and realization of potential growth, health, and autonomy

Defining characteristics
• Expressed concern about effect of environmental conditions on health status
• Expressed or observed desire for increased control of health practices
• Expressed or observed desire to seek higher level of wellness
• Expressed or observed lack of knowledge about health promotion behaviors
• Expressed or observed unfamiliarity with wellness community resources

Associated medical diagnoses (selected)
This diagnosis may coincide with any medical diagnosis, depending on the patient and the circumstances of hospitalization.

Expected outcomes
• Patient communicates understanding of benefits of an aerobic exercise program.
• Patient states guidelines for aerobic exercise.
• Patient develops exercise routine.
• Patient states proper target heart rate to be achieved during exercise (60% to 80% of 220, minus patient's age).
• Patient demonstrates ability to take pulse accurately.

Interventions and rationales

• Discuss benefits of regular exercise on the cardiovascular and respiratory systems and on mental health status *to introduce patient to the various benefits of an exercise program.*

• Review basic components of an aerobic exercise routine, including:
  – frequency (minimum of three times weekly)
  – duration (minimum of 20 minutes, not including 5 to 10 minutes of warm-up and cool-down)
  – intensity (work load should progress only according to perceived exertion and target heart rate).

This informs patient of minimum requirements needed to get aerobic benefit from exercise program.

• Discuss activities considered to be aerobic, such as walking, jogging, swimming, cycling, rowing. *Patient must build individualized program around enjoyable activity that meets aerobic criteria.*

• Recommend that patient consult with doctor before starting exercise program *so patient can have exercise stress test, if necessary, and receive medical clearance for exercise program.*

• Recommend either a supervised or unsupervised exercise program, depending on patient's motivation to continue the program. *Supervised program may help less motivated patients.*

• Review warm-up and cool-down techniques, *which prevent abrupt changes in heart rate,* and stretch working muscles *to avoid injuries and an overworked heart.*

• Instruct patient on independent pulse-taking techniques and monitor accuracy. *Patient must know how to take pulse to maintain correct heart rate range.*

• Instruct patient to notify doctor of any adverse symptoms experienced while exercising *to detect any adverse effects early.*

• Provide patient with literature on exercise guidelines and community exercise programs *to reinforce teaching and provide references following discharge.*

Evaluations for expected outcomes

• Patient lists several benefits of aerobic exercise program.

• Patient outlines basic aerobic exercise program.

• Patient provides example of individualized exercise routine.

• Patient states personal target heart rate range.

• Patient demonstrates accurate pulse-taking techniques.

Documentation

• Patient's expression of concern about promoting a higher level of wellness

• Patient's response to nursing interventions

• Instructions given and patient's understanding of the instructions

• Patient's plan of exercise after discharge from the hospital

• Patient's ability to take and record pulse

• Literature provided and referrals made to resources in the community

• Evaluations for each expected outcome.

Health-seeking behaviors

related to elevated serum cholesterol level as a risk factor for coronary artery disease

Definition

State in which a patient in stable health actively seeks ways to alter personal health habits or the environment in order to move toward optimal health

Assessment

- Risk factor analysis, including age, diabetes, elevated cholesterol level, family history, lack of exercise, obesity, sex, smoking, stress
- Current health status
- Psychosocial status, including lifestyle and motivation
- Recognition and realization of potential growth, health, and autonomy

Defining characteristics

- Expressed concern about effect of environmental conditions on health status
- Expressed or observed desire for increased control over health practices
- Expressed or observed desire to seek higher level of wellness
- Expressed or observed lack of knowledge about health promotion behaviors
- Expressed or observed unfamiliarity with wellness community resources

Associated medical diagnoses (selected)

This diagnosis may coincide with any medical diagnosis, depending on the patient and the circumstances of hospitalization.

Expected outcomes

- Patient states personal cholesterol level.
- Patient reports that an elevated cholesterol level is a risk factor for coronary artery disease.
- Patient states an appropriate dietary intake of fat and cholesterol to reduce cholesterol level.
- Patient identifies ways to decrease cholesterol level.
- Patient's cholesterol level declines to desired level.
- Age-appropriate illness is prevented or signs and symptoms of disease, if present, are controlled.

Interventions and rationales

- Discuss patient's cholesterol level *to inform patient of desirable level.*
- Discuss patient's understanding of cholesterol and its sources, *to increase understanding of the intrinsic and extrinsic sources, and the connection between high levels and coronary disease.*
- Discuss ways to lower cholesterol level *to encourage compliance with post-discharge diet plan.*
- Provide literature on cholesterol *to reinforce teaching after discharge.*
- Have patient meet with dietitian *to correct any dietary imbalances and reinforce healthy eating habits.*
- Review outside resources available to patient *to provide follow-up and reinforcement after discharge.*
- Review patient's dietary habits, foods high in cholesterol and saturated fats, and the importance of adhering to a low-cholesterol, low-fat diet *to reinforce dietary teaching and healthy eating habits.*

Evaluations for expected outcomes

- Patient states cholesterol level.

• Patient states that elevated cholesterol level is risk factor for coronary artery disease.
• Patient communicates understanding of how diet affects cholesterol level.
• Patient describes other factors, such as exercise, that can decrease cholesterol level.
• Follow-up laboratory tests reveal reduction in patient's serum cholesterol level.
• Patient does not exhibit signs or symptoms of disease associated with elevated cholesterol level.

Documentation
• Patient's expression of concern about promoting a higher level of wellness
• Patient's response to nursing interventions
• Instructions provided and patient's understanding of instructions
• Literature recommended to or provided for the patient
• Evaluations for each expected outcome.

Health-seeking behaviors

related to hypertension as a risk factor for coronary artery disease

Definition
State in which a patient in stable health actively seeks ways to alter personal health habits or the environment in order to move toward optimal health

Assessment
• Risk factor analysis, including age, diabetes, elevated cholesterol level, family history, lack of exercise, obesity, sex, smoking, stress
• Current health status
• Psychosocial status, including lifestyle and motivation
• Recognition and realization of potential growth, health, autonomy

Defining characteristics
• Expressed concern about current environmental conditions on health status
• Expressed or observed desire for increased control over health practices
• Expressed or observed desire to seek higher level of wellness
• Expressed or observed lack of knowledge about health promotion behaviors
• Expressed or observed unfamiliarity with wellness community resources

Associated medical diagnoses (selected)
This diagnosis may coincide with any medical diagnosis, depending on the patient and the circumstances of hospitalization.

Expected outcomes
• Patient expresses an interest in learning new behaviors to help reduce blood pressure.
• Patient states an understanding of hypertension and that it is a risk factor for coronary artery disease.
• Patient identifies and demonstrates appropriate interventions for lowering blood pressure.
• Patient states own blood pressure range.
• Patient expresses and demonstrates appropriate dietary measures used to reduce high blood pressure.
• Patient maintains blood pressure within desired limits.
• Age-appropriate illness is prevented or signs and symptoms of disease, if present, are controlled.

Interventions and rationales

- Discuss patient's understanding of hypertension and how it affects the body. Clarify any misconceptions. *This increases patient's awareness of hypertension's dangers.*
- Inform patient of blood pressure reading each time it's taken *to reiterate range and give patient responsibility for maintaining it.*
- Provide patient with pamphlets on hypertension *for reinforcement and easy reference after discharge.*
- Encourage patient to continue prescribed antihypertensives, as ordered, *to control blood pressure.*
- Teach patient how to monitor own blood pressure *to help maintain normal pressure.*
- Instruct patient on methods to lower blood pressure *using simple exercise and dietary guidelines.*
- Have patient meet with dietitian *to discuss low-sodium diet, assess eating habits, and make appropriate modifications.*

Evaluations for expected outcomes

- Patient expresses desire to control blood pressure.
- Patient communicates an understanding of hypertension and that it is a risk factor for coronary artery disease.
- Patient reports at least three methods to help control blood pressure.
- Patient states blood pressure range.
- Patient demonstrates use of appropriate dietary measures to reduce high blood pressure.
- Patient's blood pressure remains within desired limits.
- Patient does not exhibit signs or symptoms of disease associated with hypertension.

Documentation

- Patient's expression of concern about promoting a higher level of wellness
- Patient's response to nursing interventions
- Instructions provided and patient's understanding of instructions
- Literature recommended or provided to the patient
- Referrals made to community resources
- Evaluations for each expected outcome.

Health-seeking behaviors

related to smoking as a risk factor for coronary artery disease

Definition

State in which a patient in stable health actively seeks ways to alter personal health habits or the environment in order to move toward optimal health

Assessment

- Risk factor analysis, including age, diabetes, elevated cholesterol level, family history, lack of exercise, obesity, sex, smoking, stress
- Current health status
- Psychosocial status, including lifestyle and motivation
- Recognition and realization of potential growth, health, autonomy

Defining characteristics

- Expressed concern about current environmental conditions on health status
- Expressed or observed desire for increased control over health practices

• Expressed or observed desire to seek higher level of wellness
• Expressed or observed lack of knowledge about health promotion behaviors
• Expressed or observed unfamiliarity with wellness community resources

Associated medical diagnoses (selected)
This diagnosis may coincide with any medical diagnosis, depending on the patient and the circumstances of hospitalization.

Expected outcomes
• Patient states need to stop or decrease smoking.
• Patient states the hazards of smoking and how it affects the body.
• Patient understands ways to stop or decrease smoking.
• Patient chooses which alternative to implement.
• Patient stops smoking or enters a program to stop smoking.
• Age-appropriate illness is prevented or signs and symptoms of disease, if present, are controlled

Interventions and rationales
• Determine patient's capability and motivation to promote a higher level of wellness. *Patient cannot be forced to change, but rather must have inherent desire.*
• Discuss with patient the hazards of smoking *to emphasize nicotine's long-term detriment to body; support behavior change.*
• Assess patient's understanding of how smoking affects the body (blood pressure, cholesterol, clotting, heart rate). Clarify any misconceptions. *This reinforces patient's desire to change behavior.*
• Emphasize benefits of stopping smoking *to reinforce behavior changes.*
• Review with patient past methods used to decrease or stop smoking (successful or not) *to discover most effective methods for patient.*
• Suggest ways for patient to decrease or stop smoking, including the following:
  – List reasons to stop.
  – Set dates to stop.
  – Get support.
  – Switch brands.
  – Cut down on number smoked.
  – Perform alternative activities.

These measures provide patient with methods that can be individually implemented.
• Provide literature on smoking cessation *to reinforce teaching and provide easy reference after discharge.*
• Discuss resources available *to support patient's attempts to stop smoking after discharge.*

Evaluations for expected outcomes
• Patient voices desire to stop or decrease smoking.
• Patient lists several hazards associated with smoking.
• Patient lists several options for assistance with efforts to stop smoking (self-help group, smoking cessation class, hypnosis).
• Patient chooses a method to stop smoking and signs a self-contract (including rewards for smoking cessation) to commit to program.
• Patient implements chosen option to stop smoking.
• Patient is free of signs and symptoms of disorders associated with smoking.

Documentation
• Patient's expression of concern about promoting a higher level of wellness
• Patient's response to nursing interventions

• Instructions provided and patient's understanding of instructions
• Referrals made to smoking cessation programs available in the hospital and community
• Evaluations for each expected outcome.

Health-seeking behaviors

related to stress as a risk factor for coronary artery disease

Definition
State in which a patient in stable health actively seeks ways to alter personal health habits or the environment in order to move toward optimal health

Assessment
• Risk factor analysis, including age, diabetes, elevated cholesterol level, family history, sex, lack of exercise, obesity, smoking, stress
• Current health status
• Psychosocial status, including lifestyle and motivation
• Recognition and realization of potential growth, health, autonomy

Defining characteristics
• Expressed concern about effect of current environmental conditions on health status
• Expressed or observed desire for increased control over health practices
• Expressed or observed desire to seek higher level of wellness
• Expressed or observed lack of knowledge about health promotion behaviors
• Expressed or observed unfamiliarity with wellness community resources

Associated medical diagnoses (selected)
This diagnosis may coincide with any medical diagnosis, depending on the patient and the circumstances of hospitalization.

Expected outcomes
• Patient states that stress is a risk factor for coronary artery disease.
• Patient identifies and lists factors that create stress in life.
• Patient voices understanding of how stress affects body.
• Patient states ways to maximize positive aspects and minimize negative aspects of stress.

Interventions and rationales
• Inform patient that stress is a risk factor for many major health problems, including coronary artery disease. *Patient may be unaware that stress can contribute to disease and death.*
• Review stressors in patient's personal and professional life and mechanisms used to cope with them. *This increases patient's awareness of stressors and provides baseline for stress management tools.*
• Discuss how stress affects patient's body and how decreasing stress changes these effects. *This encourages patient to manage stress as a way to improve quality of life.*
• Discuss the difference between type A and type B personalities. *Type A and B behaviors define personality type and provide framework for dealing with stress.*
• Discuss with patient stress management techniques, including:
  – perceiving situation differently
  – managing time
  – taking a mental health day or evening periodically
  – practicing relaxation techniques

– being assertive when faced with unreasonable demands
– improving self-image and self-esteem
– exercising
– facing problems and discussing alternatives with family or friends
– setting realistic goals
– relaxing standards of living.

These measures provide tools to manage stress.

• Review available community resources for stress management and provide literature *to reinforce teaching after discharge.*

Evaluations for expected outcomes

• Patient states that stress contributes to coronary artery disease.
• Patient identifies habits and situations that create stress.
• Patient identifies physiologic responses to stress.
• Patient states methods to minimize harmful stressors and ways to cope better with daily stress.

Documentation

• Patient's expression of concern about promoting a higher level of wellness
• Patient's response to nursing interventions
• Instructions provided and patient's understanding of the instructions
• Referrals made and literature provided about stress management courses available in the community
• Evaluations for each expected outcome.

Home maintenance management impairment

related to impaired cognitive or emotional functioning

Definition

Inability to meet self-care needs adequately because of cognitive or emotional dysfunction of patient or family member

Assessment

• Home environment
• Financial resources
• Patient's and family's knowledge of self-care requirements
• Patient's and family's psychological status, including perception of reality, communication patterns, assignment of responsibilities, degree of awareness and concern, history of psychiatric illness
• Drug or alcohol abuse
• Support systems, including close friends, organizations with which patient is affiliated, community resources

Defining characteristics

• Household disrepair, marked by excessive clutter, unwashed clothing and cooking equipment, offensive odors, presence of rodents and insects, accumulation of dirt and food wastes
• Household members' emotional state hinders their ability to maintain home
• Household members express difficulty in maintaining a sanitary home
• Household members request assistance with home maintenance
• Household members sustain infections or injuries

Associated medical diagnoses (selected)
Anxiety disorders (phobias, panic disorder, posttraumatic stress disorder), bipolar disorder, borderline personality, delusional (paranoid) disorder, dissociative disorders (depersonalization disorder, multiple personality disorder, psychogenic fugue), substance abuse disorders, major depressive disorder, schizophrenia

Expected outcomes
- Patient and family members express concern about poor home maintenance.
- Patient and family members verbalize plan to correct health and safety hazards in home.
- Patient and family members identify community resources available to help maintain home.

Interventions and rationales
- Discuss obstacles to effective home maintenance management with patient and family *to develop understanding of potential and actual health and safety hazards.*
- Help family members assign responsibilities for household care and establish appropriate expectations *to aid communication and help set realistic goals.*
- Help family members establish daily and weekly home maintenance activities and assignments *to impose structure on the family's routine and set standards for measuring progress.*
- Encourage weekly discussions about progress in maintaining home maintenance schedule *to develop family unity and allow members to address problems before they become overwhelming.*
- Help family members contact community resources that can assist them in their efforts to improve home maintenance management, such as self-help groups, cleaning services, and exterminators. *Community resources can lesson a family's burden while members learn to function independently.*

Evaluations for expected outcomes
- Family establishes and follows daily and weekly schedule for home management.
- Family members clear the home of clutter, debris, and waste.
- Family contacts community resources.

Documentation
- Patient's and family members' expressions of difficulty in maintaining household
- Patient's and family members' mental status
- Presence of health hazards, such as filth, rodents, waste matter
- Presence of safety hazards, such as faulty wiring
- Presence of offensive odors
- Patient's and family members' understanding of home maintenance management and resources
- Interventions to improve home maintenance skills
- Patient's and family members' responses to nursing interventions
- Evaluations for each expected outcome.

■ Home maintenance management impairment

related to inadequate support system

Definition
Insufficient resources available to meet self-care needs adequately and safely in the patient's home

Assessment
- Psychosocial status
- Support systems, including family in the home, close friends, organizations with which the patient is affiliated; if patient lives alone, access to family, friends, pets
- Financial resources
- Home environment
- Patient's and family's or significant other's knowledge of disease and self-care requirements

Defining characteristics
- Household members describe outstanding debts or financial crisis
- Household members or patient express difficulty in maintaining a comfortable home
- Household members request assistance with home maintenance
- Lack of needed equipment or aids
- Overtaxed family members

Associated medical diagnoses (selected)
This diagnosis may coincide with any medical diagnosis and frequently occurs in geriatric or impoverished patients.

Expected outcomes
- Patient and family or significant other express need to make adjustments in home to help manage patient's condition.
- Patient and family or significant other identify individuals or organizations that may provide assistance.

Interventions and rationales
- Help patient and family or significant other explore available resources *to help identify discharge problems and ease transition from hospital to home.*
- Provide sufficient information to patient and family or significant other *to ensure knowledge necessary for them to make appropriate decisions.*
- Refer patient to social service department, *which can assist with follow-up care after discharge.*
- Suggest referral to home health agency, homemaker service, Meals On Wheels, or other appropriate outside agencies for assistance and follow-up. *The patient's various needs may be met best by a range of community services.*

Evaluations for expected outcomes
- Patient and family or significant other describe changes needed to promote maximum health and safety at home.
- Patient and family or significant other list agencies that can assist with home care.

Documentation
- Patient's and family's or significant other's perception of the problem
- Observations regarding the problem's magnitude
- Interventions performed to alleviate the problem
- Responses of others asked to assist with the problem
- Evaluations for each expected outcome.

■ Hopelessness

related to chronic illness

Definition
Subjective state in which an individual sees few or no available alternatives or personal choices and cannot mobilize energy on own behalf

Assessment
- Nature of chronic illness

- Patient's, family's, or significant other's knowledge of illness
- Mental status, including cognitive functioning, affect, mood, stage in grieving process
- Communication, including verbal (speech content, quality, quantity), nonverbal (body positioning, eye contact, facial expression), quality of interactions with others
- Nutritional status, including alteration in appetite or body weight
- Motivation level, including personal hygiene, therapies (physical and occupational), use of diversional activities, sense of control over current life situation
- Developmental stage, including age and role in family
- Disruption in usual roles and activities, losses (real, perceived)
- Actual or perceived self-care deficits (specify)
- Number and types of stressors
- Coping mechanisms and decision-making ability
- Support systems, including clergy, family, friends
- Spiritual values or religious beliefs

Defining characteristics
- Decreased affect
- Decreased involvement in care
- Decreased verbalization
- Despondent mood
- Inability to concentrate
- Increased sleep
- Lack of attention to personal grooming
- Lack of spontaneity, initiative, interest, motivation
- Limited contact with others
- Loss of faith and spiritual values
- Low self-esteem
- Nonverbal cues, such as minimal eye contact, shrugging in response to questions, turning away from speaker
- Progressively deteriorating condition
- Verbal cues, including frequent sighing and responses with hopeless content

Associated medical diagnoses (selected)
Addison's disease, acquired immunodeficiency syndrome, bipolar disorder (depressive phase), burns, cancer, cardiovascular disease, diabetes, chronic respiratory disease, chronic renal disease, depression, Cushing's disease, diseases of pancreas and liver, endocrine disorders, hepatitis, leukemia and related lymphomas, lupus erythematosus, multiple sclerosis, Parkinson's disease, schizophrenia, transplantation

Expected outcomes
- Patient expresses feelings of hopelessness.
- Patient recognizes and accepts limitations of chronic illness.
- Patient works through stages of grief.
- Patient develops coping mechanisms to deal with feelings of hopelessness.
- Patient recognizes the benefit of positive social interactions.
- Patient participates in self-care activities and in decisions regarding care planning.
- Patient resumes and maintains as many former roles as possible.
- Patient regains and maintains self-esteem.
- Patient begins to develop feelings of hope.

Interventions and rationales
- Assess for evidence of self-destructive behavior. *Assessment for suicide potential in a depressed patient is a nursing care priority.*
- If possible, assign a primary nurse to patient *to encourage establishment*

of a therapeutic relationship between patient and nurse.

• Allow for specific amount of uninterrupted, non-care-related time each shift to talk with patient. Encourage verbal response with open-ended statements and questions. If patient chooses not to talk, spend time in silence. *This establishes rapport with depressed patient even if patient talks little.*

• Provide for appropriate physical outlets for expression of feelings (punching bag, walking) *to help patient release hostilities, thereby decreasing tension and anxiety.*

• Convey belief in patient's ability to develop and use coping skills *to increase patient's self-esteem and reduce feelings of dependence.*

• Acknowledge patient's pain. Encourage patient to express feelings of depression, anger, guilt, and sadness. Convey to the patient that all these feelings are appropriate. *This will help patient work through the stages of coming to terms with chronic illness.*

• Identify patient's strengths and encourage putting strengths to use *to maintain optimal functioning.*

• Encourage patient's participation in self-care to the fullest extent possible *to reduce feelings of helplessness.*

• Help patient to participate in usual activities as strength, energy, and time permit. *Patient needs to maintain a sense of being connected to others.*

• Encourage patient to identify enjoyable diversions and to participate in them *to decrease negative thinking and enhance self-esteem.*

• Encourage positive thinking. Convey a sense of confidence in the patient's ability to cope with illness *to promote an optimistic outlook.*

• Provide positive reinforcement for patient's efforts to participate in self-care activities *to encourage patient to participate in self-care.* Encourage patient to establish self-care schedule *to enhance feelings of usefulness and control.*

• Assist patient with hygiene and grooming needs *to help enhance patient's self-esteem.*

• Offer patient and family a realistic assessment of the present situation, and communicate hope for the immediate future. *This facilitates acceptance, helps promote patient safety and security, and allows planning of future health care.*

• Encourage patient to identify spiritual needs and facilitate the fulfillment of those needs *to help patient come to terms with chronic illness and its limitations.*

• Involve patient and family or significant other in care planning, and allow patient to choose degree of self-involvement on a continuing basis. Begin by offering patient a choice between two alternatives. Increase alternatives as initiative improves. *Cognitive disturbances associated with anxiety or depression often prevent patient from making healthy decisions.*

• Teach patient and family how to manage illness, prevent complications, and control factors in the environment that affect the patient's health. *Education enables family members to become resources in the patient's care.*

• Refer patient and family or significant other to other caregivers (dietitian, social worker, clergyman, mental health clinical nurse specialist) or support groups as necessary. *Referrals to outside specialists ensure continuity of care. Support groups give patient chance to discuss illness with others similarly affected.*

Evaluations for expected outcomes

- Patient talks about negative feelings instead of acting on them.
- Patient expresses understanding of life-style changes imposed by chronic illness.
- Patient discusses impact of illness and sees the future realistically.
- Patient demonstrates the ability to solve problems and make decisions.
- Patient acknowledges a belief in self and demonstrates increased energy and will to live.
- Patient states that feelings of hopelessness are less frequent.
- Patient interacts with others and regains involvement in life experiences.
- Patient demonstrates involvement in own general health.
- Patient demonstrates understanding that involvement in self-care is necessary to maintain optimal functioning.

Documentation

- Patient's perception of chronic illness
- Patient's responses to treatment regimen
- Patient's mental and emotional status (baseline and ongoing)
- Patient education, counseling, and precautions taken to maintain or enhance patient's level of functioning
- Interventions to help patient deal with daily stressors
- Interventions to protect patient from harming self
- Patient's response to nursing interventions
- Evaluations for each expected outcome.

Hopelessness

related to failing or deteriorating physiologic condition

Definition

Subjective state in which an individual sees few or no available alternatives or personal choices and cannot mobilize energy on own behalf

Assessment

- Nature of current medical diagnosis
- Patient's and family's or significant other's knowledge of diagnosis and prognosis
- Actual or perceived self-care deficits (specify)
- Mental status, including cognitive functioning, affect, mood
- Communication, including verbal (speech content, quality, quantity) and nonverbal (body positioning, eye contact, facial expression)
- Available support systems, including clergy, family, friends
- Past experience with loss, including body part or function, death, residence, employment
- History of depression, bipolar disease, other psychiatric illness
- Coping mechanisms and decision-making ability
- Nutritional status, including alteration in appetite or body weight
- Sleep pattern
- Motivation level, including personal hygiene, therapies (physical and occupational therapy), and use of diversional activities
- Developmental stage (Erikson's model), including age and role in family

Defining characteristics

- Decreased affect

- Decreased appetite
- Decreased initiative and involvement in care
- Decreased verbalization
- Increased sleep
- Nonverbal cues, such as minimal eye contact, shrugging in response to questions, turning away from speaker
- Verbal cues, including frequent sighing and hopeless responses, such as "I can't" and "What's the use."

Associated medical diagnoses (selected)
Acquired immunodeficiency syndrome, amyotrophic lateral sclerosis, Alzheimer's disease, carcinomas, cerebrovascular accident, chronic congestive heart failure, chronic obstructive pulmonary disease, Crohn's disease, end-stage renal disease, multiple sclerosis, muscular dystrophy, psychiatric illness, rheumatoid arthritis, spinal cord injuries with paralysis

Expected outcomes
- Patient identifies feelings of hopelessness regarding current situation.
- Patient demonstrates more effective communication skills, including direct verbal responses to questions and increased eye contact.
- Patient resumes appropriate rest and activity pattern.
- Patient participates in self-care activities and in decisions regarding care planning.
- Patient uses diversional activities (specify).
- Patient identifies social and community resources for continued assistance.

Interventions and rationales
- Follow medical regimen *to manage patient's physiologic condition and increase potential for patient's physiologic recovery.*
- Allow specific amount of uninterrupted, non-care-related time each shift to talk with patient. If patient chooses not to talk, spend time in silence. *This establishes rapport with depressed patient even if patient talks little.*
- Encourage patient to talk about personal assets and accomplishments and about improvements in condition, no matter how small. Give positive feedback. *Conversation will help in evaluating patient's self-concept and adaptive abilities; positive feedback reinforces patient's healthy perceptions.*
- Direct patient's focus beyond current state. For example, "Your nasogastric tube will come out tomorrow and you'll feel more comfortable." *This helps instill hope in a depressed patient with no time perspective.*
- Encourage patient to identify enjoyable diversions and to participate in them. *Lack of pleasurable activity can increase potential hazard of crisis situation.*
- Keep patient informed of what to expect and when to expect it. *Accurate information reduces patient's anxiety.*
- Involve patient and family or significant other in care planning, and allow patient to choose degree of self-involvement. Begin by offering patient a choice between two alternatives. Increase alternatives as initiative improves. *Cognitive disturbances associated with anxiety or depression often prevent patient from making healthy decisions.*
- Use comfort measures (give back rub, dim room light, reduce noise level, minimize procedures) in addition to prescribed sleep medication, *to help induce sleep.*
- Refer patient and family or significant other to other disciplines (dieti-

tian, social worker, clergy, mental health clinical nurse specialist) or support groups (I Can Cope, Ostomy Support Group, Reach For Recovery) as necessary. *These groups give patient chance to discuss illness with others similarly afflicted.*
- Help patient mobilize resources before discharge, including contacting family and follow-up appointments to referral groups. *This helps give patient a sense of future direction.*

Evaluations for expected outcomes
- Patient voices feelings of hopelessness.
- Patient responds to questions and, at least once each day, participates in a conversation.
- Patient sleeps at least 6 hours per night and remains awake during day, except for two rest periods.
- Patient performs self-care measures and makes decisions related to care.
- Patient engages in diversional activity (specify) at least twice daily.
- Patient identifies factors that make him feel more hopeful (specify).
- Patient seeks out help from social support groups and professional agencies.

Documentation
- Patient's and family's knowledge of current condition
- Patient's mental status
- Patient's verbal and nonverbal behaviors
- Interventions to increase patient's feelings of hope, self-worth, and initiative in self-care
- Patient's and family's responses to nursing interventions
- Evaluations for each expected outcome.

Hopelessness

related to prolonged activity restriction, creating isolation

Definition
Subjective state in which an individual sees few or no available alternatives or personal choices and cannot mobilize energy on own behalf

Assessment
- Nature of illness or injury
- Activity or rest pattern before illness or injury
- Past experience with prolonged inactivity
- Actual or perceived self-care deficit (specify)
- Mental status, including affect, cognitive functioning, mood
- Communication, including verbal (speech content, quality, quantity) and nonverbal (body positioning, eye contact, facial expression)

Defining characteristics
- Absence of diversion
- Decreased affect
- Decreased appetite
- Despondent mood
- Frequent crying
- Increased sleep
- Lack of attention to personal grooming
- Poor eye contact
- Verbal cues with hopeless content

Associated medical diagnoses (selected)
Cardiovascular disease, orthopedic injuries requiring skeletal traction, pulmonary disease requiring ventilatory support, vertebral fracture requiring prolonged bed rest, spinal cord injuries

Expected outcomes

- Patient identifies feelings of hopelessness regarding current situation.
- Patient demonstrates more effective communication.
- Patient initiates self-involvement in care.
- Patient describes persons, events, and interventions that instill hope.
- Patient joins in diversional activities.
- Patient resumes appropriate sleep pattern and dietary intake.
- Patient mobilizes support systems as necessary.
- Patient begins to make plans regarding activity after discharge.

Interventions and rationales

- Follow medical regimen *to manage patient's physiologic condition and increase potential for patient's physiological recovery.*
- Visit frequently, allowing for specific amount of uninterrupted, non-care-related time each shift to talk with patient. Encourage verbal response with open-ended statements and questions. *This establishes rapport with a depressed patient even if patient talks little.*
- Provide structured schedule of daily routine, including morning care, meals, therapies, and rest periods; post schedule within patient's range of vision. *A structured environment helps patient move beyond emotional self-absorption and focus on external factors.*
- Encourage patient's participation in self-care to the extent possible *to reduce patient's feeling of helplessness.*
- Ask patient to identify support systems and enjoyable diversions and encourage their use. *Absence of supportive persons or pleasurable diversions increases potential hazard of a crisis situation.*
- Ask family member or significant other to bring patient a few personal belongings from home, such as a radio, family photographs, clock, or pillow. *A familiar environment will reduce patient's stress.*
- Assist patient with plans for resuming activity after discharge. *As feelings of hopelessness subside, patient will be more willing to discuss future plans.*

Evaluations for expected outcomes

- Patient voices feelings of hopelessness.
- Patient responds to questions and engages in conversation at least once daily.
- Patient performs self-care measures without prompting.
- Patient identifies factors that make him feel more hopeful (specify).
- Patient engages in diversional activity (specify) at least once daily.
- Patient sleeps at least 6 hours per night and maintains caloric intake appropriate for age and sex.
- Patient seeks out support persons or agencies for assistance.
- Patient discusses plans for resuming activity after discharge.

Documentation

- Patient's perception of current situation
- Patient's previous rest or activity pattern
- Patient's mental status
- Patient's verbal and nonverbal behavior
- Interventions to increase patient's hope, initiative, and involvement in self-care and diversional activities
- Patient's response to nursing interventions
- Evaluations for each expected outcome.

Hyperthermia

related to dehydration

Definition

Elevation of body temperature above normal range

Assessment

- History of pathologic conditions known to cause dehydration, such as anorexia nervosa or infection
- Medications (diuretics, for example)
- Physiologic manifestations of fever, including vital signs
- Skin temperature
- Skin color
- Fluid and electrolyte status, including blood urea nitrogen, creatinine, intake and output, mucous membranes, serum electrolytes, skin turgor, urine specific gravity
- Neurologic status, including level of consciousness, mental status, orientation
- Nutritional status, including current weight, dietary pattern, normal weight
- Psychosocial status, including change in financial status, coping skills, recent traumatic event

Defining characteristics

- Fever
- Flushed skin
- Increased respiratory rate
- Seizures
- Skin warm to touch
- Tachycardia

Associated medical diagnoses (selected)

Anorexia nervosa, depression, diabetes mellitus (uncontrolled), drug toxicity, GI dysfunction (involving vomiting, diarrhea, anorexia), heat exhaustion, infection, postoperative status.

Expected outcomes

- Temperature remains normal.
- Fluid balance remains stable (intake equal to or greater than output).
- Patient states increased comfort.
- Complications, such as seizures, are avoided.
- Patient identifies risk factors that exacerbate the problem.
- Patient states measures to prevent dehydration.

Interventions and rationales

- Monitor body temperature every 4 hours, or more often if indicated, *to evaluate effectiveness of interventions.* Identify and record route *to ensure accurate data comparison.*
- Administer antipyretic medication as ordered *to reduce fever.* Record effectiveness.
- Employ measures to reduce excessive fever, such as removing blankets and placing loin cloth over patient, applying ice bags to axilla and groin, sponging with tepid water, and using hypothermia blanket for temperature greater than ____. *These measures promote patient comfort and lower body temperature.*
- Monitor and record heart rate and rhythm, central venous pressure, blood pressure, respiratory rate, level of responsiveness, and skin temperature at least every 4 hours. *Increased heart rate, decreased central venous pressure, and decreased blood pressure may indicate hypovolemia, which leads to decreased tissue perfusion. Cool and blanched or mottled skin may also indicate decreased tissue perfusion. Increased respiratory rate compensates for tissue hypoxia.*
- Observe patient for confusion or disorientation. Report changes in

mentation to doctor. *Changed levels of consciousness may result from tissue hypoxia.*
- Determine patient's preference for liquids (specify). *Using them facilitates adequate hydration.*
- Keep liquids at bedside and within reach *to allow patient easy access.*
- Encourage patient to drink as much fluid as possible unless contraindicated. *Vigorous fluid intake can cause fluid overload or cardiac decompensation that may worsen patient's condition.*
- Treat patient for dehydration:
  - Monitor and record intake and output accurately.
  - Administer I.V. fluids as ordered.

These measures avoid excessive loss of water, sodium chloride, and potassium.
- Discuss precipitating factors with patient, if known, *to develop recommendations for keeping cool and avoiding heat-related illnesses.*
- Encourage adherence to other aspects of health care management, including dietary habits *to help reduce fever.* Patient should drink plenty of fluids *to replace losses from sweating.* Water, fruit juices, vegetable juices, or iced tea are recommended.

Evaluations for expected outcomes
- Patient's temperature remains within normal range.
- Patient's fluid intake is approximately equal to output.
- Patient indicates increased comfort, either through verbal reports or behavior.
- Patient avoids complications of hyperthermia.
- Patient lists risk factors that exacerbate hyperthermia.
- Patient identifies measures to prevent dehydration associated with hyperthermia.

Documentation
- Physical findings
- Nursing interventions carried out
- Effectiveness of medications
- Patient's response to nursing actions (behavioral, cognitive, physiologic)
- Evaluations for each expected outcome.

Hypothermia

related to exposure to cold or cold environment

Definition
State in which body temperature is reduced below normal range

Assessment
- History of present illness
- Circumstances surrounding development of hypothermia
- Age
- Medication history
- Neurologic status, including level of consciousness, mental status, motor status, sensory status
- Cardiovascular status, including blood pressure, capillary refill time, ECG, heart rate and rhythm, pulses (apical, peripheral), temperature
- Respiratory status, including arterial blood gases, breath sounds, and role, depth, and character of respirations
- Integumentary status, including color, temperature, and turgor
- Nutritional status, including current weight and dietary pattern
- Fluid and electrolyte status, including blood urea nitrogen, intake and

output, serum electrolytes, and urine specific gravity
• Psychosocial status, including behavior, financial resources, mood, and occupation

Defining characteristics

Major characteristics include cool skin, mild shivering, and moderate pallor. Minor characteristics include cyanotic nail beds, hypertension, piloerection, slow capillary refill time, and tachycardia.

Associated medical diagnoses (selected)

Addison's disease, alcohol intoxication, cerebrovascular accident, cirrhosis, drug overdose, frostbite, hypoglycemia, myocardial infarction, myxedema, pancreatitis, pituitary insufficiency, perioperative reaction (especially after general anesthesia), Wernicke's encephalopathy

Expected outcomes

• Body temperature is normal.
• Skin feels warm and dry.
• Heart rate and blood pressure remain within normal range.
• Patient does not shiver.
• Patient expresses feelings of comfort.
• Patient shows no complications associated with hypothermia, such as soft tissue injury, fracture, dehydration, hypovolemic shock if warmed too quickly.
• Patient understands how to prevent recurrent episodes of hypothermia.

Interventions and rationales

• Monitor body temperature at least every 4 hours or more frequently, if indicated, *to evaluate effectiveness of interventions.* Record temperature and route *to allow accurate data comparison. Baseline temperatures vary, depending on route used. If temperature is ≤ 95° F (35° C), low-reading thermometer should be used.*
• Monitor and record neurologic status at least every 4 hours. *Falling body temperature and metabolic rate reduce pulse rate and blood pressure, which reduces blood perfusion to brain, resulting in disorientation, confusion, and unconsciousness.*
• Monitor and record heart rate and rhythm, blood pressure, and respiratory rate at least every 4 hours. *Blood pressure and pulse decrease in hypothermia. During rewarming, patient may develop hypovolemic shock. During warming, ventricular fibrillation and cardiac arrest may occur, possibly signaled by irregular pulse.*
• Provide supportive measures, such as placing patient in warm bed and covering with warm blankets; removing all wet or constrictive clothing; covering all metal or plastic surfaces that contact patient's body. *These measures protect patient from heat loss.*
• Follow the prescribed treatment regimen for hypothermia:
  – As ordered, administer medications to prevent shivering *to avoid overheating.* Monitor effectiveness and record.
  – As ordered, administer analgesic *to relieve pain associated with warming.* Monitor effectiveness and record.
  – Use hypothermia blanket *to warm patient* if temperature drops below _____. Warm patient to _____.
  – Fluids may be needed during rewarming *to prevent hypovolemic shock.* If administering large volumes of I.V. fluids, consider using a fluid warmer *to avoid heat loss.*

• Discuss precipitating factors with patient, if indicated. *Factors may include living conditions, finances, and medications (such as sedatives and alcohol).*
• Instruct patient in precautionary measures to avoid hypothermia, such as dressing warmly even when indoors, eating proper diet, remaining as active as possible. *Precautions avoid accidental hypothermia.*

Evaluations for expected outcomes
• Patient's temperature remains within the normal range.
• Patient's skin is warm and dry.
• Patient's heart rate and blood pressure remain within normal range.
• Patient does not shiver.
• Patient voices feelings of comfort.
• Patient does not develop any complications associated with hypothermia.
• Patient describes measures to prevent recurrent episodes of hypothermia.

Documentation
• Patient's complaints of coldness, shivering
• Observations of physical findings
• Interventions carried out to resolve the nursing diagnosis
• Patient's response to interventions, including physiologic, behavioral, and cognitive
• Evaluations for each expected outcome.

■ Incontinence, bowel

related to neuromuscular involvement

Definition
Involuntary passage of stool

Assessment
• History of neuromuscular disorder
• Bowel elimination status, including usual bowel pattern, history of bowel disorder (laxative or enema use), incontinence characteristics (frequency, awareness of need to defecate, precipitating factors), presence or absence of anal sphincter reflex, bowel sounds
• Fluid and electrolyte status, including intake and output, urine specific gravity, skin turgor, mucous membranes
• Nutritional status, including usual dietary pattern, appetite, tolerance or intolerance for foods, current weight, change from normal weight
• Activity status, including type of exercise, frequency, duration

Defining characteristics
• Clinical evidence of neuromuscular deficits
• Involuntary passage of stool

Associated medical diagnoses (selected)
Amyotrophic lateral sclerosis, brain or spinal cord tumor, cerebrovascular accident, diabetic neuropathy, Guillain-Barré syndrome, hemorrhoidectomy, Huntington's disease, multiple sclerosis, myasthenia gravis, spinal cord injury

Expected outcomes
• Patient establishes and maintains a regular pattern of bowel care.
• Patient states understanding of bowel care routine.
• Patient or caregiver demonstrates skill in carrying out bowel care routine with help from nurse.
• Patient or caregiver demonstrates increasing skill in performing bowel care routine independently.
• Patient participates in social activities.

Interventions and rationales

- For upper motor neuron lesion (anal reflex intact):
  - Establish regular pattern for bowel care; for example, after breakfast every other day, maintain patient in upright position after inserting suppository and allow ½ hour for suppository to melt and maximum reflex response to occur. *Regular pattern encourages adaptation and routine physiologic function.*
  - Discuss bowel care routine with patient and family *to promote feelings of safety, adequacy, and comfort.*
  - Demonstrate bowel care to patient and caregivers *to reduce anxiety from lack of knowledge or involvement in care.*
  - Observe return demonstration of bowel care routine by patient and caregivers *to check skills and establish a therapeutic relationship.*
  - Establish a date when patient or caregivers will carry out bowel routine independently, with supportive assistance, *to reassure patient of dependable care.*
  - Instruct patient and family on need to regulate foods and fluids that cause diarrhea or constipation *to encourage good nutritional habits.*
  - Maintain dietary intake diary *to identify irritating foods;* instruct patient to avoid foods that are spicy, rich, or produce gas, *to prevent painful flatulence.*
  - Obtain order allowing modified bowel preparations for tests and procedures *to avoid interrupting routine and to encourage regular bowel function.*
  - Encourage patient to use protective padding under clothing, changing it as necessary *to prevent odor, skin breakdown, or embarrassment, and to promote positive self-image.*
- For lower motor neuron lesion (flaccid sphincter):
  - Establish regular pattern for bowel care; for example, after breakfast every other day, turn patient on left side, put waterproof pads under buttocks, administer prescribed enema and allow to remain in place 2 to 5 minutes. Then perform digital removal of stool, clean perianal area, and remove soiled pads. *These procedures encourage regular physiologic function, stimulate peristalsis, minimize infection, and promote comfort and elimination.*
  - Follow interventions for upper motor neuron lesion.

Evaluations for expected outcomes

- Patient establishes and maintains a regular pattern of bowel care.
- Patient states understanding of bowel care routine.
- Patient and caregiver demonstrate competence in performing bowel care routine with assistance from nurse.
- Patient and caregiver carry out bowel routine independently.
- Patient attends social events without experiencing bowel incontinence.

Documentation

- Patient's feelings about the problem and the bowel routine
- Bowel care routine and administration of suppositories and enemas
- Description of incontinent episodes, including known precipitating factors, time of day, etc.
- Patient's and caregivers' skills in bowel care

• Evaluations for each expected outcome.

Incontinence, bowel

related to perceptual or cognitive impairment

Definition

Involuntary passage of stool

Assessment

• History of neurologic or psychiatric disorder
• Fluid and electrolyte status, including intake and output, skin turgor, urine specific gravity, and mucous membranes
• Gastrointestinal status, including usual bowel habits, change in bowel habits, stool characteristics (color, amount, size, consistency), pain or discomfort, inspection of abdomen, auscultation of bowel sounds, palpation for masses and tenderness, percussion for tympany and dullness, laxative and enema use
• Characteristics of incontinence, including frequency, time of day, before or after meals, relationship to activity, behavior pattern (restlessness, etc.)
• Neurologic status, including orientation, level of consciousness, memory, cognitive ability

Defining characteristics

• Involuntary passage of stool
• Lack of awareness of need to defecate
• Lack of awareness of passage of stool

Associated medical diagnoses (selected)

Alzheimer's disease, brain tumor, cerebrovascular accident, coma, head injury, meningitis, organic brain syndrome

Expected outcomes

• Patient experiences bowel movement every ____ day(s) when placed on commode or toilet at ____ a.m./p.m.
• Patient's skin remains clean and intact.
• Patient gains or improves control of incontinent episodes.
• Caregiver states understanding of bowel routine.
• Caregiver demonstrates skill in placing patient on commode.
• Caregiver demonstrates skill in use of suppository, if indicated.
• Caregiver understands and explains relationship of food and fluid regulation to promotion of continence.
• Patient maintains self-respect and dignity through participation and acceptance within group.

Interventions and rationales

• Establish a regular pattern for bowel care; for example, after breakfast every other day, place patient on commode chair 1 hour after inserting suppository; allow patient to remain upright for 30 minutes for maximum response; then cleanse anal area. *Procedure encourages adaptation and routine physiologic function.*
• Monitor and record incontinent episodes; keep baseline record for 3 to 7 days *to track effectiveness of toileting routine.*
• Discuss bowel care routine with family or caregiver *to foster compliance.*
• Demonstrate bowel care routine to family or caregiver *to reduce anxiety from lack of knowledge or involvement in care.*
• Arrange for return demonstration of bowel care routine *to help establish*

therapeutic relationship with patient and family or caregiver.
• Establish a date when family or caregiver will carry out bowel care routine with supportive assistance; *this will assure patient of dependable care.*
• Instruct family or caregiver on need to regulate foods and fluids that cause diarrhea or constipation *to encourage helpful nutritional habits.*
• Maintain a diet log *to identify irritant foods,* and then eliminate them from patient's diet.
• Cleanse and dry perianal area after each incontinent episode *to prevent infection and promote comfort.*
• Maintain patient's dignity by using protective padding under clothing, by removing patient from group activity after incontinent episode, and by cleansing and returning patient to group without undue attention. *These measures prevent odor, skin breakdown, and embarrassment, and promote patient's positive self-image.*

Evaluations for expected outcomes
• Patient has one soft bowel movement every _____ day(s).
• Patient's skin remains clean, dry, and intact.
• Episodes of incontinence decrease by 50%.
• Caregiver can explain bowel routine.
• Caregiver successfully demonstrates placing patient on commode.
• Caregiver successfully demonstrates insertion of suppositories.
• Caregiver explains the relationship between the food and fluid intake and the regulation of continence, and plans appropriate diet for patient.
• Patient expresses positive self-image.

Documentation
• Patient's level of awareness, response to incontinent episodes, and acceptance of bowel care routine
• Family's or caregiver's response to incontinence and to establishment and implementation of a bowel care routine
• Observation of effects of bowel care routine, episodes of incontinence, stool characteristics, and condition of skin
• Family's or caregiver's skill in carrying out bowel routine and modifying diet
• Evaluations for each expected outcome.

Incontinence, functional

related to cognitive deficits

Definition
Involuntary and unpredictable passage of urine in socially unacceptable situations, where patient usually does not recognize warning signs of bladder fullness

Assessment
• History of mental illness
• Age
• Sex
• Vital signs
• Genitourinary status, including frequency, voiding pattern
• Fluid and electrolyte status, including blood urea nitrogen, creatinine, intake and output, mucous membranes, serum electrolytes, skin turgor
• Neuromuscular status, including daily living activities, mental status, mobility, sensory ability to perceive bladder fullness

• Psychosocial status, including behavior before and after voiding, support from family or significant other, impact of incontinence on self and others, stressors (family, job, change in environment)

Defining characteristics
• Incontinence
• Lack of awareness of need to control voiding
• Voiding that occurs in socially unacceptable situations

Associated medical diagnoses (selected)
Alzheimer's disease, cerebrovascular accident, dementia, emotional illness (anxiety, depression, schizophrenia, withdrawal, manipulative behavior), toxic confusional states (infection, myxedema, uremia, hepatic dysfunction, drug overdose)

Expected outcomes
• Patient voids in appropriate situations.
• Patient does not void in unacceptable situations.
• Complications are avoided or minimized.
• Patient and family or significant other demonstrates skill in managing incontinence.
• Patient discusses impact of incontinence on self and family or significant other.
• Patient and family or significant other identifies resources to assist with care following discharge.

Interventions and rationales
• Monitor and record patient's voiding patterns *to ensure correct fluid replacement therapy.*
• Assist with specific bladder elimination procedures, such as:
  – bladder training. Place patient on commode or toilet every 2 hours while awake and once during the night. *Successful bladder training revolves around adequate fluid intake, muscle-strengthening exercises, and carefully scheduled voiding times.*
  – rigid toilet regimen. Toilet patient at specific intervals (every 2 hours or after meals). Note whether patient was wet or dry and whether voiding occurred at each interval. *This helps patient adapt to routine physiologic function.*
  – behavior modification. Reward continence or voiding in lavatory. Do not punish unwanted behavior, such as voiding in the wrong place. Reinforce behavior consistently, using social or material rewards. *This helps patient learn alternatives to maladaptive behaviors.*
  – insertion of external catheter. Apply according to established procedure and maintain patency. Observe condition of perineal skin and cleanse with soap and water at least twice daily. *This ensures effective therapy and prevents infection and skin breakdown.*
  – application of protective pads and garments. Use only when interventions have failed, *to prevent infection and skin breakdown and promote social acceptance.* Allow at least 4 to 6 weeks for trial period. *Establishing continence requires prolonged effort.*
• Maintain continence based on patient's voiding patterns and limitations.
  – Use reminders.
  – Orient patient to toileting environment, time, activity, and

place. *A structured environment offers security and helps patient with elimination problems.*
- Stimulate patient's voiding reflexes (give patient drink of water while on toilet; stroke area over bladder; pour water over perineum). *External stimulation triggers bladder's spastic reflex.*
- Provide hyperactive patient with distractor, such as magazine, to occupy attention while on toilet. *This reduces anxiety and eases voiding.*
- Provide privacy and adequate time to void *to allow patient to void easily without anxiety.*
- Praise successful performance *to give patient a sense of control and to encourage compliance.*
- Change wet clothes *to accustom patient to dry clothes.*
- Teach family members and support personnel to assist, *thus reducing anxiety that results from noninvolvement and increasing chances for successful treatment.*
- Respond to patient's call light promptly *to avoid delays in voiding routine.*
- Choose patient's clothing to promote easy dressing and undressing. (For example, use Velcro fasteners and gowns instead of pajamas.) *This reduces patient's frustration with voiding routine.*

• Schedule patient's fluid intake to encourage voiding at convenient times. Maintain adequate hydration up to 3,000 ml daily, unless contraindicated. *Optimum time interval between voiding is based on reasonable distention of bladder.* Limit fluid intake to 150 ml after dinner *to reduce need to void at night.*

• Instruct patient and family or significant other on continence techniques to be used at home, *to increase chances of successful bladder retraining.*

• Encourage patient and family or significant other to share feelings related to incontinence. *This allows specific problems to be identified and resolved. Attentive listening conveys recognition and respect.*

• Refer patient and family or significant other to psychiatric liaison nurse, visiting nurse's association, or support group *to provide access to additional community resources.*

Evaluations for expected outcomes

• Record of voiding pattern indicates that patient voids at appropriate intervals and that episodes of incontinence are minimized.

• Patient does not experience urinary tract infection, skin breakdown, or other complications related to incontinence.

• Patient recognizes urge to void, undresses without assistance, and walks to toilet.

• Patient and family or significant other demonstrate the proper procedures for managing incontinence.

• Patient expresses feelings about condition and its effect on family. Patient and family members are neither overwhelmed nor excessively optimistic about patient's condition.

• Patient and family or significant other contact support group or visiting nurse's association, if needed.

Documentation

• Observations of incontinence and response to treatment regimen

• Interventions to provide supportive care and patient's response to supportive care

• Instructions given to patient and family or significant other; return demonstration of knowledge and

skills needed to carry out continence management techniques
• Patient's expression of concern about incontinence and motivation to participate in self-care
• Evaluations for each expected outcome.

Incontinence, functional

related to sensory or mobility deficits

Definition

Involuntary and unpredictable passage of urine in socially unacceptable situations, where patient usually does not recognize warning signs of bladder fullness

Assessment

• History of mental retardation, trauma, alcohol abuse
• Medication history
• Age
• Sex
• Vital signs
• Genitourinary status, including amount, extent of clothing wetness due to urine, frequency, palpation of bladder, urine leakage when standing or sitting, voiding pattern
• Fluid and electrolyte status, including blood urea nitrogen, creatinine, intake and output, mucous membranes, serum electrolytes, skin turgor, urine specific gravity
• Neuromuscular status, including manual dexterity, mental status, mobility, motor ability to start and stop urine stream, rectal exam (muscle tone, prostate size, fecal impaction), sensory ability to perceive bladder fullness
• Psychosocial status, including behavior before and after voiding, coping skills, support from family or significant other, perception of health problem, self-concept, stressors (finances, job, change in environment)

Defining characteristics

• Incontinence
• Nocturia
• Voiding that occurs before reaching an appropriate site or receptacle
• Warning signals of bladder fullness usually not recognized

Associated medical diagnoses (selected)

Alcohol abuse, Alzheimer's disease, closed head injuries, episodic loss of consciousness (seizures, hypoglycemia, dementia), mental retardation, toxic confusional states (infection, myxedema, uremia, hepatic dysfunction, drug overdose)

Expected outcomes

• Patient voids in appropriate situation using suitable receptacle.
• Patient voids at specific times.
• Patient has no wet episodes.
• Patient maintains fluid balance; intake equals output.
• Complications are avoided or minimized.
• Patient and family or significant other demonstrate skill in managing incontinence.
• Patient discusses impact of incontinence on self and significant other.
• Patient and family or significant other identifies resources to assist with care following discharge.

Interventions and rationales

• Monitor patient's voiding pattern; document and report intake and output *to ensure correct fluid replacement therapy.*
• Assist with specific bladder elimination procedures, such as:

– bladder training. Place patient on commode or toilet every 2 hours while awake and once during the night. *Successful bladder training revolves around adequate fluid intake, muscle-strengthening exercises, and carefully scheduled voiding times.*
– rigid toilet regimen. Toilet patient at specific intervals (every 2 hours or after meals). Note whether patient was wet or dry and whether voiding occurred at each interval. *This helps patient adapt to routine physiologic function.*
– insertion of external catheter. Apply according to established procedure and maintain patency. Observe condition of perineal skin and cleanse with soap and water at least twice daily. *This ensures effective therapy and prevents infection and skin breakdown.*
– application of protective pads and garments. Use only after incontinence management procedures have failed, *to prevent infection and skin breakdown and promote social acceptance.* Allow at least 4 to 6 weeks for trial period. *Establishing continence requires prolonged effort.*

• Maintain continence based on patient's voiding patterns and limitations.
– Use reminders.
– Orient patient to toileting environment, time, and place of activity. *A structured environment offers security and helps patient with elimination problems.*
– Stimulate voiding reflexes. Give patient a drink of water while on the toilet; stroke the area over the bladder; pour water over the perineum. *External stimulation triggers bladder's spastic reflex.*
– For hyperactive patients, provide a distractor, such as a magazine, to occupy attention while on the toilet. *This reduces anxiety and eases voiding.*
– Provide privacy and adequate time to void *to allow patient to void easily without anxiety.*
– Praise successful performance *to give patient a sense of control and encourage compliance.*
– Change wet clothes *to accustom patient to dry clothes.*
– Teach family members and support personnel to assist, *thus reducing anxiety that results from noninvolvement and increasing chances for successful treatment.*
– Respond quickly to patient's call light *to avoid delays in voiding routine.*
– Choose patient's clothing to promote ease in dressing and undressing. (For example, use Velcro fasteners and gowns instead of pajamas.) *This reduces patient's frustration with voiding routine.*

• Schedule patient's fluid intake to encourage voiding at convenient times. Maintain adequate hydration up to 3,000 ml daily, unless contraindicated. *Optimum time interval between voidings is based on reasonable distention of bladder.* Limit fluid intake to 150 ml after supper *to reduce need to void at night.*

• Decrease patient's use of alcohol *to reduce sensory or mobility deficits.*

• Instruct patient and family or significant other on continence techniques to be used at home. Have patient and family or significant other return demonstrations. *This will*

increase the chances for successful bladder retraining.
- Encourage patient and family or significant other to share feelings related to incontinence. *This allows specific problems to be identified and resolved. Attentive listening conveys recognition and respect.*
- Refer patient and family or significant other to psychiatric liaison nurse, Visiting Nurses Association, support group, and similar resources when appropriate *to provide access to additional community resources.*
- Keep skin as clean and dry as possible. Use mild soap and water *to cleanse urea burns and prevent skin breakdown.*

Evaluations for expected outcomes
- Patient voids in appropriate situation using suitable receptacle.
- Record of voiding pattern indicates that patient voids at appropriate intervals and episodes of incontinence are minimized.
- Patient maintains fluid balance with intake approximately equal to output.
- Patient does not experience urinary tract infection, skin breakdown, or other complications related to incontinence.
- Patient and family or significant other demonstrate the proper procedures for managing incontinence.
- Patient expresses feelings about condition and its effect on family. Patient and family members are neither overwhelmed nor excessively optimistic about patient's condition.
- Patient and family or significant other contact support group or visiting nurse's association, if needed.

Documentation
- Observations of incontinence and response to treatment regimen
- Interventions to provide supportive care and patient's response
- Instructions given to patient and family or significant other; return demonstration of knowledge and skills needed to carry out continence management techniques
- Patient's expression of concern about incontinence problem and motivation to participate in self-care
- Evaluations for each expected outcome.

Incontinence, reflex

related to sensory or neuromuscular impairment

Definition

Involuntary loss of urine, controlled by spinal cord reflex, occurring at somewhat predictable intervals when a specific bladder volume is reached

Assessment
- History of sensory or neuromuscular impairment
- History of urinary tract disease, trauma, surgery, or infection
- Genitourinary status, including bladder palpation, residual urine volume after voiding, urinalysis, urine characteristics, urine culture and sensitivity, voiding patterns
- Neuromuscular status, including anal sphincter tone, motor ability to start and stop urine stream, neuromuscular function, sensory ability to perceive bladder fullness and voiding, and involuntary voiding after stimulation of skin on abdomen, thighs, or genitals
- Fluid and electrolyte status, including blood urea nitrogen, creatinine, intake and output, medication history, mucous membranes, serum

electrolytes, skin turgor, urine specific gravity
• Sexuality status, including capability, concerns, and habits
• Psychosocial status, including coping skills, self-concept, and perception of problem by patient and family or significant other

Defining characteristics
• Frequency
• Interrupted, involuntary, or incomplete voiding
• Involuntary bladder contractions, which may occur with involuntary spasms of lower extremities
• No awareness of bladder filling
• No feelings of fullness or urge to void
• Normal or increased anal sphincter tone
• Reduced bladder capacity
• Voiding and involuntary contractions of the extremities triggered by stimulation of skin on the abdomen, thighs, genitals

Associated medical diagnoses (selected)
Cerebrovascular accident, multiple sclerosis, Parkinson's disease, prolapsed intervertebral disk, upper motor neuron damage resulting from spinal cord tumor, spinal cord trauma, arteriosclerosis of spinal cord.

Expected outcomes
• Patient maintains fluid balance; intake equals output.
• Complications are avoided or minimized.
• Patient achieves urinary continence.
• Patient and family or significant other demonstrate skill in managing urinary incontinence.
• Patient discusses impact of incontinence on self, family, and significant others.
• Patient and family or significant other identify resources to assist with care following discharge.

Interventions and rationales
• Monitor intake and output, *to ensure correct fluid replacement therapy.* Report output greater than intake.
• Implement and monitor effectiveness of specific bladder elimination procedure, such as:
  – stimulating reflex arc. Patient who voids at somewhat predictable intervals may be able to regulate voiding by reflex arc stimulation. Voiding should be triggered at regular intervals (for example, every 2 hours) by stimulating skin of abdomen, thighs, or genitals to initiate bladder contractions. Avoid stimulation at nonvoiding times. Stimulate primitive voiding reflexes by giving patient water to drink while he sits on the toilet, or pouring water over the perineum. *External stimulation triggers bladder's spastic reflex.*
  – applying external catheter according to established procedure and maintaining patency. Observe condition of perineal skin and cleanse with soap and water at least twice daily. *Cleanliness avoids skin breakdown or infection. External catheter protects surrounding skin, promotes accurate output measurement, and keeps patient dry. Applying foam strip in spiral fashion increases adhesive surface and cuts risk of impaired circulation.*
  – inserting indwelling (Foley) catheter. Monitor patency and keep tubing free of kinks *to avoid drainage pooling and assure accurate therapy.* Keep

drainage bag below level of bladder *to avoid urine reflux into bladder.* Perform catheter care according to established procedure. Maintain closed drainage system *to prevent bacteriuria.* Secure catheter to leg (female) or abdomen (male) *to avoid tension on bladder and sphincter.*
– applying suprapubic catheter. Change dressing according to established procedure *to avoid skin breakdown.* Monitor patency and keep tubing free of kinks *to avoid drainage pooling in loops of catheter.* Keep drainage bag below bladder level *to avoid urine reflux into badder.* Maintain closed drainage system *to prevent bacteriuria.*
– changing wet clothes *to prevent patient from becoming accustomed to wet clothes.*

- Encourage high fluid intake (2,500 ml daily, unless contraindicated) *to stimulate micturition reflex.* Limit fluid intake after 7 p.m. *to prevent nocturia.*
- Instruct patient and family or significant other on continence techniques to be used at home. Have patient and family member or significant other return demonstrations until procedure can be performed well. *Patient education begins with assessment and depends on nurse's establishing therapeutic relationship with patient and family.*
- Encourage patient and family or significant other to share feelings and concerns regarding incontinence. *A trusting environment allows nurse to make specific recommendations to resolve patient's problems.*
- Refer patient and family or significant other to psychiatric liaison nurse, visiting nurse's association, support group, other resources as appropriate. *Community resources often provide health care not available from other health agencies.*

Evaluations for expected outcomes

- Records indicate that fluid intake equals output. Patient maintains fluid balance.
- Patient avoids complications associated with incontinence, such as infections, swelling of penis (because of external catheter), skin breakdown, catheter obstruction, and urine odor. Results of urinalysis are normal.
- Patient achieves urinary continence.
- Patient and family or significant other successfully demonstrate chosen technique for bladder control.
- Patient expresses both positive and negative feelings about condition. Patient is able to cope with dependence brought on by condition.
- Patient and family or significant other initiate contact with a support group or visiting nurse.

Documentation

- Observations of urologic condition and response to treatment regimen
- Interventions to provide supportive care and patient's response
- Instructions given to patient and family or significant other; return demonstration of knowledge and skills needed to carry out continence management techniques
- Patient's expression of concern about incontinence and its impact on body image and life-style; patient's motivation to participate in self-care
- Evaluations for each expected outcome.

Incontinence, stress

related to weak pelvic musculature

Definition
Loss of urine (less than 50 ml) resulting from increased abdominal pressure

Assessment
- History of long-term use of tranquilizers, multiple pregnancies, prolonged or difficult labor, surgery, trauma, vaginal infections
- Age
- Sex
- Vital signs
- Genitourinary status, including inspection of abdomen for scars from previous surgeries, rectal examination, vaginal examination, voiding pattern, and leakage of urine during sneezing, laughing, vomiting, coughing, defecating, physical exertion, or change from prone to upright position
- Fluid and electrolyte status, including creatinine, blood urea nitrogen, estrogen levels, intake and output, mucous membranes, serum electrolytes, skin turgor
- Nutritional status, including appetite, dietary habits, present weight
- Neuromuscular status, including degree of neuromuscular function, motor ability to start or stop urine stream, sensory ability to perceive fullness
- Sexuality status, including capability, concerns, habits, and patterns
- Psychosocial status, including coping skills, self-concept, stressors (finances, family, job), and perception of problem by family members or significant others

Defining characteristics
- Dribbling with increased abdominal pressure
- Frequency
- Incontinence
- Urgency

Associated medical diagnoses (selected)
Atrophic senile vaginitis, atrophic urethritis secondary to estrogen deficiency, cystocele, gravid uterus, multiple pregnancies, obesity, pelvic fracture, pelvic tumor, disorders requiring radical prostatectomy or sphincterostomy; urethrocele, uterine prolapse

Expected outcomes
- Patient maintains continence.
- Patient states increased comfort.
- Patient states understanding of treatment.
- Patient states understanding of surgical procedure.
- Patient and family or significant other demonstrate skill in managing urinary elimination problems.
- Patient and family or significant other identify resources to assist with care following discharge.

Interventions and rationales
- Observe patient's voiding patterns, time of voiding, amount voided, and whether voiding is provoked by stimuli. *Accurate, thorough assessment forms the basis of an effective treatment plan.*
- Provide appropriate care for the urologic condition present, monitor progress, and report patient's responses to treatment. *Patient expects to receive adequate care and to participate in decisions regarding care.*
- Help patient to strengthen pelvic floor muscles by Kegel exercises for sphincter control. *Exercises increase*

muscle tone and restore cortical control.

- Promote patient's awareness of condition through education *to help patient understand illness as well as treatment.*
- Help patient reduce intra-abdominal pressure by:
  - weight reduction
  - avoiding heavy lifting
  - avoiding chairs or beds that are too high or too low.

These measures reduce intraabdominal pressure and bladder pressure.

- Provide supportive measures:
  - Respond to call light quickly, assign patient to bed next to bathroom, put night light in bathroom, and have patient wear clothing that's easily removed (gown rather than pajamas, Velcro fasteners rather than buttons or zippers). *Early recognition of problems promotes continence; easily removed clothing reduces patient frustration and helps achieve continence.*
  - Provide privacy during toileting *to reduce anxiety and promote elimination.*
  - Have patient empty bladder before meals, at bedtime, and before leaving accessible bathroom area *to promote elimination, avoid accidents, and help relieve intraabdominal pressure.*
  - Limit fluids to 150 ml after dinner *to reduce patient's need to void at night.*
  - Encourage high fluid intake, unless contraindicated, *to moisten mucous membranes and maintain hydration.*
  - Before going on a long trip, patient may eat increased amount of salty food (unless contraindicated). *Increased sodium decreases urine production.*
  - Make protective pads available for patient's undergarments, if needed, *to absorb urine, protect skin, and control odors.*
- If surgery is scheduled, give attentive, appropriate preoperative and postoperative instructions and care *to reduce patient's anxiety and build trust in caregivers.*
- Encourage patient to ventilate feelings and concerns related to urologic problems. *This helps patient focus on specific problem.*
- Refer patient and family or significant other to psychiatric liaison nurse, support group, or other resources, as appropriate. *Community resources often provide health care not available from other health agencies.*
- Alert patient and family or significant other to need for toilet schedule. Prepare for discharge according to individual needs *to ensure that patient will receive proper care.*

Evaluations for expected outcomes

- Patient maintains continence.
- Patient expresses satisfaction with progress in overcoming stress incontinence.
- Patient expresses understanding of techniques to reduce intra-abdominal pressure and other supportive measures.
- Patient explains surgical procedure, including risks and expected outcome.
- Patient and family or significant other demonstrate all procedures and supportive measures to enable patient to remain continent. They also make arrangements for home care, such as providing bedroom near bathroom and purchasing easily removable clothing.

- Patient and family or significant other make contact with appropriate community resources.

Documentation
- Observations of urologic condition and patient's response to treatment regimen
- Interventions to provide supportive care and patient's response to interventions
- Instructions given to patient and family or significant other on urologic problem present, their response to instructions, and demonstrated ability to carry out self-care management
- Patient's expression of concern about the urologic problem and its impact on body image and life-style
- Patient's motivation to participate in self-care
- Evaluations for each expected outcome.

Incontinence, total

related to neurologic dysfunction

Definition
Continuous and unpredictable passage of urine

Assessment
- History of trauma, sensory or neuromuscular impairment, surgery, congenital anomalies
- Vital signs
- Age
- Sex
- Genitourinary status, including palpation of bladder, previous bladder elimination procedures, urinalysis, urine characteristics, use of urinary assistive devices, voiding pattern
- Fluid and electrolyte status, including BUN, creatinine, intake and output, mucous membranes, skin turgor, serum electrolytes
- Neuromuscular status, including degree of neuromuscular function, motor ability to start or stop urine stream, sensory ability to perceive bladder fullness
- Sexuality status, including capability, concerns, and sexual partner
- Psychosocial status, including patient's perception of health problem, coping skills, family or significant other, self-concept

Defining characteristics
- Constant flow of urine occurs at unpredictable times without distention or uninhibited bladder contractions or spasms
- Incontinence refractory to treatments
- Lack of awareness of incontinence, perineal fullness, or bladder filling
- Nocturia

Associated medical diagnoses (selected)
Cerebral tumor; cerebrovascular accident; congenital anomalies, such as bladder exstrophy, ectopic ureters, and epispadias; diabetes mellitus; fistulas secondary to trauma, gynecologic procedures, long labor, or radiation therapy; multiple sclerosis; neuromuscular trauma related to abdominal perineal resections or retropubic prostatectomy; and spinal cord injury or tumor

Expected outcomes
- Patient maintains fluid balance; intake equals output.
- Patient states increased comfort.
- Complications are avoided or minimized.
- Patient contains urine.

- Patient and family or significant other demonstrate skill in managing incontinence.
- Patient and family or significant other discuss impact of incontinence on their lives.
- Patient and family or significant other identify resources to assist with care following discharge.

Interventions and rationales

- Monitor patient's voiding pattern; document and report intake and output *to ensure correct fluid replacement therapy.*
- Assist with specific bladder elimination devices, such as:
  - external catheter. Apply according to established procedure and maintain patency. Avoid constriction. Observe condition of perineal area and cleanse with soap and water at least twice daily. Reusable penile sheaths are available for long-term use. *Cleanliness prevents skin breakdown or infection. External catheter protects surrounding skin, promotes accurate output measurement, and keeps patient dry. Applying foam strip in spiral fashion increases adhesive surface and cuts risk of impaired circulation.*
  - indwelling (Foley) catheter. Monitor patency and keep tubing free of kinks *to avoid drainage pooling and assure accurate therapy.* Keep drainage bag below level of bladder *to avoid urine reflux into bladder.* Cleanse urinary meatus according to established procedure *to reduce risk of infection.* Maintain closed drainage system *to prevent bacteriuria.* Secure catheter to leg (female) or abdomen (male) *to avoid tension on bladder and sphincter.*
  - suprapubic catheter. Monitor patency, change dressing, and cleanse catheter site according to established policy *to avoid skin breakdown.* Keep tubing free of kinks; keep drainage bag below level of bladder *to prevent urine reflux into bladder.* Maintain closed drainage system *to prevent bacteriuria.*
  - body-worn appliances. These are body-worn "urinals" to fit over the penis, a drainage bag, and waist and leg straps for body attachment, *to protect skin and keep patient dry.* Selection depends on patient's self-help skills. Appliances need regular, careful washing *to protect skin and keep patient dry.*
  - incontinence aids. (1) Pad and pants: absorbent pad with protective waterproof shield. (2) Drip collector: absorbent pouch fits over penis. (3) Bed protector: absorbent pad protects bed. *These aids trap urine to keep it away from patient's skin.*
- Disguise urinary bag by placing it in shopping bag or tote bag *to enhance patient's self-image.*
- Provide supportive measures:
  - Regulate fluid intake on a specific schedule *to encourage voiding at convenient times.* Maintain adequate hydration up to 3,000 ml daily, unless contraindicated. Limit fluid intake to 150 ml after dinner *to reduce need to void at night.*
  - Clothe patient to promote ease in dressing and undressing, and to accommodate appliance. (For example, use Velcro fasteners and gowns rather than pajamas.) *Unwieldy clothing increases pa-*

tient frustration with voiding routine.
  - Keep skin as clean and dry as possible *to promote skin integrity.* Treat urea burns by cleansing with mild soap and water.
- Instruct patient and family or significant other on continence techniques for home use. Provide for return demonstrations. *Patient education begins with assessment and depends on nurse's establishing therapeutic relationship with patient and family.*
- Encourage patient and family or significant other to share feelings and concerns related to incontinence. *A trusting environment allows nurse to make specific recommendations to resolve patient's problems.*
- Refer patient and family or significant other to psychiatric liaison nurse, visiting nurse's association, support group, or other resources, as appropriate. *Community resources often provide health care not available from other health agencies.*

Evaluations for expected outcomes
- Patient takes in enough fluid to void approximately eight times each day.
- Patient remains dry, maintains usual life-style, and does not experience skin breakdown or infection. Patient expresses increased comfort.
- Complications are avoided or minimized.
- Patient contains urine.
- Before discharge, patient and family or significant other demonstrate skill in managing incontinence.
- Patient and family or significant other discuss openly the impact of incontinence on their lives.
- Patient and family or significant other identify two resources in the community to assist with care following discharge.

Documentation
- Observations of incontinence and response to treatment regimen
- Interventions to provide supportive care and patient's response to interventions
- Instructions given to patient and family or significant other, their understanding of information, and their demonstrated ability to carry out continence management techniques
- Patient's expressions of concern about incontinence and motivation to participate in self-care
- Evaluations for each expected outcome.

■ Incontinence, urge

related to decreased bladder capacity

Definition

Involuntary passage of urine occurring shortly after a strong sense of urgency to void

Assessment
- History of cerebrovascular accident, urinary tract disease, spinal cord injury, surgery, infection
- Medication history
- Vital signs
- Genitourinary status, including cystometrogram, pain or discomfort, urinalysis, urine specific gravity, use of urinary assistive devices, voiding pattern
- Fluid and electrolyte status, including blood urea nitrogen, creatinine, intake and output, mucous membranes, postvoiding residual volume, skin turgor, serum electrolytes

- Neuromuscular status, including ambulation ability, degree of neuromuscular function, dexterity, and sensory ability to perceive fullness
- Sexuality status, including capability, concerns, habits, and sexual partner
- Psychosocial status, including coping skills, self-concept, stressors (finances, family, job), and perception of health problem by patient, family, or significant other

Defining characteristics
- Bladder contraction or spasm
- Dysuria
- Frequency
- Hesitancy
- Incontinence
- Loss of urine regardless of position
- Nocturia
- Sensory or neuromuscular impairment of urinary tract
- Urgency

Associated medical diagnoses (selected)
Acute bladder infection, Alzheimer's disease, bladder cancer, brain trauma or tumor, cerebrovascular accident, dementia, incomplete supraspinal cord injury, interstitial cystitis, multiple sclerosis, outlet obstruction, Parkinson's disease, spinal compression, transverse myelitis, urethritis

Expected outcomes
- Episodes of incontinence occur less frequently.
- Patient states increased comfort.
- Patient states understanding of treatment.
- Complications are avoided or minimized.
- Patient discusses impact of urologic disorder on self and family or significant other.
- Patient and family or significant other demonstrate skill in managing incontinence.

Interventions and rationales
- Observe voiding pattern; document intake and output. *This ensures correct fluid replacement therapy and provides information about patient's ability to void adequately.*
- Provide appropriate care for urologic condition present, monitor progress, and report patient's responses to treatment. *Patient should receive adequate and qualified care, and be allowed to understand and participate in care as much as possible.*
- Provide supportive measures:
  - Administer medication and monitor effectiveness. *Patient's knowledge that pain can be alleviated reduces tension and anxiety.*
  - Prepare pleasant toilet environment that's warm, clean, and free of odors *to promote continence.*
  - Place commode to the right of bed, or assign a bed next to the bathroom. *A bedside commode or convenient bathroom requires less energy expenditure than bedpan.*
  - Keep bed and commode at same level *to facilitate patient's movements.*
  - Provide good lighting from bed to bathroom *to reduce sensory misinterpretation.*
  - Remove all obstacles between bed and bathroom *to reduce chance of falling.*
  - Provide clock *to help patient maintain voiding schedule through self-monitoring.*
  - Unless contraindicated, maintain fluids to 3,000 ml daily *to*

moisten mucous membranes and ensure hydration; limit patient to 150 ml after supper *to reduce need to void at night.*
 – Have patient wear clothes that are easily removed (gown instead of pajamas, Velcro fasteners instead of buttons or zippers) *to reduce frustration and delay in voiding routine.*
 – If caught short on way to bathroom, instruct patient to stop and take a deep breath. *Anxiety and rushing caused by anxiety may strengthen bladder contractions.*

- Assist with specific bladder elimination procedures:
  – bladder training. Place patient on commode every 2 hours while awake and once during the night. Provide privacy. Gradually increase intervals between toileting. *These measures aim to restore a regular voiding pattern.*
  – rigid toilet regimen. Toilet patient at specific times (for example, every 2 hours). *This aids adaptation to routine physiological function.* Keep baseline micturition record for 3 to 7 days *to monitor toileting effectiveness.*
- Encourage patient to ventilate feelings and concerns related to his or her urologic problem *to identify patient's fears.*
- Explain urologic condition to patient and family or significant other; include instructions on preventive measures and established bladder schedule. *Patient education begins with educational assessment and depends on establishing a therapeutic relationship with patient and family.* Prepare patient for discharge according to individual needs, *so patient can practice under supervision.*
- Instruct patient and family or significant other on continence techniques for home use. *This reduces fear and anxiety resulting from lack of knowledge of patient's condition, and reassures patient of continuing care.*
- Refer patient and family or significant other to psychiatric liaison nurse, support group, or other resources, as appropriate. *Community resources often provide health care not available from other health agencies.*

Evaluations for expected outcomes

- Patient maintains continence.
- Patient expresses increased comfort and reduces requests for pain medication.
- Patient expresses understanding of treatment.
- Patient does not experience nighttime incontinence or other complications.
- Patient expresses feelings about condition.
- Patient and family or significant other discuss treatment of urologic condition and home bladder schedule. They also demonstrate necessary skills.

Documentation

- Observations of urologic condition and patient's response to treatment regimen
- Interventions to provide supportive care
- Patient's response to nursing interventions
- Instruction given to patient and family or significant other on urologic problem, their response to instructions, and their demonstrated ability to carry out self-care management

• Patient's expression of concern about the urologic problem and its impact on body image and life-style; patient's motivation to participate in self-care
• Evaluations for each expected outcome.

Infection, high risk for

related to external factors

Definition

Presence of internal or external hazards that threaten physical well-being

Assessment

• Health history, including accidents, allergies, falls, hyperthermia, hypothermia, poisoning, seizures, trauma, exposure to pollutants
• Sensory or perceptual changes (auditory, gustatory, kinesthetic, olfactory, tactile, visual)
• Circumstances of present situation that could lead to infection
• Neurologic status, including level of consciousness, mental status, orientation
• Laboratory studies, including clotting factors, hemoglobin and hematocrit, platelet count, serum albumin, white blood cell count, and cultures of blood, body fluid, sputum, urine, wounds

Risk factors

• Admission to hospital
• Age (over 65)
• Chemotherapy
• Hemodialysis
• Hospitalized longer than 1 month
• Immobility
• Indwelling urinary catheter
• Intravenous catheter
• Invasive monitoring procedures
• Obesity
• Prophylactic antibiotic therapy
• Respiratory treatments (endotracheal or tracheostomy tube, humidifier or nebulizer, ventilator)
• Steroid therapy
• Surgical procedure

Associated medical diagnoses (selected)

Although any patient can develop a nosocomial infection, debilitated, elderly, and postoperative patients (especially transplantation patients) are at greatest risk. Associated medical diagnoses include acquired immunodeficiency syndrome, acute renal failure, acute respiratory failure, cancer, cirrhosis, congestive heart failure, diabetes mellitus, hepatitis, multiple sclerosis, multisystem trauma, spinal cord injury.

Expected outcomes

• Temperature stays within normal range.
• White blood cell count and differential stay within normal range.
• No pathogens appear in cultures.
• Patient maintains good personal and oral hygiene.
• Respiratory secretions are clear and odorless.
• Urine remains clear yellow, odorless, with no sediment.
• Patient shows no evidence of diarrhea.
• Wounds and incisions appear clean, pink, and free of purulent drainage.
• I.V. sites show no signs of inflammation.
• Patient shows no evidence of skin breakdown.
• Patient takes _____ ml of fluid and _____ g of protein daily.
• Patient states infection risk factors.
• Patient identifies signs and symptoms of infection.

• Patient remains free of all signs and symptoms of infection.

Interventions and rationales

• Minimize patient's risk of infection by:
  – washing hands before and after providing care. *Handwashing is the single best way to avoid spreading pathogens.*
  – wearing gloves to maintain asepsis when providing direct care. *Gloves offer protection when handling wound dressings or carrying out various treatments.*

• Monitor temperature at least every 4 hours and record on graph paper. Report elevations immediately. *Sustained temperature elevation after surgery may signal onset of pulmonary complications, wound infection or dehiscence, urinary tract infection, or thrombophlebitis.*

• Monitor white blood cell (WBC) count, as ordered. Report elevations or depressions. *Elevated total WBC count indicates infection. Markedly decreased WBC count may indicate decreased production resulting from extreme debilitation or severe lack of vitamins and amino acids. Any damage to bone marrow may suppress white blood cell formation.*

• Culture urine, respiratory secretions, wound drainage, or blood according to hospital policy and doctor's order. *This identifies pathogens and guides antibiotic therapy.*

• Help patient wash hands before and after meals and after using the bathroom, bedpan, or urinal. *Hand washing prevents spread of pathogens to other objects and food.*

• Assist patient when necessary to ensure that the perianal area is clean after elimination. *Cleaning perineal area by wiping from area of least contamination (urinary meatus) to area of most contamination (anus) helps prevent genitourinary infections.*

• Instruct patient to report incidents of loose stools or diarrhea. Inform the doctor immediately. *Diarrhea or loose stools may indicate the need to discontinue or change antibiotic therapy. It may also indicate the need to test for* Clostridium difficile.

• Offer oral hygiene to the patient every 4 hours to prevent colonization of bacteria and reduce the risk of descending infection. *Disease and malnutrition may reduce moisture in mucous membranes of mouth and lips.*

• Use strict aseptic technique when suctioning the lower airway, inserting indwelling urinary catheters, inserting I.V. catheters, and providing wound care *to avoid spreading pathogens.*

• Change I.V. tubing and give site care every 24 to 48 hours or as institutional policy dictates *to help keep pathogens from entering the body.*

• Rotate I.V. sites every 48 to 72 hours or as institutional policy dictates *to reduce chances of infection at individual sites.*

• Have patient cough and deep-breathe every 4 hours after surgery *to help remove secretions and prevent pulmonary complications.*

• Provide tissues and disposal bag for expectorated sputum. *Convenient disposal encourages expectoration; sanitary disposal reduces spread of infection.*

• Help patient turn every 2 hours. Provide skin care, particularly over bony prominences, *to help prevent venous stasis and skin breakdown.*

• Use sterile water for humidification or nebulization of oxygen. *This prevents drying and irritation of respiratory mucosa, impaired ciliary action,*

and thickening of secretions within respiratory tract.
• Encourage fluid intake of 3,000 to 4,000 ml daily, unless contraindicated, *to help thin mucous secretions.*
• Ensure adequate nutritional intake. Offer high-protein supplements unless contraindicated. *This helps stabilize weight, improves muscle tone and mass, and aids wound healing.*
• Arrange for reverse isolation if patient has compromised immune system. Monitor flow and number of visitors. *These measures protect patient from pathogens in the environment.*
• Educate the patient regarding:
  – good hand-washing technique
  – factors that increase infection risk
  – infection signs and symptoms.

These measures allow patient to participate in care and help patient modify life-style to maintain optimum health level.

Evaluations for expected outcomes
• Patient's temperature remains within normal range.
• Patient's WBC count and differential remain within normal range.
• Cultures do not exhibit pathogen growth.
• Patient demonstrates appropriate personal and oral hygiene.
• Patient's respiratory secretions remain clear and odorless.
• Patient's urine remains clear, yellow, odorless, and free of sediment.
• Patient's bowel patterns remain normal.
• Patient's incisions or wounds remain clear, pink, and free of purulent drainage.
• Patient's I.V. sites do not show signs of inflammation.
• Patient's skin does not exhibit signs of breakdown.
• Patient's fluid intake remains at specified level.
• Patient consumes specified amount of protein daily.
• Patient lists risk factors for infection.
• Patient lists signs and symptoms of infection.
• Patient remains free of signs and symptoms of infection.

Documentation
• Temperature
• Dates, times, and sites of all cultures
• Dates, times, and sites of all catheter insertions
• Appearance of all invasive catheter sites, tube sites, and wounds
• Interventions performed to reduce infection risk
• Patient's response to nursing interventions
• Evaluations for each expected outcome.

■ Infection, high risk for

related to surgical incision

Definition
Accentuated risk of invasion of a surgical wound by a pathogenic organism (bacteria, virus, fungus, protozoa, parasite) from either endogenous or environmental sources

Assessment
• Age
• Sex
• Weight
• Reason for surgery
• Type of surgery
• Current health status, including vital signs, temperature, nutritional status, integumentary status

- Laboratory studies, including hematocrit and hemoglobin, complete blood count, electrolytes, urinalysis, blood cultures, blood coagulation studies, immunologic and serologic tests, liver function tests
- Presence of infection (urinary, respiratory, oral)
- Health history, including drug allergies, recent infection, substance abuse, chronic metabolic or systemic disease (diabetes mellitus; cardiovascular, hepatic, or renal disease; coagulation disorders; splenic or bone marrow disorders)
- Mobility status
- Anticipated length of surgery
- Current medical treatments, including radiation therapy, chemotherapy, antibiotic or antifungal therapy, steroid treatment, anticoagulant or thrombolytic therapy, immunosuppressive therapy
- Presence of invasive devices, including indwelling urinary (Foley) catheter, endotracheal tube, tracheostomy tube, I.V. lines, central venous and arterial lines, drains, gastric feeding tubes
- Wound classification (clean, clean-contaminated, contaminated, dirty)

Risk factors
- Altered immune function
- Chronic illness
- Immobility
- Impaired cardiovascular functioning leading to decreased oxygen transport
- Malnutrition
- Substance abuse

Associated medical diagnoses (selected)
Acquired immunodeficiency syndrome, anemia, blood dyscrasia, cancer, cardiovascular disease, chronic obstructive pulmonary disease, diabetes mellitus, emphysema, hepatitis, leukemia, liver cirrhosis, malnutrition, multiple myeloma, open wounds or lesions, peripheral vascular disease, portal hypertension, rheumatoid arthritis, substance abuse, systemic lupus erythematosus, thrombocytopenia

Expected outcomes
- Vital signs, temperature, and laboratory values remain within the patient's normal limits.
- Incision site remains free of signs and symptoms of infection.
- Dehiscence does not occur.

Interventions and rationales
- Document and report results of preoperative nursing assessment. Identify risk factors predisposing the patient to infection. *A complete nursing assessment allows development of an individualized plan of care.*
- Make sure all surgical team members wear appropriate operating room (OR) attire. *The human body is a major source of microbial contamination.*
- Inspect the OR for cleanliness before opening supplies and instruments *to provide a safe environment.*
- Perform a surgical hand scrub. Put on sterile gown and gloves. Place sterile drapes on the patient, furniture, and equipment. *The surgical hand scrub minimizes the number of microorganisms on the skin. Sterile gown and gloves protect against contamination. Sterile drapes create the sterile field.*
- Check the package integrity, chemical indicator, and, if appropriate, the expiration date on all sterile items before dispensing them onto the sterile field. *All items used within the field must be sterile.*
- Closely monitor the sterile field and initiate corrective measures when a

break in technique occurs. *Contamination of the sterile field may lead to wound contamination and subsequent infection.*

- Use proper technique when opening items onto the sterile field *to avoid contamination.*
- Perform preoperative skin preparation of the surgical site. *Skin preparation reduces the resident microbial count to subpathogenic amounts and inhibits rapid rebound growth of microbes.*
- Keep OR doors closed at all times and minimize traffic in and out. *Air turbulence caused by movement and the mixing of corridor air with room air can sharply increase OR bacterial counts.*
- Maintain room temperature of 68° to 75° F (20° to 23.9° C) and the relative humidity at 50% ± 10, unless contraindicated. *Cooler air temperature and lower humidity inhibit microbial growth.*
- Classify the surgical wound according to the degree of contamination of the wound and surrounding tissue. *Classification helps to assess the risk of wound infection from an endogenous source and determine the need for antibiotic therapy.*
- Wash hands following contact with the patient or any object contaminated with blood or body fluids. *Handwashing is the most effective means for preventing microbial transmission.*
- Administer antibiotics, as ordered. *Intraoperative administration of antibiotics can decrease the incidence of wound infection and lessen its severity.*
- Disinfect and sterilize all instruments and equipment before and immediately after the surgical procedure. *All instruments and equipment used during surgery must be free of microorganisms. Sterilizing instruments and equipment after use prevents growth and spread of microorganisms during storage.*
- Promptly clean areas outside the sterile field that become contaminated by blood, tissue, or body fluids with an approved disinfectant *to prevent the distribution of microbes into the environment.*
- Apply sterile dressing to the surgical wound before removing the surgical drapes *to avoid wound contamination and subsequent infection.*

Evaluations for expected outcomes

- Patient's oral temperature remains below 100° F (37.8° C). Postoperative vital signs and laboratory values (especially white blood cell count) are consistent with preoperative values.
- Patient's incision site remains free of erythema, edema, undue tenderness, warmth, induration, foul odor, purulent drainage, or other signs and symptoms of infection.
- Wound edges are approximated and evidence of dehiscence is absent.

Documentation

- Results of preoperative nursing assessment
- Operative procedure
- Type of anesthesia
- Surgical times (time patient entered OR, time incision was made, time incision was closed, time patient left OR)
- Wound classification
- Intraoperative administration of antibiotics
- Presence of packing, drains, Foley catheter, or other invasive devices
- Intraoperative insertion of permanent or temporary implants
- Type of wound closure method

- Type of dressing applied
- Estimated intraoperative blood loss
- Evaluations for each expected outcome.

Injury, high risk for

related to lack of awareness of environmental hazards

Definition
Accentuated risk of physical harm caused by lack of awareness of dangers in the environment

Assessment
- Age
- Health history, including accidents, falls, exposure to environmental hazards
- Environmental factors, including household layout, electrical wiring, lighting, utilities, fire precautions, presence of toxic or noxious substances, medications, special safety needs, childproofing
- Mental status, including mood, affect, thought processes, thought content, orientation, judgment, ability to perform activities of daily living
- Knowledge, including understanding of household safety precautions, automobile safety
- Participation in recreational activities, such as swimming, diving, motorcycling, bicycling, contact sports

Risk factors
- Access to poisons or toxins
- Age (infant, child, over 65)
- Evidence of environmental hazards
- History of household or automobile accidents
- Improper use of toys
- Lack of knowledge of environmental hazards
- Lack of knowledge of household safety precautions

Associated medical diagnoses (selected)
Burns, inhalation injuries, poisoning, psychiatric disorders, suffocation, trauma

Expected outcomes
- Patient and family acknowledge presence of environmental hazards in their everyday surroundings.
- Patient and family practice safety and take safety precautions in the home.
- Adults in household instruct children in safety habits.
- Adults in household childproof the house to ensure safety of young children and cognitively impaired adults.

Interventions and rationales
- Help patient identify situations and hazards that can cause accidents *to increase the patient's awareness of potential dangers.*
- Encourage patient to make repairs and remove potential safety hazards from the environment *to decrease the possibility of injury.*
- Encourage adults to discuss safety rules with children, for example:
  - Don't play with matches.
  - Use electrical equipment carefully.
  - Know location of fire escape route.
  - Don't speak to strangers.
  - Dial 911 in an emergency.

Teaching by parents fosters household safety.
- Refer patient to appropriate community resources for more information about identifying and removing safety hazards. *This enables patient and family to alter environment to achieve optimal safety level.*

Evaluations for expected outcomes
- Patient and family identify and eliminate safety hazards in their surroundings.
- Patient and family members demonstrate prevention and safety measures.
- Children describe safety measures they have learned.
- Patient and family point out evidence of childproofing measures in the home.

Documentation
- Patient's statements about situations that cause accidents and injuries
- Patient's lack of awareness of, or disregard for, safety hazards
- Patient's cognitive deficits that inhibit learning or attention to safety hazards
- Interventions to help patient recognize and eliminate safety hazards
- Patient's or family's response to nursing interventions
- Evaluations for each expected outcome.

Injury, high risk for

related to sensory or motor deficits

Definition
Accentuated risk of physical harm caused by sensory or motor deficits

Assessment
- Age
- Nature of sensory or motor deficit
- Health history, including cerebral function, mobility, sensory function, use of adaptive devices
- Psychological status, including substance abuse, familiarity with surroundings, mental status, coping skills, self-concept
- Medication use, including understanding of medications, compliance with prescribed regimen, use of over-the-counter medications, interactions
- Knowledge, including understanding of safety precautions
- Medication history
- Pain or fatigue
- Laboratory studies, complete blood count and differential, coagulation studies
- Diagnostic tests, including chest X-ray, cranial X-ray
- Sensory status, including hearing, vision, touch, taste

Risk factors
- Brain injury
- Contractures
- Developmental disability
- History of accidents (falls, burns, cuts, bruises, scrapes)
- Impaired mobility (immobilization, limited or restricted movement, pain with movement, vertigo)
- Inflamed joints
- Injuries in various stages of healing
- Misuse of adaptive devices or equipment (wheelchairs, crutches, walkers, grabbers, canes)
- Muscle spasticity
- Paralysis
- Paresis
- Polypharmacy or medication overdose
- Sensory deficits (decreased or absent vision, hearing, thermal perception)
- Skeletal deformities
- Substance abuse
- Unsteady gait

Associated medical diagnoses (selected)
Cardiac disorders, blindness, deafness, hallucinations, hematologic disorders, limb amputation, muscular disorders, neural disorders, organic

brain syndromes, posttraumatic head injury (closed head injury), pulmonary disorders, skeletal disorders, syncope, tinnitus, tissue hypoxemia or hypoperfusion, vertigo

Expected outcomes

- Patient identifies factors that increase potential for injury.
- Patient assists in identifying and applying safety measures to prevent injury.
- Patient and family or significant other develop strategy to maintain safety.
- Patient optimizes activities of daily living within sensorimotor limitations.

Interventions and rationales

- Observe for factors that may cause or contribute to injury *to increase awareness of patient, significant other, and caregivers.*
- Improve environmental safety, as needed:
  - Orient patient to environment. Assess patient's ability to use call bell, side rails, and bed positioning controls. Keep bed at lowest level and conduct close night watch. *These measures will help patient cope with unfamiliar surroundings.*
  - Teach patient and family about need for safe illumination. Advise patient to wear sunglasses to reduce glare. Advise using contrast colors in household furnishings. *These measures will enhance visual discrimination.*
  - Test heating pads and bath water before using; assess extremities daily for injury *to assist patient with decreased tactile sensitivity.*
  - For the patient with hearing loss, encourage use of hearing aid *to minimize deficit.*
  - Teach patient with unstable gait correct use of adaptive devices *to decrease potential for injury.*
- Provide additional patient teaching as needed. Possible topics may include household, automobile, and pedestrian safety. Refer patient to appropriate resources (police, fire, visiting nurses association) for more information. *Health education can help patient take steps to prevent injury.*

Evaluations for expected outcomes

- Patient identifies two factors that increase risk for injury.
- Patient cooperates with nurse during assessment of sensorimotor function.
- Patient and family describe and demonstrate preventive measures to minimize potential for injury.
- Patient increases self-care activities within limits posed by sensorimotor limitations.

Documentation

- Statements by patient and family or significant other about potential for injury due to sensory or motor deficits
- Manifestations of deficit
- Observation or knowledge of unsafe practices
- Interventions to decrease risk of injury to patient
- Patient's responses to nursing interventions
- Evaluations for each expected outcome.

Injury secondary to perioperative positioning, risk for

related to surgical positioning

Definition

Accentuated risk of tissue injury, neuromuscular impairment, vascular compromise, or impaired gas exchange during surgery

Assessment

- Reason for surgery
- Type of surgery and its expected length
- Health status, including age, weight, vital signs, nutritional status, integumentary status, musculoskeletal status, hydration status, temperature, peripheral vascular status, neurologic status, smoking history
- Laboratory studies, including hematocrit and hemoglobin, complete blood count, electrolytes, urinalysis, blood coagulation studies, liver function tests
- Mobility status, including range of motion; presence of prosthesis; limb abnormality, impairment, or injury
- Current medical treatments, including radiation therapy, chemotherapy, steroid therapy

Risk factors

- Altered circulation or sensation
- Altered metabolic or nutritional state (obesity, emaciation)
- Anesthesia (general, regional)
- Bony prominences
- Broken skin
- Cardiovascular, hepatic, renal, or respiratory disease; diabetes mellitus; musculoskeletal disorders
- Edema
- Extended surgery
- Hypovolemia
- Immobility
- Mechanical factors, including friction, pressure, or shearing force

Associated medical diagnoses (selected)

Any disease that may require surgery.

Supine position: Abdominal aortic aneurysm resection, appendectomy, arthroscopy, arthrotomy, bowel resection, bronchoscopy, cholecystectomy, colostomy, coronary artery bypass grafting, cystectomy, exploratory laparotomy, gastrectomy, hernia repair, ileal conduit, mediastinoscopy, splenectomy, total abdominal hysterectomy, pacemaker insertion, rotator cuff repair

Prone position: Achilles tendon repair, anal fissurectomy or fistulectomy, hemorrhoidectomy, laminectomy, pilonidal cyst excision, posterior cervical fusion, spinal fusion with Harrington rods

Lateral position: Descending thoracic aortic aneurysm resection, nephrectomy, nephrolithotomy, thoracotomy, total hip arthroplasty

Lithotomy position: Anterior or posterior vaginal repair, conization of the cervix, dilatation and curettage, hemorrhoidectomy and other rectal procedures, laparoscopy, perineal condyloma, low anterior bowel resection, rectovaginal or vesicovaginal fistulectomy, total vaginal hysterectomy, uterine or bladder suspension

Expected outcomes

- Patient maintains effective breathing patterns.
- Patient maintains adequate cardiac output.
- Surgical positioning facilitates gas exchange.
- Patient shows no evidence of neurologic, musculoskeletal or vascular compromise.

- Patient maintains tissue integrity.

Interventions and rationales

- Document and report results of preoperative nursing assessment. Identify factors predisposing the patient to pressure tissue injury. *This information guides interventions.*
- Use appropriate mode of patient transportation (stretcher, patient bed, wheel chair, crib) *to ensure patient safety.*
- Make sure an adequate number of staff assist with transferring patient. A minimum of two staff are needed for moving the patient onto the operating room (OR) bed. A minimum of four staff are needed for moving the anesthetized patient off the OR bed. *Adequate staffing enhances safety.*
- Check the OR bed preoperatively for proper functioning. *Intraoperative bed malfunction can result in increased anesthesia time and a more difficult surgical approach.*
- Ensure proper positioning.

Supine:
  - Check neck and spine for proper alignment.
  - Check that legs are straight and uncross ankles. *Crossed ankles cause pressure on tissue, vessels, and nerves.*
  - Place safety strap 2″ above the knees, tight enough to restrain without compromising superficial venous return. *Applied too tightly, safety strap may cause venous thrombosis or compression of the tibial, peroneal, or sciatic nerves.*
  - Secure arms at sides with draw sheet, palms down, making sure no part of arm or hand extends over mattress. Alternatively, secure arms on padded arm boards at less than 90-degree angle from body, palms supinated. *Hyperextension can cause injury to the brachial plexus. Supination of palms minimizes pressure.*
  - Apply eye pads if eyelids will not remain closed or if surgery is being performed on head, neck, or chest. *If allowed to remain open, the eye may dry out and become infected. Corneal abrasions may result from drapes and other foreign material rubbing against eye.*
  - If surgery is expected to last more than 2 hours or if patient is predisposed to pressure injury, place padding under occiput, scapulae, olecranon, sacrum, coccyx, and calcaneus *to protect potential pressure points.* Apply a padded foot board *to support the feet, avoid plantar flexion, and prevent stretching of the tibial nerve and subsequent foot drop.*
  - Unless contraindicated, place a foam doughnut or small pillow under head *to prevent stretching of the neck muscles.*

Prone:
  - Make sure at least four staff members assist when turning the patient *to assure safety.*
  - Place a foam doughnut or small pillow under head. Check lower eye and ear for excessive pressure. Apply eye pads. *Head support assists in maintaining cervical and thoracic spine alignment. Checking dependent ear and eye lowers risk of pressure injury. Pads protect eyes.*
  - Place arms on armboards extended in front beside head with elbows slightly flexed and palms pronated *to prevent strain on shoulder, elbows, and wrist joints.*

– Check for proper alignment of neck and spine.
– Check female patient's breasts and male patient's genitalia for excessive pressure from chest rolls or laminectomy brace *to avoid soft tissue and nerve injury.*
– Check bilateral pulses of upper and lower extremities. *Top and bottom edges of chest rolls or laminectomy brace may compress radial and femoral arteries.*
– Place padding under knees *to avoid injury to soft tissue and knee joint.*
– Place a pillow under ankles *to avoid putting pressure on toes and feet, stretching the tibial nerve, or causing plantar flexion.*
– Place safety strap 2″ above the knees, securely but not too tightly *to restrain patient without compromising superficial venous return.*
– If surgery is expected to last more than 2 hours or if patient is predisposed to pressure injury, place padding under acromion process, olecranon, and anterior iliac spine *to protect pressure points.*

Lateral:

– Make sure at least four staff members assist when turning patient *to ensure safety.*
– Check neck and spine for proper alignment.
– Place a foam doughnut or small pillow under patient's head. Check dependent eye and ear for excessive pressure. Apply eye pads. *Head supports assist in maintaining cervical and thoracic spine alignment. Checking dependent ear and eye lowers risk of pressure injury. Pads protect patient's eyes.*
– Place a small roll under dependent lower axilla *to relieve pressure on the chest and axilla, allow for adequate chest expansion, and prevent compression of the brachial plexus by the humeral head.*
– Place lower arm on arm board less than 90-degree angle from body, palm supinated. Place upper arm on an elevated padded support, less than 90-degree angle from body, palm pronated, and apply restraints *to avoid injury to the brachial plexus.*
– Place bottom leg flexed at the hip and knee and the top leg straight. *Flexing the bottom leg provides greater stability for the torso, decreases the pressure on the lateral aspect of lower leg, and prevents the bony areas of the knees and ankles from pressing against each other.*
– Place pillows between knees and ankles *to support the top leg, prevent strain on the top hip, and pad pressure points on medial aspects of both legs.*
– Place padding under lateral aspects of bottom knee and ankle *to reduce risk of tissue injury to the area over the lateral malleolus of the ankle and peroneal nerve damage (foot drop).*
– Place safety strap across upper thighs or wide tape over hips. Attach strap or tape to bed *to assure safety.*
– If surgery is expected to last more than 2 hours or if patient is predisposed to pressure injury, place padding under acromion process, ilium, and greater trochanter *to protect pressure points.*

Lithotomy:
- Secure arms on armboards or at sides. If arms are placed at sides, position fingers away from the break in the table *to prevent fingers from becoming compressed in bed mechanism.*
- Check neck and spine for proper alignment.
- Position stirrups at equal height and attach them to bed securely *to prevent accidental movement. Uneven leg flexion and hip abduction can cause strain on lumbar and sacral areas.*
- Place the loop straps of post stirrup behind the ankle and under the foot. Pad the post portion of stirrup if it could come in contact with the leg. *Loop straps support and secure the legs.*
- Pad popliteal knee support stirrups *to prevent possible thrombosis of superficial vessels and pressure injury to the femoral and obturator nerves.*
- If surgery is expected to last more than 2 hours or if patient is predisposed to pressure injury, place padding under occiput, scapulae, olecranon, and sacrum *to protect potential pressure points.*
- With the help of a co-worker, raise and lower patient's legs simultaneously and slowly *to prevent ankle and knee injury and hip dislocation. Lowering the legs too quickly may cause sudden hypotension.*

• Assess patient position following each positional change *to ensure proper body alignment and adequate padding and support.*
• Apply restraints after positioning patient *to prevent falls and injury.*

Evaluations for expected outcomes

• Patient maintains effective breathing patterns. Patient's position does not restrict ventilation. Chest expansion is adequate.
• Cardiac output remains adequate. Patient does not experience any significant episodes of hypertension or hypotension.
• Positioning allows for adequate gas exchange, as evidenced by patient's ventilation-perfusion ratio and oxygen saturation.
• Evidence of neurologic, musculoskeletal, or vascular compromise is absent. Patient's mobility status and range of motion remain at preoperative levels. Patient does not experience pain, numbness, tingling, or weakness in positioned body parts.
• Patient's tissue integrity remains intact; skin does not become reddened, discolored, ulcerated, edematous, or excoriated.

Documentation

• Results of preoperative nursing assessment
• Operative procedure, type of anesthesia, and surgical positioning
• Surgical times, including time patient entered OR, time incision was made, time incision was closed, time patient left OR
• Method of patient transport and transfer
• Estimated intraoperative blood loss
• Types and placement of padding, restraints, and positional devices
• Intraoperative repositioning of the patient
• Intraoperative insertion of permanent or temporary implants
• Peripheral pulses
• Evaluations for each expected outcome.

Knowledge deficit

related to cognitive impairment

Definition

Inadequate understanding of information or inability to perform skills needed to practice health-related behaviors

Assessment

- Psychosocial status, including age, learning ability (affective domain, cognitive domain, psychomotor domain), decision making, developmental stage, financial resources, interest in learning, knowledge and skills related to current health problem, obstacles to learning, support systems (willingness and capability of others to help patient), usual coping pattern
- Neurologic status, including level of consciousness, memory, mental status, orientation

Defining characteristics

- Cognitive impairment
- Inaccurate follow-up on previous instruction
- Inadequate performance of a test or demonstration of a skill
- Inappropriate or exaggerated behaviors (hysteria, hostility, agitation, apathy)
- Patient's statements indicating insufficient recall of information, poor understanding, misinterpretation, or misconception

Associated medical diagnoses (selected)

Alzheimer's disease, brain tumor, cerebrovascular accident, head injury, mental retardation, organic brain syndrome

Expected outcomes

- Patient demonstrates ability to perform simple self-care measures, such as feeding, maintaining hygiene, dressing, toileting.
- Family or significant other communicates understanding of patient's cognitive impairment.
- Family or significant other expresses willingness to help patient maintain maximum independence.
- Family or significant other demonstrates method being used to teach patient.

Interventions and rationales

- Provide all equipment needed for each self-care measure patient must learn. *This reduces frustration, aids learning, and minimizes dependence by promoting self-care.*
- When teaching self-care measures, go slowly and repeat frequently. Offer small amounts of information and present it in various ways. *By building cognition, patient will be better able to complete self-care measures.*
- Have patient practice each task. Provide positive reinforcement each time task is performed correctly. *This encourages desired behavior.*
- Discuss patient's limitations with family or significant other. *Communication promotes working relationship and reduces fear and anxiety.*
- Demonstrate to family or significant other how each self-care measure is broken down into simple tasks *to enhance patient's success and foster sense of control.*
- Encourage family or significant other to participate in patient's learning process *to help create an encouraging, therapeutic climate after discharge.*
- Have family or significant other give return demonstration of patient's methods of performing self-care

measures. *This provides hands-on experience with equipment, builds confidence, and encourages compliance.*
- Refer family or significant other to outside agencies, such as a home health care organization, for assistance after patient's discharge. *This ensures continuity of care and assistance with follow-up after discharge.*

Evaluations for expected outcomes
- Patient practices simple self-care measures.
- Patient demonstrates ability to perform activities of daily living.
- Family member or significant other describes cause of patient's cognitive impairment.
- Family member or significant other demonstrates willingness to help patient learn to perform self-care measures.
- Family member or significant other provides return demonstration of patient's methods of performing self-care measures.

Documentation
- Patient's abilities and limitations in performing self-care measures
- Progress made by patient in learning each specific task
- Information imparted to family or significant other concerning patient's limitations and progress in learning tasks
- Family's or significant other's participation in the learning process
- Referrals to outside agencies
- Evaluations for each expected outcome.

Knowledge deficit

related to lack of exposure

Definition
Inadequate understanding of information or inability to perform skills needed to practice health-related behaviors

Assessment
- Psychosocial status, including age, learning ability (affective domain, cognitive domain, psychomotor domain), decision making ability, developmental stage, financial resources, health beliefs and attitudes, interest in learning, knowledge and skill regarding current health problem, obstacles to learning, support systems (willingness and capability of others to help patient), usual coping pattern
- Neurologic status, including level of consciousness, memory, mental status, orientation

Defining characteristics
Patient's requests for information, expressions of problem, and lack of familiarity with informational resources

Associated medical diagnoses (selected)
This nursing diagnosis can occur in association with any medical diagnosis

Expected outcomes
- Patient communicates a need to know.
- Patient states or demonstrates understanding of what has been taught.
- Patient demonstrates ability to perform new health-related behaviors as they are taught, and lists specific

skills and realistic target dates for each.
• Patient sets realistic learning goals.
• Patient states intention to make needed changes in life-style, including seeking help from health professional when needed.

Interventions and rationales
• Establish an environment of mutual trust and respect to enhance learning. *Comfort with growing self-awareness, ability to share this awareness with others, receptiveness to new experiences, and consistency between actions and words form the basis of a trusting relationship.*
• Negotiate with patient to develop goals for learning. *Involving patient in planning meaningful goals encourages follow-through.*
• Select teaching strategies (discussion, demonstration, role-playing, visual materials) appropriate for patient's individual learning style (specify), *to enhance teaching effectiveness.*
• Teach skills that patient must incorporate into daily life-style. Have patient give return demonstration of each new skill *to help gain confidence.*
• Have patient incorporate learned skills into daily routine during hospitalization (specify skills). *This allows patient to practice new skills and receive feedback.*
• Provide patient with names and telephone numbers of resource people or organizations *to provide continuity of care and follow-up after discharge.*

Evaluations for expected outcomes
• Patient expresses a desire to overcome lack of knowledge.
• Patient demonstrates newly learned health-related behaviors.
• Patient performs new skills by target date.
• Patient develops realistic learning goals.
• Patient identifies specific changes in life-style needed to promote optimal health.

Documentation
• Patient's statements of information and skills known or unknown
• Expressions of need to know, motivation to learn
• Learning objectives
• Methods used to teach patient
• Information imparted
• Skills demonstrated
• Patient's responses to teaching
• Evaluations for each expected outcome.

Knowledge deficit

related to lack of motivation

Definition
Inadequate understanding of information or inability to perform skills needed to practice health-related behaviors

Assessment
• Psychosocial status, including age, learning ability (affective domain, cognitive domain, psychomotor domain), decision-making, developmental stage, financial resources, interest in learning, knowledge and skills related to current health problem, obstacles to learning, support systems (willingness and capability of others to help patient), usual coping pattern
• Neurologic status, including level of consciousness, memory, mental status, orientation

Defining characteristics

- Behavior that indicates failure to adhere
- Failure to learn new skills
- Inaccurate follow-up of instruction
- Inappropriate or exaggerated behavior
- Unwillingness to set goals

Associated medical diagnoses (selected)

This nursing diagnosis may coincide with any medical diagnosis but most commonly accompanies chronic diseases requiring major changes in health-related behaviors or life-style, such as cardiovascular disease, chronic obstructive pulmonary disease, diabetes mellitus, hypertension, and end-stage renal disease.

Expected outcomes

- Patient expresses interest in learning new behaviors.
- Patient gradually sets realistic learning objectives (specify).
- Patient strives to meet each objective by target date.
- Patient practices new health-related behaviors during hospitalization; for example, selects appropriate diet, self-medicates, weighs self daily, monitors intake and output.
- Patient develops realistic plan for maintaining new skills at home.

Interventions and rationales

- Provide uninterrupted time for patient to state reasons for not wanting to learn or practice new health-related behaviors. *Attentive listening conveys caring attitude, encouraging patient to talk.*
- Avoid nonconstructive criticism. Rather, encourage expression of feelings. *Nonjudgmental approach encourages patient to express feelings more freely.*
- Ascertain what patient already knows *to determine what patient needs to know. Building on known information leads to successful learning.*
- Explore with patient the impact of behavior on self and family or significant other. *Learning is more effective if patient recognizes a need to know.*
- Urge patient to ask questions *to help clarify information and evaluate patient's comprehension.*
- Determine whether patient enjoys learning through such media as videotapes, audiotapes, books, and discussions *to discover most effective teaching tools.*
- Begin negotiating learning objectives with patient. *Involving patient in defining goals increases understanding and encourages compliance.*
- Be patient; offer praise when patient attempts new behaviors *to motivate patient to learn more.*
- Provide emotional support as patient attempts distasteful or anxiety-producing behaviors. *Support will help patient perform tasks successfully.*
- Suggest that patient discuss situation with a person who has developed skill in managing a similar health problem *to encourage patient to air feelings and concerns.*
- Help patient plan realistically for continuing new behaviors, which may include teaching family or significant other. *Realistic goals increase probability of compliance. Involving others adds support after discharge.*

Evaluations for expected outcomes

- Patient expresses desire to change behavior.
- Patient participates in development of educational goals.

• Patient displays motivation to attain goal by target date.
• Patient practices new health-related behaviors.
• Patient states plans for inclusion of new activities into daily routine after discharge.

Documentation
• Statements of motivation or lack of interest in learning
• Observations that indicate readiness or lack of readiness to learn
• Goals set by patient
• Methods used to teach patient
• Information imparted
• Skills demonstrated
• Patient's responses to trying new behaviors
• Evaluations for each expected outcome.

Management of therapeutic regimen, ineffective

related to health beliefs

Definition
Failure to integrate program for treating illness into daily living

Assessment
• Medical history
• Physical examination
• Prescriptions for treatment, including medications, activity, diet, other
• Current medication schedule, including medications used at home (prescribed and over-the-counter)
• Activities of daily living and exercise pattern
• Nutrition pattern, including 3-day diet history or 1-day diet recall
• Weight
• Patient's and family members' health-related goals
• Self-care abilities and resources, including presence of family members or significant other
• Health beliefs, including perceived susceptibility to illness, perceived seriousness of illness, perceived effectiveness of treatment, perceived barriers to managing regimen
• Other influences on health-related behavior, including age, sex, knowledge, social pressures

Defining characteristics
• Exacerbation (expected or unexpected) of illness
• Inappropriate choices with regard to meeting the goals of treatment or prevention program
• Patient expresses difficulty with integrating prescribed treatment regimen into life-style
• Patient reports failure to include treatment regimen in daily routine
• Patient reports failure to take action to reduce risk factors for illness

Associated medical diagnoses (selected)
Any illness has potential to be managed ineffectively by the patient. Common examples include acquired immunodeficiency syndrome (AIDS), asthma, chronic fatigue and immune dysfunction syndrome, chronic obstructive pulmonary disease, chronic renal failure, coronary artery disease, diabetes mellitus, hypertension, multiple sclerosis, Parkinson's disease, rheumatoid arthritis, spinal cord injury

Expected outcomes
• Patient expresses personal beliefs about illness and its management.
• Patient and family members develop plan for integrating components of therapeutic regimen, such as medications, activity, and diet, into pattern of daily living.

- Patient selects daily activities to meet the goals of treatment or prevention program.
- Patient expresses intent to reduce risk factors for progression of illness.
- Patient and family members use available support services.

Interventions and rationales

- Discuss patient's personal beliefs about illness and review relevant information *to establish common understanding for development of a plan to improve management of therapeutic regimen.*
- Educate patient about pathophysiology of illness and explain relationship between pathophysiology and therapeutic regimen. *A patient who knows the reasons for specific behaviors may be more willing to adjust life-style.*
- Help patient and family members clarify values associated with life-style *to enhance understanding of conflicts between life-style and demands of therapeutic regimen.*
- Work with patient and family members to develop a daily routine for managing the therapeutic regimen that fits with life-style. *Collaboration with patient and family members makes it possible to combine scientific knowledge of the illness with life-style factors such as culture, family dynamics, and finances.*
- Correct patient's misconceptions about susceptibility to and seriousness of illness. *Misconceptions may undermine treatment.*
- Assist patient and family members in modifying factors (such as social pressures, lack of family support, or previous behavior patterns) that interfere with treatment management *to enhance the level of care.*
- Provide verbal reminders to reinforce health-promoting behaviors. For example, remind patient with heart disease to stop smoking. *Verbal cues may stimulate patient to take action – if not immediately, then at a later point in time.*
- Provide clearly written literature about treatment regimen *to reinforce patient's knowledge.*
- Assist patient and family members in selecting appropriate options for managing the therapeutic regimen *to help patient and family members integrate potentially complicated and disruptive therapeutic interventions into their life-style.*
- Refer patient or family members to support groups or self-help organizations *to empower patient and family members to continue effective management of therapeutic regimen.*
- Help patient and family members plan for future course of illness. For example, patient or family members may need to make structural changes at home to accommodate a wheelchair or hospital bed. *Planning enhances the patient's and family members' abilities to develop appropriate management strategies.*

Evaluations for expected outcomes

- Patient expresses personal beliefs about illness and therapeutic regimen.
- Patient and family members successfully incorporate components of the therapeutic regimen into daily activities.
- Patient carries out therapeutic regimen.
- Patient describes daily activities that will help him achieve the goals of treatment or prevention program.
- Patient states intent to reduce risk factors for illness.
- Patient and family members contact appropriate support services.

Documentation
- Patient's knowledge and beliefs about illness and therapeutic regimen
- Patient's explanation of values and life-style
- Information provided to clarify misconceptions
- Actions taken to modify patient's environment or behavior
- Written materials given to patient
- Referrals to support services
- Evaluations for each expected outcome.

Mobility impairment

related to neuromuscular impairment

Definition
Limitation of physical movement

Assessment
- History of neuromuscular disorder or dysfunction
- Musculoskeletal status, including coordination, gait, muscle size and strength, muscle tone, range of motion, and functional mobility as follows:
  - 0 = completely independent
  - 1 = requires use of equipment or device
  - 2 = requires help, supervision, or teaching from another person
  - 3 = requires help from another person and equipment or device
  - 4 = dependent; does not participate in activity
- Neurologic status, including level of consciousness, motor ability, sensory ability

Defining characteristics
- Decreased muscle strength, control, mass, endurance
- Impaired coordination
- Inability to purposefully move within the physical environment, including bed mobility, transfer, and ambulation
- Limited range of motion
- Reluctance to attempt movement

Associated medical diagnoses (selected)
Amyotrophic lateral sclerosis, cerebral palsy, cerebrovascular accident, multiple sclerosis, muscular dystrophy, myasthenia gravis, Parkinson's disease, poliomyelitis, rheumatoid arthritis, spinal cord injury (paraplegia, quadriplegia), tetanus

Expected outcomes
- Patient maintains muscle strength and joint range of motion.
- Patient shows no evidence of complications, such as contractures, venous stasis, thrombus formation, or skin breakdown.
- Patient achieves highest level of mobility (transfers independently, is wheelchair-independent, ambulates with such assistive devices as walker, cane, braces).
- Patient or significant other carries out mobility regimen.
- Patient or significant other makes plans to use resources to help maintain level of functioning, such as physical therapist, Stroke Program, American Heart Association, or National Multiple Sclerosis Society.

Interventions and rationales
- Perform range-of-motion exercises to joints, unless contraindicated, at least once every shift. Progress from passive to active, as tolerated. *This prevents joint contractures and muscular atrophy.*
- Turn and position patient every 2 hours. Establish turning schedule for dependent patients; post at bedside

and monitor frequency of turning. *This prevents skin breakdown by relieving pressure.*

- Place joints in functional position, use trochanter roll along thigh, abduct thighs, use high-top sneakers, and put small pillow under head. *These measures maintain joints in functional position and prevent musculoskeletal deformities.*
- Identify level of functioning using a functional mobility scale (see Assessment). Communicate patient's skill level to all staff *to provide continuity and preserve identified level of independence.*
- Encourage independence in mobility by assisting patient in using trapeze and side rails, in using unaffected leg to move affected leg, and in performing such self-care activities as combing hair, feeding, dressing, etc. *This increases muscle tone and patient's self-esteem.*
- Place items within reach of unaffected arm if one-sided weakness or paralysis is present *to promote patient's independence.*
- Monitor and record daily any evidence of immobility complications (contractures, venous stasis, thrombus, pneumonia, urinary tract infection). *Patients with history of neuromuscular disorders or dysfunctions may be more prone to develop complications.*
- Carry out medical regimen to manage or prevent complications; for example, prophylactic heparin for venous thrombosis. *This promotes patient's health and well-being.*
- Provide progressive mobilization to limits of patient's condition (bed mobility to chair mobility to ambulation) *to maintain muscle tone and prevent complications of immobility.*
- Refer to physical therapist for development of mobility regimen *to help rehabilitate musculoskeletal deficits.*
- Encourage attendance at physical therapy sessions and support activities on unit by using same equipment and technique. Request written mobility plans and use as reference. *All members of health care team should reinforce learned skills in same manner.*
- Instruct patient and family or significant other in range-of-motion exercises, transfers, skin inspection, mobility regimen *to help prepare patient for discharge.*
- Demonstrate mobility regimen and note date. Have patient and family or significant other return mobility regimen demonstration and note date. *This ensures continuity of care and use of proper technique.*
- Assist in identifying resources to carry out mobility regimen, such as Stroke Program, American Heart Association, or National Multiple Sclerosis Society. *This helps provide comprehensive approach to rehabilitation.*

Evaluations for expected outcomes

- Patient maintains muscle strength and joint range of motion.
- Patient shows no evidence of contractures, venous stasis, thrombus formation, skin breakdown, hypostatic pneumonia, or other complications.
- Patient achieves highest mobility level possible identified by health care team (specify).
- Patient or significant other carries out mobility regimen.
- Patient or significant other identifies and contacts at least one resource person or group to help maintain level of functioning.

Documentation

- Patient's expression of concern about the loss of mobility, current status of functional abilities, and goals set for self
- Observations of the patient's mobility status, presence of complications, and response to mobility regimen
- Instruction and demonstration of skills in carrying out mobility regimen
- Patient's response to nursing interventions
- Evaluations for each expected outcome.

Mobility impairment

related to pain or discomfort

Definition

Limitation of physical movement

Assessment

- History of recent surgery, injury, or disorder causing pain or discomfort
- Medication history
- Musculoskeletal status, including coordination, gait, muscle size and strength, muscle tone, range of motion, and functional mobility as follows:
  - 0 = completely independent
  - 1 = requires use of equipment or device
  - 2 = requires help, supervision, or teaching from another person
  - 3 = requires help from another person and equipment or device
  - 4 = dependent; does not participate in activity
- Pain, including environmental and cultural influences, intensity, location, quality, temporal factors
- Psychosocial status, including coping mechanisms, family or significant others, life-style, personality, stressors (disease process, finances, job, marital discord)

Defining characteristics

- Clinical evidence or verbal complaint of pain on movement
- Decreased muscle strength, control, mass, or endurance
- Impaired coordination
- Imposed restriction of movement, including mechanical; medical protocol
- Inability to move purposefully within the physical environment, including bed mobility, transfer, and ambulation
- Limited range of motion
- Reluctance to attempt movement

Associated medical diagnoses (selected)

Ankylosing spondylitis, arthritis (all types), bursitis, dermatomyositis, dislocation, epicondylitis, fractures, gout, herniated disk, osteochondrosis, osteomyelitis, Paget's disease, peripheral neuritis, peripheral vascular disease, polymyositis, sickle-cell crisis, sprains, systemic lupus erythematosus, tendinitis, trauma

Expected outcomes

- Patient states relief from pain.
- Patient displays increased mobility.
- Patient shows no evidence of such complications as contractures, venous stasis, thrombus formation, or skin breakdown.
- Patient attains highest degree of mobility possible within confines of disease.
- Patient or significant other demonstrates mobility regimen.
- Patient states feelings about limitations.

Interventions and rationales

- Observe patient's functional ability daily; document and report any changes using functional mobility scale (see Assessment). *Changes may indicate progressive decline or improvement in underlying disorder.*
- Encourage patient to verbalize pain and discomfort. Observe for nonverbal cues of pain, including favoring a body part, grimacing, etc. *This aids assessment of location, quality, and intensity of pain.*
- Perform prescribed treatment regimen for underlying condition producing pain or discomfort. Monitor progress and report favorable and adverse response to treatment *to assess effectiveness of treatment.*
- Provide supportive measures as indicated:
  - Administer pain medication and assess nonverbal cues, verbal reports, and vital signs *to monitor effectiveness.*
  - Ensure patient comfort by padding extremities prone to skin breakdown (heels, elbows), ensuring correct measurement of crutches, and using convoluted foam mattress on bed. *These measures prevent skin breakdown.*
  - Encourage patient's active movement by using assistive devices *to increase muscle tone and increase patient's feelings of self-esteem;* promote joint rest between activities.
  - Implement range-of-motion exercises every shift after pain medication, unless medically contraindicated; progress from passive to active, as tolerated. *This prevents joint contracture and muscle atrophy.*
  - Reposition patient every 2 hours and provide meticulous skin care *to prevent skin breakdown.*
  - Promote progressive mobilization to maximum, within limits of patient's tolerance for pain (bed mobility to chair mobility to ambulation). *This maintains muscle tone and prevents complications of immobility.*
- Discuss use of distraction and other nonpharmacologic pain-relief methods with patient. Instruct patient and family or significant other on the preferred method and monitor effectiveness. Encourage patient to choose an alternative if ineffective. Document response. *In addition to providing pain relief, nonpharmacologic techniques may help patient achieve sense of control. Documentation helps ensure continuity of care.*
- Explain necessity of movement even during painful periods, unless contraindicated, to prevent greater pain, such as occurs in arthritic conditions and after surgery. Let patient know when to expect to move; provide pain-relief measures before moving patient. *Movement alleviates effects of immobility. Medication alleviates pain and maintains patient's functional activity level.*
- Instruct patient and significant other in range-of-motion exercises, transfers, skin inspection, and mobility regimen. Have patient and significant other return mobility demonstration under supervision. *Education will enable patient and significant other to prevent complications of immobility.*
- Encourage patient to discuss feelings and concerns about altered state of mobility *to reduce anxiety and promote compliance.*
- Encourage adherence to other aspects of health care management *to*

control or minimize effects on mobility. This promotes health and well-being by alleviating pain and preventing complications.
- Refer to psychiatric liaison nurse, social service agency, support group, or other resources as appropriate *to provide patient with alternative approaches to care.*

Evaluations for expected outcomes
- Patient expresses relief from pain.
- Patient demonstrates increased mobility.
- Patient shows no evidence of contractures, venous stasis, thrombus formation, skin breakdown, hypostatic pneumonia, or other complications.
- Patient attains highest mobility level possible as determined by health care team (specify).
- Patient or significant other carries out mobility regimen.
- Patient begins to accept limitations imposed by immobility and accompanying life-style changes.
- Patient expresses willingness to participate in care.

Documentation
- Patient's expression of feelings and concerns about immobility, impact on life-style, and willingness to participate in care
- Observations of patient's impaired mobility, pain, and response to treatment
- Interventions to provide supportive care
- Instructions to patient and significant other, their understanding of instructions, and demonstrated skill in carrying out the prescribed mobility and pain-relief program
- Patient's response to nursing interventions
- Evaluations for each expected outcome.

■ Mobility impairment

related to perceptual or cognitive impairment

Definition
Limitation of physical movement

Assessment
- History of neurologic, sensory, or psychological disorder with impaired movement
- Musculoskeletal status, including coordination, gait, muscle size and strength, muscle tone, range of motion, and functional mobility as follows:
  - 0 = completely independent
  - 1 = requires use of equipment or device
  - 2 = requires help, supervision, or teaching from another person
  - 3 = requires help from another person and equipment or device
  - 4 = dependent; does not participate in activity
- Neurologic status, including cognition, communication skills, insight and judgment, level of consciousness, memory, motor ability, orientation, sensory ability
- Psychosocial status, including coping mechanisms, family or significant others, life-style, personality, stressors (disease process, finances, job, marital discord)

Defining characteristics
- Clinical evidence of impaired memory or intellectual capacity
- Decreased muscle strength, control, mass

- Impaired coordination
- Inability to move purposefully within the physical environment, including bed mobility, transfer, ambulation
- Limited range of motion
- Reluctance to attempt movement
- Restriction of movement, including mechanical, imposed by medical protocol

Associated medical diagnoses (selected)
Alcoholism, Alzheimer's disease, bipolar disease (manic or depressive phase), blindness, brain tumor, central nervous system infections, cerebrovascular accident, head injury, Huntington's disease, Laennec's cirrhosis, Ménière's disease, myxedema, pellagra, Reye's syndrome, vitamin B_1 deficiency

Expected outcomes
- Patient maintains functional mobility.
- Complications are avoided or minimized.
- Patient states feelings about impairment.
- Family or significant other communicates understanding of mobility regimen.
- Family or significant other demonstrates skill in carrying out mobility regimen.
- Family or significant other obtains support necessary to continue care.

Interventions and rationales
- Observe patient's functional ability daily; document and report any changes using functional mobility scale (see Assessment). *Changes may indicate progressive decline or improvement in underlying disorder.*
- Determine patient's degree of perceptual or cognitive impairment and ability to follow directions *to determine presence of deficits. Modify interventions accordingly.*
- Perform prescribed treatment regimen for the underlying condition producing pain or discomfort. Monitor progress, reporting favorable and adverse response to treatment, *to assess effectiveness of treatment.*
- Allow patient and family or significant other to ventilate frustration and other negative feelings regarding difficulty in performing mobility tasks. *Expressing feelings helps patient and family or significant other cope with impaired mobility.*
- Ask patient to perform one task at a time; offer encouragement and provide simple, direct instructions ("walk to the bathroom") to avoid confusion. *Limiting new skills to small, critical units enhances learning.*
- Provide patient with ample time to perform each new mobility-related task. *Patient may need extensive supervision and repetition to master new tasks.*
- Provide supportive measures as indicated:
  - Perform range-of-motion exercises to joints (unless medically contraindicated) every shift; progress from passive to active, as tolerated, and monitor progress. *This prevents joint contracture and muscle atrophy.*
  - Turn and position patient every 2 hours; establish a turning schedule for dependent patients. Post at bedside and monitor effectiveness. *Regular turning and positioning prevents skin breakdown.*
  - Place joints in functional position (for example, trochanter roll along thigh) on an alternating schedule. *This prevents musculoskeletal deformities.*

– Encourage patient's active movement by use of trapeze and side rails, using unaffected leg to move affected leg, and performance of self-care activities. Provide frequent reinforcement and demonstrations. *This increases muscle tone and feelings of self-esteem and reinforces learning.*
– Walk patient with one or two assistants on regular schedule, if possible. *This preserves muscle tone, has positive psychological effect on patient and family, and prevents complications of immobility.*

• Teach patient (if capable) and family or significant other how to perform range-of-motion exercises, transfers, skin inspection and mobility regimen; provide time for return demonstrations with supervision. *Informed patient and significant other will be better prepared to prevent complications of immobility.*
• Encourage adherence to other aspects of health care management to control or minimize effects on mobility. *This promotes health and well-being by alleviating pain and preventing complications.*
• Refer to psychiatric liaison nurse, social service agency, support group, or other resources as appropriate *to provide patient with alternative approaches to care.*

Evaluations for expected outcomes
• Patient maintains functional mobility.
• Patient shows no evidence of skin breakdown, contractures, venous stasis, thrombus formation, hypostatic pneumonia, or other complications of impaired physical mobility.
• Patient begins to accept limitations imposed by mobility impairment and impact on life-style.
• Family or significant other communicates understanding of purpose and principles of mobility regimen.
• Family or significant other successfully demonstrates range-of-motion exercises, transfers, skin inspection, and other aspects of mobility regimen.
• Family or significant other identifies and contacts at least two sources for support.

Documentation
• Observations of patient's impaired mobility, perceptual or cognitive status, and response to treatment
• Interventions to provide supportive care
• Instructions to patient and family or significant other, their understanding of instructions, and demonstrated skill in carrying out the prescribed mobility program
• Patient's response to nursing interventions
• Patient's and family's or significant other's expressions of feelings and concern about immobility, impact on life-style, and capacity for participating in care
• Evaluations for each expected outcome.

Neglect, unilateral

related to neurologic illness or trauma

Definition
Lack of awareness of a body part

Assessment
• History of neurologic impairment
• Age

• Neurologic status, including awareness of body parts, cognition, level of consciousness, mental status, memory, sensory function, orientation, position sense, visual acuity, visual fields, ability to communicate (verbally and nonverbally), bowel and bladder control
• Musculoskeletal status, including coordination, muscle size and strength, muscle tone, range of motion, and functional mobility as follows:
  0 = completely independent
  1 = requires use of equipment or device
  2 = requires help, supervision, or teaching from another person
  3 = requires help from another person and equipment or device
  4 = dependent; does not participate in activity
• Integumentary status, including color, texture, turgor, temperature, elasticity, sensation, moisture, hygiene, lesions
• Psychosocial status, including coping mechanisms, support systems (family, significant other), life-style, understanding of physical condition
• Self-care abilities, including preparation of equipment and supplies, technical or mechanical skills, use of assistive devices

Defining characteristics
• Consistent inattention to stimuli on affected side
• Denial of body part affected by neurologic illness or trauma, either by refusing to acknowledge the paralysis, by neglecting the involved side, or by attributing ownership of paralyzed limb to someone else
• Inadequate self-care
• Lack of awareness of body part

Associated medical diagnoses (selected)
Bell's palsy, body image agnosia, cerebrovascular accident, head injury, hemianopsia, neoplastic brain disease

Expected outcomes
• Patient avoids injury to affected body part.
• Patient avoids skin breakdown.
• Patient avoids contractures.
• Patient recognizes neglected body part.
• Patient and family or significant other demonstrate measures to protect affected body part.
• Patient and family or significant other demonstrate exercises for affected body part.
• Patient and family or significant other express feelings about altered state of health and neurologic deficits.
• Patient and family or significant other identify community resources and support groups to help cope with the effects of illness.

Interventions and rationales
• Place sling on affected arm *to prevent dangling or injury.* Support affected leg and foot while in bed, place foot strap on wheelchair, and perform other measures as appropriate *to keep limbs in functional position and avoid contractures.* Use draw sheet to move patient up in bed *to avoid skin abrasions.*
• Touch and rub affected limb. Describe it in conversation with patient *to remind patient of neglected body part.*
• Direct patient to perform activities that require use of affected limb. *A patient who experiences usefulness of paretic or paralyzed limb will more easily integrate affected limb into his body image.*

- Encourage patient to check position of affected body part with each repositioning or transfer *to reestablish awareness of body part.*
- Establish and follow a regular turning schedule *to maintain skin integrity.*
- Request consultations with occupational and physical therapists regarding adaptive equipment, exercise program, and other recommendations *to increase awareness of affected limb.*
- Use safety belts or protective devices according to hospital policy. *Safety devices remind patient of limitations and help prevent falls.*
- Remove splints and other devices at least every 2 hours. Inspect skin for pressure areas. Reapply splint. *Proper use of splints and other devices prevents deformities and maintains skin integrity.*
- Perform range-of-motion exercises to the affected side at least once every shift, unless medically contraindicated, *to maintain joint flexibility and prevent contractures.*
- Instruct family and nursing personnel to observe position of affected body part frequently. Remove food or drainage from face if unnoticed by patient. Place arm or leg in proper position as often as necessary *to prevent injury.*
- Arrange environment for maximum functioning; for example, place water, TV controls, and call light within reach. *These measures enhance orientation and encourage independence.*
- Assist with activities of daily living or provide supervision as appropriate *to protect patient's affected side.*
- Encourage patient and family members or significant others to express feelings regarding the patient's condition and level of functioning *to release tension and enhance coping.*
- Refer patient and family or significant other to appropriate support groups and other community resources *to assist patient and family in adjusting to altered state of health.*

Evaluations for expected outcomes

- Patient does not experience injury.
- Patient's skin does not show signs of breakdown.
- Patient does not show evidence of contractures.
- Patient recognizes and protects neglected body part when carrying out activities of daily living.
- Patient and family or caregiver demonstrate exercise routine and program for protecting affected body part.
- Patient's environment is arranged for maximum functioning.
- Patient and family or significant other openly express fear and other feelings associated with patient's neurologic deficits and altered level of functioning.
- Patient and family or significant other identify and contact appropriate community resources and support groups.

Documentation

- Patient's expressions of feelings about neglected side of body
- Safety measures taken to prevent injury
- Patient's ability to perform activities of daily living and nursing measures taken to overcome deficits
- Observations of patient's and family's coping skills
- Patient's response to nursing interventions, including verbal expressions or behavior that indicate increased awareness of affected limb

• Evaluations for each expected outcome.

■ Noncompliance

related to patient's value system

Definition
Unwillingness to practice prescribed health-related behaviors

Assessment
• Age
• Health beliefs
• Patient's perceptions of health problem, treatment regimen, and importance of complying with treatment regimen
• Patient's ability to learn and perform prescribed treatment (activity, diet, medications)
• Financial resources
• Cultural and ethnic influences
• Religious influences
• Educational and language background

Defining characteristics
• Challenged beliefs and value systems
• Evidence of complications
• Evidence of symptom exacerbation
• Failure of objective tests
• Failure to adhere to treatment regimen, indicated either through direct observation of behavior or statements by the patient, family, or significant other
• Failure to keep appointments
• Failure to progress
• Inability to set or attain mutual goals

Associated medical diagnoses (selected)
This nursing diagnosis can occur in association with any medical diagnosis and depends upon the patient's value system.

Expected outcomes
• Patient identifies factors that influence noncompliance.
• Patient demonstrates a level of compliance that does not interfere with physiologic safety.
• Patient contracts with nurse to perform _____ (specify behavior and frequency).
• Patient uses support systems to modify noncompliant behavior.

Interventions and rationales
• Listen to patient's reasons for noncompliance. *Active listening may reveal concerns not clearly stated in words and helps individualize teaching process.*
• Approach patient in a nonjudgmental manner. *This demonstrates unconditional positive regard for the patient.*
• Identify specific areas of patient's noncompliant behavior *to help develop appropriate interventions.*
• Attempt to identify influencing factors associated with noncompliant behaviors, such as lack of understanding, unrealistic expectations, or cultural differences. *Reasons for noncompliance may range widely and include lack of knowledge, forgetting, feeling better or worse, and getting contradictory advice from family, friends, and health care providers.*
• Emphasize the positive aspects of compliance; *it can reduce risk factors, prevent complications, and help manage certain chronic diseases.*
• Assist patient with values clarification process *because values have both intellectual and emotional components and form a basis for patient's behavior.*

• Acknowledge patient's right to choose against carrying out the prescribed regimen. *Patient's autonomy must be respected; control over patient's action is legitimate only if needed to prevent harm to the patient, to others, or to yourself.*
• Contract with patient for behaviors that are not threatening. *This involves both patient and caregiver in formal commitment and gives patient sense of personal control.*
• Use support systems to enforce or reinforce negotiated behaviors. *Support from patient's family helps foster compliance.*
• Give positive reinforcement for compliant behavior *to encourage the patient to continue such behavior.*

Evaluations for expected outcomes
• Patient describes factors that influence noncompliance with health care regimen.
• Patient performs daily self-care in compliance with health care regimen.
• Patient performs behaviors agreed upon in contract with nurse.
• Patient uses available support resources as needed.

Documentation
• Patient's statements that indicate noncompliant behavior
• Direct observation of noncompliant behavior
• Statements by patient that provide insight into causes of noncompliant behavior
• Terms agreed upon by the patient in performing negotiated behaviors
• Patient's daily progress in complying with treatment regimen
• Evaluations for each expected outcome.

■ Nutrition alteration, high risk for: More than body requirements

related to excessive intake

Definition
Accentuated risk of change in normal eating pattern that results in increased body weight

Assessment
• Nutritional history, including financial resources, height and weight, hereditary influences, history of obesity, meal preparation, sociocultural influences, usual dietary pattern, weight fluctuations over past year
• Eating patterns, including internal and external cues that trigger desire to eat, rate of food consumption, stated food preferences
• Psychosocial status, including behavior, mood, stressors (finances, job, marital discord), coping mechanisms, sources of support (family, friends, others), life-style, knowledge level, hobbies, interests
• Activity levels
• Body image, including perception of observer and self-perception
• Additional circumstances which may lead to excessive intake

Risk factors
• Cognitive or emotional difficulties, such as perfectionism, dichotomous thinking, negative self-talk, isolation from support person or group
• Dysfunctional eating patterns, such as concentrating food intake at end of day, eating in response to internal cues other than hunger (guilt, anger, depression), pairing food with other activities, hiding food away for later

use, eating in response to external cues (time of day, social situations, television advertisements)
- Excessive preoccupation with food
- History of obesity
- Immobility
- Obesity in one or both parents
- Reduced motor ability
- Sedentary life-style
- Use of food to stave off boredom or relieve stress or as a reward or comfort measure

Associated medical diagnoses (selected)
Anxiety, depression, diabetes mellitus

Expected outcomes
- Patient expresses need to maintain or stabilize weight within 5 to 10 pounds of target weight.
- Patient plans to monitor weight and sustain target weight.
- Patient expresses feelings regarding dietary regimen and current weight.
- Patient identifies internal and external cues which lead to increased food consumption.
- Patient plans menus appropriate for prescribed diet.
- Patient adheres to prescribed diet.
- Patient participates in selected exercise program every week (specify).

Interventions and rationales
- Weigh patient weekly or as prescribed *to monitor effectiveness of diet.*
- Work with patient to establish realistic target weight. Instruct patient how to record weight. *Involvement in nursing care plan improves compliance.*
- Instruct patient to keep food diary. *This helps patient confront actual intake, break through denial, and achieve a more objective view of eating habits.*
- Monitor fluid intake and output and assess for edema. *Fluid retention may increase body weight.*
- Encourage patient to express feelings about dietary restrictions *to assess patient's perception of problem.* Help patient identify emotions associated with food and situations which trigger eating episodes. *Permanent weight maintenance requires an understanding of risk factors that contribute to weight gain.*
- Determine patient's food likes and dislikes *to evaluate eating habits and include preferred foods in patient's diet.*
- Encourage consumption of foods low in calories and fat, and high in complex carbohydrates and fiber. Have patient meet with dietitian to discuss meal planning. *These steps will help patient plan nutritious, well-balanced meals.*
- Refer patient to appropriate resource for behavior modification and cognitive therapy *to prevent relapse into high-risk eating behaviors.*
- Give patient emotional support and positive feedback for adhering to prescribed diet. *This will foster compliance and help ensure adherence to regimen.*
- Recommend patient explore group diet therapies, such as Weight Watchers or Overeaters Anonymous *to provide additional sources of information and encouragement.*
- Discuss importance of incorporating exercise into life-style. Help patient select a program with a variety of activities (swimming, walking, aerobics, biking) appropriate for age and physical condition. *Besides burning calories, exercise offers an alternative to eating to alleviate stress and fosters a sense of accomplishment.*

Evaluations for expected outcomes

- Patient expresses need to maintain or stabilize weight.
- Patient states plan to maintain food diary, weighs self weekly, and expresses motivation to sustain current weight.
- Patient expresses feelings regarding dietary regimen and current weight.
- Patient identifies at least three internal and three external cues that lead to increased food consumption.
- When filling out menus, patient selects low-fat, high-complex carbohydrate, high-fiber food.
- Patient adheres to prescribed diet, as evidenced by selection of well-balanced meals and low-calorie snacks.
- Patient selects at least two activities for exercise program.

Documentation

- Patient's expression of feelings about weight, eating, and dietary regimen
- Patient's weight
- Ability of patient to maintain target weight
- Foods consumed by patient
- Behaviors that facilitate or impede weight maintenance
- Evaluations for each expected outcome.

■ Nutrition alteration: Less than body requirements

related to inability to digest or absorb nutrients because of biological factors

Definition

Change in normal eating pattern that results in changed body weight

Assessment

- GI assessment, including antibiotic therapy, auscultation of bowel sounds, change in bowel habits, stool characteristics (color, amount, size, consistency), history of GI disorder or surgery, inspection of abdomen, pain or discomfort, usual bowel pattern, palpation for masses and tenderness, and percussion for tympany, dullness, nausea and vomiting
- Nutritional status, including change in type of food tolerated, financial resources, height and weight, meal preparation, serum albumin level, sociocultural influences, usual dietary pattern, weight fluctuations over past 10 years
- Change in intrapersonal or interpersonal factors, including internal or external cues that trigger desire to eat, rate of food consumption, and stated food preference
- Psychosocial status
- Activity level
- Coping behaviors
- Body image, including perception of observer and self-perception

Defining characteristics

- Abdominal pain with or without pathologic condition
- Body weight 20% or more under ideal weight for height and frame
- Diarrhea, steatorrhea
- Halitosis, coated tongue
- Hyperactive bowel sounds
- Loss of body weight with adequate food intake
- Pale conjunctivae and mucous membranes
- Perceived inability to digest food
- Poor muscle tone
- Poor skin turgor
- Pressure ulcers
- Reported inadequate food intake (less than recommended daily allowances)

• Sore, inflamed buccal cavity
• Weakness of muscles required for chewing or swallowing

Associated medical diagnoses (selected)
Acute gastritis, bleeding esophageal varices, cholecystitis, cirrhosis, Crohn's disease, diverticulitis, dumping syndrome, hepatitis, intestinal obstruction, malabsorption syndrome, pancreatitis, paralytic ileus, peptic ulcer, peritonitis, pressure ulcers, tumors of GI tract, ulcerative colitis

Expected outcomes
• Patient shows no further evidence of weight loss.
• Patient tolerates oral, tube, or I.V. feedings without adverse effects.
• Patient takes in _____ calories daily.
• Patient gains _____ lb weekly.
• Patient and family or significant other communicate understanding of preoperative instructions.
• Patient and family or significant other communicate understanding of special dietary needs.
• Patient and family or significant other demonstrate ability to plan diet after discharge.

Interventions and rationales
• Obtain and record patient's weight at the same time every day *to obtain the most accurate readings.*
• Monitor fluid intake and output *because body weight may decrease as a result of fluid loss.*
• Maintain parenteral fluids, as ordered, *to provide patient with needed fluids and electrolytes.*
• Provide diet prescribed for patient's specific condition, *to improve patient's nutritional status and increase weight.*
• Determine food preferences and provide them within limitations of patient's prescribed diet. *This enhances compliance with diet regimen.*
• Monitor electrolytes and report abnormal values. *Poor nutritional status may cause electrolyte imbalances.*
• If patient vomits, record amount, color, and consistency. Keep a record of all stools. *Vomitus and stool characteristics indicate status of nutrient absorption.*
• Refer to dietitian or nutritional support team for dietary management (possible regimens include yogurt feedings or low-bulk diet.) *Dietitian or nutritional support team can help patient and health team individualize diet within prescribed restrictions.*
• If patient is receiving tube feeding:
  – Add food coloring if patient has an altered state of consciousness or diminished gag reflex *to help detect aspiration.*
  – If possible, use continuous infusion pump *to avoid diarrhea.*
  – Begin regimen with small amount and diluted concentration *to decrease diarrhea and improve absorption.* Increase volume and concentration as tolerated.
  – Keep head of bed elevated during feeding *to reduce risk of aspiration.*
  – Check feeding tube placement each shift *to verify placement in GI tract rather than in lungs.*
• If patient receives total parenteral nutrition:
  – Ensure delivery as prescribed. *Electrolytes, amino acids, and other nutrients must be tailored to patient's needs.*
  – Monitor blood glucose levels and urine specific gravity at least once each shift. *Since glucose is the main component of hyperalimentation, patient may become hyperglycemic if not carefully monitored.*

• Monitor bowel sounds once a shift. *Normal active bowel sounds may indicate readiness for enteral feedings; hyperactive sounds may indicate poor absorption and may be accompanied by diarrhea.*
• Reinforce medical regimen by explaining to patient and family or significant other the reasons for present regimen. *Collaborative practice enhances patient's overall care.*
• Teach principles of good nutrition for the specific condition. *This encourages patient and significant others to participate in patient's care.*
• Provide or assist with oral hygiene *to help keep patient comfortable.*
• Provide preoperative teaching, if needed, *to reduce patient's fear and anxiety and promote understanding.*
• Involve family and significant other in meal planning *to encourage them to help patient comply with diet regimen after discharge.*

Evaluations for expected outcomes

• Patient remains at or above specified weight.
• Patient does not develop adverse reactions from feedings, such as aspiration of food particles into lungs, diarrhea, or hyperglycemia.
• Patient's weight increases by specified amount weekly.
• Patient consumes specified number of calories daily.
• Patient and family communicate understanding of preoperative instructions, either verbally or through behavior.
• Patient and family communicate understanding of special dietary needs, either verbally or through behavior.
• Patient and family plan appropriate diet for patient to follow after discharge.

Documentation

• Daily weight
• Mouth care
• Maintenance of nasogastric tube
• Intake and output
• Bowel sounds
• Blood glucose levels
• Urine specific gravity
• Patient's ability to eat
• Incidence of vomiting or diarrhea
• Presence of other complications
• Patient's statements of understanding of dietary education
• Evaluations for each expected outcome.

Nutrition alteration: Less than body requirements

related to inability to ingest foods

Definition

Change in normal eating pattern that results in changed body weight

Assessment

• GI assessment, including auscultation of bowel sounds; change in bowel habits; characteristics of stool (color, amount, size, consistency); history of GI disorder or surgery; inspection of abdomen; pain or discomfort; palpation for masses, tenderness; percussion for tympany, dullness; nausea, vomiting; usual bowel pattern
• Nutritional status, including financial resources, height, meal preparation, serum albumin level, sociocultural influences, usual dietary pattern, weight, weight fluctuations over past 10 years
• Intrapersonal and interpersonal factors, including internal and external cues that trigger desire to eat, rate of

food consumption, stated food preference
- Psychosocial status
- Activity level
- Coping behaviors
- Body image, including perception of observer, self-perception

Defining characteristics
- Abdominal pain with or without pathologic condition
- Body weight 20% or more under ideal weight for height and frame
- Diarrhea or steatorrhea
- Hyperactive bowel sounds
- Loss of body weight with adequate food intake
- Poor muscle tone
- Reported inadequate food intake: less than recommended daily allowances
- Sore, inflamed buccal cavity
- Weakness of muscles required for swallowing or mastication

Associated medical diagnoses (selected)
Acute gastritis, Alzheimer's disease, bleeding esophageal varices, cerebrovascular accident, cholecystitis, cirrhosis, Crohn's disease, diverticulitis, dumping syndrome, dysphagia, head injury, hepatitis, intestinal obstruction, malabsorption syndrome, pancreatitis, paralytic ileus, peptic ulcer, peritonitis, pressure ulcers, tumors of GI tract, ulcerative colitis

Expected outcomes
- Patient shows no further evidence of weight loss.
- Patient tolerates _____ ml of nasogastric or gastrostomy tube feedings.
- Patient avoids aspiration.
- Patient avoids episodes of diarrhea.
- Patient gains _____ lb weekly.
- Patient avoids skin breakdown or infection around tube site.
- Patient and family or significant other communicate understanding of special dietary needs.
- Patient and family or significant other demonstrate correct tube feeding procedures.

Interventions and rationales
- Obtain and record patient's weight at the same time every day *to obtain the most accurate readings.*
- Monitor fluid intake and output *because body weight may increase as a result of fluid retention.*
- Administer prescribed amount of tube feeding *to provide patient with needed nutrition.*
  - Begin regimen with small amount and diluted concentration *to decrease diarrhea and improve absorption.* Increase volume and concentration as tolerated.
  - Elevate head of bed during infusion *to reduce risk of aspiration.*
  - Check feeding tube placement at least once every shift *to verify placement in GI tract rather than in lungs.*
  - Give water and juices, as needed, *to maintain adequate hydration.*
  - If possible, use continuous infusion pump *to avoid diarrhea.*
  - Put food coloring in tube feeding *to monitor for aspiration.*
- Provide nares care every 4 hours *to prevent ulceration and skin breakdown.* Tape nasogastric tube *to prevent visual obstruction.* Use hypoallergenic tape *to minimize skin reactions.*
- Change gastrostomy dressing daily or according to institutional protocol.
- Ensure proper temperature of feeding (room temperature); change feeding tube bags and tubing according to institutional protocols.

• Assess and record bowel sounds once a shift *to monitor for an increase or decrease.*
• Auscultate and record breath sounds every 4 hours *to monitor for aspiration.* Report wheezes, rhonchi, crackles, or decreased breath sounds. If aspiration is suspected, stop tube feeding. Keep suction apparatus at bedside and suction as needed. Turn patient on side *to avoid further aspiration.*
• Instruct patient and family or significant other in tube feeding procedures. Supervise return demonstrations until competence is achieved. *This encourages patient and significant others to participate in patient's care.*

Evaluations for expected outcomes

• Patient shows no further evidence of weight loss.
• Patient tolerates nasogastric or gastrostomy tube feedings without adverse effects.
• Patient does not exhibit signs of aspiration, diarrhea, or hyperglycemia.
• Patient gains specified amount of weight weekly.
• Patient consumes specified amount of calories daily.
• Patient avoids skin breakdown or infection around tube site.
• Patient and significant other communicate understanding of special dietary needs and plan appropriate diet.
• Patient and significant other demonstrate correct tube feeding procedures.

Documentation

• Daily weights
• Intake and output
• Tolerance of tube feeding
• Incidents of vomiting, aspiration, diarrhea
• Bowel sounds
• Breath sounds
• Response to instructions
• Demonstration of feeding procedures
• Evaluations for each expected outcome.

■ Nutrition alteration: Less than body requirements

related to psychological factors

Definition

Change in normal eating pattern that results in changed body weight

Assessment

• Nutritional history, including financial resources, height and weight, hereditary influences, meal preparation, sociocultural influences, usual dietary pattern, weight fluctuations over past 10 years
• Change in intrapersonal or interpersonal factors, including internal and external cues that trigger desire to eat, rate of food consumption, stated food preference
• Activity level
• Coping behaviors
• Body image, including perception of observer and self-perception

Defining characteristics

• Abdominal pain with or without pathologic condition
• Aversion to eating
• Body weight 20% or more under ideal weight for height and frame
• Diarrhea
• Lack of interest in food
• Pale conjunctiva and mucous membranes
• Perceived inability to ingest food
• Poor muscle tone

• Reported inadequate food intake; less than recommended daily allowances

Associated medical diagnoses (selected)
Anorexia nervosa, bipolar disease (manic or depressive phase), bulimia, depression

Expected outcomes
• Patient consumes at least _____ calories daily.
• Patient gains _____ lb weekly.
• Patient eats independently, without being prodded.
• Patient identifies emotional and psychological factors that interfere with eating.
• Patient develops a plan to monitor and maintain target weight at discharge.
• Patient plans to use mental health resources to help resolve psychological problems.

Interventions and rationales
• Provide opportunities for patient to discuss reasons for not eating *to help assess causes of eating disorder.*
• Observe and record patient's intake (both liquid and solid) *to assess which nutrients are consumed and which supplements are needed.*
• Determine patient's food preferences and attempt to obtain these foods. Offer foods that appeal to olfactory, visual, and tactile senses *to enhance patient's appetite.*
• Offer high-protein, high-calorie supplements, such as milk shakes, custard, or ice cream. *Such foods prevent body protein breakdown and provide caloric energy.*
• Serve foods that require little cutting or chewing *to help prevent malingering at meals.*
• Provide a pleasant environment at mealtime *to enhance patient's appetite.*
• Keep snacks at bedside *to give patient some control over eating time.*
• With some patients, begin with nutritious liquids and gradually introduce solids. *A severely malnourished patient may not be able to chew solid foods immediately.*
• Avoid asking whether patient is hungry or wants to eat. Be positive in offering food. *A positive, undemanding attitude avoids confrontation with patient.*
• Whenever possible, sit with patient for predetermined length of time during meal. *This inhibits patient from dawdling during meal, or from hiding or hoarding food.*
• Monitor and record elimination patterns. *Patient may be taking laxatives or diuretics to keep weight low in spite of eating.*
• Weigh patient at the same time every day. Reinforce weight gain with privileges or rewards. *This yields accurate data and gives patient some control over food eaten and privileges or rewards gained.*
• Set target weight and have patient record daily weight, *to involve patient in treatment.*
• Refer patient and significant others to appropriate mental health professional. *Most eating disorders are psychological. Patient and significant others must be followed and treated to prevent recurrence.*

Evaluations for expected outcomes
• Patient consumes specified number of calories daily.
• Patient gains specified amount of weight weekly.
• Patient eats independently without constant encouragement.

- Patient lists emotional and psychological factors that interfere with eating.
- Patient states plan to monitor and maintain specific target weight after discharge.
- Patient contacts support groups and mental health resources as needed.

Documentation

- Patient's expressed attitudes toward food and eating at the present time
- Patient's expressed feelings about weight, body image, emotional status
- Patient's daily intake (liquid and solid) and output (urine, stool, vomitus)
- Daily weights; progression of weight gain
- Interventions to feed patient adequately
- Emotional support provided
- Patient's response to nursing interventions
- Evaluations for each expected outcome.

Nutrition alteration: More than body requirements

related to excessive intake

Definition

Change in normal eating pattern that results in changed body weight

Assessment

- Nutritional history, including financial resources, height and weight, hereditary influences, history of obesity, meal preparation, sociocultural influences, usual dietary pattern, weight fluctuations over past 10 years
- Change in intrapersonal or interpersonal factors, including internal and external cues that trigger desire to eat, motivation to lose weight, rate of food consumption, stated food preference
- Psychosocial status
- Activity level
- Coping patterns
- Body image, including perception of observer and self-perception

Defining characteristics

- Body weight 10% or more over ideal weight for height and frame
- Clinical obesity
- Dysfunctional eating patterns, such as concentrating food intake at end of day, eating in response to internal cue other than hunger (anxiety, for example), eating in response to such social cues as time of day and social situation, pairing food with other activities
- Observed use of food as a reward or comfort measure
- Reported or observed obesity in one or both parents
- Triceps skin fold greater than 15 mm in men and 25 mm in women

Associated medical diagnoses (selected)

Anxiety, depression, diabetes mellitus, Pickwickian syndrome

Expected outcomes

- Patient voices feelings about present weight.
- Patient identifies internal and external cues that increase food consumption.
- Patient states need to lose weight.
- Patient sets a weight-loss goal of _____ lb weekly.
- Patient plans menus appropriate to prescribed diet.
- Patient adheres to prescribed diet.
- Patient loses at least _____ lb weekly.

- Patient sets target weight before discharge.
- Patient states plan to monitor and maintain target weight.
- Patient participates in selected exercise program _____ times weekly.

Interventions and rationales

- Help patient identify the problem, feelings associated with eating, and circumstances in which patient turns to food. *Permanent weight loss starts with examination of factors contributing to weight gain.*
- Discuss patient's normal food preferences *to evaluate eating habits and include preferred foods in patient's diet.*
- Have dietician discuss meal planning with patient during hospitalization *to help patient plan nutritious, satisfying meals.*
- If resource is available, refer patient to a mental health professional for behavior modification *to help patient change poor eating habits and ensure permanent weight loss.*
- Teach patient about low-calorie, nutritious foods. *This encourages patient to eat foods that provide energy without causing weight gain.*
- Help patient set realistic goals for losing weight. *This aids positive reinforcement and reduces frustration.*
- Give patient emotional support and positive feedback for adhering to prescribed dietary regimen *to promote compliance.* Encourage nondietary rewards, such as purchase of a new accessory or book, *to promote continuation of dietary plan and help patient avoid using food as a reward.*
- Weigh patient weekly or as prescribed *to monitor effectiveness of diet plan.*
- Set target weight with patient and have patient record weight. *This involves patient in plan and provides positive reinforcement.*
- Explore feasibility of having patient participate after discharge in Weight Watchers, Overeaters Anonymous, or other group or individual diet therapies. *Such resources provide reinforcement and information.*
- Help patient select an exercise program (walking, jogging, aerobics, swimming) appropriate to age and physical condition. *Besides aiding weight loss, activities offer an alternative to eating to alleviate stress.*

Evaluations for expected outcomes

- Patient expresses feelings about present weight.
- Patient identifies cues that increase food consumption.
- Patient expresses desire to lose weight.
- Patient and health care professional establish weekly weight loss goal.
- Patient and family plan menus within parameters of prescribed diet.
- Patient adheres to prescribed diet.
- Patient loses specified amount of weight weekly.
- Patient and health care professional set target weight before discharge.
- Patient summarizes plan to monitor and maintain specified target weight.
- Patient participates in specific number of selected exercise activities weekly.

Documentation

- Patient's expressions of feelings about weight, eating, food, dieting
- Goals set by patient
- Record of weight
- Foods consumed by patient
- Behaviors that facilitate or impede weight reduction
- Evaluations for each expected outcome.

Oral mucous membrane alteration

related to dehydration

Definition
Altered mouth integrity

Assessment
- History of pathologic conditions known to cause dehydration, such as diabetes
- Medications such as diuretics and antihistamines
- Vital signs
- Fluid and electrolyte status, including blood urea nitrogen, creatinine, intake and output, mucous membranes, serum electrolytes, skin turgor, urine specific gravity
- Oral status, including inspection of oral cavity (gums and tongue), pain or discomfort, salivation
- Nutritional status, including current weight, change from normal weight, and dietary pattern
- Psychosocial status, including change in financial status, coping skills, habits (smoking, alcohol intake), patient's perception of health problem, recent traumatic event

Defining characteristics
- Clinical evidence of dehydration
- Coated tongue
- Decreased or absent salivation
- Dry mouth
- Halitosis
- Oral lesions or ulcers
- Oral pain or discomfort
- Oral plaque
- Stomatitis
- Thirst

Associated medical diagnoses (selected)
Alcoholism, anorexia nervosa, depression, diabetes insipidus, diabetes mellitus (uncontrolled), drug-induced stomatitis, fever, GI dysfunction involving vomiting or diarrhea, heat exhaustion, heat stroke, hemorrhage, hypovolemic shock, NPO status, oxygen therapy, postoperative status, radiation therapy

Expected outcomes
- Patient maintains fluid balance (intake equals output).
- Patient states increased comfort.
- Oral mucous membranes are pink and moist.
- Complications are avoided or minimized.
- Patient correlates precipitating factors with appropriate oral care.
- Patient demonstrates oral hygiene practices.

Interventions and rationales
- Inspect patient's oral cavity every shift. Describe and document condition; report any change in status. *Regular assessments can anticipate or alleviate problems.*
- Perform prescribed treatment regimen, including administering I.V. or oral fluids, *to improve condition of patient's mucous membranes.* Monitor progress, reporting favorable and adverse responses to treatment regimen.
- Provide supportive measures, as indicated:
  - Assist with oral hygiene before and after meals *to promote feeling of comfort and well-being.*
  - Use a toothbrush with suction if patient cannot spit out water *to minimize risk of aspiration.*
  - Provide mouthwash or gargles, as ordered, *to increase patient*

comfort and maintain moisture in mouth.
 - Lubricate patient's lips frequently with water-based lubricant *to prevent cracked, irritated skin.*
- Instruct patient in oral hygiene practices, if necessary. Have patient return demonstration of oral care routine.
 - Use soft-bristled toothbrush.
 - Brush with circular motion downward from the gums.
 - Include the tongue when brushing.
 - Review need for routine visits to dentist (annually for adults).

These measures increase patient's awareness of oral hygiene practices and reduce discomfort, resulting in increased nutrition and hydration.
- Tell patient to chew gum or suck on sugarless hard candy *to stimulate salivation.*
- Discuss precipitating factors, if known, and work to prevent future episodes. For example, encourage patient to avoid exercising in heat and to report effects of medication. *Patient's increased awareness of causative factors will help prevent recurrence.*
- Encourage adherence to other aspects of health care management (controlling diabetes, changing dietary habits, avoiding alcoholic beverages) *to control or minimize effects on mucous membranes.*

Evaluations for expected outcomes
- Patient's total daily fluid intake equals total output.
- Patient chews and swallows without discomfort.
- Patient's mucous membranes remain moist, pink, and free of cuts and abrasions.
- Patient does not develop complications related to extended dehydration of mucous membranes.
- Patient discusses possible causes of alteration in oral mucous membranes, such as heat exhaustion or reactions to medication.
- Patient discusses preventive measures, such as regular oral hygiene.
- Patient demonstrates prescribed oral hygiene measures.

Documentation
- Observations of condition, healing, and response to treatment
- Interventions to provide supportive care and patient's response to supportive care
- Instructions given, patient's understanding of instructions, and patient's demonstrated skill in carrying out prescribed oral care measures
- Evaluations for each expected outcome.

Oral mucous membrane alteration

related to mechanical trauma

Definition
Altered mouth integrity

Assessment
- History of oral surgery, dentures, braces, or dental problems
- Medications such as diuretics or antihistamines
- Vital signs
- Fluid and electrolyte status, including blood urea nitrogen, creatinine, intake and output, mucous membranes, serum electrolytes, skin turgor, urine specific gravity

- Oral status, including inspection of oral cavity (with gums and tongue), pain or discomfort, salivation
- Nutritional status, including current weight, change from normal weight, dietary pattern
- Psychosocial status, including coping skills, patient's perception of health problem, recent traumatic event

Defining characteristics
- Braces
- Decreased or absent salivation
- Dry mouth
- Halitosis
- Ill-fitting dentures
- Leukoplakia
- Oral lesions or ulcers
- Oral pain or discomfort
- Oral plaque

Associated medical diagnoses (selected)
Abscessed tooth, facial fracture, hemorrhagic gingivitis, impacted wisdom teeth, jaw fracture, other conditions requiring oral surgery

Expected outcomes
- Patient maintains fluid balance (intake equals output).
- Oral mucous membranes are pink and moist.
- Patient states increased comfort.
- Complications are avoided or minimized.
- Patient correlates precipitating factors with appropriate oral care.
- Patient demonstrates correct oral hygiene practices.

Interventions and rationales
- Inspect patient's oral cavity every shift. Describe and document condition and report any status change. *Mechanical trauma can be caused by ill-fitting dentures, jagged teeth, braces, oral surgery, and insertion of endotracheal tube. Regular assessments can anticipate or alleviate problems.*
- Establish and follow routine oral hygiene schedule. For example, soak dentures every evening, cleanse with denture cream, rinse, and keep in properly labeled container at patient's bedside. *Routine oral hygiene can improve condition of mucous membranes.*
- Provide supportive measures, as indicated:
  - Assist with oral hygiene before and after meals *to promote feeling of comfort and well-being.*
  - Use a toothbrush with suction if patient cannot spit out water *to minimize risk of aspiration.*
  - Provide mouthwash or gargles, as ordered, *to increase patient comfort.*
  - Lubricate patient's lips frequently with water-based lubricant. *Fluid and food intake increases when comfort is increased.*
- Instruct patient in oral hygiene practices, if necessary. Have patient return demonstration of oral care routine. Tell patient to stimulate saliva by chewing gum or sucking on sugarless hard candy. *These measures increase patient's awareness of oral hygiene practices and reduce discomfort, resulting in increased nutrition and hydration.*
- Discuss precipitating factors, if known, and work to prevent future episodes (for example, weight loss may change contours of oral cavity). *Patient's increased awareness of causative factors will help prevent recurrence.*
- Encourage adherence to other aspects of health care management *to control or minimize effects on mucous membranes.* For example, encourage

patients with braces to avoid popcorn, chewing gum, caramels. *These measures reduce risk of trauma to oral mucous membrane.*
- Refer patient to dentist, dental hygienist, or other appropriate resource to correct ill-fitting dentures, modify braces, adjust jaw wires, etc. *Regularly scheduled dental follow-up reduces risk of trauma to oral mucous membranes.*

Evaluations for expected outcomes
- Patient's total daily fluid intake equals output.
- Patient's mucous membranes remain moist, pink, and free of cuts and abrasions.
- Patient chews and drinks without discomfort.
- Patient does not exhibit complications related to trauma to oral mucous membranes.
- Patient discusses possible causes of alteration in oral mucous membrane, such as ill-fitting dentures or braces.
- Patient discusses preventive measures, such as regular oral hygiene, including cleaning of dentures.
- Patient demonstrates prescribed oral hygiene measures.

Documentation
- Observations of condition, healing, and response to treatment
- Interventions to provide supportive care and patient's response to supportive care
- Instructions given, patient's understanding of instructions, and demonstrated skill in carrying out prescribed oral care measures
- Evaluations for each expected outcome.

■ Oral mucous membrane alteration

related to pathologic condition

Definition
Altered mouth integrity

Assessment
- History of oral cavity disorder or surgery
- Medication history
- Oral status, including condition of teeth, inspection of oral cavity (including gums and tongue), oral hygiene routine, pain or discomfort, palpation of buccal mucosa, salivation
- Nutritional status, including current weight, change from normal weight, dietary pattern, vitamin intake
- Psychosocial status, including coping skills, family or significant other, habits (smoking, alcohol intake), patient's perception of health problem, self-concept, stressors (finances, family, job)

Defining characteristics
- Carious teeth
- Clinical evidence of pathology affecting oral mucous membranes
- Coated tongue
- Decreased or absent salivation
- Desquamation
- Dry mouth
- Gum hypertrophy or recession
- Halitosis
- Hyperemia
- Inflammation of gums or mucous membranes
- Leukoplakia
- Oral edema, bleeding, exudates
- Oral lesions, vesicles, ulcers
- Oral pain or discomfort
- Oral plaque

Associated medical diagnoses (selected)
Aphthous ulcers, bleeding disorders, cardiovascular disease with anticoagulant therapy, carious teeth, dental surgery, fractured jaw, gingivitis (all types), head and neck cancer with irradiation or chemotherapy, leukemia, malnutrition, oral cancer, oral candidiasis, oral trauma, periodontal disease, scurvy, stomatitis, terminal cancer

Expected outcomes
- Lesions or wounds show improvement or heal.
- Complications are avoided or minimized.
- Patient voices increased comfort.
- Patient demonstrates understanding of surgical measures.
- Patient voices feelings about condition.
- Patient explains oral care routine.
- Patient demonstrates oral hygiene practices.

Interventions and rationales
- Inspect patient's oral cavity every shift. Describe and document condition, reporting any status change. *Regular assessment prevents recurrence or exacerbation of problems.*
- Perform prescribed treatment regimen for the underlying pathologic condition. Report favorable and adverse responses to treatment regimen. *Treating underlying condition improves condition of oral mucous membranes.*
- Encourage patient to state feelings and concerns about oral condition and its impact on body image, *to help him accept changes in body image.*
- Provide supportive measures as indicated:
  - Assist with oral hygiene before and after meals. Use soft-bristled toothbrush or cotton applicator and nonalcoholic mouthwash, *to minimize trauma to damaged tissues.*
  - Lubricate patient's lips frequently *to prevent cracking and irritation.*
  - Use artificial saliva solution if mouth remains dry *to restore normal moisture.*
  - Avoid serving hot, cold, spicy, fried, or citrus foods, *which irritate damaged tissue.*
  - Suction oral cavity to prevent drooling and aspiration of accumulated secretions. *Aspiration may lead to pneumonia or coughing and further trauma.*
  - To reduce pain, give soft or pureed foods, *which don't irritate tissues.*
- If oral surgery is scheduled, give appropriate preoperative and postoperative instruction and care. Document response. *Instruction enhances compliance with therapy.*
- Instruct patient in oral hygiene practices and have patient give return demonstration. Suggest referral to dentist or dental hygienist. *This increases patient's awareness of oral hygiene and reduces discomfort, resulting in increased nutrition and hydration.*
- Encourage patient to stop smoking. *Smoking has been linked to mucous membrane breakdown and cancer.*
- Refer to psychiatric liaison nurse or support group, *to help patient cope with altered body image.*

Evaluations for expected outcomes
- Lesions or wounds are absent or cause the patient less discomfort.
- Patient does not exhibit complications related to trauma to oral mucous membranes.

• Patient chews and swallows without discomfort.
• Patient discusses impending surgical procedures.
• Patient discusses fears of oral surgery and outcomes.
• Patient discusses postoperative oral care routine.
• Patient demonstrates oral hygiene practices, including treatments and medications.

Documentation
• Patient's expression of concern about oral condition and its impact on body image
• Patient's willingness to join in own care
• Observations of condition, healing, and response to treatment
• Interventions to provide supportive care and patient's response to supportive care
• Instructions given, patient's understanding of instructions, and demonstrated skill in carrying out prescribed oral care measures
• Evaluations for each expected outcome.

■ Pain

related to physical, biological, or chemical agents

Definition
Subjective sensation of discomfort derived from multiple sensory nerve interactions generated by physical, chemical, biological, or psychological stimuli

Assessment
• Descriptive characteristics of pain, including location, quality, intensity on a scale of 1 to 10, temporal factors, sources of relief
• Physiologic variables, such as age and pain tolerance
• Psychological variables, such as body image, personality, previous experience with pain, anxiety, and secondary gain
• Sociocultural variables, including cognitive style, culture or ethnicity, attitude and values, sex, and birth order
• Environmental variables, such as the setting and time

Defining characteristics
• Alteration in muscle tone (may range from listless to rigid)
• Autonomic responses not seen in chronic stable pain (diaphoresis, blood pressure and pulse rate change, dilated pupils, and increased or decreased respiratory rate)
• Communication (verbal or coded) of pain description
• Distracting behavior, such as moaning, crying, and seeking out other people or activities
• Facial mask of pain, characterized by lackluster eyes, a "beaten" look, fixed or scattered movement, or grimacing
• Guarding or protective behavior, such as favoring a body part
• Narrowed focus, including altered time perception, withdrawal from social contact, and impaired thought process
• Self-focusing

Associated medical diagnoses (selected)
Pain can be experienced with most medical diagnoses. The following represent diagnoses in which pain is severe: angina pectoris, burns, migraine headache, myocardial infarction, pancreatitis, renal colic, thoracic surgery

Expected outcomes

- Patient identifies pain characteristics.
- Patient articulates factors that intensify pain and modifies behavior accordingly.
- Patient expresses a feeling of comfort and relief from pain.
- Patient states and carries out appropriate interventions for pain relief.

Interventions and rationales

- Assess patient's physical symptoms of pain and administer pain medication as prescribed. Monitor and record medication's effectiveness and side effects. *Assessment allows for care plan modification as needed.*
- Perform comfort measures to promote relaxation, such as massage, bathing, repositioning, relaxation techniques. *These measures reduce muscle tension or spasm, redistribute pressure on body parts, and help patient focus on non-pain-related subjects.*
- Plan activities with the patient to provide distraction, such as reading, crafts, television, or visits, *to help patient focus on non-pain-related matters.*
- Provide the patient with information to help increase pain tolerance; for example, reasons for pain and length of time it will last. *This educates patient and encourages compliance in trying alternative pain relief measures.*
- Manipulate the environment to promote periods of uninterrupted rest. *This promotes health, well-being, and increased energy level important to pain relief.*
- Apply heat or cold as ordered (specify) *to minimize or relieve pain.*
- Help patient into a comfortable position and use pillows to splint or support painful areas, as appropriate, *to reduce muscle tension or spasm and to redistribute pressure on body parts.*
- Collaborate with patient in administering prescribed analgesics when alternative methods of pain control are inadequate. *Gaining patient's trust and involvement helps ensure compliance and may reduce medication intake.*

Evaluations for expected outcomes

- Patient's pain rating is documented (using a scale of 1 to 10) before administering medication and 30 to 45 minutes afterward.
- Patient articulates factors that intensify pain and modifies behavior accordingly.
- Patient carries out alternative pain control measures, such as heat or cold applications.
- Patient reports more than 4 hours sleep nightly (reports of less than 4 hours require further assessment).
- Patient decreases amount and frequency of pain medication within 72 hours.
- Patient expresses a feeling of comfort.

Documentation

- Patient's description of physical pain, pain relief, and feelings about pain
- Observations of patient's physical, psychological, and sociocultural responses to pain
- Comfort measures and medications provided to reduce pain; also effectiveness of interventions
- Information provided to patient about pain and pain relief
- Other interventions performed to assist patient with pain control
- Evaluations for each expected outcome.

Pain

related to psychological factors

Definition

Subjective sensation of discomfort derived from multiple sensory nerve interactions generated by physical, chemical, biological, or psychological stimuli

Assessment

- History of exposure to physical, biological, or chemical agents as a cause of pain
- Descriptive characteristics of pain, including location, quality, intensity on a scale of 1 to 10, temporal factors, and sources of provocation or relief
- Physiologic variables, such as age and pain tolerance
- Psychological variables, such as body image, personality, previous experience with pain, anxiety, and secondary gain
- Sociocultural variables, including cognitive style, culture and ethnicity, attitude and values, sex, and birth order
- Environmental variables, such as time and setting

Defining characteristics

- Absence or insufficient levels of physical, biological, or chemical agents to cause pain intensity experienced by patient
- Communication (verbal or coded) of pain description
- Distracting behavior, such as moaning, crying, pacing or restlessness, or seeking out other people or activities
- Facial mask of pain, including lackluster eyes, a "beaten" look, fixed or scattered movement, grimacing, and altered muscle tone (may range from listless to rigid)
- Guarding or protective behavior, such as favoring a body part
- Narrowed focus, including altered time perception, withdrawal from social contact, and impaired thought processes
- Pattern of pain described by patient that's difficult to associate with a physiologic process

Associated medical diagnoses (selected)

Depending on the variables present in assessment, such psychological factors as stress, depression, and ineffective coping mechanisms may intensify pain caused by physical, biological, or chemical agents. An example of psychological pain is the phantom pain often experienced following limb amputation.

Expected outcomes

- Patient identifies specific characteristics of pain.
- Patient expresses relief from pain within a reasonable time after taking prescribed medication.
- Patient helps develop a plan for pain control.
- Patient articulates possibility of physical pain being associated with emotional stressors.
- Patient requires less pain medication (specify).
- Patient states satisfaction with pain management regimen.
- Patient utilizes available resources to understand pain phenomenon and cooperates with treatment plan.

Interventions and rationales

- Assess physical symptoms that require pain medication and administer medication as prescribed. *Continuous reassessment documents patient's sub-*

jective complaints and behavior with organic pathology.
• Return to patient in 30 minutes to check medication's effectiveness. *This establishes trusting-caring relationship that encourages accurate communication.*
• Discuss with patient possible association between exacerbation of pain and patient's identified stressors. *This helps patient explore exacerbating emotional or environmental factors that may affect pain.*
• Ask patient to help establish goals and develop plan for pain control. *This gives patient sense of control.*
• Provide patient with positive feedback about progress toward reaching goals *to improve motivation and encourage compliance.*
• Spend at least 15 minutes per shift allowing patient to express feelings, *which will help give patient a sense of control.*
• Consider the services of a psychiatric mental health professional to help patient and staff establish a realistic plan to resolve the problem. *Patients who remain helpless, unmotivated, uncooperative and manipulative are self-destructive. Underlying causes should be explored.*
• Plan activities to distract the patient, such as reading, television, and family visits, *to help keep the patient from focusing on pain.*

Evaluations for expected outcomes
• Patient discusses characteristics of pain, including location, duration, and frequency.
• Patient reports achieving pain relief with analgesia or other measures.
• Patient participates in development of health care plan and discusses modifications.
• Patient acknowledges that pain may be related to emotional factors and lists stressors that may exacerbate pain.
• Patient achieves reduction in use of pain medication.
• Patient states satisfaction with pain management regimen.
• Patient displays motivation by seeking out resources to explain pain phenomenon and cooperating with treatment plan.

Documentation
• Patient's expressions of physical pain and well-being, and emotional pain and well-being
• Observations of patient's physical well-being
• Interventions performed to assist patient in controlling pain
• Results of interventions
• Evaluations for each expected outcome.

■ Pain, chronic

related to physical disability

Definition
Pain complaints that last longer than the expected healing process, which is usually 6 to 12 weeks

Assessment
• Descriptive characteristics of pain, including location, quality, intensity on a scale of 1 to 10, temporal factors, duration, precipitating factors (food, alcohol, activity, stress), comfort factors
• Physiologic variables, such as general health state, length of pain, organ system involvement, pain tolerance, disability (work, family, social), pain interventions (injection, traction, ice, physical therapy, trans-

cutaneous electrical nerve stimulation [TENS])
- Psychological variables, such as age, self-esteem, self-worth, role (worker, husband, breadwinner), coping behavior (appropriate or inappropriate), secondary gains (disability insurance, workmen's compensation, litigation), suffering (emotional component), manipulative behavior, dependence on others or on system, previous hospital experience
- Sociocultural variables, including educational level, motivation, culture or ethnicity, sex, values and beliefs, pain behaviors, financial distress, religion
- Environmental variables, such as setting and time
- Pharmacologic variables, including type of drugs, amount used in one day, use of illicit drugs, and use of alcohol

Defining characteristics
- Autonomic responses generally absent
- Communication (verbal or coded) of pain description
- Demands for immediate relief
- Fatigue
- GI concerns or problems
- Insomnia
- Muscle tone alteration; spasm
- Narrowed perception and awareness of surroundings
- Pain behavior: crying, moaning
- Protective behavior: guarding, limping
- Self-focusing
- Sexual dysfunction
- Weight gain or loss

Associated medical diagnoses (selected)
Cervical pain, chronic low back pain, diabetic neuropathy, intermittent or chronic headaches, phantom limb, postherpetic neuralgia, postsurgical pain, reflex sympathetic dystrophy

Expected outcomes
- Patient identifies characteristics of pain and pain behaviors.
- Patient develops pain management program that includes activity and rest schedule, exercise program, and medication regimen that's not pain-contingent.
- Patient carries out resocialization behavior and activities.
- Patient states relationship of increasing pain to stress, activity, and fatigue.
- Patient states importance of self-care behavior or activities.

Interventions and rationales
- Assess patient's physical symptoms of pain, physical complaints, and daily activities. Administer pain medication as prescribed. Monitor and record effectiveness and adverse effects of medication. (Keep in mind that pain behavior and pain talk may be inconsistent.) *Correlating patient's pain behavior with activities, time of day, and visits may be useful in modifying tasks.*
- Develop behavior-oriented care plan, following activity schedule, for example. *Learned pain behaviors must be modified through behavioral-cognitive measures.*
- Instruct patient in use of relaxation techniques, music, or therapy to relieve pain, *as adjunct to medications; also to increase self-help and foster independence.*
- Teach patient and family such techniques as massage, use of ice, or exercise *to relieve pain and foster independence.*
- Work closely with staff and patient's family *to achieve pain man-*

agement goals and maximize patient's cooperation.

- Use behavior modification; for example, spend time with patient only if discussion includes no pain talk. Use contingency rewards for decreasing pain talk and pain behavior. *Reducing pain talk helps patient refocus on other, more important, matters.*
- Encourage self-care activities. Develop a schedule. *This helps patient gain sense of control and reduces dependence on caregivers and society.*
- Establish a specific time to talk with patient about pain and its psychological and emotional effects *to establish a trusting, supportive relationship encompassing patient's physiologic, emotional, social, sexual, and financial concerns.*

Evaluations for expected outcomes

- Patient maintains activity diary and pain level chart that rates severity of pain on a scale of 1 to 10.
- Patient maintains a pain management program that includes activity and rest schedule, exercise program, and medication regimen.
- Patient's increased activity is documented in daily activity diary.
- Patient uses two or three alternative measures to achieve pain relief for 1 hour before asking for medication. An observer verifies and documents patient's efforts.
- Patient and family develop realistic expectations for day-to-day living.
- Patient discusses pain issue only during specified time.
- Patient discusses past relationships with family and friends and identifies new roles.
- Patient states that stress, activity, and fatigue may increase pain.
- Patient states that self-care activities are important.

Documentation

- Patient's description of physical pain, pain relief, and feelings about pain
- Pain talk and pain behavior and affect
- Relationship of reports of pain to activities
- Treatments and pain talk
- Time out of bed
- Comfort measures initiated by nurse, patient, or family
- Response to interventions
- Response to pharmacologic agents
- Interaction with staff
- Evaluations for each expected outcome.

■ Peripheral neurovascular dysfunction, high risk for

Definition

Accentuated risk of disruption in circulation or sensation in an extremity or motion of an extremity

Assessment

- History of trauma or vascular injuries
- Inspection of extremities, including signs of soft-tissue injury such as abrasions, lacerations, contusions
- Pain sensation, including characteristics (sharp, dull, constant, intermittent), precipitating factors, reaction to passive stretching of affected muscles
- Tactile sensation in areas innervated by major nerves of upper extremities, including deltoid, radial side of forearm, palmar surface of thumb, fingers, palmar surface of little finger, webbed space between thumb and index finger

- Tactile sensation in lower extremities, including medial side of foot and leg, medial side of thigh, sole of foot, lateral aspect of leg below the knee
- Motor nerve function of the upper extremities, including arm abduction at the shoulder, arm flexion at the elbow, thumb and little finger opposition, abduction and adduction of fingers, extension of wrist and fingers
- Motor nerve function of lower extremities, including knee extension, thigh adduction, plantar flexion and dorsiflexion of ankle, flexion and extension of toes
- Pulses in upper and lower extremities, including radial, ulnar, brachial, femoral, popliteal, posterior tibial, dorsalis pedis
  - bilateral comparison
  - quality using the following scale:

  0 = absent
  1 = very weak, barely palpable
  2 = weak, reduced
  3 = slightly weak, easily located
  4 = normal, easily located
- Vascular status, including capillary refill time, blanching, skin temperature, skin color
- Point tenderness, especially over bony prominences
- Edema
- Increased intracompartmental pressure
- Cranial nerves (if patient has halo cast)

Risk factors
- Fractures
- Mechanical compression, such as tourniquet, cast, brace, dressing, or restraint
- Orthopedic surgery
- Trauma
- Immobilization
- Burns
- Vascular obstruction

Associated medical diagnoses (selected)
Carpal tunnel syndrome, compartment syndrome, ganglion cyst, neurovascular compression, peripheral circulatory failure, peripheral nerve entrapment syndrome, vascular insufficiency, vascular occlusion

Expected outcomes
- Patient does not experience disability related to peripheral neurovascular dysfunction after injury or treatment.
- Patient maintains circulation in extremities.
- Patient can feel and move each toe or finger after application of cast, splint, or brace.
- Patient demonstrates correct body positioning techniques.
- Patient or significant other expresses understanding of risk for altered neurovascular status and the need to report symptoms of impaired circulation.
- If appropriate, patient enrolls in smoking cessation program.
- Symptoms of neurovascular compromise are absent.

Interventions and rationales
- Note if patient is to undergo surgery or procedure that increases his risk of peripheral neurovascular dysfunction *to anticipate complications.*
- Immobilize joints directly above and below a suspected fracture site, leaving room for pulse assessment *to facilitate monitoring of circulatory status.*
- As appropriate, assess circulation before application of cast, brace, or splint. After application of cast, brace, or splint, have patient move fingers and toes every 4 hours until

discharge *to detect signs of impaired circulation.*

- Remove clothing around suspected fracture site, clean site, apply sterile dressings to open wounds, and carefully apply cast, brace, or splint *to avoid further infection and trauma.*
- Follow institutional guidelines for the application of devices such as tourniquets, restraints, and tape *to ensure adequate circulation in affected extremity.*
- If you suspect nerve compression, assess position of extremity that has cast, brace, or splint. *Positioning of extremity may affect circulation.*
- Elevate limb above heart level after surgery or trauma *to reduce risk of edema.* If increased intracompartmental pressure is evident, maintain affected limb at heart level *to reduce pressure.*
- If edema appears in affected extremity, split, bivalve, slit, or cut a window in the cast and padding, according to institutional protocol, *to avoid neurovascular impairment.*
- Inject prescribed neurotoxic agents (such as penicillin G, hydrocortisone, tetanus toxoid, and diazepam) away from affected extremity and major nerves *to avoid injury.*
- Avoid flexing affected extremity. *Flexion may reduce venous circulation, thereby increasing risk of neurovascular complications.*
- If patient smokes, encourage him to enroll in a smoking cessation program. *Quitting smoking may enhance oxygenation and thereby decrease risk of peripheral neurovascular dysfunction.*
- Take steps to ease patient's anxiety. *Stress may lead to vasoconstriction.*
- Administer and monitor effectiveness of vasodilators, as ordered, *to control vasospasm.*
- If patient requires fasciotomy to restore circulation, provide educational material that explains this emergency procedure *to reduce patient anxiety.*
- Instruct patient or significant other in proper positioning when lying in bed and when sitting and in methods of obtaining pressure relief *to avoid pooling of blood and pressure ulcers.*
- If appropriate, discuss cause of injury and safety precautions *to avoid further injury.* Injuries to the upper extremities are usually caused by industrial accidents; injuries to the lower extremities, by automobile accidents.
- Instruct patient or significant other in recognizing signs and symptoms of peripheral neurovascular dysfunction, including numbness, pain, or tingling. Emphasize need to report symptoms to doctor *to prevent onset of neurovascular damage after discharge.*

Evaluations for expected outcomes

- Patient does not experience disability related to peripheral neurovascular dysfunction.
- Patient maintains circulation in extremities.
- Patient demonstrates ability to move each toe or finger after application of cast, brace, or splint.
- Patient demonstrates correct body positioning techniques.
- Patient or significant other expresses understanding of risk for altered neurovascular status.
- Patient enrolls in smoking cessation program.
- Symptoms of neurovascular compromise are absent.

Documentation

- Results of neurovascular assessment (baseline and ongoing)
- Nature of injury or treatment

- History of illnesses and surgeries
- Symptoms of neurovascular dysfunction reported by patient or significant other
- Patient's turning schedule
- Instructions provided to patient or significant other at discharge
- Evaluations for each expected outcome.

Personal identity disturbance

related to lowered self-esteem

Definition

Uncertainty about components of self regarding choices of vocation, intimacy and life-style

Assessment

- Choices of vocation, sexual orientation, religious orientation, friendships
- Ability to defend choices regarding long-range goals, to recognize alternatives, and appreciate consequences
- Comfort level of decisions made regarding long-range goals
- Degree of anxiety or depression regarding long-range goals
- Loss of interest, or social isolation from usual activities or friends
- Level of irritability about long-range goals
- Sleep difficulties
- Changes in eating habits
- Family status, including method of dealing with general conflicts; level of patient's communication with parents; handling of negotiations regarding restriction of freedom; degree of patient's separation from family; tolerance of patient's expressed opinions; age-appropriateness of dating, curfew regulation, money responsibilities; reaction of parents to patient's long-range goals
- Family and cultural standards related to separation issues

Defining characteristics

- Condition typically occurs in adolescence and young adulthood, but can occur later as well.
- Patient is distressed about uncertainties regarding variety of long-range goals, which may include vocation or career, relationships with friends, sexuality and sexual preferences, or religious affiliation.

Associated medical diagnoses (selected)

Identity disorder, adjustment reaction. Patient's disorder cannot result from major affective disorder, schizophrenia, or borderline personality disorder.

Expected outcomes

- Patient establishes trusting relationship with caregiver.
- Patient's issues are explored.
- Family's issues are explored.
- Patient establishes a firm, positive sense of self and personal identity.
- Patient chooses long-range goals using problem-solving techniques and is comfortable with choices.
- Family accepts patient's choices of long-range goals.

Interventions and rationales

- Assess patient alone, without family, *to gather baseline data and begin therapeutic relationship.*
- Explain your role as patient advocate; negotiate rules of interaction, including confidentiality, depth and breadth of discussion. *This establishes your role as a resource to the patient rather than as family's agent.*

• Explore personal identity issues distressing to patient *to isolate issues into smaller, more solvable units.*
• Help patient identify values, beliefs, hopes, dreams, skills, and interests. *Patient's deficits may lie in lack of self-exploration, problem-solving methods used, or separation issues with parents.*
• Integrate personal identity issues into decisions and choices *to develop skill in problem-solving methods.*
• Help patient identify likelihood and consequences of each choice. *Discussion and explanation aid problem-solving skills.*
• Promote choices with most likelihood of success. *Specific instructions can help patient gain problem-solving ability and maturity.*
• Encourage family conferences to explore potential reactions to patient's choices and promote support for patient's independent decision-making. *Meetings can help patient and family identify problems and find better ways to interact. Meetings also allow patient and family to ventilate true feelings in a safe environment.*
• Encourage peer support groups to explore and share personal identity experiences. *Adolescents and young adults often accept peer groups more than adults.*
• Promote outpatient counseling, family meetings, and peer support groups as appropriate to reinforce progress. *Establishing outpatient support systems can reduce regression.*

Evaluations for expected outcomes
• Patient openly discusses concerns with caregiver.
• Patient describes personal identity struggles.
• Family members discuss their reactions to patient's personal identity choices.
• Patient describes values, beliefs, skills, and interests in positive way.
• Patient identifies choices and possible alternatives, postulates consequences, and makes decisions about long-term goals.
• Family accepts patient's choices of long-term goals.

Documentation
• Assessment of patient's initial issues and problem-solving ability, including family's reactions as well as assessment of level of separation achieved by patient
• Patient's level of emotional distress and changes in sleep and eating, initially and as hospitalization continues
• Patient's progress in problem-solving and making choices
• Patient-family interactions, and content of family meetings
• Patient's interaction in peer-group meetings
• Outpatient resources identified and suggested to patient and family
• Evaluations for each expected outcome.

■ Poisoning, high risk for

related to external factors

Definition
Accentuated risk of accidental exposure to or ingestion of drugs or dangerous products in doses sufficient to cause poisoning

Assessment
• Health history, including accidents, allergies, exposure to pollutants, falls, hyperthermia, hypothermia, poisoning, sensory or perceptual changes (auditory, gustatory, kines-

thetic, olfactory, tactile, visual), trauma
- Circumstances surrounding the present situation that might lead to injury
- Neurologic status, including level of consciousness, mental status, orientation
- Psychosocial history, including age, habits (drug, alcohol use), occupation, personality
- Laboratory studies, including clotting factors, hemoglobin and hematocrit, platelet count, white blood cell count, toxicology screening

Risk factors
- Dangerous products stored or placed within the reach of children
- Large supplies of drugs in the environment
- Medicines stored in unlocked cabinets and accessible to confused persons
- Poisonous plants with prominent leaves or berries that entice handling and ingestion

Associated medical diagnoses (selected)
Alzheimer's disease, brain tumor, cerebrovascular accident, chronic obstructive pulmonary disease, depression with suicidal ideation or inclination, drug overdose, organic brain syndrome, posttraumatic head injury

Expected outcomes
- Patient is not exposed to and does not ingest dangerous substances.
- Patient communicates an understanding of need for self-protection.
- Patient and family or significant other state method for safekeeping of dangerous or potentially dangerous products.

Interventions and rationales
- Observe, record, and report falls, seizures, and unsafe practices *to ensure implementation of appropriate interventions. Overdose of certain medications (for example phenothiazines) can cause such neurologic problems as convulsions or seizures.*
- Monitor and record respiratory status *because certain poisons can cause respiratory depression.*
- Monitor and record neurologic status *because excessive toxic exposure can cause coma.* Pupils may be pinpoint or dilated, depending on type of drug ingested and length of time patient has been hypoxic.
- Monitor vital signs, intake and output, and level of consciousness. Record and report any changes. *Severe hypotension may develop following overdose. It may be related to central nervous system defect, direct myocardial depression, or vasodilation. Marked hyperthermia can occur with salicylate overdose, which affects metabolic rate. Dehydration may develop in some patients from increased respiratory rate, sweating, vomiting and urine losses.*
- Remove all dangerous or potentially dangerous products from the environment *to avoid injury.*
- Check settings on oxygen flow meters every ½ hour on all patients known to be carbon dioxide retainers (for example, some patients with chronic obstructive pulmonary disease). *This avoids carbon dioxide narcosis from excessive oxygen therapy in poorly ventilated patients; if unchecked, patient may stop breathing.*
- Provide patient and family or significant other with information about such specific products as medications, oxygen, and total parenteral nutrition. Tailor instructions to spe-

cific product and patient's capability for learning self-care. *This enables patient and family or significant other to identify and alter environmental or life-style factors to achieve optimum health level.*

Evaluations for expected outcomes

- Patient does not report or exhibit signs or symptoms resulting from exposure to or ingestion of dangerous substances.
- Patient requests information on protection from dangerous products.
- Patient and family or significant other describe method for safekeeping of dangerous or potentially dangerous products.

Documentation

- Patient's statements that indicate potential for injury
- Physical findings
- Observations or knowledge of unsafe practices
- Interventions performed to prevent injury
- Patient's response to nursing interventions
- Evaluations for each expected outcome.

Poisoning, high risk for

related to internal factors (biological, psychological, developmental)

Definition

Accentuated risk of accidental exposure to or ingestion of drugs or dangerous products in doses sufficient to cause poisoning

Assessment

- Health history, including accidents, allergies, exposure to pollutants, falls, hyperthermia, hypothermia, poisoning, seizures, trauma, sensory-perceptual changes (auditory, gustatory, kinesthetic, olfactory, tactile, visual)
- Circumstances of present situation that might lead to injury
- Neurologic status, including level of consciousness, mental status, orientation
- Psychosocial history, including age, habits (drug, alcohol use), occupation, personality
- Laboratory studies, including clotting factors, hemoglobin and hematocrit, platelet count, white blood cell count, toxicology screening

Risk factors

- Cognitive or emotional difficulties
- Lack of proper precautions
- Lack of safety or drug education
- Reduced vision
- Verbalization of unsafe environment

Associated medical diagnoses (selected)

Alzheimer's disease, brain tumor, cerebrovascular accident, depression with suicidal ideation or inclination, mental retardation, organic brain syndrome, posttraumatic head injury, schizophrenia

Expected outcomes

- Patient is not exposed to and does not ingest dangerous products.
- Patient communicates understanding of the need for self-protection.
- Patient and family or significant other explain method for safekeeping of dangerous products.

Interventions and rationales

- Observe, record, and report falls, seizures, and unsafe practices *to ensure implementation of appropriate interventions. Overdose of certain medications can cause such neuro-*

logic problems as convulsions or seizures.
- Monitor and record respiratory status *because certain poisons can cause respiratory depression.*
- Monitor and record neurologic status *because excessive toxic exposure can cause coma. Pupils may be pinpoint or dilated, depending on type of drug ingested and length of time patient has been hypoxic.*
- Remove dangerous or potentially dangerous products from the environment *to avoid injury.*
- Monitor vital signs, intake and output, and level of consciousness. Record and report any changes. *Severe hypotension may develop following overdose. It may be related to central nervous system defect, direct myocardial depression, or vasodilation. Marked hyperthermia can occur with salicylate overdose, which affects metabolic rate. Dehydration may develop in some patients from increased respiratory rate, sweating, vomiting, and urine losses.*
- Provide patient or significant other with information about such specific products as medications, oxygen, and total parenteral nutrition. Tailor instructions to the specific product and the patient's capability for learning self-care. *This enables patient and family or significant other to identify and alter environmental or life-style factors to achieve optimum health level.*

Evaluations for expected outcomes
- Patient does not report or exhibit signs or symptoms related to exposure to or ingestion of dangerous products.
- Patient requests information on self-protection from dangerous products.
- Patient and family or significant other state method for safekeeping of dangerous or potentially dangerous products.

Documentation
- Patient's statements about the situation that indicate potential for injury
- Physical findings
- Record of falls, seizures, and unsafe practices
- Interventions that reduce risk of injury
- Patient's response to nursing interventions
- Evaluations for each expected outcome.

■ Posttrauma response

related to accidental injury

Definition
Sustained painful response to an unexpected life event

Assessment
- History and circumstances of accident
- Physical injuries sustained, including cardiopulmonary, musculoskeletal, genitourinary, integumentary
- Neurologic status
- Emotional reactions, including grief reaction, self-concept, sleep pattern
- Cognitive reactions, including concentration, memory, orientation
- Behavioral reactions, including available support systems, clergy, coping patterns, family or significant other, problem-solving ability, social interactions

Defining characteristics
- Psychic numbing, including amnesia, constricted affect, confusion,

difficulty with interpersonal relationships, impaired reality interpretation, phobia, poor impulse control
• Reexperience of trauma, including exaggerated startle response, excessive verbalization of traumatic event, flashbacks, hyperalertness, intrusive thoughts, nightmares

Associated medical diagnoses (selected)
This nursing diagnosis can occur in any hospitalized patient seriously injured by sudden, unexpected trauma, such as a motor vehicle accident, airplane crash, train derailment, or fall.

Expected outcomes
• Patient recovers or is rehabilitated from physical injuries to the extent possible.
• Patient states feelings and fears related to traumatic event.
• Patient expresses feelings of safety.
• Patient uses available support systems.
• Patient uses effective coping mechanisms to reduce fear.
• Patient maintains or reestablishes adaptive social interactions with family or significant other.

Interventions and rationales
• Follow medical regimen to manage physical injuries. *Attention to physical needs remains primary, according to Maslow's hierarchy.*
• Provide emotional support:
  – Visit patient frequently *to reduce fear of being alone.*
  – Be available to listen *to respond empathetically to patient's feelings.*
  – Accept and encourage statement of patient's feelings *to reassure patient that feelings are appropriate and valid.*
  – Assure patient of safety and take measures needed to ensure it. *Frequent nightmares or flashbacks may cause patient to question safety of environment.*
  – Avoid care-related activities or environmental stimuli that may intensify symptoms associated with trauma (loud noises, bright lights, abrupt entrances to patient's room, painful procedures or treatment). *Environmental stimuli can easily intensify flashbacks to traumatic event.*
  – Reorient patient to surroundings and reality as frequently as necessary. *Post-trauma psychic numbing impairs orientation, memory, and reality perception.*
  – Instruct patient in at least one fear-reducing behavior, such as seeking support from others when frightened. *As patient learns to reduce fears, coping skills will increase.*
• Support patient's family or significant other:
  – Provide time for them to express feelings.
  – Help them understand patient's reactions.

This reduces their anxiety and gives them a chance to help patient.
• Offer referral to other support persons or groups, including clergy, mental health professionals, trauma support group. *Referrals help patient to cite sense of universality, reduce isolation, share fears, and deal constructively with feelings.*

Evaluations for expected outcomes
• Patient resumes usual activities of daily living to the extent possible.
• Patient expresses feelings associated with traumatic event.
• Patient expresses feeling of safety inside hospital.

• Patient interacts with support people to alleviate distress.
• Patient demonstrates use of at least one fear-reducing behavior (specify).
• Patient interacts with family or significant other in beneficial manner.

Documentation

• Patient's perception of traumatic event
• Observations of patient's behavior
• Observations of patient's social interaction with others
• Interventions
• Patient's responses to nursing interventions
• Referrals to other support persons or groups
• Evaluations for each expected outcome.

■ Posttrauma response

related to assault

Definition

Sustained painful response to an unexpected life event

Assessment

• History and circumstances of assault
• Patient's perception of event
• Physical injuries sustained, including cardiopulmonary, genitourinary, integumentary, musculoskeletal
• Neurologic status
• Emotional reactions, including grief reaction, self-concept, sleep pattern
• Cognitive reactions, including concentration, memory, orientation
• Behavioral reactions, including coping patterns, social interactions
• Available support systems

Defining characteristics

• Psychic numbing, including confusion, constricted affect, difficulty with interpersonal relationships, impaired reality interpretation, phobia, poor impulse control
• Reexperience of trauma, including exaggerated startle response, excessive or minimal verbalization of traumatic event, flashbacks, hyperalertness, intrusive thoughts, nightmares, verbal reports of guilt and self-recrimination

Associated medical diagnoses (selected)

This nursing diagnosis can occur in any hospitalized patient injured as a result of an alleged physical assault. Examples include battered wives, physically abused children and elderly persons, victims of gunshot wounds or stabbing, prisoners of war, and hostages.

Expected outcomes

• Patient recovers from physical injuries to the extent possible.
• Patient states feelings related to alleged assault.
• Patient expresses feelings of guilt.
• Patient expresses feelings of physical safety.
• Patient uses effective coping mechanisms to reduce fear.
• Patient mobilizes support systems and professional resources as necessary.
• Patient reestablishes and maintains adaptive interpersonal relationships.

Interventions and rationales

• Follow medical regimen to manage physical injuries. *This reduces anxiety as patient perceives body's ability to recover from injury.*

- Provide patient with psychological support:
  - Visit frequently *to decrease patient's fear of being left alone and to encourage trusting relationship.*
  - Be available to listen *to respond empathetically to patient's feelings.*
  - Accept patient's feelings and behaviors *to reassure patient that they're appropriate and valid.*
  - Reassure patient of safety and take appropriate measures to ensure it. *Patient's feelings of safety are compromised by fear of repeated assaults.*
- Avoid care-related activities and environmental stimuli that may intensify symptoms (loud noises, bright lights, abrupt entrances to room, painful procedures or treatments). *Patient's traumatic experience may be intensified by misinterpreting procedures or environmental factors as repeated assaults.*
- Monitor mental status, reorienting patient to surroundings and interpreting reality as often as necessary. *This alleviates psychic numbing, a characteristic symptom of assault.*
- Instruct patient in at least one fear-reducing behavior, such as seeking support from others when frightened. *This helps patient gain sense of mastery over current situation.*
- Support family or significant others:
  - Provide time for them to express feelings.
  - Help them understand phases of crisis and patient's reactions to them.

These measures help reduce anxiety.
- Offer referral to community or professional resources, including clergy, mental health professional, social service, "Victims of Assault" support groups. *Referrals help patient to cite sense of universality, decrease isolation, share fears, and deal constructively with feelings.*

Evaluations for expected outcomes
- Patient recovers from injuries to the extent possible and resumes normal or near-normal activities of daily living.
- Patient expresses feelings of anger, blame, fear, and guilt. Patient spends less time recriminating self.
- Patient reports feeling safe inside hospital.
- Patient demonstrates at least one fear-reducing behavior during times of panic (specify).
- Patient uses available support groups, such as Victims of Assault, a trauma support group, or a mental health crisis center
- Patient interacts socially with others.

Documentation
- Patient's perception of event
- Observations of patient's verbal and nonverbal behaviors
- Observations of patient's interaction with others
- Interventions
- Patient's responses to nursing interventions
- Referrals to other support systems
- Evaluations for each expected outcome.

■ Powerlessness

related to chronic illness

Definition
Perceived loss of control over what happens to oneself and one's environment

Assessment
- Nature of medical diagnosis
- Mobility
- Behavioral responses (verbal and nonverbal), including calmness, agitation, anger, anxiety, depression, independence or dependence, interest or apathy, satisfaction or dissatisfaction
- Coping strategies, including passage through the grieving process
- Past experiences with hospitalization
- Knowledge, including current understanding of physical condition; physical, mental, emotional readiness to learn
- Environment, including equipment and supplies, health care professionals and personnel, lighting, location of patient's personal belongings, noise, privacy, space
- Number and types of stressors
- Social factors
- Spiritual beliefs and value system

Defining characteristics
- Ambivalent feelings about dependence on others
- Apathy
- Depression over physical deterioration
- Doubts about ability to perform usual roles
- Fear, sadness, crying
- General discomfort or anxiety
- Passivity
- Periodic displays of irritability, resentment, anger, and guilt
- Reluctance to express true feelings because of fear of alienating caregivers
- Reluctance to participate in decisions regarding health
- Verbal expressions of dissatisfaction with management of illness and self-care
- Verbal expressions of inadequacy and self-doubt
- Verbal expressions of lack of control over current situation

Associated medical diagnoses (selected)
Acquired immunodeficiency syndrome, affective disorders, arthritis, brain tumor, burns, cerebrovascular accident, chronic congestive heart failure, chronic graft-versus-host disease, chronic mental illness, chronic obstructive pulmonary disease, chronic renal failure, cirrhosis, cranial trauma, diabetes mellitus, digestive cancers, genital herpes, Parkinson's disease, respiratory neoplasms, schizophrenia, seizure disorder, spinal cord injury

Expected outcomes
- Patient acknowledges fears, feelings, and concerns about current situation.
- Patient makes decisions regarding course of treatment.
- Patient decreases level of anxiety by changing response to stressors.
- Patient participates in self-care activities (specify).
- Patient expresses feeling of regained control.
- Patient accepts and adapts to lifestyle changes.

Interventions and rationales
- Encourage patient to express feelings and concerns. Set aside time for discussions with patient about daily events. *This helps patient bring vaguely understood emotions into focus.*
- Accept patient's feelings of powerlessness as normal. *This indicates respect for patient and enhances patient's feelings of self-worth.*
- Try to be present during situations where feelings of powerlessness are

likely to be greatest *to help patient cope.*

- Identify and develop patient's coping mechanisms, strengths, and resources for support. *By making use of coping skills, the patient can reduce anxiety and fears and successfully undergo grieving necessary to come to terms with chronic illness.*
- Discuss situations that provoke feelings of anger, anxiety, and powerlessness *to identify areas patient can control and to prevent anger from being inappropriately directed at self or others.*
- Encourage participation in self-care. Provide positive reinforcement for patient's activities. Encourage patient to take active role as member of health care team. *This enhances patient's sense of control and reduces passive and dependent behavior.*
- Provide as many opportunities as possible for patient to make decisions with regard to self-care (positioning, choosing an injection site, visiting, and so forth) *to communicate respect for patient and enhance feelings of independence.*
- Help patient learn as much as possible about health condition, treatment, and prognosis *to help patient feel in control.*
- Modify environment when possible to meet patient's self-care needs *to promote patient's sense of control over the environment.*
- Decrease unpredictable events by discussing rules, policies, procedures, and schedules with patient. *Fear of the unknown interferes with patient's ability to cope.*
- Encourage family to support patient without taking control *to increase the patient's feelings of self-worth.*
- Reinforce patient's rights as stated in the Patient's Bill of Rights *to protect the patient's right to make decisions about health care treatment.*
- Identify and arrange to accommodate patient's spiritual needs. *Spirituality enables the patient to gain courage and resist despair.*

Evaluations for expected outcomes

- Patient verbalizes positive and negative feelings about current situation.
- Patient describes strategies for decreasing anxiety.
- Patient demonstrates increased control by participating in decision making related to health care.
- Patient actively participates in planning and executing aspects of personal and health care.
- Patient communicates renewed sense of power and control of current situation.

Documentation

- Observations and interactions related to the disease process and the health care environment
- Patient's responses to opportunities to participate in own care
- Patient's feelings about chronic illness and situations that cannot be changed
- Teaching and counseling to enhance patient's decision-making ability
- Interventions to help the patient gain sense of control
- Patient's response to nursing interventions
- Evaluations for each expected outcome.

Powerlessness

related to health care environment

Definition

Perceived loss of control over what happens to oneself and one's environment

Assessment

- Nature of the medical diagnosis
- Mobility
- Behavioral responses (verbal and nonverbal), including calmness, agitation, anger, independence or dependence, interest or apathy, satisfaction or dissatisfaction
- Usual coping strategies
- Past experiences with hospitalization
- Knowledge, including current understanding of physical condition; physical, mental, emotional readiness to learn
- Environment, including equipment and supplies, health care professionals and personnel, lighting, location of patient's personal belongings, noise, privacy, space

Defining characteristics

- Apathy
- Dependence on others that may result in irritability, anger, resentment, guilt
- Discomfort or dissatisfaction with health care environment
- Expressions of dissatisfaction and frustration over inability to perform previous tasks or activities
- Expressions of doubt regarding role performance
- Fear, sadness, crying
- Passivity
- Verbal expressions of having no control or influence over self-care
- Verbal expressions of having no control or influence over situation

Associated medical diagnoses (selected)

This diagnosis is best identified by considering problems that restrict or confine patients rather than by medical diagnosis. Examples include blindness, confinement to an intensive care or cardiac care unit, isolation, language barrier, multiple I.V. lines, multisystem trauma, and restrictions caused by dependence on ventilators, paralysis, and traction.

Expected outcomes

- Patient identifies feelings of powerlessness associated with the environment.
- Patient describes modifications or adjustments to the environment that allow feelings of control.
- Patient participates in self-care activities (specify).
- Patient states feelings of regained control.

Interventions and rationales

- Visit with patient 15 minutes each shift *to allow patient to express concerns and feelings.*
- Acknowledge the importance of patient's space:
  - Verbally delineate patient's space.
  - Orient patient to space.
  - If patient is immobilized, ask for instructions regarding placement of personal belongings.
  - If possible, allow patient to walk around the space and arrange personal belongings.

These measures enhance patient's potential for regaining a sense of power.

- Place call light, TV controls, bedside table, telephone, urinal, and other items within easy reach. Im-

provise wherever possible to give control over use of these objects. Be attentive to patient's ability or inability to use hands and arms. *These measures help reduce patient's frustration over inability to reach items in immediate area.*
• Reduce irritating noises, if possible, and explain reasons for alarms and other disturbances. *Excessive sensory stimuli can cause disorientation, hallucinations, and delusional thinking.*
• Explain all treatments and procedures and encourage patient to participate in planning care. Provide choices for when and how activities will occur (bathing, eating, getting out of bed). *This increases patient's feeling of powerfulness and reduces passivity and dependence on caregiver.*
• Provide as many situations as possible where patient can take control (such as positioning, choosing an injection site, and visiting) *to help reduce potential for maladaptive coping behaviors.*
• Encourage participation in self-care. Provide positive reinforcement for patient's activities *to encourage increasing participation in self-care in the future.*
• Help patient learn as much about current health problem as possible. *The greater the understanding, the more the patient will feel in control.*

Evaluations for expected outcomes
• Patient expresses feelings of lack of control.
• Adjustments are made to the environment to enhance the patient's feelings of control.
• Patient performs self-care measures to the extent possible.
• Patient expresses feelings of regained control.

Documentation
• Patient's expressions of anger, frustration, sense of lack of control over the environment
• Patient's interest in surroundings, participation in self-care, verbalization of understanding, and demonstration of skill in relation to medical diagnosis
• Interventions to promote patent's control over the environment
• Patient's response to nursing interventions
• Evaluations for each expected outcome.

■ Powerlessness

related to illness-related regimen

Definition
Perceived loss of control over what happens to oneself and one's environment

Assessment
• Nature of medical diagnosis
• Mobility
• Behavioral responses (verbal and nonverbal), including calmness, agitation, anger, independence or dependence, interest or apathy, satisfaction or dissatisfaction
• Past experiences with hospitalization
• Environment, including equipment and supplies, health care professionals and personnel, lighting, location of patient's personal belongings, noise, privacy, space
• Knowledge, including current understanding of physical condition; physical, mental, emotional readiness to learn

Defining characteristics

- Apathy
- Dependence on others that may result in irritability, anger, resentment, guilt
- Depression over physical deterioration that occurs despite compliance with regimens
- Expressions of dissatisfaction and frustration over inability to perform previous tasks or activities
- Fear, sadness, crying
- Passivity
- Reluctance to express true feelings, fearing alienation from caregivers
- Verbal expressions of having no control or influence over self-care
- Verbal expressions of having no control over situation

Associated medical diagnoses (selected)

Acute respiratory failure, burns, cardiac disease that requires pacemaker, cerebrovascular accident, chronic obstructive pulmonary disease, chronic renal failure, diseases requiring organ transplantation, hemodialysis, insulin-dependent diabetes, neoplastic diseases requiring chemotherapy or radiation, peritoneal dialysis, spinal cord injury

Expected outcomes

- Patient acknowledges feelings of powerlessness over regimen.
- Patient participates in planning care.
- Patient participates in self-care activities (specify).
- Patient enumerates factors in the illness-related regimen over which control can be maintained.
- Patient demonstrates ability to plan for controllable factors.
- Patient communicates a sense of having regained control.

Interventions and rationales

- Encourage patient to express feelings about present situation. *This helps patient bring vaguely expressed emotions into clear awareness and acceptance.*
- Accept patient's feelings of powerlessness as normal. *This indicates respect for patient and enhances patient's feelings of self-worth.*
- Allow patient to make decisions about care (positioning, times for ambulation). *This helps patient maintain a sense of control and reduces potential for maladaptive coping behaviors.*
- Encourage participation in self-care. Provide positive reinforcement for patient's activities. *This enhances patient's sense of control and reduces passive and dependent behavior.*
- Begin teaching patient how to regain and maintain optimal health. *In this teaching relationship, the nurse presents information to the patient on a need-to-know basis.*
- Help identify specific areas where patient can maintain control *to reduce patient's feelings of helplessness.*
- Have patient demonstrate ways to consciously maintain some degree of control. *Repetitive demonstrations of skills and behaviors enhance learning.*
- Help patient learn as much as possible about present health problem. *The greater the understanding, the more the patient will feel in control.*

Evaluations for expected outcomes

- Patient expresses feelings of lack of control over health care regimen.
- Patient specifies preferences for care.
- Patient performs specified daily self-care measures.
- Patient identifies specific factors in the illness-related regimen over

which control can be maintained and plans appropriate action.
• Patient expresses feelings of regained control.

Documentation
• Patient's expressions of powerlessness
• Patient's behaviors that evidence a feeling of powerlessness
• Interventions performed to assist patient in regaining sense of control
• Patient's degree of participation in planning care
• Evaluations for each expected outcome.

Rape-trauma syndrome

Definition
Physical and emotional trauma that occurs as a result of sexual assault

Assessment
• History and circumstances of traumatic event
• Physical injuries sustained, including genitourinary, integumentary, musculoskeletal, neurologic
• Emotional reactions, including grief reaction, self-concept, spiritual distress
• Support systems available to the patient, including clergy, family or significant other, friends
• Problem-solving techniques usually employed by the patient

Defining characteristics
• Emotional reactions, including anger, embarrassment; fear of physical violence; humiliation, revenge, self-blame
• Multiple physical symptoms, including GI irritability, genitourinary discomfort, muscle tension, sleep pattern disturbances

Associated medical diagnoses (selected)
Incest, rape, spouse abuse

Expected outcomes
• Patient recovers from physical injuries.
• Patient expresses feelings and fears.
• Patient uses support systems.

Interventions and rationales
• Follow the medical regimen to manage physical injuries caused by the traumatic event. *This is first step in meeting patient's hierarchy of needs and depends on extent of patient's other injuries and intensity of psychological response.*
• Follow hospital protocol regarding legal responsibilities. Be aware of potential legal issues of rape and of role nurses may play as witnesses in legal proceedings. *These steps will help protect the patient's legal rights.*
• Provide emotional support:
  – Be available to listen. *Active listening allows empathetic response to patient's feelings while being aware of own thoughts and behaviors.*
  – Accept the patient's feelings, *to let the patient know her feelings are valid and acceptable.*
  – Approach the patient in a warm, caring manner, *to cultivate her trust and cooperation.*
  – Provide privacy during physical examination and interviewing process. *To protect patient's rights, no information should be released without prior consent.*
  – Assure patient of safety and take whatever measures are needed to ensure it. *This reduces patient's fears of repeated assault.*

• Support the patient's family or significant other in their reactions to the traumatic event:
  – Provide time for them to express their feelings and concerns.
  – Help them understand the patient's reactions.

Giving them time to talk and providing accurate information helps them support their loved one.

• Offer referral to other support persons or groups, such as clergy, crisis center, mental health professionals, rape counselors, Women Organized Against Rape. *This will help the patient express feelings and develop coping skills.*

Evaluations for expected outcomes

• Patient recovers from physical injuries.
• Patient expresses feelings common to rape victims, such as anger, blame, humiliation, and fear of disease or pregnancy.
• Patient contacts local rape-counseling or mental health crisis center.

Documentation

• Patient's expressions of feelings about self and traumatic event
• Physical findings and treatment
• Observations of family's interaction with patient
• Referrals to support persons
• Patient's response to nursing interventions
• Evaluations for each expected outcome.

Rape-trauma syndrome: Compound reaction

Definition

Trauma syndrome that develops after rape or attempted rape in which the patient undergoes an acute phase of disorganization and a long-term reorganization. In a compound reaction, the patient experiences drastic changes in behavior, psychological equilibrium, and ability to function as a consequence of rape.

Assessment

• History and circumstances of traumatic event
• Physical symptoms reported by patient
• Physical injuries sustained, including genitourinary (GU), integumentary, musculoskeletal, neurologic
• Emotional reactions
• Behavioral and cognitive changes, such as expansive mood and affect, agitation, extreme alertness, narrowed attention span
• Symptoms associated with post-trauma response, including hypervigilance, reexperience of assault
• Available support systems
• Past experience with physical or psychological trauma, including coping strategies, problem-solving skills
• Occupation, educational background, life-style

Defining characteristics

• *Acute phase:* aggressive behavior, anger, embarrassment, fear of physical violence and death, homicidal ideation, humiliation, hysterical outbursts, revenge seeking, self-blame, suicidal ideation; multiple physical signs and symptoms (GI irritability, GU discomfort, muscle tension,

sleep-pattern disturbance); reactivated symptoms of previous conditions, such as physical illness, psychiatric illness; reliance on alcohol or drugs.
• *Long-term phase:* change in lifestyle, including change of residence; repetitive nightmares, seeking support from family and social network

Associated medical diagnoses (selected)
Incest, rape, sexual assault, spouse abuse

Expected outcomes
• Patient recovers from physical injuries to the fullest extent possible.
• Patient expresses feelings about the rape.
• Patient reports feeling safe.
• Patient takes first steps toward recovery from trauma.
• Patient contacts appropriate support persons or follow-up agency.
• Patient reports a desire to reestablish and maintain interpersonal relationships.

Interventions and rationales
• Follow the medical regimen to manage physical injuries. *This is the first step in meeting the patient's needs.*
• Document and report rape or attempted rape to appropriate authorities *to help protect the patient's legal rights.*
• When interviewing the patient, use open-ended questions and listen intently *to encourage the patient to talk about the trauma and to express her feelings, both verbally and through behavior.*
• Show the patient that you accept her feelings but set limits on aggressive behavior. *Demonstrating acceptance reassures the patient that her response to trauma is valid. Setting limits on behavior provides the patient with necessary structure.*
• Take appropriate measures to reassure the patient of her safety; for example:
 – Approach the patient carefully with open hands.
 – Stay with the patient.
 – Have female staff conduct the patient interview and physical examination.

Safety measures help to decrease the patient's anxiety and reduce fears of another assault.
• Direct the patient to perform purposeful activities, such as taking medications and following instructions of health care personnel. *Completing tasks helps to reduce the patient's anxiety and restore her sense of control.*
• Educate the patient about the variety of responses to trauma. *The patient with a compound reaction may feel that the extreme emotional turmoil she experiences after rape is abnormal. Learning that others have undergone the same experience may help reassure her and may help decrease isolation.*
• Provide the patient's family or significant other with an opportunity to express their reactions to the trauma and the patient's response. Educate family members about compound reaction to rape *to help them support the patient.*
• Refer the patient to appropriate support persons, such as clergy, mental health professional, or rape counselor. Encourage the patient to participate in support groups or therapy groups offered by rape counseling center. *The patient may need long-term care to cope with the psychological consequences of rape.*
• Provide ongoing support as the patient struggles to regain psychological

equilibrium. Encourage her efforts to renew involvement in usual activities. *To achieve long-term personality reorganization, the patient will require time, consistent support, and ongoing counseling.*

Evaluations for expected outcomes
- Patient recovers from physical injuries and resumes normal or near-normal activities of daily living.
- Patient expresses feelings associated with the rape.
- Patient reports feeling safe.
- After discharge, patient participates in ongoing counseling sessions or support group.
- Patient reports increased ability to cope with psychological consequences of the rape and increased social interactions and activities.

Documentation
- Patient's expressions of feelings related to trauma
- Observations of patient's behavior and interactions with others
- Nursing interventions
- Patient's response to interventions
- Referrals accepted by patient
- Evaluations for each expected outcome.

Rape-trauma syndrome: Silent reaction

Definition
Trauma syndrome that develops after rape, attemped rape, or sexual assault, in which the patient undergoes an acute phase of disorganization and a long-term process of reorganization. In a silent reaction, the patient doesn't tell anyone about the rape or deal with her feelings about it.

Assessment
- Symptoms associated with post-trauma response
- Evidence of emotional distress, including shock, fear, anger, guilt
- Behavioral and cognitive changes, such as lack of affect, agitation, decreased alertness, narrowed attention span
- Evidence of physical injuries
- Available support systems
- Past experience with physical or psychological trauma, including coping strategies, problem-solving skills
- Laboratory studies, including tests for pregnancy or sexually transmitted diseases

Defining characteristics
- Abrupt changes in relationships with men
- Increased anxiety during interview:
  - blocking of associations
  - minor stuttering
  - physical distress
- Increase in nightmares
- No expression that rape, attempted rape, or sexual assault occurred
- Pronounced changes in sexual behavior
- Signs and symptoms of posttraumatic response, such as numbness, impaired concentration, disbelief, panic, extreme detachment, severe anxiety, anger, depersonalization
- Sudden onset of phobic reactions

Associated medical diagnoses (selected)
Incest, rape, sexual assault, spouse abuse

Expected outcomes
- Patient discloses that rape, attempted rape, or sexual assault occurred.
- Patient recovers from physical injuries to the fullest extent possible.

• Patient makes contact with appropriate sources of support.
• Patient expresses willingness to address psychosocial problems associated with traumatic experience.

Interventions and rationales

• Establish an atmosphere of trust *to help the patient overcome silence about the rape or sexual assault.*
• Confront the patient directly but gently with the question of whether she is a victim of rape or sexual assault. For example, you might say "You seem very upset and you've told me about increased nightmares and a sudden loss of interest in sexual relations. These are common characteristics of victims of sexual assault. If you've been sexually assaulted, you can tell me. I'll help you." *The patient with a silent reaction needs patience and encouragement to overcome anxiety about disclosing rape or sexual assault.*
• Clear up misconceptions the patient may have about the nature of rape or sexual assault. *If, for example, intercourse didn't take place or the attacker was a boyfriend, spouse, or family member, the patient may not believe that sexual assault occurred. Tell the patient that sexual assault can take different forms and that all can be equally traumatic.*
• If the patient remains unwilling to disclose the rape or sexual assault, tell her that you'll continue to be available to help. Encourage her to contact you if she feels the need *to provide a resource for future help and maintain communication.*
• If the patient discloses the rape or sexual assault, be careful to respond in a caring, nonjudgmental manner *to cultivate trust and cooperation.* Follow medical regimen to manage physical injuries (if rape or sexual assault was recent) and follow hospital protocol for documenting rape or sexual assault and reporting it to authorities *to ensure the patient's physical well-being and protect her legal rights.* Use open-ended questions and listen intently *to encourage the patient to talk about the trauma.* If the patient is withdrawn, be understanding and supportive when gathering information *to allow the patient to proceed at her own pace.*
• Emphasize to the patient that the attack was not her fault. *The patient with a silent reaction may feel intense guilt and shame over the assault.*
• Educate the patient about the variety of emotional responses to trauma. Rape-trauma syndrome is a variant of posttraumatic stress disorder. Responses such as suicidal ideation, disorientation, confusion, extreme detachment, nightmares, flashbacks, guilt, and depression are common. *The patient may believe that the emotional turmoil she experiences after rape or sexual assault is abnormal. Pointing out that others have undergone the same experience may lessen the patient's isolation, help her talk about her symptoms, and motivate her to seek follow-up care.*
• Offer referral to appropriate support persons or groups, such as clergy, mental health professionals, or rape counselor. Contact a local rape crisis center for information about support groups or therapy groups. Note that, if only a single assault has occurred, short-term counseling may be sufficient. However, if the patient is a survivor of several assaults or repeated incest, long-term psychotherapy may be required. *Appropriate referrals help ensure that the patient gets needed care.*

Evaluations for expected outcomes
- Patient discloses that rape, attempted rape, or sexual assault occurred.
- Patient recovers from physical injuries and resumes normal or near-normal activities of daily living.
- Patient contacts rape counselor and agrees to participate in therapy group.
- Patient acknowledges that the rape or sexual assault was not her fault and that she needs to deal with psychological consequences of trauma.

Documentation
- Evidence that the patient has been raped or sexually assaulted, including patient's behavior, physical evidence
- Efforts made to help the patient discuss rape or sexual assault and patient's response
- Nursing interventions
- Patient's response to interventions
- Referrals accepted by the patient
- Evaluations for each expected outcome.

Relocation stress syndrome

related to inadequate preparation for admission, transfer, or discharge

Definition
Physiologic or psychosocial disturbances caused by change in health care environment

Assessment
- Reason for transfer or relocation
- Past experiences with relocation
- Nature of relocation
- Physical and mental status of patient, including health condition, cognitive functioning, functional abilities
- Financial resources
- Support systems, including family and friends, health care workers
- Resources available to help prepare for relocation
- Conditions in original environment versus conditions in new environment
- Coping and problem-solving abilities, including educational level, past experiences with relocation, participation in recreational activities or hobbies

Defining characteristics
- Anxiety
- Apprehension
- Change in eating patterns
- Dependency
- Depression
- Expressions of concern or anxiety about transfer
- Expressions of unwillingness to relocate
- GI disturbances
- Increased confusion (particularly among elderly patients)
- Increased verbalization of needs
- Insecurity
- Lack of trust
- Loneliness
- Restlessness
- Sad affect
- Sleep disturbance
- Unfavorable comparison of original and new staff or environment
- Vigilance
- Weight change
- Withdrawal

Associated medical diagnoses (selected)
Any change in physical, functional, or cognitive status that also requires a change in patient's environment, such as admission to hospital, transfer from one unit or institution to another, or discharge

Expected outcomes

- Patient requests information on new environment.
- Patient communicates understanding of relocation.
- Patient and family members take steps to prepare for relocation.
- Patient utilizes available resources.
- Patient expresses satisfaction with adjustment to new environment.

Interventions and rationales

- Assign a primary nurse to patient *to provide a consistent, caring, and accepting environment that enhances patient's adjustment and well-being.*
- Help patient and family members prepare for relocation. Conduct group discussions, provide pictures of the new setting, and communicate any additional information that will ease the transition *to help patient cope with new environment.*
- If possible, allow patient and family members to visit new location and provide introductions to new staff. *The more familiar the environment, the less stress patient will experience during relocation.*
- Assess patient's needs for additional health care services before relocation *to ensure that patient receives appropriate care in new environment.*
- Communicate all aspects of patient's discharge plan to appropriate staff at the new location *to ensure continuity of care.*
- Educate family members about relocation stress syndrome and its potential effects *to encourage family members to provide needed emotional support throughout the transition period.*
- Encourage patient to express emotions associated with relocation *to provide an opportunity to correct misconceptions, answer questions, and reduce anxiety.*
- Reassure patient that family members and friends know his new location and will continue to visit *to reduce feelings of abandonment and anxiety.*

Evaluations for expected outcomes

- Patient makes request for information on new environment.
- Patient expresses understanding of relocation process.
- Patient and family members complete preparation for relocation.
- Patient makes use of available resources to smooth transition to new environment.
- Patient expresses feelings associated with adjustment to new environment.

Documentation

- Evidence of patient's emotional distress over relocation
- Patient's needs with regard to preparing for relocation
- Available resources and support systems
- Intervention to prepare patient and family members for relocation and patient's and family members' responses
- Discharge plan instructions communicated to new staff
- Evaluations for each expected outcome.

■ Role performance alteration

related to ineffective coping

Definition

Disruption in the ability to perform usual social, vocational, or family roles

Assessment

- Health history, including medical diagnosis, course and severity of illness, reason for hospitalization
- Patient's perception of illness and its effect on social and vocational roles
- Psychosocial status, including current stressors, support systems, hobbies, interests, work history, educational background, and changes in role function
- Family status, including roles of family members, effect of illness on patient's family, and family's understanding of patient's illness

Defining characteristics

- Change in perception of role (by self and others)
- Change in physical capacity to resume role
- Change in usual responsibilities
- Conflict among vocational, family, and social roles
- Denial of role or responsibility
- Lack of knowledge about roles and responsibilities

Associated medical diagnoses (selected)

This diagnosis may be associated with any illness that results in long-term disability or incapacitation. Examples include chronic obstructive pulmonary disease, coronary artery disease, dementias, personality disorders, quadriplegia, recurrent affective disorders, rheumatoid arthritis, schizophrenia, and substance abuse disorders.

Expected outcomes

- Patient expresses feelings about diminished capacity to perform usual roles.
- Patient recognizes limitations imposed by illness and expresses feelings about these limitations.
- Patient makes decisions regarding course of treatment and management of illness.
- Patient continues to function in usual roles to as great a degree as possible.

Interventions and rationales

- If possible, assign the same nurse to the patient each shift *to establish rapport and foster development of a therapeutic relationship.*
- Spend an ample amount of time with patient each shift *to foster sense of safety and decrease loneliness.*
- Provide opportunities for patient to express thoughts and feelings *to help patient identify how altered role performance has affected his life.*
- Convey belief in patient's ability to develop necessary coping skills. *By projecting a positive attitude, you can help the patient gain confidence.*
- Be aware of patient's emotional vulnerability, and allow open expression of all emotions. *An accepting attitude will help the patient deal with the effects of chronic illness and loss of functioning.*
- Provide opportunities for patient to make decisions, and encourage patient to maintain personal responsibilities. *Showing respect for the patient's decision-making ability enhances feelings of independence.*
- Encourage the patient to participate in self-care activities, keeping in mind physical and emotional limitations. *Involvement in self-care promotes optimal functioning.*
- Assess patient's knowledge of illness, and educate patient about condition, treatment, and prognosis. *Education will enable the patient to cope with the effects of illness more effectively.*
- Encourage patient to be aware of personal strengths and to use them.

This will help maintain optimal functioning and foster a healthier self-perception.
- Encourage patient to continue to fulfill life roles within constraints posed by illness. *This will help patient maintain a sense of purpose and preserve connections with other people.*
- Encourage patient to participate in care as an active member of health care team. *This will foster the establishment of mutually accepted goals between patient and caregivers. The patient who participates in care is more likely to take an active role in other aspects of life.*
- Assist family members in identifying feelings about patient's decreased role functioning. Encourage participation in a support group. *Relatives of the patient may need social support, information, and an outlet for ventilating feelings.*
- Offer patient and family a realistic assessment of patient's illness, and communicate hope for the immediate future. *Education helps promote patient safety and security and enables family members to plan for future health care requirements.*
- Educate the patient and family about managing illness, controlling environmental factors that affect the patient's health, and redefining roles to promote optimal functioning. *Through education, family members may become resources in the patient's care.*

Evaluations for expected outcomes
- Patient shares feelings about illness and altered role performance in a constructive manner.
- Patient and family understand role changes that are occurring because of chronic illness.
- Patient demonstrates increased functioning by making decisions related to health care.
- Patient participates in the planning and implementation of aspects of personal care.
- Patient demonstrates ability to perceive options and uses options to adapt to role changes and illness.
- Patient expresses feeling of having made a productive contribution to self-care, to others, or to the environment.

Documentation
- Observations of the patient's physical, emotional, and mental status
- Patient's thoughts and feelings regarding illness and diminished role capacity
- Nursing interventions performed to help patient understand change in role functioning
- Patient's response to nursing interventions
- All health teaching, counseling, and precautions taken to maintain or enhance the patient's level of functioning
- Referrals to sources of support for patient and family
- Evaluations for each expected outcome.

■ Self-care deficit: Bathing and hygiene

related to musculoskeletal impairment

Definition
Inability to carry out activities associated with bathing and hygiene

Assessment

- History of injury or disease associated with musculoskeletal impairment
- Self-care abilities, including knowledge and use of adaptive equipment, preparation of equipment and supplies, technical or mechanical skills
- Musculoskeletal status, including coordination; functional ability; gait; mechanical restriction (cast, splint, traction); muscle tone, size, and strength; range of motion; tremors
- Psychosocial status, including coping mechanisms, family or significant other, life-style, patient's perceptions of health problem and self, personality

Defining characteristics

- Clinical evidence of musculoskeletal impairment
- Inability to carry out personal hygiene
- Inability to obtain or get to water source
- Inability to regulate water temperature or flow
- Inability to wash body or body parts

Associated medical diagnoses (selected)

Amyotrophic lateral sclerosis, brain or spinal cord tumor, cerebral palsy, cerebrovascular accident, fractures, Guillain-Barré syndrome, Huntington's disease, multiple sclerosis, multiple trauma, muscular dystrophy, myasthenia gravis (crisis), Parkinson's disease, rheumatoid arthritis, spinal cord injury, terminal cancer

Expected outcomes

- Patient's self-care needs are met.
- Complications are avoided or minimized.
- Patient communicates feelings about limitations.
- Patient or significant other demonstrates correct use of assistive devices.
- Patient or significant other carries out bathing and hygiene program daily.

Interventions and rationales

- Observe patient's functional level every shift; document and report any changes. *Careful observation guides adjustment of actions to meet patient's needs.*
- Perform prescribed treatment for underlying musculoskeletal impairment. Monitor progress, reporting favorable and adverse responses to treatment. *Therapy must be consistently applied to aid patient's independence.*
- Encourage patient to voice feelings and concerns about self-care deficits *to help patient achieve highest functional level possible.*
- Monitor completion of bathing and hygiene daily. Praise accomplishments. *Reinforcement and rewards may encourage renewed effort.*
- Provide assistive devices, such as long-handled toothbrush, for bathing and hygiene; instruct on use. *Appropriate assistive devices encourage independence.*
- Assist with or perform bathing and hygiene daily. Assist only when patient has difficulty *to promote feeling of independence.*
- Instruct patient or significant other in bathing and hygiene techniques. Have patient or significant other demonstrate bathing and hygiene under supervision. Instructions to significant other can be given in writing. *Return demonstration identifies problem areas and increases significant other's self-confidence.*
- Refer patient, as needed, to psychiatric liaison nurse, support group, or

home health care agency. *These extra resources will reinforce activities planned to meet patient's needs.*

Evaluations for expected outcomes

- Patient's self-care needs are met with help of staff.
- Patient participates in activities designed to minimize the risk of such complications as infection or skin integrity alteration.
- Patient expresses feelings about self-care deficit. If unable to meet own needs, patient seeks assistance from significant other or staff within 24 hours.
- Patient or significant other demonstrates appropriate use of assistive devices.
- Patient follows daily plans for self-care. Significant other assists as needed.

Documentation

- Patient's expression of feelings and concerns about self-care limitations and their impact on body image and life-style
- Patient's willingness to participate in bathing and hygiene routine
- Observations of patient's impaired ability to perform self-care
- Patient's response to treatment for underlying condition
- Interventions to provide supportive care
- Patient's response to nursing interventions
- Instructions to patient or significant other, their understanding of instructions and demonstrated skill in carrying out self-care functions
- Evaluations for each expected outcome.

■ Self-care deficit: Bathing and hygiene

related to perceptual or cognitive impairment

Definition

Inability to carry out activities associated with bathing and hygiene

Assessment

- History of neurologic, sensory, or psychological impairment
- Age
- Self-care abilities, including knowledge and use of adaptive equipment, preparation of equipment and supplies, technical and mechanical skills
- Neurologic status, including cognition, communication ability, insight or judgment, level of consciousness, memory, motor ability, orientation, sensory ability
- Psychosocial status, including coping mechanisms, family or significant other, life-style, patient's perceptions of self, personality

Defining characteristics

- Clinical evidence of perceptual or cognitive impairment
- Impaired short-term or long-term memory
- Inability to carry out personal hygiene
- Inability to obtain or get to water source
- Inability to regulate water temperature or flow
- Inability to wash body or body parts

Associated medical diagnoses (selected)

Alcoholism, Alzheimer's disease, autism, bipolar disease (manic or depressive phase), brain tumor, cerebrovascular accident, head injury, Huntington's disease, Laënnec's cirrhosis, mental retardation, organic brain syndrome, psychoses

Expected outcomes

- Patient's self-care needs are met.
- Complications are avoided or minimized.
- Patient or significant other carries out self-care program daily.
- Patient or significant other communicates feelings and concerns.
- Patient or significant other identifies resources to help cope with problems after discharge.

Interventions and rationales

- Observe, document, and report patient's functional and perceptual or cognitive ability daily. *This allows adjustment of actions to meet patient's needs.*
- Perform prescribed treatment for underlying condition. Monitor progress and report favorable and adverse responses. *Therapy must be consistently applied to aid patient's independence.*
- Allow patient to express frustration, anger, or feelings of inadequacy. Provide emotional support *to help patient achieve highest functional level.*
- Provide privacy *to enhance patient's self-esteem.*
- Monitor completion of bathing and hygiene daily. Remind patient of what is to be accomplished. Offer praise. *Reinforcement and rewards may encourage daily activities.*
- Allow ample time for patient to perform bathing and hygiene. *Rushing creates unnecessary stress and promotes failure.*
- Encourage patient to complete bathing and hygiene regimen. Provide positive, constructive feedback during task performance. *Reinforcement and rewards may encourage daily activities.*
- Direct patient in bathing and hygiene measures, using simple instructions given one at a time, *to aid comprehension.*
- Assist with bathing and hygiene daily only when patient has difficulty *to encourage independence and self-reliance.*
- Give written instructions to significant other in bathing and hygiene techniques and supervise return demonstration. *Return demonstration identifies problem areas and increases significant other's self-confidence.*
- Discuss normal aspects of bathing. Reassure the patient with such statements as "You're in the tub" and "The water is only 3 inches deep" *to guard against panic reaction caused by fear of being drowned.*
- Refer patient to psychiatric liaison nurse, support group, or home health care agency, as needed. *These extra resources will reinforce activities planned to meet patient needs.*

Evaluations for expected outcomes

- Patient's self-care needs are met with help of staff.
- Patient does not experience infection, skin integrity alteration, or other complications of altered self-care.
- Patient or significant other becomes more active in carrying out self-care program; need for staff assistance decreases.
- Patient expresses feelings about self-care deficit. If unable to meet own needs, patient seeks assistance from significant other or staff within 24 hours.

• Patient or significant other identifies and contacts available support resources as needed.

Documentation
• Patient's or significant other's expression of feelings and concern about self-care deficits
• Observations of patient's impaired ability to perform bathing and hygiene
• Patient's response to treatment for underlying condition
• Interventions to provide supportive care
• Instructions to patient (if capable) or significant other, their understanding of the instructions, and their demonstrated skill in carrying out self-care functions
• Patient's response to nursing interventions
• Evaluations for each expected outcome.

Self-care deficit: Dressing and grooming

related to musculoskeletal impairment

Definition
Inability to perform activities associated with dressing and grooming

Assessment
• History of injury or disease associated with musculoskeletal impairment
• Self-care abilities, including knowledge and use of adaptive equipment, preparation of equipment and supplies, technical or mechanical skills
• Musculoskeletal status, including coordination; functional ability; gait; mechanical restriction (cast, splint, traction); muscle tone, size, and strength; range of motion; tremors
• Psychosocial status, including coping mechanisms, family or significant other, life-style, patient's perceptions of health problem and self, personality

Defining characteristics
• Clinical evidence of musculoskeletal impairment
• Impaired ability to fasten clothing
• Impaired ability to obtain or replace articles of clothing
• Impaired ability to put on or take off clothing
• Inability to maintain appearance at a satisfactory level

Associated medical diagnoses (selected)
Amyotrophic lateral sclerosis, brain or spinal cord tumor, cerebral palsy, cerebrovascular accident, fractures, Guillain-Barré syndrome, Huntington's disease, multiple sclerosis, multiple trauma, muscular dystrophy, myasthenia gravis (crisis), Parkinson's disease, rheumatoid arthritis, spinal cord injury, terminal cancer

Expected outcomes
• Patient's self-care needs are met.
• Complications are avoided or minimized.
• Patient communicates feelings about limitations.
• Patient or significant other demonstrates correct use of assistive devices.
• Patient or significant other carries out dressing and grooming program daily.

Interventions and rationales
• Observe patient's functional level every shift; document and report any changes. *This allows adjustment of actions to meet patient's needs.*

• Perform prescribed treatment for underlying musculoskeletal impairment. Monitor progress, reporting favorable and adverse responses to treatment. *Therapy must be consistently applied to aid patient's independence.*
• Encourage patient to voice feelings and concerns about self-care deficits *to help patient achieve highest functional level.*
• Provide enough time for patient to perform dressing and grooming. *Rushing creates unnecessary stress and promotes failure.*
• Monitor patient's abilities for dressing and grooming daily. *This identifies problem areas before they become source of frustration.*
• Encourage family to provide clothing easily managed by patient. Clothing slightly larger than regular size and Velcro straps may be helpful. *Such clothing makes independent dressing easier.*
• Provide necessary assistive devices, such as long-handled shoe horn or zipper pull, as needed. Instruct on use. *Appropriate assistive devices encourage independence.*
• Assist with or perform dressing and grooming; fasten clothes; comb hair; clean nails. *Provide help only when patient has difficulty; this promotes feeling of independence.*
• Instruct patient or significant other in dressing and grooming techniques. Instructions to significant other can be given in writing. Have patient or significant other demonstrate dressing and grooming techniques under supervision. *Return demonstration identifies problem areas and increases significant other's self-confidence.*
• Refer patient, as needed, to psychiatric liaison nurse, support group, or home health care agency. *These extra resources will reinforce activities planned to meet patient's needs.*

Evaluations for expected outcomes
• Patient's self-care needs are met with help of staff.
• Patient participates in activities designed to minimize the risk of complications, such as complying with treatment.
• Patient expresses feelings about self-care limitations.
• Patient or significant other demonstrates appropriate use of assistive devices.
• Patient follows daily plans for self-care. Significant other assists as needed.

Documentation
• Patient's expression of feelings and concerns about self-care limitations and their impact on body image and life-style
• Patient's willingness to participate in dressing and grooming
• Observations of patient's impaired ability to perform dressing and grooming
• Interventions to provide supportive care
• Patient's response to nursing interventions
• Instructions to patient or significant other, their understanding of instructions, and their demonstrated skill in carrying out self-care functions
• Evaluations for each expected outcome.

Self-care deficit: Dressing and grooming

related to perceptual or cognitive impairment

Definition

Inability to carry out activities associated with dressing and grooming

Assessment

- History of neurologic, sensory, or psychological impairment
- Age
- Self-care abilities, including knowledge and use of adaptive equipment, preparation of equipment and supplies, technical and mechanical skills
- Neurologic status, including cognition, communication ability, insight or judgment, level of consciousness, memory, motor ability, orientation, sensory ability
- Psychosocial status, including coping mechanisms, family or significant other, life-style, patient's perceptions of self, personality

Defining characteristics

- Clinical evidence of perceptual or cognitive impairment
- Impaired ability to fasten clothing
- Impaired ability to obtain or replace articles of clothing
- Impaired ability to put on or take off necessary items of clothing
- Impaired short-term or long-term memory
- Inability to maintain appearance at a satisfactory level

Associated medical diagnoses (selected)

Alcoholism, Alzheimer's disease, autism, bipolar disease (manic or depressive phase), brain tumor, cerebrovascular accident, head injury, Huntington's disease, Laënnec's cirrhosis, mental retardation, organic brain syndrome, psychoses

Expected outcomes

- Patient's self-care needs are met.
- Complications are avoided or minimized.
- Patient or significant other carries out self-care program daily.
- Patient or significant other communicates feelings and concerns.
- Patient or significant other identifies resources to help cope with problems and discharge.

Interventions and rationales

- Observe, document, and report patient's functional and perceptual or cognitive ability daily. *Careful observation guides adjustment of nursing actions to meet patient's needs.*
- Perform prescribed treatment for underlying condition. Monitor progress and report favorable and adverse responses. *Therapy must be consistently applied to aid patient's independence.*
- Allow patient to express frustration, anger, or feelings of inadequacy. Provide emotional support *to help patient achieve highest functional level.*
- Provide privacy *to enhance patient's self-esteem.*
- Monitor dressing and grooming daily. *This identifies problem areas before they become a source of frustration.*
- Provide assistive devices as needed. *Appropriate assistive devices can encourage independence.*
- Do not rush patient. *Rushing creates unnecessary stress and promotes failure.*
- Remind patient of what is to be accomplished while performing actual

task. Praise accomplishments *to foster self-confidence.*
- Assist with dressing and grooming daily: fasten clothes; clean nails; comb hair. Select clothes and hand garments to patient one at a time in appropriate order. Provide help only when patient has difficulty *to promote a feeling of independence.*
- Direct patient in grooming measures, using simple instructions given one at a time, *to aid comprehension.*
- Encourage patient to complete dressing and grooming measures. Provide positive feedback during task performance. *Reinforcement and rewards may encourage effort.*
- Encourage significant other to provide clothing easily managed by patient; clothing slightly larger than regular size and Velcro straps may be helpful. *Such clothing makes independent dressing easier.*
- Give written instructions to significant other in dressing and grooming technique, and supervise return demonstration *to identify problem areas and increase significant other's self-confidence*
- Refer patient, as needed, to psychiatric liaison nurse, support group, or home health care agency. *These extra resources will reinforce activities planned to meet patient's needs.*

Evaluations for expected outcomes
- Patient's self-care needs are met with help of staff.
- Patient does not experience infection, skin integrity alteration, or other complications of altered self-care.
- Patient or significant other becomes more active in carrying out self-care program; need for staff assistance decreases.
- Patient discusses feelings about self-care deficit. If unable to meet own needs, patient seeks assistance from significant other or staff within 24 hours.
- Patient or significant other identifies and contacts available support resources as needed.

Documentation
- Patient's or significant other's expression of feelings and concern about self-care deficits
- Observations of patient's impaired ability to perform dressing and grooming activities
- Patient's response to underlying treatment
- Interventions to provide supportive care
- Instructions to patient (if capable) or significant other, their understanding of the instructions, and their demonstrated skill in carrying out self-care functions
- Patient's response to nursing interventions
- Evaluations for each expected outcome.

Self-care deficit: Feeding

related to musculoskeletal impairment

Definition
Inability to carry out the self-care activity of feeding

Assessment
- History of injury or disease associated with musculoskeletal impairment
- Self-care abilities, including knowledge and use of adaptive equipment, preparation of equipment and supplies, technical and mechanical skills
- Musculoskeletal status, including coordination, functional ability, gait;

mechanical restriction (cast, splint, traction); muscle tone, size and strength; range of motion; tremors
• Psychosocial status, including coping mechanisms, family or significant other, life-style, motivation, patient's perception of health problem and of self, personality

Defining characteristics
• Clinical evidence of musculoskeletal impairment
• Inability to bring food from receptacle to mouth

Associated medical diagnoses (selected)
Amyotrophic lateral sclerosis, brain or spinal cord tumor, cerebral palsy, cerebrovascular accident, fractures, Guillain-Barré syndrome, Huntington's disease, multiple sclerosis, multiple trauma, muscular dystrophy, myasthenia gravis (crisis), Parkinson's disease, rheumatoid arthritis, spinal cord injury, terminal cancer

Expected outcomes
• Patient expresses feelings about feeding limitations.
• Patient maintains weight at ____.
• Patient has no evidence of aspiration.
• Patient consumes ____% of diet.
• Patient or significant other demonstrates correct use of assistive devices.
• Patient or significant other carries out feeding program daily.

Interventions and rationales
• Observe patient's functional level every shift; document and report any changes. *This allows adjustment to patient's needs.*
• Perform prescribed treatment for underlying musculoskeletal impairment. Monitor progress and report responses. *Therapy must be applied consistently to facilitate independence.*
• Weigh patient weekly and record. Report change of more than 1 lb/week *to ensure adequate nutrition and fluid balance.*
• Monitor and record breath sounds every 4 hours *to check for aspiration of food.* Report crackles, wheezes, or rhonchi.
• Encourage patient to ventilate feelings and concerns about feeding deficits *to help patient achieve highest functional level.*
• Initiate feeding program:
  – Determine types of food best handled by patient. *Easily handled foods encourage patient's feelings of independence.*
  – Place patient in high Fowler's position *to aid swallowing and digestion.* Support weakened extremities, wash patient's face and hands before meals.
  – Provide assistive devices; instruct patient on use *to allow more independence.*
  – Supervise or assist at each meal; for example, cut food into small pieces. *This aids chewing, swallowing, and digestion and reduces risk of choking or aspiration.*
  – Feed patient slowly. *Rushing causes stress in patient, reducing digestive activity and causing intestinal spasms.*
  – Keep suction equipment at bedside *to remove aspirated foods if necessary.*
  – Instruct patient or significant other in feeding techniques and equipment. *This aids understanding and encourages compliance.*
  – Record percentage of food consumed *to ensure adequate nutrition.*

• Encourage patient to carry out aspects of feeding according to abilities. *This gives patient sense of achievement and control.*
• Refer patient to psychiatric liaison nurse, support group, or such community agencies as Visiting Nurse Association and Meals on Wheels. *Additional resources reinforce activities planned to meet patient's needs.*

Evaluations for expected outcomes
• Patient expresses frustration with feeding limitations.
• Patient obtains adequate fluid and nutritional intake.
• Patient maintains weight at or above established limit.
• Patient does not experience aspiration.
• Patient consumes established percentage of diet.
• Patient adapts to use of assistive devices. Significant other can explain use of assistive devices.
• Patient follows self-care feeding program daily. Significant other provides assistance as needed.

Documentation
• Patient's expression of feelings and concern about inability to feed self
• Observations of patient's impaired ability to perform self-care
• Patient's response to treatment
• Patient's weight
• Patient's intake
• Interventions to provide supportive care
• Instructions to patient and significant other, understanding of instructions, and demonstrated skill in carrying out self-care functions
• Patient's response to interventions
• Evaluations for each expected outcome.

■ Self-care deficit: Feeding

related to perceptual or cognitive impairment

Definition
Inability to feed self

Assessment
• History of neurologic, sensory, or psychological impairment
• Age
• Self-care abilities, including knowledge and use of adaptive equipment, preparation of equipment and supplies, technical and mechanical skills
• Neurologic status, including cognition, communication ability, insight or judgment, level of consciousness, memory, motor ability, orientation, sensory ability
• Psychosocial status, including coping mechanisms, family or significant other, life-style, patient's perceptions of self, personality

Defining characteristics
• Clinical evidence of perceptual or cognitive impairment
• Impaired short-term or long-term memory
• Inability to bring food from receptacle to mouth

Associated medical diagnoses (selected)
Alcoholism, Alzheimer's disease, autism, bipolar disease (manic or depressive phase), brain tumor, cerebrovascular accident, head injury, Huntington's disease, Laënnec's cirrhosis, mental retardation, organic brain syndrome, psychoses

Expected outcomes
• Patient's self-care needs are met.

• Complications are avoided or minimized.
• Patient or significant other carries out feeding program daily.
• Patient maintains weight.
• Patient or significant other communicates feelings and concerns.
• Patient or significant other identifies resources to help cope with problems and discharge.

Interventions and rationales
• Observe, document, and report patient's functional and perceptual or cognitive ability daily. *Careful observation guides adjustment of actions to meet patient's needs.*
• Weigh patient weekly and record results. Report loss of 2 lb or more *to ensure adequate nutrition and fluid balance.*
• Perform prescribed treatment for underlying condition. Monitor progress and report favorable and adverse responses. *Therapy must be consistently applied to aid patient's independence.*
• Allow patient to express frustration, anger, or feelings of inadequacy. Provide emotional support *to help patient come to terms with self-care deficit and achieve highest functional level.*
• Determine types of food best handled by patient; for example, finger foods, soft or liquid diet. *Easily handled foods encourage patient's feelings of independence.*
• Provide assistive devices at each meal, as needed. *These allow patient to do as much as possible for self.*
• Place patient in high Fowler's position *to reduce swallowing difficulty and aid digestion.*
• Supervise or assist at each meal; for example, cut food into small pieces. *Cutting food into small bites aids chewing, swallowing, and digestion, and reduces risk of choking or aspiration.*
• Feed patient slowly. Do not rush. *Rushing causes stress in patient, reducing digestive activity and causing intestinal spasms.*
• Encourage patient to do as much for self as possible, using simple instructions given one at a time, *to aid comprehension.*
• Keep suction equipment at bedside *to remove aspirated foods if necessary.*
• Instruct patient or significant other in feeding techniques and use of equipment. Have patient or significant other give return demonstration of feeding and equipment use under supervision. *This aids understanding and encourages compliance.*
• Refer patient, as needed, to psychiatric liaison nurse, support group, or home health care agency. *These extra resources will reinforce activities planned to meet patient's needs.*

Evaluations for expected outcomes
• Patient's self-care needs are met with help of staff.
• Patient does not experience infection, skin integrity alteration, weight loss, or other complications of altered self-care.
• Patient or significant other becomes more active in carrying out self-care program; need for staff assistance decreases.
• Patient expresses feelings about self-care deficit. If unable to meet own needs, patient seeks assistance from significant other or staff within 24 hours.
• Patient or significant other identifies and contacts available support resources as needed.

Documentation
- Patient's or significant other's expression of feelings and concern about difficulty with feeding
- Observations of patient's impaired ability to feed self
- Weight
- Patient's response to treatment
- Interventions to provide supportive care
- Instructions to patient (if capable) or significant other, their understanding of the instructions, and their demonstrated skill in carrying out instructions
- Patient's response to nursing interventions
- Evaluations for each expected outcome.

Self-care deficit: Toileting

related to musculoskeletal impairment

Definition
Inability to carry out toileting routine

Assessment
- History of injury or disease associated with musculoskeletal impairment
- Self-care abilities, including knowledge and use of adaptive equipment, preparation of equipment and supplies, technical or mechanical skills
- Musculoskeletal status, including coordination; functional ability; gait; mechanical restriction (cast, splint, traction); muscle tone, size, and strength; range of motion; tremors
- Psychosocial status, including coping mechanisms, family or significant other, life-style, patient's perceptions of health problem and self, personality

Defining characteristics
- Clinical evidence of musculoskeletal impairment
- Inability to carry out proper toilet hygiene
- Inability to flush toilet or empty commode
- Inability to get to toilet or commode
- Inability to manipulate clothing for toileting
- Inability to sit on or rise from toilet or commode

Associated medical diagnoses (selected)
Amyotrophic lateral sclerosis, brain or spinal cord tumor, cerebral palsy, cerebrovascular accident, fractures, Guillain-Barré syndrome, Huntington's disease, multiple sclerosis, multiple trauma, muscular dystrophy, myasthenia gravis (crisis), Parkinson's disease, rheumatoid arthritis, spinal cord injury, terminal cancer

Expected outcomes
- Patient's self-care needs are met.
- Complications are avoided or minimized.
- Patient communicates feelings about limitations.
- Patient maintains continence.
- Patient or significant other demonstrates correct use of assistive devices.
- Patient or significant other carries out toileting program daily.

Interventions and rationales
- Observe patient's functional level every shift; document and report any changes. *Careful observation guides adjustment of interventions to meet patient's needs.*
- Perform prescribed treatment for underlying musculoskeletal impairment. Monitor progress, reporting favorable and adverse responses to

treatment. *Therapy must be consistently applied to aid patient's independence.*
• Encourage patient to voice feelings and concerns about self-care deficits *to help patient achieve highest functional level possible.*
• Monitor intake and output and skin condition; record episodes of incontinence. *Accurate intake and output records can identify potential imbalances.*
• Use assistive devices as needed, such as external catheter at night, bedpan or urinal every 2 hours during day, and adaptive equipment for bowel care. Instruct on use. As control improves, reduce use of assistive devices. *Assisting at appropriate level helps maintain patient's self-esteem.*
• Assist with toileting if needed. *Allow patient to perform independently as much as possible.*
• Perform urinary and bowel care if needed. Follow urinary or bowel elimination plans. *Monitoring success or failure of toileting plans helps identify and resolve problem areas.*
• Instruct patient or significant other in toileting routine. Instructions to significant other can be given in writing. Have patient or significant other demonstrate toileting routine under supervision. *Return demonstration identifies problem areas and increases significant other's self-confidence.*
• Refer patient, as needed, to psychiatric liaison nurse, support group, or home healthc care agency. *These extra resources will reinforce activities planned to meet patient's needs.*

Evaluations for expected outcomes
• Patient's self-care needs are met with help of staff.
• Patient does not experience constipation, infection, skin integrity alteration, weight loss, or other complications of altered self-care.
• Patient maintains continence.
• Patient expresses feelings about self-care deficit. If unable to meet own needs, patient seeks assistance from significant other or staff within 24 hours.
• Patient or significant other demonstrates appropriate use of assistive devices.
• Patient follows daily plans for self-care. Significant other assists as needed.

Documentation
• Patient's expression of feelings and concerns about self-care limitations and their impact on body image and life-style
• Patient's willingness to participate in self-care
• Observations of patient's impaired ability to perform toileting routine and patient's response to treatment
• Intake and output
• Interventions to provide supportive care
• Instructions to patient or significant other, their understanding of instructions, and their demonstrated skill in carrying out self-care functions
• Patient's response to nursing interventions
• Evaluations for each expected outcome.

■ Self-care deficit: Toileting

related to perceptual or cognitive impairment

Definition
Inability to carry out toileting routine

Assessment

- History of neurologic, sensory, or psychological impairment
- Age
- Self-care abilities, including knowledge and use of adaptive equipment, preparation of equipment and supplies, technical or mechanical skills
- Neurologic status, including cognition, communication ability, insight or judgment, level of consciousness, memory, motor ability, orientation, sensory ability
- Psychosocial status, including coping mechanisms, family or significant other, life-style, patient's perceptions of self, personality

Defining characteristics

- Clinical evidence of perceptual or cognitive impairment
- Impaired short-term or long-term memory
- Inability to carry out proper toilet hygiene
- Inability to flush toilet or empty commode
- Inability to get to toilet or commode
- Inability to manipulate clothing for toileting
- Inability to sit on or rise from toilet or commode

Associated medical diagnoses (selected)

Alcoholism, Alzheimer's disease, autism, bipolar disease (manic or depressive phase), brain tumor, cerebrovascular accident, head injury, Huntington's disease, Laënnec's cirrhosis, mental retardation, organic brain syndrome, psychoses

Expected outcomes

- Patient's self-care needs are met.
- Complications are avoided or minimized.
- Patient or significant other carries out toileting program daily.
- Patient maintains continence.
- Patient or significant other communicates feelings and concerns.
- Patient or significant other identifies resources to help cope with problems and discharge.

Interventions and rationales

- Observe, document, and report patient's functional and perceptual or cognitive ability daily. *This allows adjustment of actions to meet patient's needs.*
- Perform prescribed treatment for underlying condition. Monitor progress and report favorable and adverse responses. *Therapy must be consistently applied to aid patient's independence.*
- Allow patient to express frustration, anger, or feelings of inadequacy. Provide emotional support *to help patient achieve highest functional level.*
- Monitor intake and output; record episodes of incontinence. *Accurate intake and output records can identify potential imbalances.*
- Use assistive devices as needed, such as external catheter at night, bedpan or urinal every 2 hours during day, and adaptive equipment for bowel care. As control improves, reduce use of assistive devices. *Assisting at appropriate level helps maintain patient's self-esteem.*
- Assist with toileting, if needed, using visual and auditory cues to stimulate urination. *This allows patient to perform independently as much as possible.*
- Allow ample time for patient to perform toileting routine. *Rushing creates unnecessary stress and promotes failure.*

• Provide positive, constructive feedback when assisting with toileting. *Reinforcement and rewards may enhance self-esteem.*
• Assist with toileting, using simple instructions given one at a time, *to aid comprehension.*
• Complete urinary and bowel care if patient is unable to do so. Follow urinary and bowel elimination plans. *Monitoring success or failure of toileting plans helps identify and resolve problem areas.*
• Give written instructions in toileting routine to significant other, and supervise return demonstration. *Return demonstration identifies problem areas and increases significant other's self-confidence.*
• Refer patient to psychiatric liaison nurse, support group, or community agency, as needed. *These extra resources will reinforce activities planned to meet patient's needs.*

Evaluations for expected outcomes

• Patient's self-care needs are met with help of staff.
• Patient does not experience constipation, infection, skin integrity alteration, weight loss, or other complications of altered self-care.
• Patient or significant other becomes more active in carrying out self-care program; need for staff assistance decreases.
• Patient maintains continence.
• Patient expresses feelings about self-care deficit. If unable to meet own needs, patient seeks assistance from significant other or staff within 24 hours.
• Patient or significant other identifies and contacts available support resources as needed.

Documentation

• Patient's or significant other's expression of feelings and concern about self-care deficits
• Observations of patient's impaired ability to perform toileting routine
• Intake and output
• Patient's response to treatment for underlying condition
• Interventions to provide supportive care
• Instructions to patient (if capable) or significant other, their understanding of the instructions, and their demonstrated skill in carrying out self-care functions
• Patient's response to nursing interventions
• Evaluations for each expected outcome.

Self-esteem, chronic low

Definition

Long-standing negative self-evaluation or feelings about self or capabilities

Assessment

• Reason for hospitalization or outpatient treatment
• Age
• Sex
• Developmental stage
• Family system, including: marital status, role in the family, sibling position
• Perception of health problem
• Past experience with health care system
• Mental status, including abstract thinking, affect, communication, general appearance, judgment or insight, memory, mood, orientation, perception, thinking process

- Belief system, including norms, religion, values
- Social interaction pattern
- Social and occupational history
- Perception of self (past and present), including body image, coping mechanisms, problem-solving ability, self-worth
- Past experience with crisis
- Past history of treatment for psychosocial disturbance, including hospitalization, medication, psychotherapy, suicidal ideation, plans, past attempts
- Neurovegetative signs, including ability to experience pleasure, appetite, energy level, sleep

Defining characteristics
- Difficulty making decisions
- Exhibition of need for excessive reassurance
- Exhibition of nonassertive or passive tendencies
- Expressions of shame or guilt
- Extreme conformity or dependency on others' opinions
- Frequent expression of self-negating thoughts
- Hesitation to try new things or situations
- Perception of self as unable to deal with events

Associated medical diagnoses (selected)
Medical diagnoses include cardiovascular disease, chronic illnesses requiring lifelong treatment (such as hemophilia, chronic obstructive pulmonary disease, Crohn's disease, diabetes mellitus, end-stage renal disease, seizure disorders), endocrine or metabolic disorders, neurologic or neuromuscular disease, and any illness or injury resulting in chronic pain, permanent disability, or disfigurement. *Psychiatric diagnoses* include anxiety, bipolar disorder, depression, panic state, self-destructive behaviors (anorexia nervosa, bulimia, substance abuse, attempts at suicide), and personality disorders (borderline, dependent, obsessive-compulsive, passive-dependent).

Expected outcomes
- Patient voices feelings related to self-esteem.
- Patient reports feeling safe in hospital environment.
- Patient makes verbal contract not to harm self while in hospital.
- Patient joins gradually in self-care and decision making process.
- Patient engages in social interaction with others.
- Patient demonstrates verbally and behaviorally a decrease in negative self-evaluation.
- Patient voices acceptance of positive and negative feedback without exaggeration.

Interventions and rationales
- Provide for a specific amount of uninterrupted non-care-related time to engage patient in conversation. *This gives patient time for self-exploration.*
- Listen to patient with understanding, responding with nonjudgmental acceptance, genuine interest, and sincerity. *This expands patient's self-awareness and reduces element of threat.*
- Assess patient's mental status through interview and observation at least once weekly. *High anxiety from self-rejection may cause cognitive, sensory, or perceptual disturbances.*
- Assess suicide risk and lethal potential, as indicated. *Extremely low levels of self-esteem may lead to suicide.*
- Institute suicidal precautions according to protocol. *Patient's behav-*

ior must be supervised until self-control is adequate for safety.
• Provide patient with simple, structured daily routine. *Structured activity sets limits to patient's anxious behaviors.*
• Encourage patient to care for self to the extent possible. *Patient may neglect or reject aspects of self-care, from feelings of self-hate.*
• Involve patient in decisions about care on a gradual basis, *to reduce feelings of ambivalence, procrastination and lack of confidence in decision making.*
• Arrange situations to encourage social interaction between patient and others. *Disturbed interpersonal relationships are a direct expression of self-hate.*
• Provide patient with positive feedback for verbal reports and behaviors indicative of improved self-esteem. *This encourages future adaptive coping behaviors.*
• Help patient mobilize resources for assistance when discharged, *to help patient replace maladaptive coping behaviors with more adaptive ones.*
• Refer patient to mental health professional as indicated. *Severity of symptoms accompanying chronic low self-esteem may require long-term psychotherapy.*

Evaluations for expected outcomes
• Patient expresses feelings about self.
• Patient does not feel threatened by hospital environment.
• At least once daily, patient reiterates commitment not to harm self.
• Patient participates in at least one aspect of self-care daily.
• Patient converses with others on daily basis.
• Patient states at least two positive aspects about self.
• Patient accepts constructive criticism.

Documentation
• Patient's verbal expressions and behaviors indicative of low self-esteem
• Mental status examination (baseline and ongoing)
• Suicide assessment, interventions, and patient's response
• All nursing interventions implemented to facilitate improved self-esteem
• Patient's response to interventions
• Evaluations for each expected outcome.

Self-esteem, situational low

Definition
Negative self-evaluation or feelings about self that develop in response to a loss or change in an individual who previously had a positive self-evaluation

Assessment
• Age
• Sex
• Developmental stage
• Family system, including marital status, role in family, sibling position
• Reason for hospitalization
• Mental status, including affect, general appearance, mood
• Cognitive ability
• Behavior
• Past perception of self
• Current perception of self

Defining characteristics
• Difficulty making decisions
• Episodic occurrence of negative self-appraisal in response to life events in a person with a previously positive self-evaluation

- Evaluation of self as unable to handle situational events
- Verbalization of negative feelings about self (helplessness, uselessness)

Associated medical diagnoses (selected)
This nursing diagnosis can be used with any patient experiencing an anticipated or actual loss (body part, normal body function, control over environment, threat to life). Examples include carcinoma; cerebrovascular accident; communicable diseases; conditions requiring amputation, hysterectomy, mastectomy, or ostomy; immunosuppressive conditions; myocardial infarction; or any injury or illness resulting in prolonged hospitalization.

Expected outcomes
- Patient voices feelings related to current situation and its effect on self-esteem.
- Patient verbally describes appraisal of self before current health problem.
- Patient participates in decisions related to care and therapies.
- Patient reports a sense of control over life events.
- Patient articulates a return to previous positive feelings about self.

Interventions and rationales
- Encourage patient to express feelings about self (past and present). *Self-exploration encourages patient to consider future change.*
- Provide for a specific amount of uninterrupted non-care-related time to engage patient in conversation. *Mutuality helps patient assume ultimate responsibility for coping responses.*
- Assess patient's mental status through interview and observation at least once daily. *If anxiety resulting from self-rejection becomes severe, patient may experience disorientation, psychotic symptoms.*
- Involve patient in decision-making process. *Expressions of low self-esteem include ambivalence and procrastination.*
- Provide patient with positive feedback for verbal reports or behaviors indicative of a return to positive self-appraisal. *This gives patient feelings of significance, approval and competence to cope effectively with stressful situations.*

Evaluations for expected outcomes
- Patient expresses feelings about self in relation to recent stressful events.
- Patient describes how feelings about self have changed since current health problem began.
- Each day, patient makes decisions related to care.
- Patient reports feeling more self-confident in managing current situation.
- Patient states at least two positive feelings about self.

Documentation
- Patient's expressions of lowered self-esteem
- Mental status assessment (baseline and ongoing)
- Nursing interventions directed toward a return to previous positive self-esteem
- Patient's response to interventions
- Evaluations for each expected outcome.

Self-esteem disturbance

Definition
Negative self-evaluation or feelings about self or self capabilities that may be directly or indirectly expressed

Assessment
- Age
- Developmental stage
- Sex
- Family system, including: marital status, sibling position
- Reason for hospitalization or outpatient treatment
- Patient's perception of health problem
- Past experience with health problems
- Mental status, including affect, behavior, cognitive ability, general appearance, mood
- Usual coping behaviors during stress
- Social interaction pattern

Defining characteristics
- Denial of problems that are evident to others
- Exhibitions of grandiosity
- Expressions of shame or guilt
- Frequent expression of self-negating thoughts
- Hesitation to try new things or situations
- Hypersensitivity to slight or criticism
- Perceptions of self as unable to deal with events
- Projection of blame or responsibility for problems onto others
- Tendency to rationalize away or reject positive feedback and exaggerate negative feedback about self
- Tendency to rationalize personal failures

Associated medical diagnoses (selected)
Self-esteem is an essential issue affecting all hospitalized clients. Examples include the following physical and emotional conditions: amputation, anxiety, burns, commmunicable diseases, congenital anomalies, depression, immunosuppressive conditions, infertility, mastectomy, menopause or hysterectomy, narcissistic or borderline personality disorder, ostomy, sexual dysfunction, and substance abuse.

Expected outcomes
- Patient voices feelings related to self-esteem.
- Patient participates in decisions related to care and therapies.
- Patient engages in social interaction with others.
- Patient voices an acceptance of positive or negative feedback without exaggeration.
- Patient initiates action to attain higher level of wellness, physically and emotionally.
- Patient articulates at least two positive qualities about self.

Interventions and rationales
- Encourage patient to express feelings about self. *Active listening is the most basic therapeutic skill.*
- Allow a specific amount of uninterrupted, non-care-related time to engage patient in conversation. *This creates environment that encourages patient to ventilate feelings at own pace.*
- Assess patient's mental status through interview and observation at least once daily. *This helps detect abnormal feelings and behaviors.*

• Involve patient in decision making process, *to reduce patient's feelings of dependence on others.*
• Arrange situations to encourage social interaction between patient and others. *Improving social environment helps restore confidence and self-esteem.*
• Provide patient with positive feedback for verbal reports or behaviors indicating improved self-esteem. *This encourages future effective coping behaviors.*
• Refer patient to mental health professional if indicated. *Consultation can ease frustration, increase objectivity and foster collaborative approach to patient's care.*

Evaluations for expected outcomes

• Patient expresses feelings about self.
• Patient makes at least two care-related decisions daily.
• Patient interacts with others at least once daily.
• Patient accepts responsibility for behavior and is open to constructive criticism.
• Patient performs self-care activities and undergoes therapy without prompting.
• Patient states at least two personal assets.

Documentation

• Patient's expressions of lowered self-esteem
• Mental status assessment (baseline and ongoing)
• Interventions directed toward improved self-esteem
• Patient's response to nursing interventions
• Evaluations for each expected outcome.

Self-mutilation, high risk for

related to emotional illness

Definition

State in which an individual is at risk for performing a deliberate act of self-harm that's intended to produce immediate tissue damage

Assessment

• Age
• Sex
• Developmental history
• Current stress level and coping behaviors
• Mental status, including judgment, thought content, mood
• Family history, including abusive behavior
• Previous episodes of self-mutilation, suicide attempts
• Substance abuse history
• Social history, including sexual activity, aggression within peer group

Risk factors

• Borderline personality disorder (especially in females ages 16 to 25)
• Childhood emotional disturbances or abuse
• Command hallucinations
• Dissociative episodes
• Emotional deprivation by parents
• Expressions of self-hatred
• Feelings of depression or emptiness
• History of dysfunctional family upbringing
• History of physical or sexual abuse
• Inability to cope with increased stress
• Lability of affect
• Lack of sensory stimuli
• Low self-esteem

• Psychotic state (especially in young males)

Associated medical diagnoses (selected)
Autism, borderline personality disorder, developmental disability, factitious disorder with physical symptoms, malingering, multiple personality disorder, sexual masochism

Expected outcomes
• Patient doesn't harm himself while in the hospital.
• Patient expresses increased sense of security.
• Patient reports being able to cope better with disorganization, aggressive impulses, anxiety, or hallucinations.
• Patient no longer experiences dissociative states or experiences fewer of them.
• Patient participates in therapeutic milieu.
• Patient reports suicidal thoughts to staff.

Interventions and rationales
• Limit the number of staff members interacting with the patient *to provide continuity of care and increase the patient's sense of security.*
• Have staff make frequent, short contacts with the patient *to reassure the patient without stifling independence.*
• Remove all dangerous objects from the patient's environment *to promote safety.*
• Make short-term verbal "contracts" with the patient stating that the patient won't harm himself *to make the patient aware that he is ultimately responsible for his own safety and that he is capable of guaranteeing it.*
• Administer psychotropic medications, as ordered, *to reduce tension, impulsive behavior, hallucinations, and panic.*
• If the patient enters a dissociative state or hallucinates, move him to a quiet room with reduced stimuli. If restraints must be used, remain with the patient and provide reassurance *to calm the patient and orient him to reality.*
• As ordered, place the patient under observation *to provide protection and increase the patient's sense of security.* If hospitalized, the patient can be "zoned" or asked to remain in areas within sight of staff.
• If the patient is participating in therapeutic milieu, discuss the patient's risk of self-harm with community members *to provide enhanced protection and psychological support.*
• If the patient harms himself, care for the injuries in a calm, nonjudgmental manner. Encourage the patient to talk about the feelings that prompted the self-mutilation. *Discussion may help the patient connect self-destructive behavior to the feelings that preceded it. Discussion may also provide an opportunity to explore alternative ways of dealing with negative thoughts and feelings.*
• If self-destructive acts persist, consider developing a behavior-modification program, where periods of self-control are rewarded through benefits such as personal attention or material items *to reinforce self-control.*
• Ask the patient directly if he is thinking of suicide and, if so, what plan he has. *A self-destructive patient may become suicidal and, therefore, require additional precautions.*
• Hold frequent treatment team meetings *to ensure consistent care that is appropriate to the patient's current behavior.*

Evaluations of expected outcomes

- Patient keeps terms of verbal "contracts" stating that he won't harm himself.
- Patient doesn't incur any injury.
- Patient expresses increased sense of security.
- Patient describes coping skills that enable him to deal better with disorganization, aggressive impulses, anxiety, or hallucinations.
- Patient experiences fewer dissociative states.
- Patient participates in therapeutic milieu.
- Patient tells staff member about suicidal thoughts.

Documentation

- Nursing interventions performed and the patient's response
- Contracts between the patient and nurse
- Patient's responses to medication and behavioral modification program
- Revisions to treatment plan
- Drawing of self-inflicted injuries
- Evidence of suicidal ideation
- Evaluations for each expected outcome.

■ Sensory or perceptual alteration (auditory)

related to altered sensory reception, transmission, or integration

Definition

Change in the characteristics of auditory stimuli

Assessment

- History of ear disorders, trauma, surgery
- Age
- Auditory status, including ear position, size, and symmetry; skin color and texture; tympanic membrane (cerumen, color of canal, deformities, discharge, intactness or tension, landmarks); use of hearing aid
- Rinne test
- Weber's test
- Communication status, including adaptive responses (gestures, lipreading, signing), level of comprehension and expression, speech pattern
- Environmental factors; for example, factory noise
- Activities of daily living
- Behavioral assessment, including coping mechanisms, willingness to cooperate with treatment

Defining characteristics

- Altered communication pattern, reduced facial expression
- Altered conceptualization
- Anger
- Apathy or passiveness
- Auditory distortion
- Change in behavior pattern, decreased social interaction
- Change in response to auditory stimuli
- Clinical evidence of impaired (decreased) hearing ability
- Depression
- Disorientation
- Hallucinations
- Reported or measured change in auditory activity
- Restlessness

Associated medical diagnoses (selected)

Acoustic neuroma, auditory nerve damage, chronic suppurative otitis media, deafness (uncompensated), drug-induced deafness, otosclerosis, presbycusis

Expected outcomes

- Patient discusses impact of auditory loss on life-style.
- Patient maintains orientation to person, place, and time.
- Patient expresses feeling of comfort and security.
- Patient shows interest in external environment.
- Patient compensates for auditory loss by use of signing, gestures, lipreading, hearing aid, and other measures.
- Patient plans to use community resources to assist with auditory deficit.

Interventions and rationales

- Allow patient to express feelings about hearing loss. Convey a willingness to listen, but do not pressure patient to talk. *Giving patient chance to talk about hearing loss enhances acceptance of loss.*
- Determine how to communicate effectively with patient, using gestures, written words, signing, lipreading. If patient has a hearing aid, encourage its use. *Planned communication with patient improves care delivery.*
- Give patient clear, concise explanations of treatments and procedures. Avoid information overload. Face patient when speaking; enunciate words clearly, slowly, and in normal speaking voice; avoid putting hands to mouth when speaking. Wearing red lipstick helps to define the mouth. *Patient will be better able to join in care with better understanding of treatment plan.*
- Provide sensory stimulation by using tactile and visual stimuli to help compensate for hearing loss. Encourage family to bring familiar objects from home. *Sensory stimulation of patient's other senses helps compensate for hearing loss.*
- Provide reality orientation if patient is confused or disoriented *to permit more effective patient-staff interaction.*
- Make sure other staff members are aware of patient's hearing deficit. Record information on patient's Kardex and chart cover. *This ensures effective nursing care delivery by staff.*
- Respond to call light by going to patient's room as soon as possible. If feasible, assign same staff members to care for patient. *These measures reduce patient's fears.*
- Educate patient in alternative ways of coping with hearing loss; care of hearing aid, if prescribed; and safety and protective measures to avoid harm or injury (use of amplifier or signal devices on telephone, visual cues in environment). *Knowledgeable patient will be better able to cope with hearing loss.*
- Refer to appropriate community resources, such as American Organization for the Education of the Hearing Impaired, to help patient adapt to loss. Involve family or significant other in planning and encourage participation. *These measures help patient and family cope better with hearing loss.*

Evaluations for expected outcomes

- Patient discusses impact of hearing loss on life-style.
- Patient demonstrates ability to recognize people and places and to identify the time and past and present events.
- Because of reduction in environmental risk factors, patient expresses comfort in surroundings.
- Patient expresses interest in interacting with others.
- Patient begins to come to terms with change in sensory perception.

• Patient identifies and uses alternative methods to facilitate communication.
• Patient recognizes need for support during transition from hospital to outside environment.

Documentation
• Patient's statement of feelings about auditory loss
• Observations of patient's behavior or response to auditory loss and use of adaptive aids
• Instructions regarding safety and protective measures and patient's intent to use appropriate resources
• Patient's response to nursing interventions
• Evaluations for each expected outcome.

■ Sensory or perceptual alteration (gustatory)

Definition
Change in the sense of taste

Assessment
• Taste sensation, including change from baseline, ability to differentiate sweet, salty, sour, and bitter taste
• Health history, including trauma, infection, vitamin or mineral deficiency, neurologic or oral disorders, chemotherapy or radiation therapy
• Medication history, including use of certain antidepressants (such as clomipramine), antineoplastics, penicillamine, captopril, lithium, interferon alfa-2a, levamisole, zidovudine
• Evidence of loss of appetite
• Weight change from baseline
• Mouth dryness
• Smoking history
• Sense of smell

Defining characteristics
• Altered taste sense
  – complete loss of taste (ageusia)
  – distorted sense of taste (dysgeusia)
  – partial loss of taste (hypogeusia)
• Loss of appetite
• Weight loss

Associated medical diagnoses (selected)
Basilar skull fracture, Bell's palsy, brain stem lesions, chemotherapy, common cold, influenza, oral cancer, radiation therapy, Sjögren's syndrome, thalamic syndromes, viral hepatitis (acute), vitamin B_{12} deficiency, zinc deficiency

Expected outcomes
• Patient reports changes in sense of taste.
• Patient identifies ways to enhance enjoyment of food.
• Patient consumes __% of diet.
• Patient maintains weight.

Interventions and rationales
• Assess changes in sense of taste *to establish a baseline.*
  – Gently raise the patient's tongue slightly with a gauze sponge. Use a moistened applicator to place a few crystals of salt or sugar on one side of the tongue. Wipe the tongue clean and ask the patient to identify the taste sensation.
  – Apply a tiny amount of quinine to the base of the tongue *to test bitter taste sensation.*
  – Place a small piece of sour pickle on the patient's tongue *to test sour taste sensation.*
• Pinch off one nostril and ask the patient to close his eyes and sniff through the open nostril to identify nonirritating odors, such as coffee, lime, and wintergreen, *to evaluate sense of smell; much of what consti-*

tutes taste is actually smell. Repeat the test on the opposite nostril.
- Monitor and record the patient's weight each week *to detect signs of weight loss.*
- Modify the patient's diet *so he can distinguish and enjoy as many tastes as possible.* Identify ways to emphasize smell and enhance flavor of food, such as using herbs and spices, *to compensate for loss of taste.*
- Serve food in attractive surroundings. Prepare meals in an attractive manner, using a variety of different colored foods, *to appeal to the patient's visual sense.*

Evaluations for expected outcomes
- Patient reports changes in sense of taste.
- Patient identifies ways to make meals more appealing.
- Patient consumes __% of diet.
- Patient maintains weight.

Documentation
- Evidence of changes in patient's sense of taste
- Patient's weight
- Techniques used to modify patient's diet
- Evaluations for each expected outcome.

Sensory or perceptual alteration (kinesthetic)

Definition
Diminished ability to perceive position or location of body parts, especially changes in the angles of joints

Assessment
- Health history, including presence of neurologic or musculoskeletal conditions
- Musculoskeletal status, including motor coordination, muscular weakness
- Use of safety devices
- Presence of other sensory impairments
- Neurologic status, including cognition (insight, judgment, memory), level of consciousness, orientation
- Coping behaviors
- Emotional response to illness
- Self-concept, including self-esteem, body image

Defining characteristics
- Diminished motor coordination
- Inability to identify position or location of body parts
- Inability to perceive changes in the angles of joints
- Muscular weakness, flaccidity, rigidity or atrophy
- Paralysis

Associated medical diagnoses (selected)
Cerebral palsy, multiple sclerosis, muscular dystrophy, rhizotomy, spinal trauma, spinal tumors, surgical joint replacement

Expected outcomes
- Patient expresses feelings associated with changes in kinesthetic perception.
- Patient implements safety precautions.
- Skin breakdown is avoided, especially in areas around vulnerable joints.
- Patient participates in self-care activities to maximum ability.
- Patient participates in an appropriate exercise program.
- Patient does not experience injury.

Interventions and rationales

- Encourage patient to express feelings related to diminished kinesthetic perception *to promote acceptance of perceptual impairment.*
- Assess changes in motor coordination, paralysis, or muscular weakness and report observations to health care team *to ensure appropriate care.*
- Implement appropriate safety measures, such as installing padded bed rails, maintaining bed in low position, or using wheelchair lapboard, *to avoid patient injury.*
- Remind patient to regularly observe how hands and feet are placed *to avoid injury.*
- Teach staff members to remind patient of need to check positioning of hands and feet *to ensure safety.* Emphasize the importance of communicating a supportive and accepting attitude *to enhance patient's emotional well-being.*
- Inspect skin daily, especially areas around vulnerable joints, *to detect signs of skin breakdown.*
- Encourage use of letter board, electric wheelchair, and feeding and dressing devices *to promote independence.*
- Provide patient with an exercise program that includes active and passive range-of-motion routines *to maintain range of motion and prevent musculoskeletal degeneration.*

Evaluations for expected outcomes

- Patient describes feelings brought on by changes in kinesthetic perception.
- Patient implements safety precautions.
- Patient does not exhibit signs of skin breakdown.
- Patient participates in self-care activities to maximum ability.
- Patient participates in selected exercise program.
- Patient does not experience injury.

Documentation

- Observations of diminished kinesthetic perception
- Evidence of patient's understanding of instructions regarding safety and protective measures and intent to use appropriate safety devices
- Patient's response to nursing interventions
- Evaluations for each expected outcome.

Sensory or perceptual alteration (olfactory)

Definition

Change in the sense of smell

Assessment

- Alterations in olfactory sense and related symptoms, including nosebleeds, foul taste in mouth, sneezing, postnasal drip, dry or sore mouth or throat, loss of sense of taste or appetite, excessive tearing, facial pain, eye pain
- Nutritional status, including weight, usual dietary intake, nausea
- Medication history, including use of phenothiazines, estrogen, metronidazole, antineoplastics, or prolonged use of nasal decongestants or topical anesthetics
- History of intranasal drug abuse, such as cocaine, amphetamines
- Respiratory status, including nasal drainage, sputum characteristics, history of colds, hay fever, or polyps
- Health status, including presence of any condition that causes irritation and swelling of the nasal mucosa and

obstruction of the olfactory area (such as nasal disease or allergies) or any condition that may cause a lesion in the olfactory nerve pathway (such as head trauma)
- Smoking history
- Inhalation of irritants, such as chlorine fumes
- Physical examination, including inspection and palpation of nasal structures, contour and color of nasal mucosa, size and color of turbinates, presence of polyps, source and character of nasal discharge, olfactory nerve (cranial nerve I) function
- Home environment, including presence of gas or propane heating systems, smoke detectors, chemical substances

Defining characteristics
- Altered sense of smell
  - diminished sense of smell (hyposmia)
  - absent sense of smell (anosmia)
- Diminished sense of taste and loss of appetite
- Weight changes

Associated medical diagnoses (selected)
Anterior cerebral artery occlusion, brain stem lesions, diabetes mellitus, head trauma, lead poisoning, lethal midline granuloma, nasal polyps, nasal or sinus neoplasms, nasopharyngitis, olfactory meningioma, pernicious anemia, rhinitis, septal fracture, septal hematoma, sinusitis

Expected outcomes
- If appropriate, patient states that decreased olfactory perception is temporary.
- If appropriate, patient reports improvements in olfactory perception.
- Patient maintains weight.
- Patient describes how to identify noxious odors and maintain a safe home environment.

Interventions and rationales
- Assess patient's ability to smell and document findings *to establish a baseline.*
- Prepare foods that patient likes and serve them in an attractive manner *to stimulate patient's appetite.* Use a variety of different colored foods with each meal *to appeal to patient's visual sense.*
- Weigh patient weekly *to detect weight loss and monitor for possible malnutrition.*
- If altered olfactory perception results from nasal congestion, take the following steps:
  - Reassure patient that condition is temporary and sense of smell should return *to diminish anxiety.*
  - Tell patient with nasal packing that sense of smell will return after packing is removed and swelling decreases *to provide reassurance.*
  - Administer prescribed medications, such as antihistamines and nose drops or sprays, *to relieve nasal congestion.*
  - Monitor laboratory values and vital signs *to detect signs of infection.*
  - Record nasal drainage characteristics, including amount, color, consistency, and odor, *to assess for changes in olfactory condition.*
  - Ensure adequate hydration and provide for humidification in patient's room *to prevent drying of mucous membranes.*
- If altered olfactory perception doesn't result from simple nasal congestion, prepare patient for diagnostic tests, such as sinus transillumination, skull X-ray, or computed

tomography scan, as ordered, *to guide further treatment.*

- Provide home care instructions as necessary. Teach patient to:
  - contact utility company *to implement measures for protecting against possible gas leaks.*
  - place smoke detectors throughout home *to signal danger of fire.*
  - discard food according to dates on packages rather than relying on sense of smell *to avoid eating spoiled food.*

Evaluations for expected outcomes

- Patient expresses understanding of the fact that change in olfactory perception is temporary.
- Patient reports improvement in olfactory perception.
- Patient's weight stabilizes.
- Patient demonstrates ability to identify noxious odors and maintain a safe home environment.

Documentation

- Evidence of changes in patient's olfactory perception
- Nursing interventions performed and patient's response
- Patient's dietary preferences
- Patient's weight
- Instructions for home care and patient's or caregiver's response
- Evaluations for each expected outcome.

Sensory or perceptual alteration (specify)

related to hallucinations

Definition

Perceptions of images or sensations that occur in the absence of external stimuli

Assessment

- Age
- Sex
- Reason for hospitalization, including patient's perception of problem, recent stressors, changes in somatic functioning, circumstances surrounding onset of hallucinations, duration and diurnal nature of experiences, delusional beliefs
- Mental status, including insight regarding current situation, judgment, abstract thinking, general information, mood, affect, recent and remote memory, thought processes, thought content, orientation to time, place, and person
- Physical characteristics, including manner of dress, personal hygiene, posture, gait
- Communication skills, including attitude toward interviewer, body language, facial expressions
- Psychosocial assessment, including coping mechanisms, support systems, willingness to cooperate with treatment, ability to perform activities of daily living, social interactions
- Health history, including medication history (response, effectiveness, adverse reactions), substance abuse history (type, effect on mental status), sleep habits, dietary and nutritional status
- Laboratory studies, including blood chemistry, toxicology screening
- Diagnostic tests, including computed tomography scan, EEG

Defining characteristics

- Acting out hallucinatory experience (command hallucinations)
- Images that occur in absence of external stimuli (visual hallucinations)
- Perceived odors of specific or unknown origin (olfactory hallucinations)

- Perceived taste sensations with no basis in reality (gustatory hallucinations)
- Perceived voices or sounds not heard by others and unrelated to objective reality (auditory hallucinations)
- Preoccupation, lack of awareness of surroundings
- Strange body sensations, including misperceptions about body parts (tactile hallucinations)
- Talking to self
- Watchfulness and listening in absence of external stimuli

Associated medical diagnoses (selected)
Affective disorders, amnestic syndrome, delirium, dementia, intoxication and withdrawal, mixed organic brain syndromes, organic affective syndrome, organic delusional syndrome, organic hallucinosis, personality disorders (borderline, schizoid, paranoid, schizophreniform), schizophrenia

Expected outcomes
- Patient reports decrease in number of hallucinatory experiences.
- Patient reports decrease in anxiety levels that lead to hallucinations.
- Patient demonstrates increased ability to test reality at onset of hallucinations.
- Patient can meet interpersonal needs in realistic ways.

Interventions and rationales
- Provide a safe and structured environment. Identify and reduce as many stressors as possible. Be honest and consistent in all interactions with patient. *These measures will help decrease patient's anxiety.*
- Encourage patient to identify and initiate anxiety-reducing measures *to give the patient a sense of control.*
- In organic hallucinations, use reality orientation and factual information to help the patient cope. Tell the patient that the hallucination results from organic causes and can be reversed. *This will reduce anxiety.* In nonorganic hallucinations, do not attempt to reason with the patient or challenge the hallucination. Instead, provide comfort and support. *Attempts at reasoning only increase anxiety, which exacerbates hallucinations.*
- When speaking to the patient, use directive statements, such as "Look at me and listen; try not to pay attention to the voices right now." *Reacting verbally forces the patient to focus on you rather than on internal stimuli.*
- Provide regular physical activity that requires use of concentration and large muscles *to distract the patient from internal stimuli.*
- Help patient to identify situations that evoke hallucinatory experiences *to enable the patient to anticipate hallucinations and possibly prevent their onset.*
- Teach patient to intervene in the hallucinatory experience. Encourage patient to speak out against the hallucination, using such statements as "Go away; you're not real." *Such responses foster a sense of control and help distract the patient, thereby reducing frequency and duration of hallucinations.*
- Teach patient to use consensual validation of perceptual experiences to test reality. *Having other people validate experiences will increase the patient's orientation to reality.*
- As the patient's anxiety level decreases, encourage participation in group-oriented activities and involvement in the community *to increase the patient's level of functioning.*

• Refer patient to psychiatric liaison nurse, social service, or support group, as appropriate, *to provide additional support for patient and family or significant other.*

Evaluations for expected outcomes
• Within 2 weeks, patient states that hallucinatory experiences have decreased in intensity and frequency.
• Patient describes two situations that increase anxiety.
• Patient employs self-control measures to reduce hallucinations.
• Patient demonstrates improved social skills.

Documentation
• Patient's statements regarding type, frequency, and intensity of hallucinations
• Observations about environmental factors that precipitate hallucinatory experiences
• Patient's anxiety level
• Interventions to help patient cope
• Patient's response to nursing interventions
• Referrals
• Evaluations for each expected outcome.

■ Sensory or perceptual alteration (specify)

related to sensory deprivation

Definition
Change in the characteristics of incoming stimuli

Assessment
• Nature of medical diagnosis
• Mobility
• Neurologic status, including cognition (insight or judgment, recent and remote memory); level of consciousness; orientation; sensory function
• Diagnostic tests, including electroencephalogram, computed tomography scan
• Communication status, including adaptive responses (gestures, lipreading, signing), level of comprehension and expression, speech pattern
• Environmental status, including equipment and supplies, lighting, location of patient's personal belongings, noise, privacy, space
• Psychosocial status, including alcohol and drug use, behavior and personality, coping mechanisms, history of depression, support systems

Defining characteristics
• Altered abstraction
• Altered conceptualization
• Apathy
• Change in behavior pattern
• Change in problem-solving abilities
• Disoriented to time, place, or person
• Isolation
• Reported or measured change in sensory acuity

Associated medical diagnoses (selected)
This diagnosis is often seen in elderly patients who are hospitalized or institutionalized, and in patients who are on isolation precautions. It may also occur in the following conditions: bipolar disease (depression phase), blindness, cerebrovascular accident, deafness, depression, head injury, hemianopsia, organic brain syndrome, and primary or secondary dementia.

Expected outcomes
• Patient uses adaptive equipment (glasses, hearing aid) as needed.
• Patient remains oriented to time, person, and place.

• Patient remains safe in environment.
• Patient responds to environmental stimuli.
• Patient or significant other communicates an understanding of sensory stimulation exercises.
• Patient or significant other takes active role in preventing sensory deprivation and isolation.

Interventions and rationales

• Assist or encourage patient to use glasses, hearing aid, or other adaptive devices *to help reduce sensory deprivation.*
• Reorient patient to reality:
  – Call patient by name.
  – Tell patient your name.
  – Give background information (time, place, date) frequently throughout the day.
  – Orient to environment, including sights and sounds.
  – Use large signs as visual cues.
  – Post patient's own photo on the door if patient is ambulatory and disoriented.
  – Provide for visual contrast in environment.

These measures help reduce patient's sensory deprivation.

• Arrange environment to offset deficit:
  – Place patient in room with maximal visualization of environment.
  – Encourage family to bring in personal articles, such as books, cards, and photos.
  – Keep articles in same place to promote sense of identity.
  – Use such safety precautions as a night light when needed.

These measures reduce sensory deprivation.

• Communicate patient's response level to family or significant other and staff; record on care plan and update as needed. *Sensory deprivation level can be evaluated by response to stimuli.*
• Talk to patient while providing care; encourage family or significant other to discuss past and present events with patient. Arrange to be with patient at predetermined times during the day to avoid isolation. *Verbal stimuli can improve patient's reality orientation.*
• Turn on TV and radio for short periods of time based on patient's interests *to help orient patient to reality.*
• Hold patient's hand when talking. Discuss interests with patient and family or significant other. Obtain needed items, such as talking books. *Sensory stimuli help reduce patient's sensory deprivation.*
• Assist patient and family or significant other in planning short trips outside hospital environment. Educate about mobility, toileting, feeding, suctioning, and so forth. *Trips help reduce patient's sensory deprivation.*

Evaluations for expected outcomes

• Patient uses adaptive equipment to alleviate sensory deprivation.
• Patient demonstrates ability to recall people, places, past and present events and to identify correct time.
• Patient uses safety precautions to remain free of injury.
• Patient responds to environmental stimuli.
• Patient communicates understanding of sensory stimulation exercises.
• Patient identifies and uses techniques to prevent sensory deprivation.

Documentation
- Patient's or significant other's expression of concern about sensory deprivation
- Observations of patient's orientation, response to environmental stimuli, and safety
- Patient's or significant other's response to nursing interventions
- Instructions and demonstration of skill in providing sensory stimuli
- Evaluations for each expected outcome.

Sensory or perceptual alteration (specify)

related to sensory overload

Definition
Change in the characteristics of incoming stimuli

Assessment
- History of major trauma or surgery, seizures, alcoholism, psychiatric disorder
- Mobility status
- Neurologic status, including cognition (recent and remote memory, insight or judgment); level of consciousness; orientation; sensory function
- Sleep-wake status
- Communication status, including adaptive responses (gestures, lipreading, signing), level of comprehension and expression, speech pattern
- Environmental status, including equipment and supplies, lighting, location of patient's personal belongings, noise, privacy, space
- Psychosocial status, including alcohol and drug use, behavior and personality, coping mechanisms, history of depression, support systems

Defining characteristics
- Altered abstraction
- Altered conceptualization
- Anxiety
- Bizarre thinking
- Change in behavior pattern
- Change in problem-solving abilities
- Clinical evidence of factors causing sensory overload
- Disoriented to time, place, or person
- Exaggerated emotional responses
- Hallucinations
- Irritability
- Restlessness
- Visual and auditory distortion
- Withdrawal

Associated medical diagnoses (selected)
Alcohol withdrawal syndrome, anxiety, bipolar disease (manic phase), major trauma or surgery requiring hospitalization in an intensive care unit, metabolic alkalosis

Expected outcomes
- Patient remains oriented to person, place, and time.
- Patient voices decreased anxiety and irritability.
- Patient communicates in a lucid manner.
- Patient recognizes when sensory stimuli are excessive.
- Patient reestablishes usual sleep-wake cycle.
- Patient states measures to reduce sensory overload.
- Patient demonstrates positive coping behavior when sensory overload situation arises.

Interventions and rationales

- Reorient patient to reality:
  - Call patient by name.
  - Tell patient your name.
  - Give background information (time, place, date) frequently.
  - Orient to environment, including sights, sounds, and smells.

These measures will reduce susceptibility to sensory overload.

- Provide a nonthreatening environment, reduce excessive noise and lights, keep environment uncluttered *to reduce sensory overload.*
- Accept patient's perception of stimuli. Do not challenge hallucinations or delusions; do not ridicule or tease. *Challenging patient's perceptions does not reduce sensory overload.*
- Help patient interpret environment (for example, "This is the hospital," "I am a nurse," "You are hearing the food cart go down the hall"). *This helps reduce anxiety.*
- Simulate "normal" environment: keep lights off (or dim) at night; let in light during day; provide clock and calendar; place family photos at bedside. *This reduces sensory overload.*
- Explain procedures, tests, special equipment, and unusual sounds (such as alarms). Prepare patient for procedures in advance. *Increased knowledge reduces sensory overload.*
- Cluster procedures and treatments. Avoid disturbing patient unnecessarily. Always approach in a calm, gentle manner to avoid startling patient. *Approaching patient in a compassionate manner helps reduce sensory overload.*
- Help patient use coping strategies when sensory overload occurs, such as talking to someone. *This provides a sense of control.*
- Teach patient how to limit sensory overload; for example, turning off TV, removing self from stimulating environment. *Knowledgeable patient is better able to reduce sensory overload.*
- Encourage regular sleep pattern and routines, possibly including milk or warm bath before bedtime. *Sufficient rest improves tolerance to stimuli.*
- Encourage family or significant other to visit frequently; provide reassurance and explanations to aid understanding of patient's condition. *Orientation to reality through family visits helps to promote relaxation.*

Evaluations for expected outcomes

- Patient demonstrates ability to correctly identify people, places, the time and recall past events.
- Patient reports feeling less irritable and anxious.
- Patient communicates clearly.
- Patient recognizes when sensory stimuli are becoming excessive and requests time in quiet area.
- Patient states that he feels rested.
- Patient identifies and demonstrates measures to avoid sensory overload.

Documentation

- Patient's and family's or significant other's expression of concern about sensory overload
- Observations of orientation, response to environment, anxiety level, and sleep pattern
- Patient's or significant other's response to nursing interventions
- Instructions and demonstration of skill in managing sensory overload
- Evaluations for each expected outcome.

■ Sensory or perceptual alteration (tactile)

Definition
Change in the sense of touch

Assessment
- Vital signs
- Evidence of impaired tactile perception, including complaints of tingling, pain, numbness; response to sharp and dull stimulus; signs of bruises, cuts, scrapes, or other injury
- Neurologic status, including level of consciousness; cranial nerve function; muscle strength; deep tendon reflexes; light touch, pain, temperature, vibration, and position sensation
- Skin color and temperature
- History of chemotherapy treatment
- History of alcohol abuse
- Medication history, including use of clomipramine, ceftizoxime, amiodarone, dichlorphenamide, guanadrel, anistreplase, interferon alfa-2b, zidovudine

Defining characteristics
- Altered sense of touch
  - abnormal sensation, such as numbess, prickling, tingling (paresthesia)
  - decreased sensitivity to stimulation (hypoesthesia)
  - diminished sensitivity to pain (hypalgesia)
  - impaired sense of touch (dysesthesia)

Associated medical diagnoses (selected)
Alcoholism, arterial occlusion (acute), arteriosclerosis obliterans, arthritis, brain tumor, Buerger's disease, cerebrovascular accident, chemotherapy, diabetes mellitus, Guillain-Barré syndrome, head injury, heavy metal or solvent poisoning, herniated disk, herpes zoster, hyperventilation syndrome, hypocalcemia, migraine headache, multiple sclerosis, peripheral nerve trauma, peripheral neuropathy, polyneuropathy, rabies, Raynaud's disease, seizure disorders, spinal cord lesions, tabes dorsalis, transient ischemic attack, vitamin B deficiency

Expected outcomes
- Patient expresses feelings regarding changes in tactile perception.
- Patient does not experience falls or injury.
- Patient does not experience skin breakdown.
- Patient describes safety measures to avoid injury.
- Family members or caregiver describe program to provide patient with increased tactile stimulation.

Interventions and rationales
- Allow patient to express feelings associated with altered tactile perception. Be willing to listen, but do not pressure patient to talk. *Providing a chance to talk will help patient cope with sensory deficits.*
- Teach patient to regularly observe how hands and feet are placed *to avoid injury.*
- Inspect skin daily, especially on patient's feet, *to detect signs of skin breakdown.*
- Use padded side rails or lapboard on wheelchair, if appropriate. Make any other environmental modifications as needed *to promote safe tactile experiences and prevent accidental injury.*
- Teach patient safety measures, such as testing bathwater with a thermometer, *to prevent injury.*

• Teach family members or caregiver to touch patient in areas with preserved sensation, using a variety of textures, *to promote sensory input.* For example, suggest family members provide satin pillowcase, wrap soft scarf around patient's neck, or give gentle massage with scented lotion.

Evaluations for expected outcomes
• Patient expresses feelings associated with changes in tactile perception.
• Patient does not experience falls or injury.
• Patient's skin remains intact.
• Patient lists ways to protect against risk of injury caused by diminished tactile sensation.

Documentation
• Evidence of diminished tactile sensation
• Patient's expression of feelings about diminished tactile perception
• Instructions regarding safety and protective measures
• Patient's response to nursing interventions
• Evaluations for each expected outcome.

■ Sensory or perceptual alteration (visual)

related to altered sensory reception, transmission, or integration

Definition
Change in the characteristics of visual stimuli

Assessment
• History of eye disorders, trauma, surgery
• Age
• Visual status, including corneal reflex, extraocular movement, fields of gaze, inspection of lid and eyeball, ophthalmoscopy, palpation of lid and eyeball, pupil size and accommodation, tonometry, use of glasses, visual acuity (near and distant), visual fields
• Environmental and occupational factors
• Activities of daily living
• Behavioral assessment, including coping mechanisms, support system, willingness to cooperate with treatment

Defining characteristics
• Altered conceptualization
• Anger
• Anxiety
• Apathy or passivity
• Change in behavioral pattern
• Change in problem-solving abilities
• Change in response to visual stimuli
• Clinical evidence of impaired (decreased) visual ability
• Depression
• Disoriented to time, place, person
• Reported or measured change in visual acuity
• Restlessness
• Visual distortions

Associated medical diagnoses (selected)
Albinism, blindness (uncompensated), cataracts, cerebrovascular accident, conditions requiring enucleation, detached retina, diabetes mellitus, farsightedness, glaucoma, head injury, hemianopsia, macular degeneration, multiple sclerosis, nearsightedness, optic nerve damage

Expected outcomes
• Patient discusses impact of vision loss on life-style.

- Patient expresses a feeling of safety, comfort, and security.
- Patient maintains orientation to person, place, and time.
- Patient shows interest in external environment.
- Patient regains visual functioning.
- Patient compensates for vision loss by use of adaptive devices.
- Patient plans to use appropriate resources.

Interventions and rationales

- Allow patient to express feelings about vision loss, such as its impact on life-style. Convey a willingness to listen, but do not pressure patient to talk. *Allowing patient to voice fears aids acceptance of vision loss.*
- Provide a safe environment by removing excess furniture or equipment from patient's room. Orient patient to the room. Show patient how to use call light. Do not move furniture or leave objects in hallway. *Orienting patient to surroundings reduces risk of injury.*
- If blindness is present on admission, allow patient to direct arrangement of room; walk with patient to bathroom and other key areas until he or she becomes familiar with the environment. If patient has a seeing-eye dog, make arrangements for the feeding, exercising, and elimination needs of the dog. *Maintaining patient's optimal level of independence fosters sense of control.*
- Modify the environment to maximize any vision the patient may have. For example, with hemianopsia, place patient in room to maximize visual field, approach patient from best visual angle, remind patient to scan environment to pick up visual cues, and place objects within visual field. *Modifying environment helps patient meet self-care needs.*
- If patient has diplopia, patch one eye *to ameliorate double vision.*
- Always introduce yourself or announce your presence on entering the patient's room; let patient know when you are leaving. *Familiarizing patient with caregiver aids reality orientation and conveys respect.*
- Provide sensory stimulation by using tactile, auditory, and gustatory stimuli to help compensate for vision loss. Obtain large-print books, talking books, audiotapes, or radio, as preferred by patient. *Nonvisual sensory stimulation helps patient adjust to vision loss.*
- Provide reality orientation if patient is confused or disoriented *to allow for more effective patient-staff interaction.*
- Give patient clear, concise explanations of treatments, procedures, etc. Avoid information overload. When speaking to patient, enunciate words clearly, slowly, and in normal speaking voice. *A knowledgeable patient will be better able to participate in treatment plan.*
- Encourage family and friends to visit patient and to bring familiar objects that can be left with the patient. *Presence of familiar objects aids reality orientation.*
- Make sure that health care personnel are aware of vision loss. Record information on patient's Kardex and chart cover or post in patient's room. *Nursing care is improved if staff is aware of patient's vision loss.*
- Respond to call light as soon as possible. Provide for continuity by assigning same staff members to care for patient, if possible. *These measures help reduce patient's fears.*
- If patient has had eye surgery, provide appropriate care, as indicated. Be aware of and limit activities that increase intraocular pressure, such as

bending, stooping, getting on and off bedpan, coughing, vomiting. *Avoiding postoperative activities that increase intraocular pressure helps reduce complications.*
• Administer and monitor effectiveness of medications. Report any adverse effects. *Medications help reduce pain and may control disease process.*
• Educate patient in alternative ways of coping with vision loss; care of such adaptive devices as eyeglasses, magnifying glass, contact lenses, and artificial eye; administration of eye drops and eye drop information, including name, dosage, therapeutic effects, and adverse effects. *A knowledgeable patient will be better able to cope with vision loss.*
• Refer to appropriate community resources to help patient and family adapt to vision loss—for example, American Foundation for the Blind or other community agencies or support groups. *Postdischarge support will help patient and family cope better with patient's vision loss.*

Evaluations for expected outcomes
• Patient discusses effects of vision loss on life-style.
• Patient demonstrates ability to recognize people and places and to identify the time and past and present events.
• Because of reduction in environmental risk factors, patient reports comfort in surroundings.
• Patient expresses interest in interacting with others.
• Patient regains visual functioning to the extent possible and begins to come to terms with any permanent vision loss.
• Patient identifies and uses alternative methods to facilitate communication.
• Patient recognizes need for support during transition from hospital to outside environment.

Documentation
• Patient's feelings about visual deficits
• Observations of patient's behavior and response to visual deficit and use of adaptive equipment or devices
• Instructions regarding safety and protective measures, coping strategies, postoperative management
• Patient's and family's or significant other's intent to use appropriate resources
• Patient's response to nursing interventions
• Evaluations for each expected outcome.

■ Sexual dysfunction

related to altered body structure or function

Definition
Presence of physiologic or emotional factors that alter one's usual pattern of sexual function

Assessment
• History of problem that caused a change in structure or function
• Patient's perception of the change's effect
• Marital status, significant other
• Living arrangement
• Usual sexual patterns
• Sexual problems before present health problem
• Patient's attitude toward modifying sexual patterns
• Patient's present knowledge about appropriate options available

Defining characteristics

- Actual or perceived limitation imposed by disease or therapy
- Alterations in achieving sexual satisfaction
- Alterations in relationship with spouse or significant other
- Change of interest in self and others
- Conflicts involving values
- Inability to achieve desired satisfaction
- Seeking confirmation of desirability
- Verbalization of the problem

Associated medical diagnoses (selected)

Chronic renal failure with hemodialysis; conditions requiring colostomy, coronary artery bypass, ileostomy, pelvic surgery, radiation therapy, radical abdominal surgery, or uretero-ileostomy; diabetes mellitus; drug therapy, such as antihypertensives, diuretics; endometriosis; genitourinary problems; myocardial infarction; pelvic inflammatory disease; rheumatoid arthritis; spinal cord injury

Expected outcomes

- Patient acknowledges a problem or potential problem in sexual function.
- Patient voices feelings about changes in sexual identity.
- Patient explains reason for sexual dysfunction.
- Patient expresses willingness to obtain counseling.
- Patient reestablishes sexual activity at pre-illness level.

Interventions and rationales

- Provide a nonthreatening atmosphere and encourage the patient to ask questions about personal sexuality. *This encourages patient to ask questions specifically related to current situation.*
- Allow patient to express feelings openly in nonjudgmental atmosphere. *This enhances communication and understanding between patient and caregiver.*
- Provide answers to specific questions. *This helps patient focus on specific issues, clarifies misconceptions, and builds trust in the caregiver.*
- Provide time for privacy. *This demonstrates respect for patient, allows time for introspection, and gives patient control over time spent interacting with others.*
- Suggest that patient discuss concerns with spouse or significant other. *This fosters sharing of concerns and strengthens relationships.*
- Provide support for spouse or significant other. *Supportive interventions such as active listening communicate concern, interest, and acceptance.*
- Educate patient and spouse or significant other about limitations imposed by the patient's present physical condition. *Education about limitations imposed on sexual activity by illness helps patient avoid complications or injury.*
- Suggest referral to a sex counselor or other appropriate professional for future guidance *to provide patient with a resource for postdischarge support.*

Evaluations for expected outcomes

- Patient acknowledges existence of problem or potential problem in sexual function.
- Patient expresses anxiety, anger, depression, or frustration over changes in sexual function.
- Patient explains relationship between illness or treatment and sexual dysfunction.
- Patient expresses willingness to obtain counseling.

• Patient resumes usual sexual activity.

Documentation

• Patient's perception of problem
• Subtle comments made by patient regarding inability to cope with change in structure or function
• Observations of patient's behavior
• Interventions performed to assist the patient and spouse or significant other; response to interventions
• Evaluations for each expected outcome.

Sexual dysfunction

related to decreased libido caused by depression

Definition

Presence of physiologic or emotional factors that alter one's usual pattern of sexual function

Assessment

• Comprehensive sexual history, including attitude toward sex; sexual preference; sexual desire, enjoyment, performance; sexual responsiveness of partner; previous sexual response patterns
• Psychological factors, including self-esteem, body image, guilt, symptoms of depression, suicidal ideation
• Support systems, including family, significant other, friends, clergy
• Attitudes of family and significant other
• Sociocultural factors, including educational level, socioeconomic status, ethnic group, religious beliefs and practices
• Physiologic factors, including medication history (response, effectiveness, adverse reactions), current medication regimen (including tricyclic antidepressants or monoamine oxidase [MAO] inhibitors), substance abuse history (type, effect on mental status)
• Coping and problem-solving ability, ability to concentrate

Defining characteristics

• Decreased or absent desire for sexual activity
• Decreased or absent sexual fantasies
• Symptoms of affective disorder, including depression, crying, fatigue, feelings of worthlessness, weight gain or loss, decreased pleasure in usual activities, insomnia, hypersomnia, psychomotor agitation or retardation

Associated medical diagnoses (selected)

Bipolar disorder (depressive phase), cyclothymia, dysthymia, hypoactive sexual desire disorder, major depression (single episode or recurrent), major depressive episode (melancholic type), sexual aversion disorder

Expected outcomes

• Patient acknowledges depressive episode and problem in sexual function.
• Patient voices feelings about decreases in sexual desire.
• Patient identifies ways to enhance pleasure and improve interpersonal communication with partner.
• Patient regains sexual desire with recovery from depression.
• Patient accepts referral for sex therapy if necessary.

Interventions and rationales

• Initiate a trusting therapeutic relationship with the patient. Make the purpose, nature, and parameters of

this relationship clear *to help patient feel secure and develop trust.*
- Educate patient and significant other about the nature of depression, its treatment, and its effect on sexual desire. *Understanding the link between depression and sexual desire may diminish feelings of guilt and worthlessness, and help raise self-esteem.*
- Allow patient to express feelings openly in nonthreatening, nonjudgmental atmosphere *to foster communication and help the patient cope with unresolved issues.* Offer feedback *to validate patient's feelings and promote self-esteem.*
- Include patient and significant other in planning care and interventions *to enhance feeling of control for both partners.*
- Reinforce compliance with treatment plan for depression. *Even though tricyclic antidepressants and MAO inhibitors may diminish sexual desire, compliance is necessary for resolution of depression.*
- Discuss with patient and significant other alternative expressions of affection to enhance their relationship during treatment *to help couple preserve intimacy during temporary loss of libido.*
- Refer patient for sex counseling or therapy if low sexual desire persists after resolution of depression. *Sexual desire should return to its usual level after successful treatment for depression. If it does not, professional therapy is required.*

Evaluations for expected outcomes
- Patient describes depressive episode, treatment plan, and effects on sexual desire.
- Patient expresses concerns to staff and significant other.
- Patient identifies at least three activities to enhance pleasure and communication with partner.
- Patient reports the return of sexual fantasies and desire for sexual activity.
- Patient communicates willingness to follow through with referral for sex therapy.

Documentation
- Patient's perceptions and concerns
- Observation of patient's behavior, depressive symptoms, and suicidal risk
- Interventions to assist the patient and significant other
- Patient's and significant other's responses to nursing interventions
- Evaluations for each expected outcome.

■ Sexual dysfunction

related to hypersexuality

Definition
Presence of physiologic or emotional factors that alter one's usual pattern of sexual function

Assessment
- History of behaviors indicating excessive elation, such as hypersexuality, intrusiveness, grandiose thoughts, looseness of association, flight of ideas, extreme levels of energy, lack of sleep, lack of proper nutrition, poor judgment, elevated mood, expansiveness, pressured and rapid speech, strained interpersonal relationships
- History of psychiatric illness, including personality disorders exemplified by lack of impulse control

- Sexual history, including attitude toward sex, previous sexual patterns, sexual preference, sexual response of partners, appropriateness of sexual behavior
- Sociocultural factors, including educational level, socioeconomic status, ethnic group
- Patient's perception of sexual behaviors and sexual practices
- Family's or significant other's perception of patient's sexual behaviors
- Coping and problem-solving abilities
- Health history, including medication history (response, effectiveness, adverse reactions), use of psychosis-inducing drugs (phencyclidine [PCP], amphetamines), use of disinhibiting drugs (alcohol, amphetamines, cocaine), other substance abuse (type, effect on mental status)

Defining characteristics
- Disturbances in interpersonal relationships caused by inappropriate sexual behavior
- Excessive motor activity
- Excessive sexual activity
- Frustration and anger if sexual behavior is thwarted
- General lack of impulse control
- Impulsive acting out of sexual urges
- Inability to conform sexual behavior to social norms
- Inability to control outcome of sexual encounters
- Inappropriate and provocative verbalizations that are sexual in content
- Intrusiveness with peers, including excessive physical closeness and inappropriate touching
- Periods of excessive elation or cycles of elation and depression
- Poor perception of reality caused by psychosis or organic mental disorders
- Sexual encounters that appear self-destructive in nature; inability to maintain lasting relationships because of sexual behavior

Associated medical diagnoses (selected)
Bipolar disorder (manic phase), drug-induced psychotic states, exhibitionism, fetishism, frottage, organic mental disorder, pedophilia, personality disorder, schizophrenic disorder, transvestism, sexual masochism, sexual sadism, voyeurism

Expected outcomes
- Patient meets sexual needs in a socially appropriate manner.
- Patient reduces or eliminates sexual behaviors that may harm self or others.
- Patient achieves a consistent level of sexual behavior that is satisfying, safe, and discriminating in nature.
- Patient learns how to recognize indicators of impending episodes of hypersexuality and how to prevent such episodes from occurring.

Interventions and rationales
- Help patient recognize potentially harmful sexual behavior. Set limits on high-risk sexual behavior. *Indiscriminate, impulsive sexual behavior can lead to unwanted pregnancy, sexually transmitted diseases, and physical and emotional trauma.*
- Encourage patient to express sexual urges in socially acceptable ways (including masturbation in a private setting) *to help patient discover positive methods of relieving sexual tension.*
- Discuss with patient hypersexual behaviors and feelings associated with hypersexuality *to promote insight into behavior.*
- Refer patient to medical and psychiatric specialist or sex therapist, if needed. *Indiscriminate and impulsive*

hypersexuality usually indicates physical or psychiatric illness that requires further evaluation and treatment by an appropriate professional.

Evaluations for expected outcomes
- Patient develops increased understanding of hypersexual urges and inability to cope with intense sexual desire.
- Patient states desire to express sexual drive in a socially acceptable manner.
- Patient reports sexual relationships that are not harmful to self or others.
- Patient expresses willingness to participate in psychiatric care or sex therapy, if needed.

Documentation
- Patient's perception of sexual behaviors and level of sexual activities
- Patient's statements about sexual behaviors
- Observations of patient's behavior, including inappropriate sexual expression
- Interventions to help patient set limits on hypersexuality
- Patient's response to nursing interventions
- Evaluations for each expected outcome.

Sexual dysfunction

related to impotence

Definition
Presence of physiologic or emotional factors that alter a man's usual pattern of sexual function

Assessment
- Age
- Type of impotence:
  - organic (anatomic or central nervous system defect)
  - functional (physiologic alterations in nervous and cardiovascular systems)
  - psychogenic (emotions inhibit neural transmission from brain to sexual organs)
  - primary (patient has never achieved a satisfactory erection for coitus)
  - secondary (patient has had successful coitus at least once)
- History of organic impotence or physiologic disorders that interfere with erection
- Anatomic anomalies of penis
- Psychological variables, including patient's perception of sexual performance, relationships, desire for an erection, guilt, shame, relationship with parents (presence of overbearing mother), family or social pressures
- Physiologic status, including medication history (response, effectiveness, adverse reactions), history of substance abuse (type, effect on mental status)
- Sociocultural factors, including educational level, socioeconomic status, ethnic group, religious beliefs and practices
- Sexual history, including sexual drive, sexual preference, frequency of impotence, premature ejaculation, spontaneous morning erections, positive coital experiences, types of erotic stimulation used, past professional counseling or sex therapy, homosexual experiences, affairs (other partners, prostitutes), feelings of anger, hostility, or disgust toward partner

Defining characteristics
- Expressions of concern about sexual performance
- Expressions of desire for an erection
- Inability to attain and maintain an erection throughout sexual intercourse
- Past relationships with family members or previous sexual partners that adversely affect sexuality
- Poor communication with partner
- Use of drugs that may interfere with sexual performance

Associated medical diagnoses (selected)
Alcohol or drug abuse, cardiovascular disease (penile circulatory problem), diabetes mellitus, drug therapy with antihypertensives or beta blockers, endocrine dysfunction (low testosterone or high prolactin levels), inhibited male orgasm, male erectile disorder, premature ejaculation

Expected outcomes
- Patient acknowledges a problem in sexual function.
- Patient voluntarily discusses his problem.
- Patient and partner discuss their feelings and perceptions about changes in sexual performance.
- Patient learns methods to enhance sexual pleasure for himself and his partner and incorporates them into his sexual activities.
- Patient continues to communicate with partner about sexual issues and needs.
- Patient agrees to obtain sexual evaluation and therapy, if needed.
- Patient develops and maintains a positive attitude toward his sexuality and sexual performance.

Interventions and rationales
- Establish a therapeutic relationship with the patient *to provide a safe and comfortable atmosphere for discussing sexual concerns.*
- Encourage patient to discuss feelings and perceptions about his sexual dysfunction *to help him validate perceptions and reduce emotional distress through catharsis.*
- Encourage partner to discuss feelings and perceptions *to help couple clarify issues about their relationship and improve communication.*
- Educate patient and partner about alternative methods of lovemaking and expressing affection. *Alternative expressions of love and intimacy can raise patient's self-esteem until impotence is evaluated and treated.*
- Encourage use of sexual fantasies and erotica to promote sexual stimulation and erection. *This helps patient and partner achieve sexual satisfaction and decreases "spectatoring" (watching oneself during sexual activity with a partner), which can inhibit performance.*
- Encourage the patient to seek professional evaluation and therapy *to obtain proper diagnosis and treatment.*

Evaluations for expected outcomes
- Patient states that he feels comfortable discussing his sexual concerns.
- Patient expresses feelings about diminished sexual performance.
- Patient and partner communicate with each other about their sexual relationship.
- Patient states specific ways in which he will enhance sexual pleasure with his partner.
- Patient participates in a sexual evaluation and in sex therapy, if needed.

• Patient makes positive comments about himself.

Documentation
• Patient's perception of sexual problem
• Overt and covert remarks made by patient that indicate his difficulty dealing with impotence
• Observations of patient's behavior in response to his inability to perform
• Interventions performed to assist the patient and his partner
• Responses to nursing interventions
• Evaluations for each expected outcome.

■ Sexuality pattern alteration

related to illness or medical treatment

Definition
State in which an individual expresses concern about personal sexuality

Assessment
• History of present illness
• Current treatment regimen (medications, therapies)
• Marital status, significant other
• Patient's perception of sexual identity and role
• Usual sexual activity pattern
• Patient's perception of changes in sexual activity resulting from illness or treatment
• Significance of sexual relationship to patient and spouse or significant other
• Emotional reactions (affect, mood)
• Behavioral reactions (specify)

Defining characteristics
• Emotional and behavioral reactions, including anger, constricted affect, depressed mood, noncompliance with prescribed therapies, withdrawal from social interactions
• Reported difficulties, limitations, or changes in sexual activity

Associated medical diagnoses (selected)
Acquired immunodeficiency syndrome, amputation, carcinoma, coronary disease, diabetes mellitus, end-stage renal disease with hemodialysis, genitourinary problems, gynecologic problems, hypertension treated with antihypertensives, mastectomy, ostomy (colostomy, ileoconduit, ileostomy), sexually transmitted diseases (herpes, gonorrhea, syphilis), spinal cord injury with paralysis

Expected outcomes
• Patient voices feelings about potential or actual changes in sexual activity.
• Patient expresses concern about self-concept, esteem, body image.
• Patient states at least one effect of illness or treatment on sexual behavior.
• Patient and spouse or significant other resume effective communication patterns.
• Patient and spouse or significant other use available counseling referrals or support groups.

Interventions and rationales
• Allow for specific amount of uninterrupted time to talk with patient. *This demonstrates nurse's comfort with sexuality issues and reassures patient that his or her concerns are acceptable for discussion.*
• Provide a nonthreatening, nonjudgmental atmosphere to encourage the patient to verbalize feelings about

perceived changes in sexual identity and behaviors. *This demonstrates unconditional positive regard for patient and patient's concerns about sexuality patterns.*
- Provide patient and spouse or significant other with information about illness and treatment. Answer any questions and clarify any misconceptions they may have. *This helps them focus on specific concerns, encourages questions, and avoids misunderstandings.*
- Provide time for privacy. *This demonstrates respect for patient, allows time for introspection, and gives patient control over time spent interacting with others.*
- Encourage social interaction and communication between patient and spouse or significant other. *This fosters sharing of concerns and strengthens relationships.*
- Offer referral to counselors or support persons, such as mental health professional, sex counselor, or illness-related support groups ("I Can Cope," Reach for Recovery, Ostomy Association), *to provide patient with resources for postdischarge support.*

Evaluations for expected outcomes
- Patient expresses concerns and fears related to altered sexuality pattern.
- Patient expresses feelings about change in self-image resulting from illness or medical treatment.
- Patient identifies specific physical symptom that has a negative effect on sexual behavior.
- Patient and spouse or significant other communicate effectively.
- Patient and spouse or significant other participate in therapy with an appropriate counselor.

Documentation
- Patient's perception of changes in sexual patterns
- Patient's ability to interact with others
- Interventions to support and educate patient and spouse or significant other
- Response to nursing interventions
- Evaluations for each expected outcome.

■ Sexuality pattern alteration

related to separation from significant other

Definition
State in which an individual expresses concern regarding personal sexuality

Assessment
- Reason for hospitalization
- Current and anticipated length of stay
- Marital status, significant other
- Living arrangement
- Patient's perception of sexual identity and role
- Usual sexual activity pattern
- Patient's perception of limitation on sexual activity resulting from hospitalization
- Significance of sexual relationship to patient and spouse or significant other
- Emotional reactions (affect, mood)
- Behavioral reactions (specify)

Defining characteristics
- Behavioral and emotional responses, including constricted affect, depressed mood, inappropriate sexual comments or behavior, withdrawal from social interaction

• Verbal report of limitations on usual sexual behavior or activity

Associated medical diagnoses (selected)
This nursing diagnosis can occur in any hospitalized patient separated from spouse or significant other for a prolonged period. Examples include patients with infectious diseases, neurologic illnesses, orthopedic injuries, postoperative complications, or terminal illnesses.

Expected outcomes
• Patient voices feelings about changes in usual sexual activity.
• Patient alters inappropriate behaviors, if indicated.
• Patient and spouse or significant other discuss possible realistic alternatives for intimacy within hospital setting.
• Patient and spouse or significant other use available counseling referrals.

Interventions and rationales
• Allow for a specific amount of uninterrupted, non-care-related time to talk with patient. *This demonstrates nurse's comfort with sexuality issues and reassures patient that his or her concerns are acceptable for discussion.*
• Display an accepting, nonjudgmental manner to encourage patient to discuss concerns about sexuality. Approach spouse or significant other in the same manner and include in discussions with patient, if agreeable to both. *A nonjudgmental approach demonstrates unconditional positive regard for both the patient and spouse or significant other.*
• Include patient in plan for setting limits on inappropriate behavior, if indicated by behavioral assessment.
– Explain aspects of patient's behavior that are inappropriate.
– Share proposed care plan with patient, including approaches for reducing bothersome behavior, expectations, and goals.
– Request patient's cooperation, but be willing to compromise if acceptable alternatives are presented.

In limit-setting, patients work with nurse in planning to reduce undesirable behavior.
• Discuss with patient and spouse or significant other realistic, acceptable alternatives for intimacy. *This encourages open communication between them as sexual partners.*
• Explain to patient and spouse or significant other limitations related to illness and hospital environment *to establish a standard for realistic and acceptable behavior.*
• Provide time for privacy. *This allows patient and spouse or significant other to discuss feelings regarding sexuality and to engage in alternatives for intimacy while patient is hospitalized.*
• Offer referral for counseling, such as a mental health professional or a sex counselor, if indicated. *Referrals provide opportunities for additional ongoing therapy during hospitalization and after discharge.*

Evaluations for expected outcomes
• Patient describes usual sexual activity pattern and expresses feelings resulting from changes in pattern.
• Patient demonstrates ability to decrease or eliminate inappropriate behavior. For example, patient avoids making comments with sexual or abusive overtones, maintains appropriate grooming and attire, and finds outlet for angry feelings to lessen potential for acting out.

• Patient and spouse or significant other request privacy and seek permission to use acceptable alternatives for intimacy, such as holding or kissing.
• Patient and spouse or significant other seek counseling.

Documentation
• Patient's verbal and nonverbal behaviors
• Patient's and spouse's or significant other's perception of current situation
• Specific nursing interventions to reduce emotional and behavioral reactions, such as active listening, limit setting, and counseling referrals
• Patient's and spouse's or significant other's response to nursing interventions
• Evaluations for each expected outcome.

■ Skin integrity impairment

related to external (environmental) factors

Definition
Interruption in skin integrity

Assessment
• History of skin problems, trauma, surgery, immobility
• Age
• Integumentary status, including color, elasticity, hygiene, lesions, moisture, quantity and distribution of hair, sensation, temperature and blood pressure, texture, turgor
• Musculoskeletal status, including anesthetic area, joint mobility, muscle strength and mass, paralysis, range of motion
• Nutritional status, including appetite, dietary intake, hydration, present weight and change from normal
• Hemoglobin and hematocrit
• Serum albumin
• Psychosocial status, including coping skills, family or significant other, mental status, self-concept and body image
• Occupational hazards
• Patient's current understanding of physical condition
• Patient's physical, mental, and emotional readiness to learn

Defining characteristics
• Clinical evidence of external factors adversely affecting skin integrity (chemical agents, cold, heat, pressure)
• Destruction of skin layers
• Disruption of skin surface
• Invasion of body structures

Associated medical diagnoses (selected)
Burns (chemical, thermal, electrical), extravasation from vesicants (chemotherapy, antibiotic therapy), fractures (traction, casts), hyperthermia, hypothermia, pressure ulcers, radiation therapy, surgical incision or wounds, traumatic injuries

Expected outcomes
• Patient exhibits no evidence of skin breakdown.
• Patient shows normal skin turgor.
• Patient regains skin integrity; for example, pressure ulcer decreases in size (specify).
• Surgical wound healed.
• Patient communicates understanding of skin protection measures.
• Patient demonstrates skill in care of wound or burn or incision.
• Patient demonstrates skin inspection technique.
• Patient performs skin care routine.

• Patient communicates feelings about change in body image.

Interventions and rationales

• Inspect skin every shift; describe and document skin condition; report changes. *This provides evidence of effectiveness of skin care regimen.*

• Perform prescribed treatment regimen for skin condition involved; monitor progress. Report responses to treatment regimen, *to maintain or modify current therapy.*

• Provide supportive measures, as indicated.
  – Assist with general hygiene and comfort measures *to promote comfort and sense of well-being.*
  – Administer pain medication and monitor its effectiveness. *Pain relief is needed to maintain health.*
  – Maintain proper environmental conditions *to promote sense of well-being.*
  – Use foam mattress, bed cradle, or other devices *to avoid skin breakdown.*
  – Warn against tampering with wound or dressings *to avoid potential infection.*
  – Maintain infection control standards *to reduce risk of spreading disease.*

• Position patient for comfort and minimal pressure on bony prominences. Change position at least every 2 hours. Monitor frequency of turning and skin condition. *These measures reduce pressure, promote circulation, and avoid skin breakdown.*

• Explain therapy to patient and family or significant other, *to encourage compliance.*

• Allow patient to express feelings regarding skin problem. *This helps allay anxiety and develops coping skills.*

• Instruct patient and family or significant other in skin care regimen, *to encourage compliance.*

• Supervise patient and family or significant other in skin care management. Provide feedback, *to improve skill in managing skin care.*

• Make referral to psychiatric liaison nurse, social service, or other support groups, as indicated. *These provide additional support for patient and family.*

Evaluations for expected outcomes

• Patient's skin remains intact.

• Patient's skin turgor remains normal.

• Patient's pressure ulcer heals, as evidenced by presence of granulation tissue and decreased size and depth of ulcer.

• Patient's surgical wound heals, as evidenced by clean suture line and absence of scar discoloration and skin breakdown.

• Patient understands necessity of avoiding prolonged pressure, obtaining adequate nutrition, and using protective devices.

• Patient demonstrates skill in care of wound, burn, or incision.

• Patient demonstrates skin inspection techniques.

• Patient performs skin care routine.

• Patient expresses feelings about changes in body image.

Documentation

• Patient's concerns about change in skin integrity, willingness to accept treatment, and participation in treatment regimen

• Observations of wound, pressure ulcer, and incision healing and response to treatment regimen

• Interventions to provide supportive care and prescribed treatment
• Patient's response to nursing interventions
• Patient's and family's or significant other's understanding and skill in performing skin care measures
• Evaluations for each expected outcome.

Skin integrity impairment

related to internal (somatic) factors

Definition

Interruption in skin integrity

Assessment

• History of skin problems, trauma, chronic debilitating disease, immobility
• Age
• Integumentary status, including color, elasticity, hygiene, lesions, moisture, quantity and distribution of hair, sensation, temperature and blood pressure, texture, turgor
• Musculoskeletal status, including anesthetic area, joint mobility, muscle strength and mass, paralysis, range of motion
• Nutritional status, including appetite, dietary intake, hydration, present weight or change from normal
• Hemoglobin and hematocrit
• Serum albumin
• Psychosocial status, including coping patterns, family or significant other, mental status, occupation, self-concept and body image
• Knowledge, including patient's current understanding of physical condition; patient's physical, mental, and emotional readiness to learn

Defining characteristics

• Clinical evidence of internal factors adversely affecting skin integrity
• Destruction of skin layers
• Disruption of skin surfaces
• Invasion of body structures

Associated medical diagnoses (selected)

Anasarca, anemia, chronic renal disease, dermatologic conditions (allergic or atopic dermatitis, drug-induced dermatitis), diabetes mellitus, Laënnec's cirrhosis, malnutrition, neuromuscular disorders, peripheral vascular disorders (venous and arterial ulcers), terminal cancer

Expected outcomes

• Patient exhibits improved or healed lesions or wounds.
• Patient reports increased comfort.
• Complications avoided or minimized.
• Patient correlates precipitating factors with appropriate skin care regimen.
• Patient explains skin care regimen.
• Patient and family or significant other demonstrates skin care regimen.
• Patient voices feelings about changed body image.

Interventions and rationales

• Inspect skin every shift; describe and document skin condition; report changes. *This provides evidence of effectiveness of skin care regimen.*
• Perform prescribed treatment regimen for skin condition involved; monitor progress. Report favorable and adverse responses to treatment regimen *to maintain or modify current therapies as needed.*
• Provide supportive measures, as indicated:
  – Assist with general hygiene and comfort measures *to promote*

comfort and general sense of well-being.
- Administer pain medications and monitor effectiveness. *Pain relief is needed to maintain health.*
- Maintain proper environmental conditions, including room temperature and ventilation. *Providing comfortable environment promotes sense of well-being.*
- Apply bed cradle *to protect lesions from bed covers.*
- Remind patient not to scratch *to avoid skin injury.*
- Administer and monitor effectiveness of antipruritic medications. *Antipruritics reduce itching sensation.*
- Explain dietary restrictions, for example, from skin allergy to food. *Resulting pruritus leads to skin breakdown.*

- Encourage patient to express feelings about skin condition *to enhance coping.*
- Explain therapy to patient and family, *to encourage compliance.*
- Discuss precipitating factors, if known, and the long-term effects of skin integrity interruption. *Knowledge of precipitating factors helps patients reduce their occurrence and severity.*
- Instruct patient and family in skin care regimen *to ensure compliance.*
- Supervise patient and family in skin care regimen. Provide feedback. *Practice helps improve skill in managing skin care regimen.*
- Encourage adherence to other aspects of health-care management *to control or minimize effects on skin.*
- Refer patient to psychiatric liaison nurse, social service, or support group, as appropriate. *These provide additional support for patient and family.*

Evaluations for expected outcomes
- Patient's skin remains intact.
- Patient's wounds or lesions heal.
- Patient reports feeling of comfort.
- Patient does not experience further skin breakdown.
- Patient lists factors precipitating skin breakdown.
- Patient understands and demonstrates skin integrity regimen.
- Patient expresses feelings about body image changes.

Documentation
- Patient's concerns about skin disorder and its impact on body image and life-style
- Patient's willingness to participate in care
- Observations of skin condition, healing, and response to treatment regimen
- Interventions to provide supportive care
- Instructions regarding treatment regimen
- Patient's or family's understanding of and skill in carrying out instructions
- Patient's response to nursing interventions
- Evaluations for each expected outcome.

■ Skin integrity impairment, high risk for

Definition
Presence of risk factors for interruption or destruction of skin surface

Assessment
- History of skin problems, trauma, chronic debilitating disease, immobility

• Age
• Integumentary status, including color, elasticity, hygiene, lesions, moisture, sensation, quantity and distribution of hair, temperature and blood pressure, texture, turgor
• Musculoskeletal status, including anesthetic area, muscle strength and mass, joint mobility, paralysis, range of motion
• Nutritional status, including appetite, dietary intake, hydration, present weight and change from normal
• Hemoglobin and hematocrit
• Serum albumin
• Psychosocial status, including activities of daily living, mental status, occupation (sun exposure), recreational activities

Risk factors
• External (environmental) factors, including pressure, friction, shearing forces, restraints, physical immobilization, confinement to bed or chair, excretions and secretions, hypothermia or hyperthermia
• Internal (somatic) factors, including altered nutritional status (cachexia or debilitation), decreased serum albumin, dehydration, dependence on others for self-care, skin maceration, bladder or bowel incontinence, comatose state, paralysis, skeletal prominences, decreased circulation, obesity, localized infection in pressure-supporting areas, loss of subcutaneous tissue or muscle mass, altered metabolic state, vitamin deficiency

Associated medical diagnoses (selected)
Anasarca; chronic hepatitis; chronic renal disease; cirrhosis (ascites); conditions requiring colostomy, gastrostomy, nephrostomy, or ureteroileostomy; diabetes mellitus; fractures (traction, cast); frostbite; malnutrition; neuromuscular disorders; peripheral vascular disease; spinal cord injury; sunburn; terminal cancer. This diagnosis may occur in any patient who is on prolonged bed rest or is immobilized.

Expected outcomes
• Patient experiences no skin breakdown.
• Patient maintains muscle strength and joint range of motion.
• Patient sustains adequate food and fluid intake.
• Patient maintains adequate skin circulation.
• Patient communicates understanding of preventive skin care measures.
• Patient and family demonstrate preventive skin care measures.
• Patient and family correlate risk factors and preventive measures.

Interventions and rationales
• Inspect skin every shift; document skin condition and report any status changes. *Early detection of changes prevents or minimizes skin breakdown.*
• Change patient's position at least every 2 hours; follow turning schedule posted at bedside. Monitor frequency of turning. *These measures reduce pressure on tissues, promote circulation, and avoid skin breakdown.*
• Encourage ambulation or perform or assist with active range-of-motion exercises at least every 4 hours while patient is awake. *Exercises prevent muscle atrophy and contractures; ambulation promotes circulation and relieves pressure.*
• Use preventive skin care devices as needed, such as a foam mattress, an alternating pressure mattress, sheepskin, pillows, or padding, *to avoid discomfort and skin breakdown.*

These measures do not replace need for turning.

• Keep patient's skin clean and dry; lubricate as needed. Avoid use of irritating soap; rinse skin well. *These measures alleviate skin dryness, promote comfort, and reduce risk of irritation and skin breakdown.*

• Protect bony prominences with foam padding. *Prominences have little subcutaneous fat and are prone to breakdown; using foam padding may help promote skin integrity.*

• Lift patient's body when moving; avoid shearing force. *Shearing force is caused when tissues slide against each other; a lifting sheet reduces sliding.*

• Keep linen dry, clean, and free of wrinkles or crumbs. Change wet bed linens and incontinence pads immediately. *Dry, smooth linens avoid excoriation and skin breakdown.*

• Monitor nutritional intake; maintain adequate hydration. *Anemia (< 10 mg hemoglobin) and low serum albumin concentrations (< 2 mg) are associated with development of pressure ulcers. Hydration helps maintain skin integrity.*

• Educate patient and family in preventive skin care: maintaining good personal hygiene; using nonirritating (nonalkaline) soap; patting rather than rubbing to dry skin; inspecting skin on a regular basis; avoiding prolonged exposure to water, sun, cold, wind; avoiding rubber rings; recognizing beginning of skin breakdown (redness, blisters, discoloration); and reporting symptoms. *These measures encourage compliance with skin care regimen.*

• Indicate risk factor potential on patient's chart and plan of care, and reevaluate weekly, using an accepted form such as the Braden Scale. *Risk factor score helps evaluate treatment progress.*

• Explain why preventive skin care measures are needed, *to encourage compliance with skin care regimen.*

• Supervise patient and family in preventive skin care measures. Give constructive feedback. *Practice helps improve skill in managing skin care regimen.*

Evaluations for expected outcomes

• Patient's skin remains intact.

• Patient does not show evidence of contractures or muscle atrophy.

• Patient's mucous membranes remain intact.

• Patient's weight remains within established limits.

• Patient does not show evidence of poor circulation.

• Patient lists preventive skin care measures.

• Patient and family demonstrate skin care measures.

• Patient and family understand necessity of avoiding prolonged pressure, obtaining adequate nutrition, preventing incontinence, and consistently performing skin care measures.

Documentation

• Patient's and family's expression of concern about potential skin breakdown

• Observations of risk factors and skin condition

• Use of preventive skin care devices and their effectiveness

• Instructions regarding preventive skin care; patient's and family's understanding of instructions

• Patient's and family's demonstrated skill in carrying out preventive skin care measures

• Patient's response to nursing interventions

• Evaluations for each expected outcome.

Sleep pattern disturbance

related to external factors, such as environmental changes

Definition

Inability to meet individual need for sleep or rest arising from internal or external factors

Assessment

- Daytime activity and work patterns
- Normal bedtime
- Usual number of hours of sleep required
- Problems associated with sleep, including early-morning awakening, falling asleep, nightmares, sleepwalking, staying asleep
- Quality of sleep
- Sleeping environment
- Activities associated with sleep
- Personal beliefs about sleep
- Chemical ingestion, including alcohol, caffeine, hypnotics, nicotine

Defining characteristics

- Awakening earlier or later than desired
- Changes in behavior or performance, including disorientation, increased irritability, lethargy, listlessness, restlessness
- Evidence of external factors that prevent or disrupt sleep
- Interrupted sleep
- Physical signs, including dark circles under eyes; expressionless face; frequent yawning; mild, fleeting nystagmus; ptosis of the eyelid; slight hand tremor; thick speech with mispronunciation or incorrect words
- Verbal complaints of difficulty falling asleep
- Verbal complaints of not feeling well-rested

Associated medical diagnoses (selected)

This diagnosis may affect elderly, hospitalized patients, patient sharing a room with someone confused and noisy, and patients whose treatment involves any of the following: frequent monitoring of vital signs, intensive care, mechanical ventilation, medications during the night, treatments given during the night.

Expected outcomes

- Patient identifies factors that prevent or facilitate sleep.
- Patient sleeps _____ hours without interruption.
- Patient expresses feeling of being well-rested.
- Patient shows no physical signs indicative of sleep deprivation.
- Patient alters diet and habits to promote sleep; for example, reduces caffeine, limits alcohol intake.
- Patient exhibits no sleep-related behavioral symptoms, such as restlessness, irritability, lethargy, or disorientation.
- Patient performs relaxation exercises at bedtime.

Interventions and rationales

- Ask patient what environmental factors make sleep difficult. *Sleeping in strange or new environment tends to influence both REM and NREM sleep.*
- Ask patient what changes would facilitate sleep. *This allows patient to take active role in treatment.*
- Make whatever immediate changes are possible to accommodate patient; for example, reduce noise, change lighting, close door. *These measures promote rest and sleep.*
- Plan medication administration schedules *to allow for maximum rest.* If patient requires diuretics in the

evening, give far enough in advance *to allow peak effect before bedtime.*
• Make a detailed plan to provide the patient with _____ hours of uninterrupted sleep, if possible. *This allows consistent nursing care and gives patient uninterrupted sleep time.*
• Provide patient with normal sleep aids, such as pillow, bath, back rub, food, drink. *Milk and some high-protein snacks, such as cheese or nuts, contain L-tryptophan, a sleep promoter. Personal hygiene routine precedes sleep in many patients.*
• Ask patient to describe in specific terms each morning the quality of sleep during the previous night. *This helps detect presence of sleep-related behavioral symptoms.*
• Teach patient such relaxation techniques as guided imagery, meditation, progressive muscle relaxation. Practice them with patient at bedtime. *Purposeful relaxation efforts often help promote sleep.*
• Instruct patient to eliminate caffeine from diet, limit alcohol intake, and avoid foods that interfere with sleep (for example, spicy foods). *Foods and beverages containing caffeine should be avoided for 4 to 5 hours before bedtime.*

Evaluations for expected outcomes
• Patient describes factors that prevent or facilitate sleep.
• Patient sleeps specified number of hours without interruption.
• Patient expresses feeling of being well rested.
• Patient does not exhibit physical signs indicating sleep deprivation.
• Patient reports changing diet habits and making life-style changes to promote sleep.
• Patient does not exhibit sleep-related behavioral symptoms.
• Patient performs relaxation exercises at bedtime.

Documentation
• Patient's complaints about sleep disturbances
• Patient's verbalization of feelings in relation to sleep
• Observations of behavior indicative of sleep deprivation
• Interventions to alleviate sleep disturbance
• Patient's response to nursing interventions
• Evaluations for each expected outcome.

Sleep pattern disturbance

related to internal factors, such as illness, psychological stress, drug therapy, biorhythm disturbance

Definition
Inability to meet individual need for sleep or rest arising from internal or external factors

Assessment
• Age
• Daytime activity and work patterns
• Time the patient usually retires
• Number of hours of sleep patient usually requires in order to feel rested
• Problems associated with sleep, including early-morning awakening, falling asleep, nightmares, sleepwalking, staying asleep
• Quality of sleep
• Sleeping environment
• Activities associated with sleep, including bath, drink, food, medication
• Personal beliefs about sleep

Defining characteristics
- Awakening earlier or later than desired
- Changes in behavior or performance, including disorientation, increased irritability, lethargy, listlessness, restlessness
- Evidence of internal factors that prevent or disrupt sleep
- Interrupted sleep
- Physical signs, including dark circles under eyes; expressionless face; frequent yawning; mild, fleeting nystagmus; ptosis of the eyelid; slight hand tremor; thick speech with mispronunciation and incorrect words
- Verbal complaints of difficulty falling asleep
- Verbal complaints of not feeling well rested

Associated medical diagnoses (selected)
Alcoholism, bipolar disorder (manic-depressive), chronic obstructive pulmonary disease, depression, drug addiction, pickwickian syndrome, sleep apnea

Expected outcomes
- Patient identifies factors that prevent or disrupt sleep.
- Patient sleeps _____ hours a night.
- Patient expresses feeling of being well-rested.
- Patient shows no physical signs of sleep deprivation.
- Patient exhibits no sleep-related behavioral symptoms, such as restlessness, irritability, lethargy, disorientation.
- Patient performs relaxation exercises at bedtime.

Interventions and rationales
- Allow patient to discuss any concerns that may be preventing sleep. *Active listening aids determination of causes of difficulty with sleep.*
- Plan nursing care routines to allow _______ hours of uninterrupted sleep. *This allows consistent nursing care and gives patient uninterrupted sleep time.*
- Provide patient with usual sleep aids, such as pillows, bath before sleep, food or drink, reading materials, etc. *Milk and some high protein snacks such as cheese and nuts, contain L-tryptophan, a sleep promoter. Personal hygiene routine precedes sleep in many patients.*
- Create a quiet environment conducive to sleep; for example, close the curtains, adjust the lighting, close the door. *These measures promote rest and sleep.*
- Administer medications that promote normal sleep patterns, as ordered. Monitor and record side effects and effectiveness. *A hypnotic agent induces sleep; a tranquilizer reduces anxiety.*
- Promote involvement in diversional activities or exercise program during the day. Discuss the relationship of exercise and activity to improved sleep. Discourage excessive napping. *Activity and exercise promote sleep by increasing fatigue and relaxation.*
- Ask patient to describe in specific terms each morning the quality of sleep during the previous night. *This helps detect presence of sleep-related behavioral symptoms.*
- Educate patient in such relaxation techniques as imagery, progressive muscle relaxation, meditation. *Purposeful relaxation efforts often help promote sleep.*

Evaluations for expected outcomes
- Patient identifies factors that prevent or disrupt sleep.
- Patient sleeps specified number of hours nightly.

- Patient expresses feeling of being well rested.
- Patient does not exhibit signs of sleep deprivation.
- Patient does not exhibit sleep-related behavioral symptoms.
- Patient performs relaxation exercises at bedtime.

Documentation
- Patient's complaints about sleep disturbances
- Patient's report of improvement in sleep patterns
- Observations of physical and behavioral sleep-related disturbances
- Interventions to alleviate sleep disturbances
- Patient's response to nursing interventions
- Evaluations for each expected outcome.

Social interaction impairment

related to altered thought processes

Definition
Insufficient quantity or ineffective quality of social exchange

Assessment
- Reason for hospitalization (physiologic, psychiatric)
- Usual pattern of social interaction (nonverbal behaviors, verbal communication)
- Neurologic functioning, including level of consciousness, orientation, sensory and motor ability
- Mental status, including abstract ability, affect, concentration ability, insight and judgment, memory, mood, thought content
- History of substance abuse
- Education and intelligence level
- Sociocultural background, including beliefs, norms, religion, values
- Support systems available, including clergy, family or significant other, friends

Defining characteristics
- Delusional thinking
- Observed or verbalized discomfort in social interaction skills.
- Observed use of unsuccessful or dysfunctional social interaction skills
- Sensory and perceptual alterations, including auditory, visual, or tactile hallucinations
- Verbalized or observed inability to communicate needs or to receive a sense of need-gratification from caregivers

Associated medical diagnoses (selected)
Alzheimer's disease, brain tumor, cerebrovascular accident, diabetic ketoacidosis, drug or alcohol withdrawal, head trauma, organic brain syndrome, psychiatric disorder

Expected outcomes
- Patient remains free of injury.
- Patient and family or significant other report concern about difficulties in social interaction.
- Patient maintains orientation to person, place, and time.
- Patient's perceptions are reality-based.
- Patient and family or significant other participate in care and prescribed therapies.
- Patient expresses needs and communicates whether needs are met.
- Patient regains appropriate neurologic function to the extent possible.
- Patient demonstrates effective social interaction skills in both one-on-one and group settings.

• Patient and family or significant other identify and mobilize resources for rehabilitation and discharge planning, as necessary.

Interventions and rationales

• Follow medical regimen to treat underlying condition. *Nurse is responsible for following medical regimen and working with doctor to plan appropriate care.*

• Take precautions to ensure safe and protected environment (provide side rails, assistance with out-of-bed activities, uncluttered room, physical restraints, as necessary). *This reduces potential for patient injury.*

• Assess neurologic function and mental status every shift *to monitor changes in patient's status,* and reorient patient as often as necessary:

  – Call patient by name and say your name each time you interact with patient.
  – Tell patient correct day, date, time, and place at least once a shift.
  – Teach family how to reorient patient and assist them in doing so.
  – Ask family or significant other to bring patient familiar objects from home, such as clock, radio, or photographs.
  – Post structured schedule of daily activities in patient's room within visual range.
  – Explain schedule to family or significant other and other caregivers to provide consistency and continuity.

Reorienting patient and involving family or significant other enhances patient's reality testing ability and overall mental status. Scheduling daily routine narrows patient's frame of reference, thereby decreasing potential for increased confusion.

• If delusions and hallucinations occur, do not focus on them; provide patient with reality-based information and reassure patient of safety. *This increases patient's ability to grasp reality and reduces fears associated with these disturbances.*

• Provide specific, non-care-related time with patient each shift to encourage social interaction. Begin with one-on-one interaction and increase to group interaction as patient's skills indicate. *Gradually increasing social interaction reduces patient's feeling of being overwhelmed and eliminates sensory input that may renew cognitive or perceptual disturbance.*

• Give positive reinforcement for appropriate and effective interaction behaviors (verbal and nonverbal). *This helps patient recognize progress and enhances feelings of self-worth.*

• Assist patient and family or significant other in progressive participation in care and therapies. *This reduces feelings of helplessness and enhances patient's feeling of control and independence.*

• Initiate or participate in multidisciplinary patient-centered conferences to evaluate progress and plan discharge. In addition to patient and family or significant other, conferences may include physical, occupational, and speech therapists; social worker; attending doctor; and other consultants, as necessary. *These conferences involve patient and family in cooperative effort to develop strategies for altering care plan as necessary.*

Evaluations for expected outcomes

• Patient does not exhibit physical evidence of injury.

• Patient or significant other expresses concern about patient's inability to interact normally.

- Neurologic assessment reveals that patient is oriented to time, place, and person.
- Patient's verbal responses and behavior do not indicate delusions or hallucinations.
- Patient and family or significant other perform care-related procedures to extent possible.
- Patient uses words, gestures, or writing to communicate needs and whether needs are met.
- Patient maintains appropriate cognitive and perceptual functioning to the extent possible.
- Patient communicates effectively in one-on-one and group settings.
- Patient and family or significant other identify and contact available support resources as needed.

Documentation
- Patient's verbal and nonverbal behaviors
- Neurologic and mental status assessment
- Observations of patient's social interaction skills
- Interventions to facilitate appropriate and effective social interaction
- Patient's responses to nursing interventions
- Evaluations for each expected outcome.

■ Social interaction impairment

related to sociocultural dissonance

Definition
Insufficient quantity or ineffective quality of social exchange

Assessment
- Reason for hospitalization (physiologic, psychiatric)
- Sociocultural background (beliefs, norms, rituals, values)
- Usual pattern of social interaction, including: dominant language, group participation, level of comprehension, nonverbal communication skills (drawing, gestures), speech pattern
- Patient's position in family
- Support systems available, including clergy, family or significant other, friends
- Education and intelligence level

Defining characteristics
- Observed use of unsuccessful social-interaction behavior
- Verbalized or observed discomfort in situations requiring social exchange
- Verbalized or observed inability to communicate needs or to receive a sense of need-gratification from caregivers

Associated medical diagnoses (selected)
This diagnosis can occur in any hospitalized patient separated from usual sociocultural environment. For example, in some European and Asian cultures, nonverbal means of communication (eye contact, touch) are considered an invasion of privacy; many Native Americans consider social interaction outside the family to be disloyal.

Expected outcomes
- Patient provides information concerning cultural background.
- Patient identifies needs and communicates (verbally or nonverbally) whether needs are met.
- Patient expresses an understanding of care-related instruction.

- Patient and family or significant other participate in planning care.
- Patient identifies effective coping techniques to deal with sociocultural differences.
- Patient and family or significant other express feelings of comfort and trust in interaction with caregivers.
- Patient uses resources outside normal sociocultural group, as necessary.

Interventions and rationales

- Assign a primary nurse to this patient, if possible. *Primary nursing provides consistency, enhances trust and decreases potential for fragmented care.*
- Provide specific time (for example, 10 minutes each shift) to talk with patient and family or significant other about sociocultural background. *In many cultural groups, trust is developed slowly and may be hampered by lengthy interviews.*
- Explain care-related activities clearly, answering questions as accurately as possible. *This enhances patient's understanding of care-related procedures and hospital routine.*
- Use an interpreter when necessary, *to ensure effective communication for non-English-speaking patients.*
- Involve patient and family or significant other in planning care, and encourage patient's participation in self-care on a continuing basis. *This increases their sense of control and reduces feelings of helplessness and isolation.*
- Assist patient in identifying and using effective social-interaction behaviors, such as increased eye contact, calling person by name, asking questions, etc. *Teaching patient effective intrapersonal communication is an essential part of nursing practice.*
- Demonstrate respect for patient's privacy, personal belongings, cultural norms, and religious beliefs and practices *to provide sensitive care to patients from varied cultural backgrounds.*
- Offer referral to other support systems, if indicated (such as social services, financial counseling, home health care, mental health care, professional care). *This ensures a comprehensive approach to patient's care.*

Evaluations for expected outcomes

- Patient provides information concerning culture, including values, attitudes, roles, and beliefs.
- Patient reports needs and gratification of these needs, either verbally or through behavior.
- Patient demonstrates care-related procedures.
- Patient and family or significant other develop plan of care.
- Patient specifies positive ways to cope with cultural differences.
- Patient and family communicate sense of security and demonstrate decrease in anxiety-related behaviors.
- Patient uses appropriate resources outside normal sociocultural group, as needed.

Documentation

- Patient's and family's or significant other's perception of current situation
- Interventions to facilitate effective social interaction
- Patient's verbal and nonverbal responses to nursing interventions
- Evaluations for each expected outcome.

Social isolation

related to altered state of wellness

Definition

Aloneness that the patient perceives negatively; may be self-imposed or be perceived as being imposed by others; alternatively, may result from environmental factors

Assessment

- Reason for hospitalization (physiologic, psychiatric)
- Support systems available, including clergy, family, relatives, friends
- Functional ability
- Diversional interests
- Attitudes of family or friends toward patient
- Financial resources
- Occupation
- Education level
- Coping and problem-solving ability
- Self-esteem

Defining characteristics

- Culturally unacceptable behavior
- Describes life-style as solitary or circumscribed by membership in subculture
- Evidence of physical or mental handicap or altered state of wellness
- Expresses feelings of being different from others
- Expresses feelings of rejection or aloneness
- Expresses frustration over inability to meet expectations of others
- Inappropriate or immature interests or activities
- Insecurity in public
- Lack of family, friends, social groups
- Lack of purpose in life
- Preoccupation with own thoughts
- Projection of hostility in voice and behavior
- Repetitive, meaningless actions
- Sad, dull affect
- Uncommunicative, withdrawn, poor eye contact

Associated medical diagnoses (selected)

Acquired immunodeficiency syndrome, Alzheimer's disease (early stage), cancer, depression, disorders requiring isolation precautions, genital herpes, head or neck surgery, hepatitis, organic brain syndrome, schizophrenia, spinal cord injuries, tuberculosis

Expected outcomes

- Patient expresses feelings associated with social isolation.
- Patient identifies causes of social isolation and participates in developing a plan for increasing social activity.
- Patient interacts with family or friends.
- Patient interacts with staff members.
- Patient performs self-care activities independently.
- Patient participates daily in a meaningful diversional activity (specify).
- Patient indicates social relationships have improved and negative feelings have diminished.
- Patient achieves expected state of wellness.

Interventions and rationales

- Assign a primary nurse to this patient, if possible, *to provide continuity, enhance trust, and decrease potential for fragmented care.*
- Initiate a trusting nurse-patient relationship *to help gain patient's confidence.*

• Provide honest and immediate feedback about patient's behavior *to help patient become aware of effects of behavior and to modify, verify, or correct patient's perceptions.*
• Help patient to identify causes of social isolation *to identify patient's needs and guide planning of care.* Involve patient and family or friends in setting goals and planning care *to individualize plan of care and decrease patient's feelings of helplessness and isolation.*
• Encourage patient to perform such self-care activities as bathing, grooming, dressing, eating, and ambulating *to reduce feelings of helplessness and foster independent action.*
• Spend at least 15 minutes each shift with patient. Sit with patient and listen. *Listening communicates concern, interest, and acceptance and allows time for patient to collect thoughts and express feelings.*
• Arrange with patient for specific periods of appropriate planned diversional activity *to provide pleasure, increase feelings of self-worth, and decrease negative self-absorption.*
• Allow ample private time for patient to spend with family or friends *to demonstrate respect for patient and for patient's relationships with others.*
• Identify appropriate social agencies and support groups for patient and provide referrals *to ensure ongoing opportunities for patient to increase social interaction.*
• Educate patient and family about health care needs and treatment *to promote optimal health and well-being, thereby allowing for greater social activity.*

Evaluations for expected outcomes
• Patient expresses sadness, frustration, anxiety and other feelings associated with social isolation.
• Patient identifies causes of social isolation and participates in developing a plan for increasing social activity.
• Patient interacts with family or friends.
• Patient communicates with caregivers.
• Patient initiates self-care activities, such as bathing, dressing, eating, and grooming, to extent possible.
• Patient expresses frustration over limitations and fears about loneliness.
• Patient identifies at least three activities that provide enjoyment and participates in one activity daily.
• Patient reports decreased feelings of isolation.
• Patient increases social interaction.
• Patient reports regaining physical and psychological health. Patient's reports are backed by assessment data and perceptions of doctors and other caregivers.

Documentation
• Observations of patient's social interaction skills
• Causes of social isolation identified by patient
• Resources identified to help patient increase social interaction
• Interventions to encourage social interaction and patient's response
• Evaluations for each expected outcome.

Social isolation

related to inadequate personal resources

Definition

Self-imposed or environmentally imposed lack of contact with support systems

Assessment

- Reason for hospitalization (physiologic, psychiatric)
- Support systems available, including clergy, family or significant other, friends
- Diversional interests
- Attitudes of family or significant other toward patient in this situation
- Financial resources
- Occupation
- Level of education and intelligence
- Coping and problem-solving ability
- Self-esteem

Defining characteristics

- Absence of support system, including family or significant other, friends, support group
- Displays behavior unacceptable to dominant cultural group
- Evidence of insufficient resources to meet societal expectations
- Expresses feelings of aloneness or rejection
- Projects hostility in voice, behavior
- Sad, dull affect
- Seeks to be alone or exists in subculture
- Uncommunicative, withdrawn

Associated medical diagnoses (selected)

This diagnosis occurs among elderly patients, homeless people, patients with present or past history of psychiatric disorders, and patients who have no family or friends to support them.

Expected outcomes

- Patient interacts with caregivers in a positive way.
- Patient expresses feelings about lack of supportive relationships.
- Patient expresses desire to be involved with others.
- Patient expresses desire to improve self and present condition; for example, by obtaining further education or learning how to better manage finances.
- Patient uses resources available through the agency (social services, home health care, psychology services, self-improvement classes) to establish a realistic plan for the future.
- Patient states plan to participate in social activity.

Interventions and rationales

- Assign same caregivers to patient to promote trusting relationships with staff members. *Consistent care promotes patient's ability to communicate openly.*
- Assign a primary nurse to coordinate patient's care. *This reduces potential for fragmented nursing interventions.*
- Plan a 15-minute period to sit with patient each shift. If patient does not wish to talk, remain silent. *Active listening communicates concern, allows time to collect thoughts, and encourages patient to initiate interaction.*
- Involve patient in planning care; have patient participate in self-care continuously. *This provides structure, reduces feelings of helplessness, and fosters independent action.*
- Discuss patient's living accommodations and life-style outside the hospital. *Knowledge of patient's current*

life-style and accommodations aids understanding of patient's uniqueness and helps with discharge planning.
• Refer patient to social services for follow-up, if necessary, *to ensure a comprehensive approach to care.*
• Help patient identify social outlets (peer group, associations, participation in group activity). *This draws patient's attention to specific data and promotes goal-directed interaction.*

Evaluations for expected outcomes
• Patient seeks information from and expresses feelings to caregivers.
• Patient acknowledges concern about the absence of supportive relationships.
• Patient expresses desire to develop meaningful relationships.
• Patient states at least two methods of achieving personal growth and improving current situation.
• Patient identifies and contacts social service agencies and states plan to participate in social activities.

Documentation
• Patient's perceptions of the present situation
• Patient's expressions of plans for the future
• Observations of patient's behavior
• Planning done by patient with nurse, physician, social worker, etc.
• Patient's response to nursing interventions
• Evaluations for each expected outcome.

■ Spiritual distress

related to separation from religious and cultural ties

Definition
Separation or alienation from religious traditions or values

Assessment
• Religious ties and practices
• Religious commitment
• Visits (church members, family members, or clergy)

Defining characteristics
• Can't or won't participate in usual religious practices
• Expresses concern with meaning of life and death or belief systems
• Questions meaning of own existence
• Questions meaning of suffering
• Seeks spiritual assistance
• Shows anger toward God (as defined by the patient)
• Shows displacement of anger toward religious representatives
• Voices inner conflicts about beliefs

Associated medical diagnoses (selected)
This diagnosis may be seen in any hospitalized patient, depending on the individual and the circumstances.

Expected outcomes
• Patient communicates conflict about beliefs.
• Patient identifies the source of spiritual conflict.
• Patient specifies whatever spiritual assistance is needed.
• Patient discusses beliefs regarding religious practices.
• Patient identifies coping techniques to deal with spiritual discomfort.

- Patient expresses feelings of spiritual comfort.

Interventions and rationales

- Listen for cues indicative of patient's feelings ("Why did God do this to me?" or "God is punishing me"). *Active listening demonstrates involvement with patient and allows nurse to hear important messages indicating spiritual distress.*
- Approach patient in a nonjudgmental way *to focus on patient's feelings without evaluating them as right or wrong, good or bad.*
- Acknowledge patient's spiritual concerns, and encourage expression of thoughts and feelings *to help build a therapeutic relationship.*
- Help patient define in concrete terms the problem causing the inner conflict. *This is first step in developing strategies for resolving conflicts.*
- Arrange for visits by clergy, as appropriate, *thereby using expert spiritual care resources to help the patient.*
- Encourage patient to continue religious practices during hospitalization; do whatever is necessary to facilitate this. For example:
  - If patient is accustomed to reading the Scriptures and doesn't have a Bible, make an effort to get one.
  - If Jewish male wears a yarmulke, allow him to continue wearing it if possible.
  - In cases where certain foods are prohibited or special foods are required, according to patient's religious traditions, make every effort to communicate these needs to the dietary department and see that they are honored.

  These measures demonstrate support and convey caring and acceptance to patient.
- Communicate and collaborate with patient's minister or with the hospital chaplain, when this is appropriate. *This ensures consistent care and provides more complete data base.*
- Arrange for patient to have at the bedside objects that provide spiritual comfort (Bible, prayer shawl, pictures, statues, rosary beads). *Items of spiritual significance may influence patient's ability to reduce conflict.*
- Provide privacy during patient's visits with minister or chaplain *to demonstrate respect for patient's relationship with clergy.*

Evaluations for expected outcomes

- Patient expresses feelings of uncertainty or ambivalence related to spiritual beliefs.
- Patient states specific causes of spiritual distress.
- Patient requests spiritual assistance, if needed.
- Patient discusses usual religious practices, including rituals, prayers, values, and beliefs.
- Patient reports decreased spiritual discomfort.
- Patient expresses desire to resume usual religious practices.

Documentation

- Patient's expressions of concern about spiritual matters, whether direct or subtle
- Observations about patient's spiritual distress or well-being
- Interventions carried out to promote spiritual comfort
- Observations about patient's responses to interventions
- Evaluations for each expected outcome.

Spiritual distress

related to situational crisis

Definition

Separation or alienation from religious tradition or values

Assessment

- Reason for hospitalization
- Religion or church affiliation
- Patient's usual and current perception of faith and religious practices
- Available spiritual support persons (minister, priest, rabbi)

Defining characteristics

- Demonstrates anger toward God, church, and clergy
- Engages in "bargaining" with God (as defined by individual) as stage of anticipatory grieving
- Expresses concern with meaning of life and death
- Reports ambivalence about faith and religious practices
- Verbalizes guilt about self and behavior

Associated medical diagnoses (selected)

This nursing diagnosis can apply to any hospitalized individual with strong religious beliefs and practices. It is particularly evident in those experiencing the threat of death.

Expected outcomes

- Patient expresses feelings about usual and current religious beliefs.
- Patient identifies areas of ambivalence and conflict resulting from current situation.
- Patient states an understanding of the grief process and its stages.
- Patient uses effective coping strategies to ease spiritual discomfort.
- Patient seeks appropriate support persons (family or significant other, priest, minister, rabbi) for assistance.

Interventions and rationales

- Approach patient in an accepting, nonjudgmental manner *to demonstrate unconditional positive regard for the patient.*
- Acknowledge patient's spiritual concerns and encourage expression of feelings *to help build a therapeutic relationship.*
- Encourage patient to provide information about religious beliefs and practices. *Acquiring this initial data base is first step in nursing process.*
- Instruct patient on the stages of grieving and on the emotions and behaviors common to each stage. *This promotes understanding and encourages feelings of normalcy.*
- Provide for continuation of patient's religious practices (allow for specific religious materials or clothing; respect dietary restrictions if possible). *These measures demonstrate support and convey caring and acceptance to patient.*
- Facilitate visits from clergy and provide privacy during visits *to demonstrate respect for patient's relationship with clergy.*
- Encourage patient to discuss concerns with clergy, *thereby using expert spiritual care resources to help the patient.*

Evaluations for expected outcomes

- Patient discusses feelings about spiritual or religious beliefs.
- Patient specifies areas of spiritual conflict, for example, anger toward God, questioning of usual beliefs regarding life after death, or guilt associated with loss of faith.
- Patient communicates understanding of grief process and its stages.

• Patient continues religious practices, which ease spiritual distress.
• Patient makes use of available resources for spiritual assistance.

Documentation
• Patient's verbal and nonverbal communication of spiritual discomfort
• Stage of anticipatory grief as indicated by behavior
• Interventions to promote spiritual comfort
• Patient's response to nursing interventions
• Evaluations for each expected outcome.

Suffocation, high risk for

related to external factors

Definition
Accentuated risk of accidental suffocation (inadequate air available for inhalation)

Assessment
• Health history, including accidents, allergies, exposure to pollutants, falls, hyperthermia, hypothermia, poisoning, seizures, sensory or perceptual changes (auditory, gustatory, kinesthetic, olfactory, tactile, visual), trauma
• Circumstances of present situation that might lead to injury
• Neurologic status, including level of consciousness, mental status, orientation
• Laboratory studies, including clotting factors, hemoglobin and hematocrit, platelet count, white blood cell count

Risk factors
• Alarms turned off on ventilators
• Immobile patient incorrectly positioned on abdomen
• Pillows placed incorrectly under the head of patient who has a compromised airway
• Ventilator connections improperly monitored

Associated medical diagnoses (selected)
Acute respiratory failure, chronic obstructive pulmonary disease, drug overdose, inhalation injuries, head injury, multisystem trauma, near-drowning episode, sedation or placement under general anesthesia

Expected outcomes
• Patient's airway remains patent at all times.
• Patient's vital signs remain within normal parameters.
• Patient and family or significant other demonstrate knowledge of safety measures to prevent suffocation.

Interventions and rationales
• Monitor and record respiratory status. *Changes in parameters (such as respiratory rate, cough, sputum production, skin color) may indicate airway obstruction.*
• Monitor and record neurologic status. *Symptoms of hypoxia include headache, depression, apathy, memory loss, poor muscular coordination, fatigue, stupor, loss of consciousness.*
• Monitor vital signs and report changes. *Changes with hypoxia include tachycardia and slight rise in blood pressure. Advanced hypoxia reduces heart rate and causes loss of consciousness.*
• Position patient on side or position head and neck to prevent relaxed neck muscles from obstructing the airway. *This allows maximal chest*

expansion and prevents aspiration and airway obstruction.
- Check all ventilator connections every 30 minutes on patient being mechanically ventilated *to ensure patient receives proper amount of oxygen at appropriate volume and rate.*
- Check ventilator alarms every 30 minutes and after suctioning *to ensure proper alarm function.*
- Suction airway as needed *to prevent secretion accumulation. Do this only as needed to prevent tracheal irritation.*
- Provide patient and family or significant other with information about safety practices *to enable patient and significant other to take active role in care and ensure performance of safety measures.*

Evaluations for expected outcomes
- Patient's airway remains free of obstruction.
- Patient's vital signs remain within normal parameters.
- Patient or caregiver demonstrates safety measures to prevent suffocation.

Documentation
- Patient's statements that indicate potential for injury
- Physical findings
- Observations or knowledge of unsafe practices
- Interventions performed to prevent injury
- Patient's response to nursing interventions
- Evaluations for each expected outcome.

■ Suffocation, high risk for

related to internal factors

Definition
Accentuated risk of accidental suffocation (inadequate air available for inhalation)

Assessment
- Health history, including accidents, allergies, exposure to pollutants, falls, hyperthermia, hypothermia, poisoning, seizures, sensory or perceptual changes (auditory, gustatory, kinesthetic, olfactory, tactile, visual), trauma
- Circumstances of present situation that might lead to injury
- Neurologic status, including level of consciousness, mental status, orientation
- Laboratory studies, including clotting factors, hemoglobin and hematocrit, platelet count, white blood cell count

Risk factors
- Cognitive or emotional difficulties
- Injury or disease process
- Lack of safety education
- Lack of safety precautions
- Reduced motor abilities
- Reduced olfactory sensation

Associated medical diagnoses (selected)
Multisystem trauma, sedation, or placement under general anesthesia

Expected outcomes
- Patient avoids accidental suffocation.
- Patient's vital signs remain within normal parameters.
- Patient and family or significant other demonstrate knowledge of

safety measures to prevent suffocation.

Interventions and rationales

- Observe, record, and report falls, seizures, and unsafe practices *to ensure implementation of appropriate interventions.*
- Monitor and record respiratory status. *Changes in parameters (such as respiratory rate, cough, sputum production, skin color) may indicate airway obstruction.*
- Monitor and record neurologic status. *Symptoms of hypoxia include headache, depression, apathy, memory loss, poor muscular coordination, fatigue, stupor, loss of consciousness.*
- Monitor vital signs and report changes. *Hypoxic changes include tachycardia and slight rise in blood pressure. Advanced hypoxia reduces heart rate and causes loss of consciousness.*
- Position patient on side or position head and neck to prevent relaxed neck muscles from obstructing the airway. *This allows maximal chest expansion and prevents aspiration and airway obstruction.*
- Obtain suction equipment, assemble, and keep at the bedside *to assure equipment readiness in case of need.*
- Suction as needed *to keep upper and lower airways clear and to stimulate cough reflex to enhance sputum removal. Do this only as needed, to prevent tracheal irritation.*
- Provide patient and significant other with information about safety practices *to enable patient and significant other to take an active role in care and ensure performance of safety measures.*

Evaluations for expected outcomes

- Patient does not experience accidental suffocation.
- Patient's vital signs remain within normal parameters.
- Patient or caregiver demonstrates safety measures that prevent suffocation.

Documentation

- Patient's statements about the situation that indicate potential for injury
- Physical findings
- Record of falls, seizures, and unsafe practices
- Interventions that reduce risk of injury
- Patient's response to nursing interventions
- Evaluations for each expected outcome.

Swallowing impairment

related to neuromuscular impairment

Definition

Inability to move food, fluid, or saliva from the mouth through the esophagus

Assessment

- History of neuromuscular, cerebral, or respiratory disease
- Age
- Sex
- Nutritional status, including appetite, dietary intake, hydration, current weight, and change from normal weight
- Neurologic status, including barium swallow; chest X-ray; cognition; esophageal video fluoroscopy; gag reflex; level of consciousness; memory; motor ability; orientation; sym-

metry of face, mouth, and neck; sensory function; tongue movement

Defining characteristics

- Evidence of aspiration
- Observed evidence of difficulty in swallowing, including choking, coughing, stasis of food in oral cavity

Associated medical diagnoses (selected)

Bell's palsy, cerebrovascular accident, head injury, laryngectomy, maxillofacial trauma, tracheostomy

Expected outcomes

- Patient shows no evidence of aspiration pneumonia.
- Patient achieves adequate nutritional intake.
- Patient maintains weight.
- Patient maintains oral hygiene.
- Patient and family or significant other demonstrate correct eating or feeding techniques to maximize swallowing.

Interventions and rationales

- Elevate head of bed 90 degrees during mealtimes and for 30 minutes after completion of meal *to decrease risk of aspiration.*
- Position patient on side when recumbent *to decrease risk of aspiration.*
- Keep suction apparatus at bedside; observe and report instances of cyanosis, dyspnea, or choking. *Symptoms indicate presence of material in lungs.*
- Monitor intake and output and weight daily until stabilized. Establish intake goal—for example, "Patient consumes _____ ml of fluid and _____% of solid food." Record and report any deviation from this. *Evaluating calorie and protein intake daily allows any necessary modifications to begin quickly.*
- Consult with dietitian to modify patient's diet, and conduct calorie count as needed *to establish nutritional requirements.*
- Consult with dysphagia rehabilitation team, if available, *to obtain expert advice.*
- Provide mouth care three times daily *to promote comfort and enhance appetite.*
- Keep oral mucous membrane moist by frequent rinses; use bulb syringe or suction, if necessary, *to promote comfort.*
- Lubricate patient's lips *to prevent cracking and blisters.*
- Encourage patient to wear properly fitted dentures *to enhance chewing ability.*
- Serve food in attractive surroundings; encourage patient to smell and look at food. Remove soiled equipment, control smells, and provide a quiet atmosphere for eating. *A pleasant atmosphere stimulates appetite; food aroma stimulates salivation.*
- Instruct patient and family in positioning; dietary requirements; specific feeding techniques, including facial exercises (such as whistling), using a short straw to provide sensory stimulation to lips, tipping head forward to decrease aspiration, applying pressure above lip to stimulate mouth closure and swallowing reflex, checking oral cavity frequently for food particles (remove if present). *These measures allow patient to take an active role in maintaining health.*

Evaluations for expected outcomes

- Patient shows no evidence of aspiration pneumonia. Breath sounds remain bilaterally clear; fever, chills, purulent sputum, and rapid shallow respirations are absent.

- Patient's fluid and dietary intake remains within established daily limits.
- Patient's weight remains stable.
- Patient's mucous membranes remain pink and moist.
- Patient demonstrates appropriate oral hygiene practices.
- Patient and caregiver demonstrate feeding techniques to maximize swallowing and minimize risk of complications.
- Patient and caregiver communicate understanding of how eating and immediately lying down may lead to pulmonary problems.
- Patient and caregiver list strategies to prevent aspiration.

Documentation
- Patient's expressions of feelings about current situation
- Observations of weight, swallowing ability, intake and output, oral hygiene
- Patient's response to nursing interventions
- Instructions about diet monitoring and feeding techniques
- Evaluations for each expected outcome.

Thermoregulation, ineffective

related to trauma or illness

Definition
Fluctuations in body temperature caused by thermoregulatory disturbances

Assessment
- History of present illness
- Medication history
- Neurologic status, including level of consciousness, mental status, motor status, sensory status
- Cardiovascular status, including blood pressure, capillary refill, electrocardiogram, heart rate and rhythm, pulses (apical and peripheral), temperature
- Respiratory status, including arterial blood gas measurements; breath sounds; and rate, depth, and character of respirations
- Integumentary status, including color, temperature, turgor
- Fluid and electrolyte status, including blood urea nitrogen, intake and output, serum electrolytes, urine specific gravity
- Laboratory studies, including clotting factors, hemoglobin and hematocrit, platelet count, white blood cell count

Defining characteristics
- Fever or hypothermic condition refractory to antipyretic therapy
- Fluctuations in body temperature above or below the normal range
- Flushed or mottled skin
- Increased or decreased respiratory and heart rates
- Mild to severe dehydration
- Possible seizures or convulsions
- Skin warm or cool to touch

Associated medical diagnoses (selected)
Brain tumor, especially if located in hypothalamus, pituitary or medulla; burns; central nervous system dysfunction related to head trauma via surgery or injury; cerebral edema; cerebral hemorrhage; cerebrovascular accident; chemical toxicity (including pharmacologic or anesthesia reaction); congestive heart failure; dehydration; head injury; heat stroke; herniation syndrome; near-drowning; smoke inhalation or other anoxic

events; temperature regulation affected by diseases causing pathologic changes in blood flow (Buerger's disease, congestive heart failure, diseases of hypothalamus and medulla, encephalitis, Raynaud's disease); untreated infection

Expected outcomes

- Patient maintains body temperature at normothermic levels.
- Patient demonstrates no signs of shivering.
- Patient expresses feelings of comfort.
- Patient has warm, dry skin.
- Patient maintains heart rate and blood pressure within normal range.
- Patient exhibits no signs of compromised neurologic status.
- Patient and family or significant other voice an understanding of the health problem.

Interventions and rationales

- Monitor body temperature every 4 hours, more often if indicated. Record temperature and route. *Monitoring determines effectiveness of therapy or if intervention is required, and facilitates accurate comparison of data. (Baseline normals vary with route.)*
- Monitor and record neurologic status every 8 hours. Report any changes to physician. *Changes in level of consciousness can result from tissue hypoxia related to altered tissue perfusion. Hyperthermia increases cerebral edema and thus intracranial pressure; hypothermia depresses metabolic rate.*
- Monitor and record heart rate and rhythm, blood pressure, and respiratory rate every 4 hours. *Hyperthermia may create hypoxia by increasing oxygen demand, which results from increased tissue metabolism (metabolism increases 7% with each 1° F increase). This also means faster breathing and rising pulse rate.*
- Administer analgesics, antipyretics, and medications that prevent shivering, as indicated. Monitor effectiveness and record. *Antipyretics help reduce fever. Shivering tends to retard lowering of body temperature.*
- If the patient develops excessive fever, take the following steps:
  - Remove blankets; place loincloth over patient.
  - Apply ice bags to axilla and groin.
  - Initiate tepid water sponge bath.
  - Use cooling blanket if temperature rises above _____. Cool patient to _____.

These measures help to reduce excessive fever.

- Maintain hydration:
  - Monitor intake and output.
  - Administer parenteral fluids as ordered.
  - Determine patient's fluid preference. Keep oral fluids at bedside and encourage patient to drink.

These measures help maintain fluid balance. Keeping fluid preferences at bedside allows patient to actively participate in prescribed treatment.

- Maintain environmental temperature at a comfortable setting:
  - Ensure that all metal and plastic surfaces that come into contact with patient's body are covered.
  - Use warm blankets.
  - Ensure that linen and clothing are clean and dry.

Temperature of external environment affects ease of body temperature regulation.

- Instruct patient and family or significant other regarding:
  - signs and symptoms of altered body temperature

– precautionary measures to avoid hypothermia or hyperthermia
– adherence to other aspects of health care management to help normalize temperature (such as dietary habits, measures to prevent increased intracranial pressure)
– rationale for treatment.

These measures allow patient to take active role in health maintenance.

Evaluations for expected outcomes

- Patient's temperature remains within normal parameters.
- Patient's skin remains warm and dry.
- Patient's heart rate and blood pressure remain within normal parameters.
- Patient does not exhibit signs of shivering.
- Patient indicates a feeling of comfort, either verbally or through behavior.
- Patient does not exhibit signs or symptoms of neurologic complications associated with extremes in temperature.
- Patient and family state understanding of health problem.

Documentation

- Patient's needs and perceptions of current problem
- Physical findings
- Intake and output
- Patient's response to nursing interventions
- Evaluations for each expected outcome.

Thought process alteration

related to loss of memory

Definition

Inability to process thoughts accurately and correctly

Assessment

- History of neurologic disorder, head injury, or psychiatric disorder
- Neurologic status, including cognition, insight and judgment, memory, motor ability, orientation, sensory ability
- Self-care status, including ability to perform activities of daily living; safety practices
- Psychosocial status, including coping mechanisms, family or significant other, occupation, personality, stressors (finances, job, marital discord)

Defining characteristics

- Altered attention span
- Clinical evidence of impaired neurologic or psychiatric functioning
- Decreased ability to grasp ideas
- Disorientation to time, place, person, circumstances, and events
- Impaired ability to abstract or conceptualize
- Impaired ability to calculate
- Impaired ability to make decisions
- Impaired ability to reason
- Impaired ability to solve problems
- Inability to follow instructions
- Inappropriate social behavior
- Memory deficit or problems

Associated medical diagnoses (selected)

Alzheimer's disease, anoxic encephalopathy, anxiety states, cerebrovascular accident, head injury, Korsakoff's psychosis, organic brain syndrome, psychiatric disorders

Expected outcomes

- Patient maintains orientation to person, place, and time.
- Patient sustains no harm or injury.
- Patient maintains current health status.
- Patient and family or significant other voice feelings and concerns.
- Family or significant other communicates an understanding of care required by patient.
- Family or significant other demonstrates appropriate coping skills.
- Family or significant other identifies available health resources.

Interventions and rationales

- Observe patient's thought processes every shift. Document and report any changes. *Changes may indicate progressive improvement or decline in underlying condition.*
- Perform prescribed treatment for underlying condition; monitor progress. Report any favorable or adverse responses to treatment *to assess effectiveness of treatment.*
- Orient patient to reality as needed.
  - Call patient by name.
  - Tell patient your name.
  - Provide background information (place, time, date) frequently throughout the day. Reinforce verbal reports with visual aids, such as a reality orientation board.
  - Orient patient to environment, including sights, sounds, and smells.
  - Use TV or radio purposefully to augment orientation.

Reality orientation techniques foster patient's awareness of self and environment.

- Keep items in the same places. *Consistent, stable environment reduces confusion, decreases frustration, and aids successful completion of activities of daily living.*
- Ask family or significant other to provide patient with photos (labeled with name and relationship on back), favorite belongings, and cards. *Belongings promote sense of continuity and memory, and create sense of security and comfort.*
- Protect patient from sensory overload; allow frequent rest periods. *Sensory overload may increase confusion; frequent rest periods help avoid fatigue.*
- Provide structured environment for patient. List daily routine and post in patient's room *to provide continuity of care.*
- Communicate patient's skill level to all personnel *to preserve level of independent functioning.*
- Spend time daily with patient to encourage memories and discussion of past events. Encourage patient's participation in reminiscence groups. *Remote memory may be intact. Discussion of past events promotes sense of continuity, aids memory, and promotes feelings of security. Joining in reminiscence groups provides diversional activity and may increase socialization skills.*
- Correct patient privately for inappropriate behavior; walk patient to room or initiate another behavior. *This avoids feelings of embarrassment and frustration. Redirection and engagement in previously successful activities increase patient's sense of accomplishment and reinforce desirable behavior.*
- Provide close supervision *to prevent patient from wandering off or incurring harm.* Instruct family or significant other on how to maintain a safe

home environment for patient. *Patient may be unable to consider own safety needs or risks.* Place patient's photo or name on door to room *to aid memory and help patient find room.*

• Encourage patient to voice feelings and concerns about loss of memory. *This helps reduce anxiety and ventilate frustrations, and promotes acceptance of need for supervision and treatment regimen.*

• Help family or significant other develop the necessary coping skills to deal with patient. *These are needed to deal with patient's neurologic or psychiatric impairment and the potential for deterioration in the patient's condition.*

• Demonstrate reorientation techniques to family or significant other and provide time for supervised return demonstrations. *Informed family or significant other will be better prepared to cope with patient with altered thought processes.*

• Help family identify (or refer family to) community support group (stroke club, Alzheimer's group) *to assist in coping with the effects of illness.*

Evaluations for expected outcomes

• Neurologic assessment indicates that patient is oriented to person, place, and time.

• Patient does not show evidence of harm or injury.

• Patient maintains current health status.

• Patient and family express concerns about loss of memory and effect on patient's life-style.

• Family member or significant other reports understanding of care required by patient.

• Family member or significant other demonstrates appropriate interventions, reorientation techniques, and coping skills.

• Family member or significant other identifies and contacts at least one support group to assist in coping with effects of illness.

Documentation

• Patient's and family's or significant other's expressions of concern and feelings about patient's altered thought processes

• Observations of patient's altered thought processes and response to treatment for underlying condition

• Patient's response to nursing interventions

• Instructions to family or significant other; their understanding of instructions and demonstrated ability to care for patient

• Referrals made for the patient and family or significant other

• Evaluations for each expected outcome.

■ Thought process alteration

related to physiologic causes

Definition

Inability to process thoughts accurately and correctly

Assessment

• Reason for hospitalization

• Mental status, including abstract thinking (ask patient to interpret a proverb); general information (ask patient to name five states); insight concerning the present situation; judgment (ask patient to solve a simple problem); memory for recent and remote past; orientation to person, place, and time

- Neurologic status, including level of consciousness, motor ability, sensory ability
- Sleep habits
- Ability to perform activities of daily living
- Safety hazards
- Medication history
- Dietary and nutritional status
- History of alcohol consumption

Defining characteristics
- Altered attention span
- Altered sleep patterns
- Changes in remote, recent, or immediate memory
- Cognitive dissonance
- Confabulation
- Decreased ability to grasp ideas
- Delusions
- Disorientation in time, place, person, circumstances, or events
- Distractibility
- Hallucinations
- Impaired ability to make decisions
- Impaired ability to reason, abstract, or conceptualize
- Impaired ability to solve problems
- Inaccurate interpretation of the environment
- Inappropriate affect
- Inappropriate social behavior
- Presence of a physiologic cause for altered thought processes
- Verbal report of limitations on usual thought processes

Associated medical diagnoses (selected)
Brain tumor; diabetic ketoacidosis; drug or alcohol withdrawal; drug intoxication; head trauma; hypoxemia or hypercarbia of acute respiratory failure; malnutrition; sensory deprivation from isolation, prolonged bed rest, or traction; septicemia

Expected outcomes
- Patient remains safe and protected from injury.
- Patient maintains awareness of the need for assistance.
- Patient maintains orientation to person, place, and time.
- Patient performs activities of daily living with assistance.
- Laboratory values stay within normal range.
- Physiologic causes receive treatment, resulting in restoration of thought processes.
- Family or significant other identifies partial or complete confusion.
- Family or significant other makes arrangements for home care.

Interventions and rationales
- Monitor the following and record: vital signs every 4 hours; neurologic status every shift; laboratory values as ordered (blood glucose and alcohol, arterial blood gases, electrolytes). *Vital signs assess patient for signs and symptoms of infection or complication. Neurologic assessment and laboratory studies may reveal progressive improvement or decline of underlying condition.*
- Carry out medical regimen to treat underlying causes of mental status deterioration. *Medical regimen aims to alleviate causes of mental status deterioration.*
- Address patient by name. Tell patient your name. *Reality orientation techniques foster patient's awareness of self and environment.*
- Give short, simple explanations to patient each time you do something *to avoid confusion and aid successful task completion.*
- Schedule nursing care to provide quiet times. *Rest periods help avoid sensory overload.*

• Mention time, place, and date frequently throughout the day. Have a clock and a calendar where patient can easily see them; refer to these aids when orienting patient. *Reality orientation techniques foster patient's awareness of self and environment.*
• Keep patient's things in the same places to the extent possible. *A consistent, stable environment reduces confusion and frustration, and aids successful completion of activities of daily living.*
• Use appropriate safety measures to protect patient from injury. Avoid physical restraints if possible. *Patient may be unable to consider own safety needs or risks. Restraints may agitate patient.*
• Ask family or significant other to bring photos (label with name and relationship on back), favorite articles, and cards. *Familiar items help create a more secure environment for patient.*
• Plan patient's routine and be as consistent as possible in following it. *A consistent daily plan aids task completion, and reduces confusion and frustration.*
• Speak slowly and clearly. Allow ample time for patient to respond. *This reduces confusion and frustration, and aids task completion.*
• Encourage patient to perform activities of daily living. Be patient and specific in providing instructions. Allow time for patient to perform each task. *This enhances patient's self-esteem and helps prevent complications of inactivity. New skills or tasks should be limited to small, critical units to aid learning. Patient may need extensive supervision and repetition to master new tasks.*
• Encourage family or significant other to share stories and discuss familiar things with patient. *Remote memory often remains intact. Sharing stories and familiar things promotes sense of continuity, aids memory, and creates a sense of security and comfort.*
• Support family or significant other in attempts to interact with patient. *Family or significant others need positive reinforcement for visiting and attempting to interact with patient.*
• Allow time before and after visits for spouse or significant other to express feelings. *Expression of feelings in a supportive environment is important in helping spouse or significant other cope with patient's illness.*
• Refer family or significant other to appropriate resources to plan for patient care after discharge. *This helps provide a comprehensive approach to postdischarge care.*

Evaluations for expected outcomes
• Patient remains free of injury.
• Patient maintains awareness of need for assistance.
• Neurologic assessment reveals that patient is oriented to person, place, and time.
• Patient performs activities of daily living with assistance.
• Patient's laboratory values remain within set limits.
• Physiologic causes of altered thought processes receive treatment.
• Family member or significant other identifies partial or complete confusion as indicator of patient's changing physiologic state.
• Family member or significant other contacts appropriate resource to arrange for home care.

Documentation
• Patient's verbal responses
• Observations of patient's behavior indicative of altered thought processes

• Interventions that focus on helping patient maintain reality orientation
• Responses of patient to nursing interventions
• Evaluations for each expected outcome.

Thought process alteration

related to psychological causes

Definition
Inability to process thoughts accurately and correctly because of a fixed, false belief that cannot be corrected by logic

Assessment
• Age
• Reason for hospitalization, including patient's perception of problem, recent stressors, changes in somatic functioning
• Mental status, including insight regarding present situation, judgment (ask patient to solve a simple problem), abstract thinking (ask patient to interpret a proverb), general information (ask patient to name five states), mood, affect, recent and remote memory, thought processes, thought content, orientation to person, place, and time
• Physical appearance, including manner of dress, personal hygiene, posture, gait
• Communication status, including attitude toward interviewer, body language, facial expressions
• Sleep habits
• Self-care status, including ability to perform activities of daily living, safety practices
• Physiologic status, including medication history (response, effectiveness, adverse reactions), history of substance abuse (type, effect on mental status)
• Dietary and nutritional status
• Laboratory studies, including toxicology screening, blood chemistry
• Diagnostic tests, including computed tomography scan, EEG

Defining characteristics
• Behavior based on delusional beliefs—for example, nonverbal cues that indicate suspiciousness or mistrust
• Behavioral manifestations of anxiety
• Delusions (erotomanic, grandiose, jealous, persecutory, somatic, unspecified)
• Disorientation to time, place, person, circumstances, and events
• Exaggeration
• Impaired ability to reason, abstract, or conceptualize
• Inability to distinguish delusion from reality
• Inappropriate interpretation of the environment
• Incorporation of mental health professionals, family, or other patients into delusional belief system
• Misinterpretation of words and actions of others
• Thoughts and beliefs not based in reality and not consensually validated

Associated medical diagnoses (selected)
Acute infection, affective disorders, atypical psychosis, brief reactive psychosis, drug toxicity, metabolic disorders, paranoid disorders, schizophrenia, substance abuse disorders

Expected outcomes
• Patient identifies internal and external factors that trigger delusional episodes.

• Patient identifies and performs activities that decrease delusions.
• Patient practices distraction techniques to reduce anxiety before the onset of delusion.
• Patient interacts with others without becoming delusional.
• Patient considers an alternative interpretation of situation without becoming unduly hostile or anxious.
• Patient recognizes how delusional system meets his interpersonal needs.
• Patient recognizes symptoms and complies with medication regimen.

Interventions and rationales

• Project a nonjudgmental and trusting attitude toward the patient through active listening. *The patient must trust you in order to talk openly about delusions and feelings.*
• Orient patient to reality as needed.
 – Call patient by name.
 – Tell patient your name.
 – Provide background information (place, time, date) frequently throughout the day, verbally and visually, using a reality orientation board.
 – Orient patient to environment, including sights, sounds, and smells.

Reality orientation techniques foster patient's awareness of self and environment.
• Explain to patient with organic delusions that distorted thinking is caused by temporary biochemical changes *to help decrease patient's anxiety level.*
• Do not argue, reason with, or challenge a patient with nonorganic delusions; instead, provide comfort and support. *Attempts to correct delusional beliefs will increase anxiety.*
• Explore events that trigger delusions. Discuss anxiety associated with triggering events. *Exploring these topics will help you understand the dynamics of the patient's delusional system.*
• Without arguing or agreeing, acknowledge the plausible elements of the delusion. Make such statements as, "I don't doubt that your family brought you to the hospital. However, I have no reason to believe that they are cooperating with the CIA to kill you." *Delusions usually have some basis in reality. By conveying acceptance of delusions but not belief in them, you can better help patient.*
• Once dynamics of delusions are understood, discourage repetitious talk about delusions and refocus conversation on patient's underlying feelings. *As patient begins to learn to cope with underlying feelings, delusions will become less necessary.*
• Help patient find other means to meet emotional needs that patient attempts to fulfill through delusions. *Delusions usually decrease when needs are met in other ways.*
• Educate patient and family or significant other about signs and symptoms of illness and the effects of medication. *Collaboration with family members promotes continuity of care.*
• Refer family or significant other to appropriate resources to plan for patient care after discharge. *This helps provide a comprehensive approach to postdischarge care.*

Evaluations for expected outcomes

• Patient describes at least two situations that increase delusions.
• Patient describes two self-initiated activities to decrease delusions.
• Patient gives two concrete examples of anxiety-reducing techniques.
• Patient interacts with primary nurse 30 minutes per day, 5 days per week, without delusional content.

• Patient discusses two reality-based interpretations of events that are consensually validated by others.
• Patient directly communicates both negative and positive feelings.
• Patient and family members discuss delusional symptoms and adverse effects of medication.

Documentation
• Patient's statements indicating type, number, and intensity of delusions
• Observations about environmental factors that precipitate delusional behavior
• Interventions that focus on helping patient maintain reality orientation
• Patient's response to nursing interventions
• Referrals
• Evaluations for each expected outcome.

Tissue integrity impairment
related to peripheral vascular changes

Definition
Damage to mucous membranes or to corneal, integumentary, or subcutaneous tissue

Assessment
• History of peripheral vascular disease or surgery
• Age
• Sex
• Integumentary status, including color, skin care practices, temperature, tenderness, texture, turgor, edema
• Cardiovascular status, including blood pressure, cardiac output, occupation, patient and family history of cardiovascular disease, peripheral pulses, smoking history
• Nutritional status, including dietary patterns, laboratory tests, serum lipids level, serum protein level, weight change from normal
• Neurologic status, including motor function, sensory pattern

Defining characteristics
• Arterial insufficiency, including bruits, coolness, cyanosis or mottling; decreased or absent peripheral pulses; delayed capillary filling; exertional limb pain relieved with rest; loss of hair on limbs; pallor on elevation of limbs; redness (rubor) on lowering of limbs; sensitivity to cold; thin, tight, shiny skin; thickened, brittle nails; ulceration on extremity
• Neurologic changes, including paresis, paresthesias
• Venous insufficiency, including atrophy of skin and soft tissue; coldness and pallor of extremities; edema of lower extremities; gangrenous changes; leg pain during menstruation; nocturnal cramping; swollen, ropelike, or ruptured superficial leg veins

Associated medical diagnoses (selected)
Buerger's disease (thromboangiitis obliterans), chronic or acute arterial insufficiency, pregnancy, Raynaud's phenomenon, venous insufficiency or venous stasis

Expected outcomes
• Patient attains relief from immediate symptoms (pain, ulcers, color changes, edema).
• Patient maintains collateral circulation.
• Patient voices intent to stop smoking.
• Patient voices intent to follow specific management routines after discharge.

Interventions and rationales

- Provide scrupulous foot care. Administer and monitor treatments according to institutional protocols. *Foot care prevents fungal infections and ingrown toenails, stimulates circulation, and promotes awareness of signs and symptoms that should be reported to doctor immediately.*
- Instruct patient to avoid pressure on popliteal space. For example, say "Do not cross your legs or wear constrictive clothing." *This avoids reducing arterial blood supply and increasing venous congestion.*
- Encourage adherence to exercise regimen as tolerated. *Exercise improves arterial circulation and venous return by promoting muscle contraction-relaxation.*
- Educate patient about risk factors and prevention of injury. Refer patient to smoking cessation program. *Teaching about factors influencing peripheral vascular disease and prevention of tissue damage helps prevent complications.*
- Maintain adequate hydration. Monitor intake and output; record daily weights. *Adequate hydration reduces blood viscosity and decreases risk of clot formation.*
- With venous insufficiency, apply antiembolism stockings or intermittent pneumatic compression stockings, removing them for 1 hour every 8 hours or according to institutional protocol. Elevate patient's feet when sitting and elevate foot of bed 6 inches to 8 inches when lying down. *These measures promote venous return and decrease venous congestion in lower extremities.*
- With arterial insufficiency, elevate head of bed 6 inches to 8 inches when lying down. *This increases arterial blood supply to extremities.*

Evaluations for expected outcomes

- Patient attains relief from immediate symptoms:
  - Patient's feet do not show signs of infection, ingrown toenails, or impaired circulation.
  - Patient maintains normal skin turgor.
  - Patient's mucous membranes remain moist.
  - Patient maintains balanced intake and output.
  - Patient's weight remains stable.
  - Patient's vital signs remain within normal parameters.
- Patient uses interventions (antiembolism stockings or intermittent pneumatic compression stockings, elevation of feet, elevation of head of bed) to facilitate arterial and venous circulation.
- Patient follows prescribed exercise program.
- Patient states intent to avoid activities that contribute to vascular compression (such as popliteal compression, leg crossing, and wearing constrictive clothing).
- Patient states rationale for quitting smoking and begins program to stop smoking.
- Patient communicates understanding of exercise program, foot care, and avoiding risk factors and plans to incorporate these measures into postdischarge routine.

Documentation

- Patient's expressions of feelings about current situation
- Observations of skin color, turgor, temperature, ulcer size
- Patient's response to nursing interventions
- Evaluations for each expected outcome.

■ Tissue integrity impairment

related to physical, chemical, or electrical hazards during surgery

Definition

Damage to mucous membranes or to corneal, integumentary, or subcutaneous tissue

Assessment

- Reason for surgery
- Type of surgery
- Anticipated length of surgery
- Health status, including age, sex, weight, vital signs, temperature, nutritional status, integumentary status, cardiovascular status, neurologic status, respiratory status, psychosocial status
- Mobility status, including range of motion
- Patient's description of pain, numbness, tingling
- Laboratory studies, including hematocrit and hemoglobin, complete blood count, blood coagulation studies, immunologic and serologic tests, electrolytes, urinalysis, liver function tests, serum protein levels
- Wound classification (clean, clean-contaminated, contaminated, dirty)
- Allergies to medications, irrigation solutions, cleansing solutions
- Health history, including altered immunologic status, malnutrition, chronic metabolic or systemic disease (diabetes mellitus; cancer; cardiovascular, renal, or hepatic diseases; coagulation disorders; blood dyscrasias; or hematopoietic diseases)
- Current medical treatments, including radiation therapy, chemotherapy, steroid therapy, immunosuppressive therapy, anticoagulant or thrombolytic therapy, antibiotic therapy
- Presence of infection, draining wounds, bruises, shear ulcers, pressure ulcers

Defining characteristics

- Blisters or blebs
- Discoloration
- Disrupted tissue
- Edema
- Erythema
- Eschar
- Exudate
- Itching
- Odor
- Pain

Associated medical diagnoses (selected)

Acquired immunodeficiency syndrome; alcoholism; anemia; cancer; cardiovascular disease; dermatitis; diabetes mellitus; infection; leukemia; liver cirrhosis; neurologic disorders affecting sensory-motor function; obesity; respiratory disease; skin lesions

Expected outcomes

- Patient expresses feelings of comfort.
- Patient remains free from alteration in tissue integrity related to physical hazards.
- Patient remains free from alteration in tissue integrity related to chemical hazards.
- Patient remains free from alteration in tissue integrity related to electrical hazards.

Interventions and rationales

- Document and report results of preoperative nursing assessment. Identify factors that predispose patient to impaired tissue integrity. *A complete nursing assessment allows for devel-*

opment of an individualized care plan.

• Classify the surgical wound according to the degree of contamination of wound and surrounding tissue. *Classifying the surgical wound facilitates assessment of risk of wound infection and subsequent tissue injury.*

• Use padding, special mattresses, and support devices during surgery. *These measures reduce undue pressure and decrease risk of impaired tissue integrity.*

• Maintain environmental temperature at a comfortable setting. Offer blankets, if needed. *A comfortable environment reduces shivering, muscle tension, and reactive pain. These metabolic stressors can affect the rate of cellular repair.*

• Monitor patient for signs of hypothermia (shivering, cool skin, pallor, piloerection, increased heart rate) *to determine the need to implement warming measures.*

• Warm prepping and irrigation solutions *to prevent reduction in patient's temperature.*

• For infants (1 year old or less), use warming unit and head covering. *Infant thermoregulatory mechanisms are immature and do not retain adequate body heat.*

• When using pneumatic tourniquets, pad skin, place cuff so skin is free of wrinkles, set to proper pressure, and monitor inflation time. *Improper tourniquet use can impair circulatory status of affected limb.*

• Check patient history for sensitivity or allergy to prepping solution. Clean and prepare skin incision site with nonirritating solutions. *Nonallergenic, physiologic prepping and cleansing solutions reduce risk of tissue reaction and injury.*

• To avoid pooling of solutions, use towels or pads during prep. When using sprays, shield patient's face and eyes. *Pooled solutions can produce skin maceration. Sprays may damage cornea and mucous membranes.*

• Ensure adequate aeration of items sterilized by ethylene oxide gas. *Residual gas is toxic to tissue.*

• Rinse chemosterilized items adequately. *Residual chemosterilization solutions are toxic to tissue.*

• Remove powder from gloves. *Glove powder may cause granulomas and other reactions.*

• Perform sponge, sharp, and instrument counts according to protocol; account for other items (bulldogs, umbilical tapes, vessel loops); and document results. *Retained objects may produce foreign body reaction or injury to tissue.*

• Follow manufacturer's instructions for applying medications and chemical agents such as glutaraldehyde and methylmethacrylate. *Agents may be toxic when applied directly to tissue.*

• Use physiologic solutions or prescribed medications for irrigation or topical application. *Nonphysiologic solutions may cause interstitial edema and cellular injury or death.*

• Check label, route, dose, and expiration date of each medication with scrub nurse *to reduce risk of error.*

• When administering medications, record drug, dosage, and route. Document verbal orders and have physician cosign. *Documentation helps to reduce medication errors.*

• Inspect all electrical, mechanical, and air-powered equipment before use. Operate equipment according to manufacturers' instruction *to reduce chances of patient injury.*

• Apply electrosurgical dispersive pad to clean, dry skin near operative site. Avoid bony prominences, hairy surfaces, scar tissue, or areas of poor

circulation. *Proper placement reduces risk of burn injury.*
• When using hypothermia or hyperthermia blanket avoid creases, place sheet between skin and blanket, set and maintain correct temperature. Pad extremities during hypothermia therapy. *Proper use protects against tissue injury.*

Evaluations for expected outcomes
• Shivering, muscle tension, and reactive pain are minimal or absent.
• Patient does not develop rash, edema, bruises, discoloration, redness, skin breakdown, or other signs of altered tissue integrity related to physical hazards.
• Patient does not develop allergic or toxic reaction to sterilizing agents, glove powder, irrigating solutions, medications, or chemical agents. Reaction to cleansing procedure is minimal or absent.
• Patient does not develop reddened or discolored areas at site of electrosurgical grounding pad or adjacent tissue. Other signs of postoperative alteration in tissue integrity related to electrical hazards do not occur.

Documentation
• Results of preoperative nursing assessment
• Surgical procedure
• Type of anesthesia
• Preoperative and postoperative diagnosis
• Wound classification
• Preexisting conditions that increase risk of tissue injury
• Nursing interventions performed to protect tissue integrity
• Medications administered
• Patient's status on discharge to post anesthesia care unit
• Skin condition on discharge to post anesthesia care unit
• Presence of lines, tubes, catheters, and drains
• Type of wound closure and dressing
• Evaluations for each expected outcome.

Tissue integrity impairment

related to radiation

Definition
Damage to mucous membranes or to corneal, integumentary, or subcutaneous tissue

Assessment
• History of radiation therapy or exposure
• Age
• Sex
• Integumentary status, including color, distribution of hair, mucous membranes, skin care practices, temperature, tenderness, texture, turgor, scars, lesions, wounds
• Nutritional status, including dietary patterns, weight change from normal

Defining characteristics
• Skin: blistered, dry, edemic, hairless, itchy (pruritus), moist, reddened, scaly, ulcerated, warm

Associated medical diagnoses (selected)
Radiation exposure occurring during cancer or keloid reduction therapy or accidental radiation exposure

Expected outcomes
• Irritation and breakdown of irradiated areas avoided.
• Ulcerated areas healed.
• Patient maintains adequate fluid and nutritional intake.
• Patient and family or significant other communicate understanding of

skin care regimen, medication use, and need for adequate fluid and nutritional intake.

Interventions and rationales

- Keep skin clean, dry, and exposed to air as much as possible *to promote healing of excoriated areas and prevent infection.*
- Avoid constrictive clothing *to reduce risk of friction and decreased blood flow.* Avoid exposure to sun *to reduce risk of sunburn and possible skin cancer.*
- Avoid nonprescribed ointments, creams, and warm packs *because they may increase skin irritation and possible radiation (if they contain heavy metals).*
- Avoid extremes of hot and cold on affected skin areas *to prevent further irritation and skin breakdown.*
- Avoid vigorous scrubbing of irradiated areas *to minimize skin breakdown.*
- Use nonadhesive dressings *to avoid pulling on affected skin.*
- Provide oral hygiene as indicated *to promote comfort and reduce risk of infection.* Use soft toothbrush *to reduce risk of bleeding.*
- Use cornstarch over unbroken areas *to decrease itching and friction.*
- Provide regular change of position, bed cradle, or pressure-relieving devices, when indicated. *These measures reduce friction and risk of skin breakdown on affected body parts.*
- Inspect skin every shift. Report areas of breakdown and signs of infection *to ensure early treatment.*
- Follow institutional protocol for treating infected lesions. Administer creams, antibiotic ointments, and irrigation solutions, as ordered, and monitor effectiveness. *Protocols are established to meet specific patient needs.*
- Administer analgesics as ordered, and monitor effectiveness. *Analgesics reduce pain resulting from skin problems.*
- Consult dietitian to assist with diet, emphasizing high protein, calories, vitamins, and minerals to promote tissue repair and prevent catabolism. *Positive nitrogen balance promotes wound healing.*
- Administer antiemetics as ordered *to promote patient comfort and adequate nutrition.* Monitor effectiveness.
- Educate family and patient in skin care regimen, medication administration, and nutritional needs *to promote compliance and maintain tissue integrity.*

Evaluations for expected outcomes

- Irradiated areas do not show signs of cracking, oozing, sloughing, or infection.
- Patient's ulcerated areas heal.
- Patient maintains adequate fluid and nutritional intake.
- Patient and caregiver demonstrate proper skin care and medication administration techniques.
- Patient and caregiver communicate understanding of importance of maintaining nutritional intake.

Documentation

- Patient's expression of feelings
- Physical findings
- Interventions performed to prevent irritation or breakdown or to promote healing
- Patient's response to nursing interventions
- Patient's and family's or significant other's response to education
- Evaluations for each expected outcome.

Tissue perfusion alteration (cardiopulmonary)

related to decreased cellular exchange

Definition

Decrease in cellular nutrition and respiration because of decreased capillary blood flow

Assessment

- Health history, including presence of diabetes mellitus, high cholesterol, hypertension, obesity, smoking, stressful life-style, family history of heart disease
- Neurologic status, including level of consciousness, mental status, orientation
- Cardiovascular status, including blood pressure; heart rate and rhythm; heart sounds; peripheral pulses; skin color, temperature, and turgor; hepatojugular reflux; jugular vein distention; history of congenital heart disease or valvular disorder
- Diagnostic tests, including chest X-ray, ECG, exercise ECG, echocardiogram, nuclear isotope studies, cardiac angiography
- Respiratory status, including arterial blood gas (ABG) levels, auscultation of breath sounds, respiratory rate and depth
- Renal status, including intake and output, urine specific gravity, weight
- Integumentary system, including cyanosis, pallor, peripheral edema

Defining characteristics

- Abnormal ABG levels
- Arrhythmias; ECG changes
- Chest pain with or without activity
- Cold, clammy skin
- Crackles
- Cyanosis
- Decreased or absent urine output
- Decreased peripheral pulses
- Elevated cardiac enzymes and isoenzymes
- Fatigue
- Hypotension
- Mental status changes
- Pallor of skin and mucous membranes
- Palpitations
- Peripheral edema
- Rhonchi
- Shortness of breath
- Slow capillary refill time
- Tachycardia
- Variations in hemodynamic readings

Associated medical diagnoses (selected)

Adult respiratory distress syndrome, anaphylactic shock, anemia, aortic stenosis or insufficiency, arteriosclerotic heart disease, cardiac tamponade, cardiogenic shock, chronic obstructive pulmonary disease, congestive heart failure, coronary artery spasm, hypovolemic shock, lung abscess, mitral stenosis or insufficiency, neurogenic shock, pericarditis, pneumonia, pulmonary artery infarct, pulmonary emboli, respiratory failure, septic shock

Expected outcomes

- Patient attains hemodynamic stability. Pulse not less than _____ beats/minute and not greater than _____ beats/minute. Blood pressure not less than _____ mm Hg and not greater than _____ mm Hg.
- Patient does not exhibit arrhythmias.
- Skin remains warm and dry.
- Patient's heart rate remains within prescribed limits while he carries out activities of daily living.
- Patient maintains adequate cardiac output.

• Patient modifies life-style to minimize risk of decreased tissue perfusion.

Interventions and rationales

• Monitor and document vital signs (heart rate, blood pressure, and central venous pressure) every 1 hour until stable, then every 2 hours. Report any findings outside prescribed limits *Decreased heart rate, central venous pressure, and blood pressure may indicate increased arteriovenous exchange, which leads to decreased tissue perfusion.*
• Monitor skin color and temperature every 2 hours. Assess for signs of skin breakdown. *Cool, blanched, mottled skin and cyanosis may indicate decreased tissue perfusion.*
• Monitor respiratory rate and breath sounds. Document findings. *Increased respiratory rate may indicate that the patient is compensating for tissue hypoxia.*
• Monitor ECG for changes in heart rate and rhythm. *Altered heart rate and rhythm may affect tissue perfusion and possibly indicate a life-threatening crisis.*
• Maintain oxygen therapy, as ordered, *to maximize oxygen exchange in alveoli and at cellular level.*
• Encourage patient to change position and participate in activity, as condition permits, *to enhance vital capacity and avoid lung congestion and skin breakdown.*
• Encourage frequent rest periods *to conserve energy and maximize tissue perfusion.*
• Monitor creatine phosphokinase, lactic dehydrogenase, and ABG levels. *Abnormal findings may indicate tissue damage or decreased oxygen exchange in lungs.*
• Inform patient about:
  – risk factors for heart and lung disease
  – proper use of nitroglycerin
  – proper use of medications and possible adverse reactions
  – the benefits of a low-fat, low-cholesterol diet
  – the need to avoid straining with bowel movements
  – the benefits of quitting smoking.

Effective teaching encourages patient to take an active role in health maintenance.

Evaluations for expected outcomes

• Patient attains hemodynamic stability.
• Patient shows no signs of arrhythmias.
• Skin remains warm, dry, and intact.
• Patient's heart rate remains within prescribed parameters while he carries out activities of daily living.
• Patient maintains adequate cardiac output.
• Patient describes plans to modify life-style to minimize cause of decreased tissue perfusion.

Documentation

• Observations of physical findings
• Observation of patient's response to activity
• Verbal statements and behavior indicating patient's perception of health problems and health needs
• Nursing interventions performed and patient response
• Patient demonstration of skills associated with maintaining diet, adhering to medication regimen, maintaining activity level, and managing stress
• Evaluations for each expected outcome.

Tissue perfusion alteration (cerebral)

related to decreased cellular exchange

Definition

Decrease in cellular nutrition and respiration because of decreased capillary blood flow

Assessment

- Vital signs
- History of the event including the presenting problem, history of development, chief complaint, associated vascular problems, associated psychosocial problems (which may contribute to behavioral changes)
- Neurologic status, including level of consciousness; Glasgow Coma Scale score (eye response, motor response, verbal response); orientation; pupil size; response to light and accommodation; motor activity; strength, positioning, and appearance of all four extremities; presence of reflexes (corneal, gag, swallowing, Babinski's); nuchal rigidity; weakness; numbness; headaches; dizziness; dysphagia; slurred speech; seizure activity; posturing; Cushing's triad (increased systolic pressure, decreased diastolic pressure, decreased heart rate)
- Respiratory status, including shallow or irregular breathing pattern

Defining characteristics

- Behavioral changes
- Change in level of consciousness
- Change in respiratory pattern
- Dizziness
- Dysphagia
- Eye deviation
- Headaches
- Impaired gag reflex
- Irritability
- Lethargy
- Memory loss
- Nausea and vomiting
- Orthostatic hypotension
- Photophobia
- Posturing
- Pupillary changes
- Restlessness
- Seizures
- Slurred speech
- Tinnitus
- Unilateral weakness or paralysis
- Visual changes

Associated medical diagnoses (selected)

Acute head injury, cerebral edema, acute meningitis, arteriovenous malformation, cerebral aneurysm, cerebral vasospasm, cerebrovascular accident, epidural hemorrhage, subtentorial herniation, subarachnoid hemorrhage, subdural hemorrhage, supratentorial herniation, supratentorial shift, transient ischemic attack, tumors, ventricular bleed

Expected outcomes

- Patient maintains or improves current level of consciousness.
- Intracranial pressure remains between _____ mm Hg and _____ mm Hg.
- Blood pressure remains high enough to maintain cerebral perfusion pressure but low enough to prevent increased bleeding or cerebral swelling.
- Hypercarbia is prevented.
- Patient is free from pain.
- Patient stays in a quiet environment.
- Patient maintains balanced intake and output
- Patient performs activities of daily living with maximum level of mobility and independence.

- Risk factors for altered cerebral perfusion and complications are reduced as much as possible.

Interventions and rationales

- Conduct a neurologic assessment every 1 to 2 hours initially, then every 4 hours once the patient becomes stable, *to screen for changes in level of consciousness and neurologic status.*
- Take vital signs every 1 to 2 hours initially, then every 4 hours once the patient becomes stable, *to detect early signs of decreased cerebral perfusion pressure or increased intracranial pressure.*
- Take patient's temperature at least every 4 hours. *Hyperthermia causes increased intracranial pressure; hypothermia causes decreased cerebral perfusion pressure.*
- Elevate head of patient's bed 30 degrees *to prevent rise in intercerebral pressure and to facilitate venous drainage, thereby reducing cerebral edema.*
- Keep head in neutral alignment *to keep carotid flow unobstructed, thereby facilitating perfusion.*
- If patient's score on the Glasgow Coma Scale is less than 10, hyperventilate patient on a ventilator in accordance with hospital policy *to increase oxygenation and prevent cerebral swelling and hypercarbia.*
- Monitor for Cushing's triad, *which is a sign of impending herniation.*
- Keep environment and patient quiet. Sedate patient if necessary. Space nursing actions. *These measures reduce increased intracranial pressure.*
- If the patient has a potentially compromised airway, use antiemetics or nasogastric suction *to prevent nausea and vomiting, which may lead to increased intracranial pressure and aspiration.*
- Institute physical and occupational rehabilitation *to increase patient's ability for independent functioning.*
- Prepare patient's discharge plan *to make sure the patient continues to receive necessary rehabilitative care after discharge.*
- Maintain adequate nutrition *to facilitate tissue healing, oxygenation, and metabolism.*
- Maintain routine bowel and bladder function and administer diuretics such as mannitol, as ordered, *to prevent increased intracranial pressure.*
- Monitor hematocrit and hemoglobin and report abnormalities *to prevent ischemia.*
- Take measures to ward off infection *to prevent increased metabolic and oxygen demands that can interfere with the brain's metabolic needs.*
- Measure accurate intake and output *to prevent volume overload or deficit.*
- Instruct patient and family members in ways to minimize risk factors for altered tissue perfusion *to increase probability that healthy adaptation will continue.*
- Administer histamine$_2$-receptor antagonists, as ordered, *to prevent the development of stress ulcers.*

Evaluations for expected outcomes

- Patient regains sense of orientation.
- Intracranial pressure remains within prescribed limits.
- Blood pressure remains high enough to maintain cerebral perfusion pressure but low enough to prevent increased bleeding or cerebral swelling.
- Hypercarbia is prevented.
- Patient stays free from pain.
- Patient intake and output is balanced.

• Patient's environment remains quiet.
• Patient performs activities of daily living with maximum level of mobility and independence.
• Risk factors are reduced as much as possible.

Documentation
• Observations of vital signs and neurologic findings
• Intake and output
• Patient's response to treatment of underlying condition
• Medications administered and patient response
• Nursing interventions performed and patient response
• Family response to education and nursing interventions
• Patient's response to physical and occupational therapy
• Evaluation of plan of care
• Evaluations for each expected outcome.

Tissue perfusion alteration (gastrointestinal)

related to decreased cellular exchange

Definition
Decrease in cellular nutrition and respiration caused by decreased capillary blood flow

Assessment
• Vital signs
• GI status, including abdominal distention; nausea and vomiting; usual bowel habits; change in bowel habits; stool characteristics (color, consistency); presence or absence of occult blood; history of GI problems, disease, or surgery; pain; inspection of abdomen; palpation for tenderness; auscultation of bowel sounds; abdominal girth
• Nutritional status, including dietary intake, change from normal diet, current weight, change from normal weight
• Laboratory studies, including complete blood count, serum electrolytes, liver profile
• Medications (especially those with vasoconstrictive properties)

Defining characteristics
• Absence of bowel sounds or change in their sound or frequency
• Abdominal pain associated with recently eaten meals
• Ascites or fluid wave
• Constipation
• Decrease in hematocrit and hemoglobin levels
• Diarrhea
• History of recent abdominal surgery or blunt abdominal trauma
• Increase in white blood count or sedimentation rate
• Nausea
• Presence of occult blood
• Recent weight loss or gain
• Vomiting

Associated medical diagnoses (selected)
Crohn's disease, duodenal ulcers, esophageal varices, GI cancer, GI hemorrhage, hepatic failure, hypovolemic liver failure, pancreatitis, paralytic ileus, small-bowel obstruction, ulcerative colitis

Expected outcomes
• Intake and output remain within normal limits.
• Normal bowel function returns.
• Nausea and vomiting are eliminated.
• Patient and significant other express understanding of need to modify dietary habits.

- Patient discusses with doctor possible need to alter medication regimen.
- Patient expresses understanding of benefits of regular exercise in maintaining routine bowel habits.
- Abdominal pain subsides.
- Laboratory values return to normal.
- Vital signs remain stable.
- Patient expresses understanding of need to check stools for occult blood.

Interventions and rationales

- Monitor intake and output every 4 hours *to prevent hypovolemia, which may cause poor perfusion and subsequent ischemia.*
- Monitor patient's vital signs with temperature every 4 hours *to detect possible hypovolemia and screen for infection.*
- Monitor for increased abdominal tenderness *to detect early signs of increased ischemia.*
- Monitor bowel sounds and report changes. *Changes in bowel sounds may signal impending obstruction or a return to normal bowel function.*
- Monitor complete blood count, serum electrolytes, and liver functions daily, as ordered, *to detect ischemia caused by low hematocrit and hemoglobin, monitor for improvement in organ function, and screen for infection.*
- Administer prescribed pain medications sparingly. *Many narcotics decrease gastric motility.* Use pain distraction techniques if possible *to provide relief with nonpharmacologic methods.*
- Implement nasogastric suction *to eliminate nausea and vomiting, thereby reducing the risk of inflammation.*
- Establish bowel regimen *to prevent constipation.*
- When appropriate, provide alternative methods of nutrition, such as total parenteral nutrition, *to allow bowel rest and recovery and to prevent ischemic episodes after meals.*
- Start enteral feedings slowly and increase them gradually *to allow recovering bowel to adapt to increased tissue demands.*
- Teach patient and significant other about dietary habits that may have contributed to poor perfusion *to prevent future episodes of altered GI tissue perfusion.*
- Encourage patient to eat small, frequent meals to increase fluid intake and to eat more high fiber foods (such as cruciferous vegetables and whole grains) *to prevent constipation and potential obstruction.*
- Teach patient the importance of routine exercise. *Routine excercise stimulates peristalsis.*
- Instruct patient to limit alcohol and fat intake *to preserve adequate liver function.*
- Teach patient to check all stools for occult blood *to monitor for blood loss, which may indicate anemia.*
- Encourage patient to discuss with doctor the need to avoid medications with vasoconstrictive properties or which decrease peristalsis. *Such medications may contribute to decreased perfusion.*
- Teach patient to rest after meals *to allow adequate blood circulation, thereby assuring oxygen supply for increased metabolic demands.*

Evaluations for expected outcomes

- Intake and output stay within normal limits.
- Normal bowel function returns.
- Nausea and vomiting cease.
- Patient and family recognize need to modify dietary habits and medication administration.

• Patient recognizes benefits of regular exercise in maintaining routine bowel habits.
• Abdominal pain subsides.
• Laboratory values return to normal.
• Vital signs remain stable.
• Patient recognizes need to check stools for occult blood.

Documentation
• Observations of physical findings
• Results of laboratory studies
• Intake and output
• Nursing interventions to treat altered tissue perfusion
• Patient's and significant other's response to teaching
• Effectiveness of nursing interventions
• Stool characteristics, including color, consistency, and presence of occult blood
• Evaluations for each expected outcome.

■ Tissue perfusion alteration (peripheral)

related to reduced arterial blood flow

Definition
Decrease in cellular nutrition and respiration because of decreased capillary blood flow

Assessment
• History of vascular problems and disease (self or family)
• Age
• Sex
• Integumentary status, including color, condition of nails, distribution of hair, lesions, temperature, texture, edema
• Cardiovascular status, including blood pressure, capillary refill, clotting profile, Doppler studies, exercise test, heart rate and rhythm, pulses (brachial, femoral, pedal, peripheral, popliteal space, posterior tibial, radial), serum cholesterol level, triglyceride levels, venogram or arteriogram
• Neurovascular status, including activity tolerance, mobility, sensation
• Nutritional status, including dietary patterns, weight
• Psychosocial status, including alcohol intake, family support, history of smoking, occupation, stressors

Defining characteristics
• Anxiety
• Atrial arrhythmias
• Bruit(s)
• Clinical evidence of interruption or reduction in arterial blood flow
• Decreased mobility of joints
• Diminished or absent peripheral pulses
• Diminished sensitivity to pressure, temperature, tissue trauma
• Edema of extremities
• Intermittent claudication
• Irritability
• Muscle wasting or weakness
• Numbness, tingling
• Obesity
• Skin: blanched when extremity raised above level of heart, cool to touch, cyanotic with severe disease, gangrenous, glossy, hairless, pale, pruritic, slow-healing, trophic changes of skin and nails, ulcerated

Associated medical diagnoses (selected)
Acute: aortic aneurysm, atrial fibrillation, bacterial endocarditis, congestive heart failure, myocardial infarction
Chronic: Buerger's disease, diabetes mellitus, Leriche's syndrome, Raynaud's disease, Raynaud's phenomenon, rheumatoid arthritis, subclavian

steal syndrome, systemic lupus erythematosus

Expected outcomes

- Patient expresses feeling of comfort or absence of pain at rest.
- Arrhythmias are avoided.
- Peripheral pulses are present and strong.
- Skin color and temperature remain unchanged.
- Feet remain clean and free of pressure areas.
- Patient performs Buerger-Allen exercises.
- Patient loses ____ lb/week.
- Prothrombin time is 35 to 60 seconds.
- Patient practices relaxation techniques at least once every 8 hours.
- Ulcerated areas heal.
- Patient demonstrates ability to perform skills needed to follow prescribed care regimen.
- Patient identifies risk factors that exacerbate the problem.
- Patient maintains tissue perfusion and cellular oxygenation.
- Patient reduces metabolic needs.

Interventions and rationales

- Elevate head of bed 30 degrees or place head of bed on 6″ to 8″ blocks *to promote circulation to lower extremities.*
- Change patient's position every 2 hours *to reduce risk of skin breakdown.*
- Administer analgesics and monitor effectiveness *to help reduce ischemic pain. Recording effectiveness guides further analgesic administration.*
- Monitor vital signs and heart rhythm every 4 hours. Report development of rapid, irregular pulse. *Rapid, irregular pulse can cause decreased cardiac output, which results in decreased tissue perfusion.*
- Check peripheral pulses every 4 hours. Document presence or absence and intensity of each. Use an ultrasonic blood flow detector if one is available. *Palpable, strong peripheral pulses indicate good arterial flow. Documentation reveals changes from one assessment to the next.*
- Assess skin color, temperature, and texture at least every 4 hours. Note, record, and report development of mottling or black-and-blue areas. *Decreased tissue perfusion causes mottling; skin also becomes cooler and skin texture changes.*
- Do not apply direct heat to extremities. Heat may be applied to the abdomen; this causes reflex dilation of arteries of lower extremities. *Directly heating extremities causes increased tissue metabolism; if arteries do not dilate normally, tissue perfusion decreases and ischemia may occur.*
- Use light cotton blankets to cover legs. *These provide insulation from cold but do not exert pressure on extremities.*
- Use a bed cradle when patient has ulcerations or gangrene. *This helps prevent heavy sheets and blankets from resting on affected extremities.*
- Provide meticulous foot care daily: soak patient's feet in warm water; trim nails carefully; rub feet with lanolin-based lotion; dry feet thoroughly; apply heel protectors; instruct patient to wear white cotton socks. *These measures prevent cracking of dry skin and other complications.*
- Teach patient to perform Buerger-Allen exercises twice a day. Raise the affected extremity above heart level; hold for 2 minutes. Lower the extremity to a dependent position, and hold for 3 minutes. Repeat. *These exercises aid collateral circulation to the legs.*

• Encourage ambulation to level of tolerance *to encourage circulation to the extremities.*
• Provide a diet low in saturated fat *to reduce risk of atherosclerosis, which further decreases circulation and tissue perfusion.*
• Reduce patient's caloric intake to promote weight reduction. *Extra weight can stress the heart and decrease circulation.*
• Help patient set goals for weight reduction. *This gives patient sense of control and provides motivation.*
• Consult dietitian *to help patient modify eating patterns and habits.*
• Administer anticoagulants, as ordered, to prevent thrombi. *Thrombi and emboli can further reduce arterial circulation and decrease tissue perfusion.*
• Monitor clotting data *to guide administration of anticoagulants.*
• Administer vasodilators, alpha-blocking agents, and other medications, as ordered. Monitor effectiveness and document patient response. *These agents aid vessel dilation, which promotes increased circulation. They work only if vessels are capable of dilating.*
• Teach relaxation techniques *to help improve vasodilation and help prevent vasoconstriction caused by anxiety.*
• For patients with leg ulcers, follow the prescribed regimen. *Collaborative practice enhances overall patient care.*
• Educate patient about:
  – foot care
  – importance of exercise
  – need for low-cholesterol, low-caloric diet
  – need to avoid tight clothes, crossing of legs, and keeping legs dependent
  – need to avoid vasoconstrictors (cold, stress, smoking)
  – precautionary measures to prevent injury.

These measures enable the patient and family or significant other to join actively in care, and allow patient to make more informed decisions about health status.

Evaluations for expected outcomes

• Patient indicates feeling of comfort, either verbally or through behavior.
• No arrhythmias are noted during monitoring or patient examination.
• Patient's radial, brachial, pedal, and popliteal pulses are present and palpable.
• Patient's skin color remains normal. Patient's skin remains warm and dry.
• Patient's feet remain clean and do not exhibit signs of redness or breakdown.
• Patient performs Buerger-Allen exercises.
• Patient's weight decreases by established amount weekly.
• Patient's prothrombin time remains between 35 and 60 seconds.
• Patient practices relaxation techniques at least once every 8 hours.
• Patient's ulcerated areas heal and do not require dressings.
• Patient demonstrates skills needed to follow self-care regimen.
• Patient states risk factors that may exacerbate problem.

Documentation

• Patient's expressions of symptoms, such as pain, numbness, muscle weakness
• Observations of physical findings
• Nursing interventions performed for patient
• Patient's response to nursing interventions
• Patient's response to education
• Evaluations for each expected outcome.

Tissue perfusion alteration (renal)

related to decreased cellular exchange

Definition

Decrease in cellular nutrition and respiration caused by decreased capillary blood flow

Assessment

- Health history, including surgery, any condition resulting in fluid volume depletion, or use of nephrotoxic drugs
- Renal status, including color of urine, intake and output, presence of anuria or oliguria, urine specific gravity, weight
- Cardiovascular status, including blood pressure, central venous pressure, hemodynamic readings, jugular filling, and presence of dependent edema, fluid retention, or palpitations
- Respiratory status, including auscultation of breath sounds, respiratory rate and rhythm, shortness of breath
- Neurologic status including level of consciousness, mental status, orientation, and evidence of decreased tolerance to activity, fatigue, weakness
- Integumentary status, including color, moisture, and presence of edema and secondary ulcerations from edema.
- Nutritional status, including thirst, signs of anorexia
- Laboratory studies, including blood urea nitrogen (BUN), creatinine, creatinine clearance, hemoglobin, serum electrolytes, urine osmolality

Defining characteristics

- Abnormal serum electolyte levels
- Dark, concentrated urine
- Decreased hemoglobin levels
- Decreased level of consciousness
- Decreased urine osmolality
- Decreased urine output
- Elevated BUN, creatinine and creatinine clearance levels
- Increased blood pressure
- Peripheral edema
- Shortness of breath
- Weakness
- Weight gain

Associated medical diagnoses (selected)

Acute: Acute renal failure, aortic aneurysm, disseminated intravascular coagulation, hemorrhage, myocardial infarction, renal calculi, shock, sickle cell crisis.
Chronic: Chronic renal failure, diabetes mellitus, nephrotoxic drug poisoning, polycystic kidney disease.

Expected outcomes

- Patient maintains fluid balance.
- Patient maintains urine specific gravity within normal limits (specify).
- Patient's weight does not fluctuate.
- Patient reports increased comfort.
- Patient maintains hemodynamic stability.
- Patient identifies risk factors that exacerbate decreased tissue perfusion and modifies his lifestyle appropriately.
- Patient communicates understanding of medical regimen, medications, diet, and activity restrictions.

Interventions and rationales

- Monitor and document intake and output every 1 hour until output is greater than 30 ml/hour, then every 2 to 4 hours. *In the absence of previous history of renal disease, urine output is a good indicator of tissue perfusion. Decreased or absent urine*

output usually indicates poor renal perfusion.
- Document urine color and characteristics. Report any changes. *Concentrated urine may indicate poor kidney function or dehydration.*
- Measure patient's weight at a specified time each day (before breakfast) and document results. *Weighing patient helps predict overall fluid status. Weight gain may indicate fluid overload. Weighing at regular times gives better indication of weight changes.*
- Assess for presence of dependent edema. *Dependent edema may indicate lack of kidney function.*
- Observe voiding patterns *to note deviations from normal.*
- Monitor urine specific gravity, serum electrolytes, BUN, and creatinine. *Rising levels may indicate decreased kidney function.*
- Monitor hemodynamic status and vital signs. Notify doctor of any changes. *An increase from baseline may indicate fluid overload caused by lack of kidney function.*
- Explain reasons for therapy and its intended effects to patient and family *to encourage patient to take an active role in health maintenance.*
- Allow for frequent rest periods *to enable patient to conserve energy.*
- Refer patient to dietitian for special diet for renal impairment *to help patient avoid foods that place increased demands on kidneys.*
- Instruct patient to check with doctor before taking over-the-counter (OTC) medications. *OTC medications may be nephrotoxic.*
- Provide patient and family with psychological support if renal failure becomes chronic *to encourage healthy adaptation.*

Evaluations for expected outcomes
- Patient maintains fluid balance.
- Patient maintains urine specific gravity within normal limits (specify).
- Patient's weight does not fluctuate.
- Patient reports achieving increased comfort level.
- Patient maintains hemodynamic stability.
- Patient recognizes risk factors that exacerbate the problem and changes his lifestyle appropriately.
- Patient communicates understanding of medical regimen, medications, diet, and activity restrictions.

Documentation
- Patient's expressions of concern over symptoms of decreased tissue perfusion
- Vital signs, intake and output, level of consciousness and other clinical findings
- Nursing interventions performed to maintain fluid balanace and hemodynamic stability
- Patient's response to nursing interventions
- Patient's response to education
- Evaluations for each expected outcome.

Tissue perfusion alteration (specify)

related to hypovolemia

Definition

Decrease in cellular nutrition and respiration because of decreased capillary blood flow

Assessment

- History of trauma, surgery, or condition resulting in fluid volume depletion
- Cardiovascular status, including blood pressure, capillary refill time, central venous pressure, ECG, heart rate and rhythm, heart sounds, hemoglobin and hematocrit, jugular filling, peripheral pulses, tilt test
- Respiratory status, including breath sounds, respiratory rate and rhythm
- Renal status, including intake and output, urine specific gravity, weight
- Neurologic status, including level of consciousness, mental status, orientation
- Integumentary status, including color, moisture, temperature

Defining characteristics

- Absent or diminished pulses
- Anxiety
- Clinical evidence of blood and fluid volume depletion
- Cool, clammy skin
- Decreased blood pressure
- Decreased cardiac output
- Decreased central venous pressure
- Decreased urine output
- Disorientation
- Increased pulse rate
- Increased systemic vascular resistance
- Persistent bleeding
- Respiratory distress
- Rhonchi, crackles

Associated medical diagnoses (selected)

Abruptio placentae; anemia; congestive heart failure; dehydration (loss of plasma volume); disseminated intravascular coagulation; GI bleeding; hemorrhage; hemothorax; hypovolemic shock; multisystem trauma; placenta previa; postoperative hypovolemia; pulmonary edema; renal failure; septic shock; spontaneous or therapeutic abortion; third-space fluid shifts in burns, bowel obstruction, and severe peritonitis; thrombosis

Expected outcomes

- Patient maintains hemodynamic stability: pulse greater than ____, less than ____; systolic blood pressure greater than ____; central venous pressure greater than ____; mean arterial pressure greater than ____ .
- Patient maintains fluid balance; intake equals output.
- Patient maintains urine specific gravity within normal parameters.
- Patient maintains respiratory rate within ±5 of baseline.
- Patient maintains skin integrity.
- Patient remains oriented to person, place, and time.
- Crackles and rhonchi are avoided.
- Hemoglobin, hematocrit, white blood cell count, and coagulation studies remain within normal parameters.
- Patient communicates understanding of medical regimen, diet, medications, and activity restrictions.

Interventions and rationales

- Monitor heart rate and rhythm, central venous pressure, and blood pressure every hour until stable, then every 2 hours; record and report any changes above or below figures noted in Expected outcomes. Monitor skin color and temperature every 2 hours. *Decreased heart rate, decreased central venous pressure, and decreased blood pressure can indicate hypovolemia, which leads to increased tissue perfusion. Cool and blanched or mottled skin are clinical signs of decreased tissue perfusion.*

• Monitor respiratory rate and depth every hour until stable, then every 2 to 4 hours. Record and report changes as noted under "Expected outcomes." *Increased respiratory rate is a compensatory mechanism in tissue hypoxia which may result from decreased tissue perfusion.*
• Measure and record urine output every hour until greater than 30 ml/hour, then every 2 to 4 hours. *Poor renal perfusion results in decreased or no urine output. Urine output is a good indicator of tissue perfusion in absence of previous history of renal disease.*
• Perform appropriate measures to treat underlying cause of hypovolemia. *Underlying cause must be treated to prevent continued or worsening hypovolemia.*
• Administer fluid or blood as ordered. Monitor for such adverse reactions as fluid overload or transfusion reactions. *Vigorous fluid or blood resuscitation can cause fluid overload, cardiac decompensation, or both. Transfusion reactions can occur during blood administration and may further compromise the patient's condition.*
• Initiate measures to help improve perfusion:
  – Keep warm, but do not overheat. *Warmth aids vasodilation, which improves tissue perfusion.*
  – Relieve anxiety and pain. *Anxiety and pain can cause a sympathetic reaction which results in vasoconstriction and decreased tissue perfusion.*
  – Elevate lower extremities *to increase arterial blood supply and improve tissue perfusion.*
• Perform pulmonary toilet as ordered; follow institutional policies. *Properly performed pulmonary toilet helps prevent pulmonary edema, respiratory complications, and possible respiratory failure.*
• Test urine specific gravity every shift; record and report abnormalities. *Concentrated urine with an increased specific gravity is an indicator of hypovolemia.*
• Weigh patient daily before breakfast; record weight. *Weighing patient daily helps predict total fluid status; weighing at regular times gives better indication of weight changes.*
• Provide regular change of position; follow turning schedule; inspect skin every shift; record and report any potential areas of breakdown. *These measures avoid decreased tissue perfusion and risk of skin breakdown.*
• Observe patient for confusion or disorientation. Reorient to reality frequently: call patient by name, tell patient your name, orient to surroundings (sounds, smells, sights). *Change in level of consciousness may result from decreased tissue perfusion. Reorientation helps patient recall person, place, and time and may also reduce fear and anxiety.*
• Monitor hemoglobin, hematocrit, white blood cell count, and coagulation studies. Frequency will depend on the severity of the patient's problem. *Monitoring helps establish blood replacement needs, fluid status, blood viscosity level, anticoagulation therapy parameters, and possible infection.*
• Educate patient in medical regimen (diet, medications, activity restrictions). *This allows patient to take an active role in health maintenance.*

Evaluations for expected outcomes

• Patient's hemodynamic measurements remain within established limits.
• Patient's daily fluid intake equals output.

- Patient's urine specific gravity remains within normal parameters.
- Patient maintains respiratory rate within established limits.
- Patient maintains normal skin color and does not exhibit redness or skin breakdown.
- Patient can identify self and state proper time of day, date, and location.
- Auscultation reveals clear lung fields.
- Patient exhibits improved circulation as evidenced by strong, palpable peripheral pulses; normal skin color and temperature; and normal blood pressure and other hemodynamic measurements.
- Patient's hemoglobin, hematocrit, white blood cell count, and coagulations studies remain within normal parameters.
- Patient communicates understanding of medical regimen, diet, medications, and activity restrictions.

Documentation

- Patient's expression of concern about hemodynamic status
- Observations of vital signs, intake and output, status of skin, and level of orientation
- Patient's response to nursing interventions
- Instructions about diet, monitoring, and medical regimen
- Evaluations for each expected outcome.

■ Tissue perfusion alteration (venous)

related to reduced peripheral blood flow

Definition

Decrease in cellular nutrition and respiration because of decreased capillary blood flow

Assessment

- History of vascular problems or disease (self or family)
- Age
- Sex
- Medication history
- Integumentary status, including color, condition of nails, distribution of hair, lesions, temperature, texture
- Cardiovascular status, including capillary refill time, clotting profile, Doppler studies, exercise test, heart rate and rhythm, pulses (brachial, femoral, pedal, peripheral, popliteal, posterior tibial, radial), serum cholesterol level, triglyceride levels, venogram or arteriogram
- Neurovascular status, including activity tolerance, mobility, sensation
- Nutritional status, including dietary patterns, weight
- Psychosocial status, including alcohol intake, family support, history of smoking, occupation, stressors

Defining characteristics

- Clinical evidence of interruption or reduction of venous blood flow
- Positive Homans' sign
- Prominence of superficial veins
- Skin: redness along course of vein, swelling around inflamed area, warm or hot to touch
- Tenderness and pain in affected extremity

Associated medical diagnoses (selected)
Abdominal tumors, chronic venous insufficiency, cirrhosis, hepatic failure, malignant ascites, oral contraceptive use, pregnancy, pulmonary embolus, sickle-cell crisis, thrombocytopenic purpura, thrombophlebitis (superficial or deep), varicose veins. Also any condition requiring prolonged bed rest, multiple venipunctures, or long-term I.V. therapy

Expected outcomes
- Embolization of thrombi avoided.
- Inflammation lessened and venous blood flow improved.
- Clotting studies remain within therapeutic range.
- Patient explains reasons for measures being used to prevent pooling of blood in lower extremities.
- Patient moves bowels without straining.
- Patient demonstrates ability to perform skills needed for prescribed care regimen.
- Patient identifies risk factors that exacerbate the problem.

Interventions and rationales
- Monitor and record temperature, pulse, respiration, and blood pressure at least every 4 hours. *Accurate monitoring of vital signs helps identify pulmonary embolus, which may increase respiratory rate, pulse rate, and blood pressure.*
- Auscultate and record breath sounds every 4 hours. *Decreased, absent, or adventitious breath sounds may result from pulmonary embolus.*
- Observe for development of pulmonary emboli. Report immediately any increase in temperature, pulse, or respiratory rate; decrease in blood pressure; anxious, apprehensive behavior; complaints of dyspnea, cough, hemoptysis; or the development of crackles or red, frothy sputum. *Embolization of thrombi from deep veins (legs and pelvis) frequently causes pulmonary embolus.*
- Monitor clotting profile, as ordered. *This guides anticoagulant therapy and indicates potential for clot formation.*
- Administer anticoagulant therapy, monitor effectiveness, and observe for bleeding (epistaxis, bleeding gums, petechiae). *This reduces further thrombosis by preventing clot propagation.*
- Measure and compare size of calves every 4 hours. *Venous pooling and stasis can cause fluid to move into interstitial space to cause edema.*
- Apply antiembolism stockings or intermittent pneumatic compression stockings, as ordered. Remove stockings for 1 hour every 8 hours or according to policy. *These may decrease venous stasis, but they can also cause edema from constriction. Monitor their use closely.*
- Apply moist heat to affected extremity, as ordered (may be contraindicated in chronic venous insufficiency.) *Moist heat may aid vasodilation, reduce vasospasm, and enhance venous return.*
- Elevate affected extremity. Avoid using pillows under knees. *Do not* use a knee gatch, and explain the reasons for not using it to the patient. *Elevation aids venous return; pillows or knee gatch hinder venous return because they elevate knees above the feet.*
- Instruct patient not to cross legs or lie in fetal position. Explain the importance of remembering not to cross legs. *Crossing legs constricts popliteal vessels, thus reducing venous return and promoting venous stasis.*
- Increase patient's activity, as ordered. *This helps prevent venous*

pooling and stasis and promotes venous return.

- Urge patient to elevate legs when sitting in a chair; be sure to support entire length of legs. *Elevating legs aids venous return. Supporting entire leg ensures blood flow.*
- Encourage patient to walk. Discourage prolonged standing in one place. *Walking promotes venous blood flow by causing muscles to compress veins. Standing promotes venous stasis.*
- Use stool softeners to avoid constipation and straining during bowel movement. *Valsalva's maneuver, used in straining during bowel movement, decreases venous blood return.*
- Educate patient regarding the following:
  - anticoagulant therapy and the importance of having blood work done as ordered; dietary precautions while on anticoagulant therapy (for example, minimizing green leafy vegetables if on oral agent); and the need to report bleeding gums and blood in urine, secretions, etc. *Leafy vegetables contain vitamin K, which inhibits anticoagulants such as coumadin.*
  - use of antiembolism stockings or intermittent pneumatic compression stockings
  - avoidance of crossing legs, wearing constrictive clothing, or standing in one place
  - importance of protecting extremities from injury.

Education allows patient and family or significant other to take active role in health maintenance.

Evaluations for expected outcomes

- Patient does not exhibit clinical signs of embolization, such as increased respiratory rate, pulse rate, and blood pressure; decreased, absent, or adventitious breath sounds; or signs and symptoms of pulmonary embolus.
- Patient's inflammation decreases and venous blood flow improves.
- Patient's prothrombin time and partial thromboplastin time remain within established limits.
- Patient explains rationales for measures used to prevent pooling of blood in lower extremities.
- Patient moves bowels without straining.
- Patient demonstrates ability to perform skills needed for prescribed care regimen.
- Patient lists risk factors that exacerbate reduced venous blood flow or demonstrates understanding of risk factors through behavior.

Documentation

- Patient's expression of feelings about hospitalization and current situation
- Observations of physical findings
- Clotting profile
- Administration of anticoagulant therapy, including side effects
- Nursing interventions performed to promote circulation to lower extremities
- Patient's response to nursing interventions
- Patient's response to education
- Evaluations for each expected outcome.

Trauma, high risk for

related to external factors (environmental, physical, chemical agents)

Definition
Accentuated risk of accidental tissue injury such as burns or fractures

Assessment
- Health history, including accidents, allergies, exposure to pollutants, falls, hyperthermia, hypothermia, poisoning, sensory or perceptual changes (auditory, gustatory, kinesthetic, olfactory, tactile, visual), seizures, trauma
- Circumstances of present situation that might lead to injury from surgery or from chemical, physical, or human agents
- Neurologic status, including level of consciousness, mental status, orientation
- Laboratory studies, including clotting factors, hemoglobin and hematocrit, platelet count, white blood cell count

Risk factors
- Bathtub lacking handgrip or antislip equipment
- High bed
- Inappropriate or broken call-for-aid mechanism for patient on bed rest
- Litter or liquid spills on floor
- Loose connections on invasive monitoring devices
- Patient contact with intense cold
- Patient sliding on coarse bed linens or struggling with bed restraints
- Patient smoking in bed or near oxygen
- Slippery floors (wet or highly waxed)
- Unlighted rooms or corridors
- Unsteady chairs

Associated medical diagnoses (selected)
Acute head injury, Alzheimer's disease, brain tumor, burns, cerebrovascular accident, drug overdose, fractures, hemophilia, Ménière's disease, multiple sclerosis, multisystem trauma, organic brain syndrome, Parkinson's disease, posttraumatic head injury, sedation or placement under general anesthesia, spinal cord injury

Expected outcomes
- Patient avoids injury.
- Patient states understanding of safety precautions.
- Patient uses assistive devices correctly (walker or cane, for example).

Interventions and rationales
- Observe, record, and report falls, seizures, and unsafe practices. *Accurate assessment promotes appropriate interventions; documentation ensures continuity of care.*
- Monitor and record respiratory status. *Trauma increases respiratory rate; other respiratory effects depend on nature of trauma.*
- Monitor and record neurologic status. *This assessment reflects all levels of nervous system.*
- If seizure occurs, remain with the patient, loosen restrictive clothing, and protect patient from environmental hazards. Do not restrain the patient or pry the mouth open. Keep oral airway at bedside. Maintain patent airway. Turn patient to the side after the seizure stops and suction if secretions occlude the airway. Record seizure characteristics, including onset, duration, and body movements. Reorient patient to surroundings and allow a rest period.

Remaining with the patient provides safety and information for the accurate documentation of the event. Loosening the clothing and proper positioning may prevent further harm.
- Keep side rails up at all times *to protect patient and provide sense of security.*
- Keep bed in low position except when providing direct care. *This minimizes effects of a possible fall.*
- Emphasize importance of asking for help before getting up. *Patient may be weakened by illness or injury.*
- Help debilitated, weak, or unsteady patient get out of bed. Ensure that the floor is dry and that furniture and litter are out of the way. *This helps protect patient from falling.*
- When using soft restraints, do not secure them too tightly *to avoid giving patient skin burns.*
- Use leather restraints following institutional policy; pad them well before applying. Release each extremity on a rotation basis every hour; check for skin burns. *Such restraints should be used only when other kinds are ineffective.*
- Instruct patient and family or significant other in safety practices, such as correct use of walker, crutches, or cane. *These enable patient and family or significant other to take an active role in health care and maintain safe environment.*

Evaluations for expected outcomes
- Patient remains free of injury.
- Patient identifies specific safety precautions.
- Patient demonstrates proper use of assistive device (specify).

Documentation
- Patient's statements that indicate potential for injury
- Physical findings
- Observations or knowledge of unsafe practices
- Interventions performed to prevent injury
- Patient's response to nursing interventions
- Evaluations for each expected outcome.

■ Trauma, high risk for

related to internal factors

Definition
Accentuated risk of accidental tissue injury such as burns or fractures

Assessment
- Health history, including accidents, allergies, exposure to pollutants, falls, hyperthermia, hypothermia, poisoning, sensory or perceptual changes (auditory, gustatory, kinesthetic, olfactory, tactile, visual), seizures, trauma
- Circumstances of present situation that might lead to injury
- Neurologic status, including level of consciousness, mental status, orientation
- Laboratory studies, including albumin and globulin levels, clotting factors, hemoglobin and hematocrit, platelet count, white blood cell count

Risk factors
- Balancing difficulties
- Malnutrition
- Poor vision
- Reduced large or small muscle coordination
- Reduced tactile sensation
- Reduced temperature
- Weakness or fatigue

Associated medical diagnoses (selected)
Acute head injury, Alzheimer's disease, brain tumor, burns, cerebrovascular accident, hemophilia, Ménière's disease, multiple sclerosis, multisystem trauma, organic brain syndrome, osteoporosis, Parkinson's disease, posttraumatic head injury, sedation or placement under general anesthesia, seizure disorder, spinal cord injury, thrombocytopenic purpura

Expected outcomes
- Patient avoids injury.
- Patient voices need for understanding safety precautions.
- Patient uses safety devices correctly (walker or cane, for example).

Interventions and rationales
- Observe, record, and report falls, seizures, unsafe practices. *Accurate assessment promotes appropriate interventions; documentation ensures continuity of care.*
- Monitor and record respiratory status. *Trauma increases respiratory rate; other respiratory effects depend on nature of trauma.*
- Monitor and record neurologic status *to assess changes and to report deteriorated status.*
- For seizures:
  - Keep side rails up *to protect patient and provide sense of security.*
  - Pad side rails *to protect patient.*
  - Protect patient from further injury during the seizure *to ensure well-being.*
  - Position patient on side *to prevent aspiration.*
  - Record such seizure characteristics as onset, duration, and body movements. *Documenting seizure helps pinpoint involved area of brain and guides treatment.*
  - If patient is confused and walking about after a seizure ends, walk with him and guide him back to his bed. Don't try to restrain him *to prevent injury.*
- To prevent falls:
  - Keep bed rails up *to enhance safety.*
  - Maintain bed in a low position except when providing direct care *to reduce risk of injury.*
  - Emphasize importance of asking for help before getting up. *Patient may be weakened by illness or injury.*
  - Provide help in ambulating and going to the bathroom *to ensure safety.*
  - Anticipate times when falls occur (during the night, after administering a diuretic, while patient is sitting in a chair) and monitor patient closely *to prevent injuries.*
- Instruct patient and family or significant other in use of such assistive devices as cane, walker, crutches, or wheelchair *to ensure their proper use and to provide patient with feeling of security.*
- Provide patient and family or significant other with information about necessary safety precautions *to enable patient and family or significant other to take active role in health care and maintain safe environment.*

Evaluations for expected outcomes
- Patient remains free of injury during specific time frame.
- Patient identifies need for specific safety precautions.
- Patient demonstrates proper use of assistive device (specify).

Documentation
- Patient's statements about the situation that indicate potential for injury
- Physical findings
- Record of falls, seizures, and unsafe practices
- Interventions that reduce risk of injury
- Patient's response to nursing interventions
- Evaluations for each expected outcome.

Urinary elimination pattern alteration

related to obstruction

Definition
Alteration or impairment of urinary function

Assessment
- History of urinary tract disease, trauma, surgery, or previous urethral infection
- Age
- Sex
- Vital signs
- Genitourinary status, including characteristics of urine, intravenous pyelogram, pain or discomfort, palpation of bladder, urinalysis, voiding patterns
- Fluid and electrolyte status, including blood urea nitrogen, creatinine, intake and output, mucous membranes (inspection), serum electrolytes, skin turgor, urine specific gravity
- Nutritional status, including appetite, constipation, dietary intake, elimination habits, present weight and change from normal, rectal examination
- Sexuality status, including capability, concerns, habits, sexual partner
- Psychosocial status, including coping skills, patient's perception of health problem, self-concept (body image), family or significant other, stressors (finances, job)

Defining characteristics
- Clinical evidence of urinary obstruction
- Dysuria
- Frequency
- Hematuria
- Hesitancy
- Incontinence
- Nocturia
- Retention
- Urgency

Associated medical diagnoses (selected)
Benign prostatic hypertrophy, bladder cancer, hydronephrosis, ileal bladder, ileal conduit, nephrolithotomy, pelvic neoplasm, prostate cancer, renal calculi, suprapubic or transurethral prostatectomy, urethral strictures, urinary diversion, urinary tract infection

Expected outcomes
- Patient maintains fluid balance; intake equals output.
- Patient voices increased comfort.
- Patient voices understanding of treatment.
- Complications avoided or minimized.
- Patient discusses impact of urologic disorder on self and family or significant other.
- Patient and family or significant other demonstrate skill in managing urinary elimination problem.

Interventions and rationales
- Observe voiding pattern. Document urine color and characteristics, intake

and output, and patient's daily weight. Report any changes. *Accurate intake and output measurements are essential for correct fluid replacement therapy. Urine characteristics help verify diagnosis.*

- Administer appropriate care for the urologic condition; monitor progress (for example, strain urine). Report favorable and adverse responses to treatment regimen. *Patient expects to receive adequate health care from qualified caregivers and to be helped to understand the disease as well as treatment.*
- Observe bowel habits.
  - Check for constipation.
  - Check for fecal impaction; if present, disimpact and institute bowel regimen.

This promotes comfort and prevents loss of rectal muscle tone from prolonged distention.

- If surgery is to be performed, give appropriate preoperative and postoperative instructions and care. *Accurate information allows patient to deal with reality and builds trust in caregivers.*
- Explain the reasons for therapy and the intended effects to patient and family or significant other *to increase patient's understanding and build trust in caregivers.* If urinary diversion is planned, prepare patient for change in body appearance (instruct patient and family or significant other how to care for ostomy site postoperatively). *Physical need or changes in physical appearance may threaten health equilibrium. Appropriate information helps patient and family or significant other cope with problem.*
- Provide supportive measures, as indicated.
  - Administer pain medication and monitor effectiveness. *Awareness that pain can be alleviated decreases pain intensity by relieving tension produced by anxiety.*
  - Force fluids, as ordered, *to moisten mucous membranes and dilute chemical materials within the body.*
  - Refer to dietitian for instructions on diet. *Dietary changes may decrease urinary infections.*
  - Assist with general hygiene and comfort measures, as needed. *Cleanliness prevents bacterial growth and promotes comfort.*
  - Maintain patency of catheters, drainage bags, and other urinary elimination equipment *to avoid reflux and risk of infection, and ensure effectiveness of therapy.*
  - Provide meatal care according to hospital procedure *to promote cleanliness and comfort and reduce risk of infection.*
- Encourage patient to ventilate feelings and concerns related to urologic problem. *Active listening conveys respect for patient; ventilation helps pinpoint patient's fears.*
- Refer patient and family or significant other to psychiatric liaison nurse, sex counselor, or support group, when appropriate. *These resources help patient gain knowledge of self and situation, reduce anxiety, and help promote personal growth. Community resources often provide support and care not available in other health agencies.*
- Explain the urologic condition to patient and family or significant other, including instructions on preventive measures, if appropriate. Prepare for discharge according to individual needs. *Accurate health knowledge increases patient's ability to maintain health. Involving family*

or significant other assures patient that he will be cared for.

Evaluations for expected outcomes

- Patient's fluid intake is equal to output.
- Patient expresses feelings of comfort.
- Patient voices understanding of treatment, including urinary diversion therapy, if appropriate.
- Patient does not show evidence of skin breakdown, infection, or other complications.
- Patient discusses disease, symptoms, complications, treatments, and adjustments to life-style caused by altered urinary pattern.
- Patient demonstrates proficiency in steps necessary to manage urinary elimination problems.
- Patient maintains urinary continence.

Documentation

- Observations of urologic condition and response to treatment regimen
- Interventions to provide supportive care; patient's response to supportive care
- Instructions given to patient and family or significant other on the urologic problem; their response to instructions and demonstrated ability in managing urinary elimination
- Patient's expression of concern about the urologic problem and its impact on body image and life-style; patient's motivation to participate in self-care
- Evaluations for each expected outcome.

Urinary elimination pattern alteration

related to sensory or neuromuscular impairment

Definition

Alteration or impairment of urinary function

Assessment

- History of urinary tract disease, trauma, surgery, or infection
- History of sensory or neuromuscular impairment
- Vital signs
- Genitourinary status, including characteristics of urine, cystometry, pain or discomfort, palpation of bladder, postcatheterization, presence and amount of residual urine; use of urinary assistive devices, urinalysis, voiding pattern
- Fluid and electrolyte status including blood urea nitrogen, creatinine, inspection of mucous membranes, intake and output, serum electrolytes, skin turgor, urine specific gravity
- Neuromuscular status, including degree of neuromuscular function present, motor ability to start and stop urinary stream, sensory ability to perceive bladder fullness
- Sexuality status, including capability, concerns, habits, sexual partner
- Psychosocial status, including coping skills, family or significant other, patient's perception of health problem, self-concept, stressors (finances, job)

Defining characteristics

- Clinical evidence of sensory or neuromuscular impairment of urinary tract
- Dysuria

- Frequency
- Hesitancy
- Incontinence
- Nocturia
- Retention
- Urgency

Associated medical diagnoses (selected)
Cerebrovascular accident, diabetes mellitus, hydronephrosis, multiple sclerosis, peripheral vascular disease, prolapsed lumbar disc, spinal cord defect (myelomeningocele, spina bifida), spinal cord injury, spinal cord tumor

Expected outcomes
- Patient maintains fluid balance; intake equals output.
- Patient voices increased comfort.
- Complications avoided or minimized.
- Patient and family or significant other demonstrate skill in managing urinary elimination problem.
- Patient discusses impact of urologic disorder on self and family or significant other.
- Patient and family or significant other identify resources to assist with care following discharge.

Interventions and rationales
- Monitor patient's neuromuscular status and voiding pattern; document and report intake and output. *Accurate intake and output measurements are essential for correct fluid replacement therapy. Data form basis for complete evaluation to diagnose causative factors.*
- Provide appropriate care for the urologic condition; monitor progress. Report responses to treatment. *Patient expects to receive adequate health care from qualified caregivers, and to be helped to understand the disease as well as treatment.*
- Assist with ordered bladder elimination procedure, as indicated.

Bladder training:
- Place patient on commode or toilet every 2 hours while awake and once during the night. Maintain regular fluid intake while patient is awake. Provide privacy. Teach patient how to perform Kegel exercises to strengthen sphincter control. *These measures aid adaptation to routine physiologic function. Women with good muscle tone may be able to improve levator muscle action significantly if Kegel exercises done routinely.*

Intermittent catheterization:
- Catheterize patient using clean or sterile technique every ____ hours. Record amount voided spontaneously and amount obtained with catheterization (for example: 7 a.m., spontaneous void of 200 ml; catheter void of 150 ml). Record bladder balance every (day or week). *These measures promote normal voiding, prevent infection, and help maintain integrity of ureterovesical function. Catheterization schedule is based on flow sheet data and can provide a baseline chart.*

$$\text{Bladder balance} = \frac{\text{Amount of residual urine}}{\text{Amount of voided urine}}$$

External catheter (male patient):
- Monitor patency. Apply condom catheter according to established policy. *Applying foam strip in spiral fashion increases adhesive surface and reduces risk of impairing circulation.* Avoid constriction. Observe skin condition of penis, and cleanse with soap and water at least twice a day. *These measures prevent infec-*

tion, and ensure therapeutic effectiveness.

Indwelling urinary (Foley) catheter:

- Monitor patency. Keep tubing free of kinks; keep drainage bag below level of bladder *to avoid urine reflux.* Cleanse urinary meatus according to established policy, and maintain closed drainage system *to prevent skin irritation and bacteriuria.* Secure catheter to leg (female) or abdomen (male); avoid tension on sphincter. *Anchoring catheter avoids straining trigone muscle of bladder and prevents friction leading to inflammation.*

Suprapubic catheter:

- Monitor patency. Change dressing and cleanse catheter site according to policy. Keep tubing free of kinks; keep drainage bag below bladder level. Maintain closed drainage system. *Suprapubic drainage allows increased patient mobility and reduces risk of bladder infection.*

- Provide supportive measures:
  - Administer pain medication and monitor effectiveness. *Awareness that pain can be alleviated decreases pain intensity by relieving tension produced by anxiety.*
  - Encourage fluid intake to as much as 3,000 ml every 24 hours (unless contraindicated) *to moisten mucous membranes and dilute chemical materials within the body.*
  - Provide privacy during toileting procedure. *This avoids inhibiting elimination.*
  - Respond to patient's call light quickly, assign patient to bed next to bathroom, and have patient wear easily removed clothing, for example, gown rather than pajamas. *These measures reduce delay and impediments to voiding routine.*
- Alert patient and family or significant other to signs and symptoms of full bladder: restlessness, abdominal discomfort, sweating, chills. *Adequate education increases patient's and family's ability to maintain health level, and to prevent patient from harming self.*
- Instruct patient and family or significant other on catheterization techniques to be used at home; provide time for return demonstrations until procedure can be performed well. *Knowledge of procedures and rationales reduces anxiety and promotes comfort. Demonstrations may progress through several sessions until patient can perform independently.*
- Instruct patient and family or significant other on signs and symptoms of autonomic dysreflexia (headache, cold sweat, nausea, elevated blood pressure) and on management of autonomic dysreflexia (check for kinked Foley catheter, catheterize, and elevate head of bed). Instruct patient and family or significant other to call doctor or hospital immediately if symptoms do not subside with initial treatment. *Autonomic dysreflexia is a pathologic reflex condition characterized by exaggerated autonomic responses to stimuli. It is a medical emergency.*
- Encourage patient to ventilate feelings and concerns related to urologic problem. *Active listening conveys respect for patient; ventilation helps pinpoint patient's fears.*
- Refer patient and family or significant other to psychiatric liaison nurse, sex counselor, visiting nurses' society, or support group, when appropriate. *These resources help patient gain knowledge of self and situation, reduce anxiety, and help*

promote personal growth. Community resources often provide care and support not available in other health agencies.

Evaluations for expected outcomes
- Patient's fluid intake equals output.
- Patient expresses feeling of comfort.
- Patient does not develop infection, swelling of penis, skin breakdown, or other complications. Urinalysis remains normal.
- Patient and family or significant other demonstrate skill in managing urinary elimination problem, including catheterization techniques to be used at home.
- Patient expresses feelings about condition.
- Patient expresses understanding of urologic disorder and its effect on family and life-style after discharge.
- Patient and family identify and contact visiting nurse, support group, or other resources as needed.

Documentation
- Observations of urologic condition and response to treatment regimen
- Interventions to provide supportive care; patient's response to supportive care
- Instructions given to patient and family or significant other; their understanding and demonstrated ability to manage urinary elimination
- Patient's expression of concern about the urologic problem and impact on body image and life-style; patient's motivation to participate in self-care
- Evaluations for each expected outcome.

Urinary retention

related to obstruction, sensory or neuromuscular impairment

Definition
Incomplete emptying of bladder

Assessment
- History of sensory or neuromuscular impairment, prostate enlargement, surgery, urethral trauma or tumor, urinary tract disease
- Age
- Sex
- Vital signs
- Genitourinary status, including pain or discomfort, palpation of bladder, residual urine volume after voiding, urethral obstruction (prostate hypertrophy or masses, fecal impaction, masses, swelling), urinalysis, urine characteristics, voiding patterns
- Fluid and electrolyte status, including inspection of mucous membranes, intake and output, skin turgor, urine specific gravity, serum electrolytes, blood urea nitrogen, creatinine
- Medication history
- Neuromuscular status, including anal sphincter tone, motor ability to start and stop stream, neuromuscular function, sensory ability to perceive bladder fullness and voiding
- Sexuality status, including capability, concerns or partner's concerns
- Psychosocial status, including coping skills; patient's or significant other's perception of problem, self-concept, stressors (finances, job)

Defining characteristics
- Bladder distention
- Dysuria
- Hesitancy

- High residual urine
- Loss of anal sphincter tone (with sensory or neuromuscular impairment)
- Nocturia
- Overflow incontinence (continuous dribbling)
- Sensation of bladder fullness
- Slow stream of urine
- Small, frequent voiding or no urine output

Associated medical diagnoses (selected)
Diabetic neuropathy, herniated intervertebral disk, nephrolithotomy, poliomyelitis, sacral nerve trauma or tumor, spinal cord injury (lower motor neuron), suprapubic or transurethral prostatectomy, surgical urinary retention, urethral obstruction (cancer of prostate, fecal impaction, fibroids, prostatic hypertrophy, stricture, surgical swelling), vitamin B_{12} deficiency

Expected outcomes
- Patient maintains fluid balance; intake equals output.
- Patient voices increased comfort.
- Patient voices understanding of treatment.
- Complications avoided or minimized.
- Patient avoids bladder distention.
- Patient and family or significant other demonstrate skill in managing urine retention.
- Patient discusses impact of urologic disorder on self and family or significant other.
- Patient and family or significant other identify resources to assist with care following discharge.

Interventions and rationales
- Monitor intake and output. Report if intake exceeds output. *Accurate intake and output measurements are essential for correct fluid replacement therapy.*
- Monitor voiding pattern. *Data on time, place, amount, and patient's awareness of micturition are needed to establish pattern of incontinence.*
- Assist with ordered bladder elimination procedure, as follows:
  - voiding techniques. Perform Credé's or Valsalva's maneuver every 2 to 3 hours *to increase bladder pressure to pass urine.* Repeat until empty.
  - intermittent catheterization. Catheterize using clean or sterile technique every ____ hours. Record amount voided spontaneously and amount obtained with catheterization. *These measures promote normal voiding, prevent infection, and help maintain integrity of ureterovesical function.*
  - use of indwelling urinary (Foley) catheter. Monitor patency. Avoid kinks in tubing. Keep drainage bag below bladder level *to avoid urine reflux.* Perform catheter care according to established policy and maintain closed drainage system *to prevent skin irritation and bacteriuria.* Secure catheter to leg (female) or abdomen (male). Avoid tension on sphincter. *Anchoring catheter avoids straining trigone muscle of bladder and prevents friction leading to inflammation.*
  - use of suprapubic catheter. Change dressings according to hospital policy. Monitor patency. Avoid kinks in tubing. Keep drainage bag below bladder level. Maintain closed drainage system. *Suprapubic drainage allows for increased mobility*

and reduces risk of bladder infection.
• Administer pain medication, as ordered, and monitor effectiveness. *Awareness that pain can be alleviated decreases pain intensity by relieving tension produced by anxiety.*
• For fecal impaction, disimpact and institute bowel regimen. *This promotes comfort and prevents loss of rectal muscle tone from prolonged distention.*
• Encourage high fluid intake (2,500 ml/day), unless contraindicated, *to moisten mucous membranes and dilute chemical materials within the body.* Limit fluid intake after 7 p.m. *to prevent nocturia.*
• Monitor therapeutic and adverse effects of prescribed medications *for early recognition and treatment of drug reactions.*
• If surgery is to be performed, give appropriate preoperative and postoperative instructions and care *to increase patient's understanding.* If urinary diversions are planned, prepare patient for change in body image. *Changes in physical appearance may threaten health equilibrium. Appropriate information helps patient and family or significant other cope with problem.*
• Instruct patient and family or significant other on voiding techniques to be used at home. Provide for return demonstrations until procedure can be performed well. *Knowledge of procedures and rationales reduces anxiety and promotes comfort. Demonstrations may progress through several sessions until patient can perform independently.*
• Encourage patient and family or significant other to share feelings and concerns related to urologic problems. *Ventilation helps pinpoint patient's fears, and establishes environment of trust in which patient and family or significant other can begin to deal with the situation.*
• Refer patient and family or significant other to psychiatric liaison nurse, enterostomal therapist, sex counselor, support group, or visiting nurse's association, when appropriate. *These resources help patient gain knowledge of self and situation, reduce anxiety, and help promote personal growth. Community resources often provide services not available at other health agencies.*

Evaluations for expected outcomes
• Patient's intake equals output.
• Patient expresses absence of pain.
• Patient voices understanding of treatment, including ordered bladder elimination procedure and surgery, if appropriate.
• Patient does not experience skin breakdown or other complications. Urinalysis remains normal.
• Patient avoids bladder distention.
• Patient and family or significant other demonstrate skill in managing urine retention, including voiding techniques to be used at home.
• Patient expresses at least one fear, one concern, and one positive feeling about urologic problem. If appropriate, patient expresses feelings and fears about surgery.
• Patient or family contacts visiting nurse, support group, or other resources, as needed.

Documentation
• Observations of urologic condition and response to treatment regimen
• Interventions to provide supportive care and patient's response
• Instructions given to patient and family or significant other on the urologic problem; their returned re-

sponse and demonstrated ability to manage urinary elimination
• Patient's expression of concern about the urologic problem and its impact on body image and life-style; motivation to participate in self-care
• Evaluations for each expected outcome.

Ventilation, spontaneous: Inability to sustain

Definition
Inability to breathe adequately

Assessment
• Health history, including previous respiratory problems
• Respiratory status, including rate and depth of respiration, chest excursion and symmetry, presence of cyanosis, use of accessory muscles
• Effectiveness of cough in clearing secretions
• Suctioning demands, including frequency, tolerance
• Sputum characteristics, including appearance, consistency, color, odor
• Neuromuscular strength and endurance
• Mental and emotional status, including cognitive state, ability to follow directions
• Laboratory values, including arterial blood gas (ABG) levels (baseline and ongoing), complete blood count, serum electrolyte levels, coagulation studies, serum and sputum cultures, sensitivity tests
• Vital signs
• Functional status, including ability to perform activities of daily living
• Related or concurrent events that may contribute to respiratory distress, such as bleeding, hypervolemia, hypovolemia, sepsis

Defining characteristics
• Apprehension
• Decreased cooperation
• Decreased arterial oxygen saturation
• Decreased partial pressure of oxygen in arterial blood (PaO_2)
• Decreased tidal volume
• Dyspnea
• Increased metabolic rate
• Increased partial pressure of carbon dioxide in arterial blood
• Increased use of accessory muscles
• Respiratory muscle fatigue
• Tachycardia

Associated medical diagnoses (selected)
Acute streptococcus infection, adult respiratory distress syndrome, amyotrophic lateral sclerosis, chronic obstructive pulmonary disease, Guillain-Barré syndrome, hemothorax, hypervolemia, hypovolemia, multiple sclerosis, multisystem organ failure, Parkinson's disease, pneumonia, pneumothorax, sepsis, severe burns, tension pneumothorax, tracheal obstruction or stricture

Expected outcomes
• Patient's respiratory rate remains within ± 5 breaths/minute of baseline.
• Patient's ABG levels are normal.
• Patient indicates feeling comfortable and does not report pain, dyspnea, or fatigue.
• Patient carries out activities of daily living with minimal supplemental oxygen.
• Patient's breathing pattern returns to baseline.
• As patient's activity level increases, PaO_2 remains within normal limits.

• After ventilator support is withdrawn, patient breathes spontaneously.

Interventions and rationales

• Monitor patient's vital signs every 15 minutes to 1 hour *to detect tachypnea and tachycardia, early indicators of respiratory distress.*

• Monitor patient for nasal flaring, change in depth and pattern of breathing, use of accessory muscles, and cyanosis *to detect signs of severe respiratory distress.*

• Monitor ABG levels and report deviations promptly *to determine need for changes to therapeutic regimen.*

• Monitor hemoglobin level and hematocrit. *Low hemoglobin level and hematocrit indicate decreased oxygen-carrying capacity of the blood.*

• Begin oxygen support using smallest concentration needed to make patient comfortable. Monitor closely *to avoid oxygen toxicity.*

• Place patient in Fowler's position *to increase comfort and to promote adequate chest expansion and diaphragmatic excursion and thereby decrease work of breathing.*

• Help patient progress gradually from bed rest to increased activity *to improve patient's sense of well-being.* Monitor vital signs and ABG levels closely. If respiratory status is compromised, return patient to bed rest *to decrease the basal metabolic rate and lower oxygen demands.*

• Explain all procedures to patient. Describe specific sensations he may experience during each procedure *to decrease anxiety.*

• Anticipate possible complications. Keep in mind that if patient decompensates while on a 100% fraction of inspired oxygen (FIO_2) nonrebreather mask, he may require endotracheal intubation. *Anticipating complications facilitates prompt intervention.*

• If intubation is required, monitor patient for spontaneous breathing and gradually wean him from ventilator. *Progressive weaning helps patient to adjust physiologically and emotionally to increased work of breathing.*

• Avoid respiratory depressants, such as narcotics, sedatives, and paralytics, *to facilitate patient's recovery.*

Evaluations for expected outcomes

• Patient's respiratory rate is within ±5 breaths/minute of baseline.

• Patient's ABG levels are normal.

• Patient does not report pain, dyspnea, or fatigue.

• Patient carries out activities of daily living with minimal supplemental oxygen.

• Patient's breathing pattern returns to baseline.

• PaO_2 remains within normal limits when patient increases activity level.

• Patient breathes spontaneously once ventilator support is withdrawn.

Documentation

• Patient's reports of malaise, dyspnea, restlessness, chest pain, dizziness, light-headedness

• Patient's response to nursing interventions

• Patient's response to initiation of oxygen therapy and progressive changes in therapy

• Laboratory data, including ABG levels

• Respiratory status (baseline and ongoing)

• Subtle personality changes

• Changes in lung sounds revealed by auscultation

• Evaluations for each expected outcome.

Ventilatory weaning response, dysfunctional

Definition

Difficulty adjusting to lowered levels of mechanical ventilator support

Assessment

- Health history, including previous respiratory problems
- Nutritional status
- Weight
- Neurologic status, including mental status, level of consciousness
- Emotional status, including signs of anxiety or stress
- Laboratory values, including arterial blood gas (ABG) levels (baseline and ongoing), serum electrolyte levels, complete blood count, blood and sputum culture, sensitivity tests
- Weaning parameters and present ventilator settings
- Respiratory status, including respiratory rate, pattern, character, and depth; chest expansion and symmetry; sputum characteristics (color, amount, odor, and consistency); cough effectiveness; presence of cyanosis in mucous membranes and nail beds; auscultation of lung sounds
- Need for suctioning, including frequency and patient's response
- Musculoskeletal status, including muscle mass, strength, endurance level
- Cognitive state, including patient's ability to follow directions and readiness to learn
- Recent administration of potential respiratory-depressant medications, such as narcotics, sedatives, neuromuscular blockers
- Vital signs
- Pulse oximetry readings

Defining characteristics

- Mild dysfunctional weaning response:
  - breathing discomfort
  - expression of increased need for oxygen
  - fatigue
  - increased concentration on breathing
  - queries about possible machine malfunction
  - restlessness
  - warmth
- *Moderate dysfunctional weaning response:*
  - apprehension
  - changes in skin color, paleness, slight cyanosis
  - decreased air entry on auscultation
  - hypervigilance to activities related to ventilator functioning
  - inability to cooperate
  - inability to respond to coaching
  - increase in blood pressure (no more than than 20 mm Hg above baseline)
  - increase in heart rate (no more than 20 beats/minute above baseline)
  - increase in respiratory rate (no more than than 5 breaths/minute above baseline)
  - slight respiratory accessory muscle use
  - "wide-eyed" look
- Severe dysfunctional weaning response:
  - adventitious breath sounds
  - agitation
  - audible airway secretions
  - cyanosis
  - decreased level of consciousness
  - deteriorating ABG levels
  - full respiratory accessory muscle use
  - increased blood pressure (more than 20 mm Hg above baseline)

– increased heart rate (more than 20 beats/minute above baseline)
– paradoxical abdominal breathing
– profuse diaphoresis
– shallow, gasping breath
– significant increase in respiratory rate
– uncoordinated breathing with the ventilator

Associated medical diagnoses (selected)
Adult respiratory distress syndrome, amyotrophic lateral sclerosis, burns, chronic obstructive pulmonary disease, metastatic disease, esophageal or tracheal anomalies, flail chest, morbid obesity, multiple trauma, myasthenia gravis, Parkinson's disease, pulmonary edema, pulmonary effusions, pulmonary fibrosis, sepsis

Expected outcomes
- Patient maintains respiratory rate within ± 5 breaths/minute of baseline during weaning period.
- ABG levels remain within acceptable limits (specify).
- Patient's mental status and emotional state remain stable as ventilatory support is gradually withdrawn.
- Patient expresses comfort with progressive ventilator changes.
- Patient does not experience dyspnea, fatigue, or pain during progressive ventilator changes.
- Adequate weaning parameters are maintained:
  – Tidal volume is 4 to 5 cc/kg.
  – Negative inspiratory force is greater than or equal to -20 cm H_2O.
  – Vital capacity is 10 to 15 cc/kg.
  – Minute ventilation is 6 to 10 liters.
- Patient's cough is effective in clearing secretions.

Interventions and rationales
- Monitor patient's vital signs every hour when changing ventilator settings. *Fever, tachycardia, tachypnea, and elevated blood pressure may indicate hypoxemia.*
- Auscultate for lung sounds every 2 hours and report deviations. *Adventitious sounds may precede respiratory failure.*
- Place patient in comfortable position (preferably Fowler's) *to facilitate adequate chest expansion and drainage.*
- Describe all weaning procedures to patient. Explain to patient that he may experience changes in breathing rate and pattern, increased difficulty breathing, and fatigue *to decrease anxiety.*
- If patient is receiving intermittent mandatory ventilation (IMV), begin to decrease IMV by increments of 2 breaths/minute. This process may take place over days or weeks. *Lowering the IMV encourages patient to take his own breaths and thereby exercise respiratory muscles.*
- Monitor ABG levels with every ventilator change *to assess for adequate oxygenation and acid-base balance.*
- Include periods of rest between ventilator changes, especially at night, *to reduce tissue oxygen demand.*
- If patient tolerates IMV of 2 to 4 breaths/minute, try pressure support ventilation (PSV). *PSV prolongs positive airway pressure during inspiration, allowing patient to regulate his own respiratory rate and tidal volume.*
- Once patient is breathing adequately without IMV, place him on continuous positive airway pressure (CPAP) of 5 cm H_2O *to prevent alveolar collapse.*

• When patient tolerates CPAP, place him on T-piece (T-bar) of 30% to 50% FIO_2. *This allows patient to breathe on his own, continue to receive oxygen, and remain intubated in the event of respiratory compromise.*
• Once patient tolerates longer weaning periods, incorporate activities of daily living into daily routine *to increase muscular strength and endurance.*
• When respiratory status, weaning parameters, and ABG levels are satisfactory, assist with removal of ventilator tubes, and keep oxygen mask on hand *to prevent respiratory compromise.*
• Assess patient for stridor, respiratory distress, or dysphonia and report these symptoms to doctor *to monitor need for renewed ventilatory assistance.*
• Perform chest physiotherapy and suctioning as needed *to maintain a patent airway.*
• Monitor respiratory effects of medications closely and evaluate response to bronchodilators *to detect respiratory status compromise.* Avoid respiratory depressants.

Evaluations for expected outcomes
• During weaning period, patient's respiratory rate is within ±5 breaths/minute of baseline.
• ABG levels are within acceptable limits.
• Patient's mental status and emotional state are stable as ventilatory support is withdrawn.
• Patient expresses comfort with progressive ventilator changes.
• Patient does not experience dyspnea, fatigue, or pain during progressive ventilator changes.
• Adequate weaning parameters are maintained.
• Patient's cough is effective in clearing secretions.

Documentation
• Patient's reports of malaise, anxiety, restlessness, breathlessness, unusual pain
• Patient's response to ventilator changes
• Subtle changes in patient's mental or emotional status
• Laboratory data, including ABG levels
• Patient's response to nursing interventions, including positioning, chest physiotherapy, and suctioning
• Patient responses to medications, including narcotics, bronchodilators, neuromuscular blockers
• Respiratory rate, pattern, and depth, including changes from baseline
• Evaluations for each expected outcome.

Verbal communication impairment

related to decreased circulation to brain

Definition
Decreased ability to speak, understand, or use words appropriately

Assessment
• Neurologic status, including level of consciousness, orientation, cognition, memory (recent and remote), insight, and judgment
• Speech characteristics, including pattern (garbled, incomprehensible, difficulty forming words), language and vocabulary, level of comprehension and expression, ability to use other forms of communication (eye blinks, gestures, pictures, nods)

- Motor ability
- Circulatory status, including a history of cardiac and circulatory problems, pulse, blood pressure, arteriogram, electroencephalogram, and computed tomography scan
- Respiratory status, including dyspnea and use of accessory muscles

Defining characteristics
- Disorientation
- Dyspnea
- Flight of ideas
- Impaired articulation
- Inability or lack of desire to speak
- Inability to identify objects
- Inability to modulate speech
- Inability to name words
- Inability to speak in sentences
- Incessant verbalization
- Loose association of ideas
- Perseveration
- Phonation difficulties
- Reduced blood volume to the brain
- Stuttering or slurring

Associated medical diagnoses (selected)
Arteriosclerotic heart disease, arteriovenous malformation, atherosclerotic heart disease, berry aneurysm, brain tumor (benign or malignant), cerebrovascular accident, chronic obstructive pulmonary disease, shock, Wernicke's aphasia

Expected outcomes
- Patient's needs met by staff.
- Patient and significant other express satisfaction with level of communication ability.
- Patient maintains orientation.
- Patient maintains effective level of communication.
- Patient answers direct questions correctly.

Interventions and rationales
- Observe patient closely for cues to needs and desires, such as gestures, pointing to objects, looking at items, and pantomime *because nonverbal cues give meaning to actions.* Do not continually respond to gestures if potential exists to improve speech *to avoid discouraging improvement.*
- Monitor and record changes in speech pattern or level of orientation. *Changes may indicate improvement or deterioration of condition.*
- Speak slowly and distinctly in a normal tone when addressing patient; stand where patient can see and hear you. *Modified speech promotes comprehension.*
- Reorient patient to reality:
  - Call patient by name.
  - Tell patient your name.
  - Give patient background information (place, date, time).
  - Use TV or radio to augment orientation.
  - Use large calendars, reality orientation boards.

These measures develop orientation skills through repetition and recognition of the familiar.
- Use short, simple phrases and yes-or-no questions when patient is very frustrated *to reduce frustration.*
- Encourage attempts at communication and provide positive reinforcement *to aid comprehension.*
- Allow ample time for response. Do not answer questions yourself if patient has ability to respond. *This improves patient's self-concept and reduces frustration.*
- Repeat or rephrase questions if necessary *to improve communication.* Do not pretend to understand if you don't. *Reduced pressure improves comprehension.*
- Remove distractions from environment during attempts at communication. Use communication boards (including the alphabet and some

common words and pictures) if appropriate. *Reduced distractions improve comprehension.*
- Review diagnostic test results *to determine improvement or deterioration of disease process; adjust plan of care accordingly.*

Evaluations for expected outcomes
- Patient's needs are consistently met by staff.
- Patient and significant other communicate at satisfactory level.
- Patient communicates effectively _____ times every 8 hours (specify).
- Patient correctly answers _____ direct questions (specify).
- Patient consistently communicates thoughts to family and staff.

Documentation
- Patient's current level of communication, orientation, and satisfaction with communication efforts
- Observations of speech deficits, expressiveness and receptiveness, and ability to communicate
- Interventions carried out to promote effective communication
- Patient's observable response to nursing interventions
- Evaluations for each expected outcome.

■ Verbal communication impairment

related to physical barriers

Definition
Decreased ability to speak, understand, or use words appropriately

Assessment
- History of respiratory, neurologic, or musculoskeletal disorder or surgery
- Respiratory status, including dyspnea, use of accessory muscles, and respiratory pattern
- Neurologic status, including mental status (level of consciousness, orientation, cognition, memory, insight, and judgment), speech (pattern, signing, and such communication aids as an artificial larynx, computer-assisted speech device, pen and pencil, slate, picture board, and alphabet board)
- Musculoskeletal status, including range of motion and manual dexterity

Defining characteristics
- Dyspnea
- Impaired articulation
- Inability or lack of desire to speak
- Inability to modulate speech
- Inability to speak in sentences
- Phonation difficulties
- Physical barriers to communication
- Slurring

Associated medical diagnoses (selected)
Cancer (head, neck, lung), facial fractures, fractured jaw, intubation with or without mechanical ventilation, laryngeal edema, laryngectomy, laryngitis, radical head or neck surgery (such as glossectomy), tracheostomy

Expected outcomes
- Patient communicates needs and desires without undue frustration.
- Patient uses alternate means of communication.
- Patient demonstrates correct use of adaptive equipment.

• Patient expresses plans to use appropriate resources to maximize communication skills.

Interventions and rationales

• Maintain a consistent daily schedule of activities as much as possible. Observe patient closely for cues to needs and desires, such as gestures, pointing to or looking at objects, pantomime. *Nonverbal cues give meaning to actions.*
• Obtain communication aids for patient's use, such as an alphabet board, slate, pen, paper, or picture board, *to provide alternative communication methods.*
• Use short, simple phrases and yes-or-no questions *to reduce frustration and anxiety.*
• Encourage communication attempts; allow time to select or write words or pictures *to reduce pressure and improve interaction with others.*
• Allow ample time for response; do not answer questions for patient *to reduce frustration.*
• Consult with speech therapist to suggest such communication aids as an artificial larynx. Assist with use. *Appropriate early referral encourages use of communication aids.*
• Demonstrate communication techniques to patient and significant others—such as gestures, sign language, and eye blinking—*to develop alternative communication skills.*
• Assist patient in energy-conserving techniques *to allow maximum breath for speech or use of communication aids.*
• Use tracheostomy plug *to facilitate speech,* if tolerated by patient.
• Provide patient with emergency call system (bell, call light) and respond to all calls immediately and in person. Place a sign over intercom to alert all staff members of need to respond quickly. *Prompt responses reduce patient's fear and anxiety.*
• Encourage attendance at a laryngectomy club or other appropriate support groups *to provide additional support.*

Evaluations for expected outcomes

• Patient consistently communicates needs without frustration.
• Patient successfully uses alternate means of communication (specify).
• Patient uses adaptive equipment _____ times daily to improve communication (specify).
• Patient identifies and contacts appropriate support resources, such as speech therapist or laryngectomy club.

Documentation

• Patient's feelings about inability to communicate
• Observations of patient's attempts to communicate, response to and ability to use alternate communication means, and level of frustration or fatigue
• Patient's response to nursing interventions
• Patient's preferences in daily care activities, such as when to shave or bathe, what kind of razor to use
• Evaluations for each expected outcome.

■ Verbal communication impairment

related to psychological barriers

Definition

Decreased ability to speak, understand, or use words appropriately

Assessment

- Neurologic status, including a history of neurologic disorders, mental status (orientation, level of consciousness, mood or behavior, knowledge and intelligence, vocabulary, and memory), speech (pattern, language, level of comprehension and expression, ability to use other forms of communication, such as gestures, pictures, and drawings)
- Psychological status, including a history of mental or psychiatric disorders, history of alcohol or psychotoxic drug use, stressors, phobias, coping strategies

Defining characteristics

- Difficulty with phonation
- Disorientation
- Flight of ideas
- Inability or lack of desire to speak
- Inability to identify objects
- Inability to modulate speech
- Inability to name words
- Inability to speak dominant language
- Inability to speak in sentences
- Incessant verbalization
- Loose association of ideas
- Stuttering or slurring

Associated medical diagnoses (selected)

Alcohol intoxication, alcohol withdrawal syndrome, Alzheimer's disease, bipolar disease (manic or depressive phase), drug overdose, organic brain syndrome, psychosis, or anxiety states

Expected outcomes

- Patient communicates needs and desires to family, friends, or staff.
- Staff meets patient's needs.
- Patient incurs no injury or harm.
- Patient returns to baseline communication level.
- Patient explains relationship of causative factors—such as alcohol—to inability to communicate effectively.
- Patient begins to make plans to use self-help groups and other resources to improve psychological status.

Interventions and rationales

- Observe patient closely to anticipate needs; for example, restlessness may indicate need to urinate. *Nonverbal cues give meaning to actions.*
- Minimize environmental stimuli and maintain a quiet, nonthreatening environment *to reduce anxiety.*
- Introduce yourself and explain procedures in simple terms. Encourage consistent use of the same terms for common objects. *Treating patient as normal may enhance responsiveness.*
- Encourage communication attempts and allow patient time to say or write words in response *to decrease frustration.*
- Assess patient's communication status daily and record. Match communication needs to interventions: for disorientation, use reality orientation techniques; for manic state, reduce environmental stimuli, talk softly and calmly; for alcohol withdrawal syndrome, reassure patient, do not reinforce presence of hallucinations, provide quiet environment; for a stutterer, use rhythm or song. *Communication status interventions must be tailored to the patient's situation.*
- Determine patient's past interests and habits from family or significant other and discuss them with patient *to stimulate nonthreatening two-way conversation.*
- Maintain a safe environment by using side rails, soft restraint or Posey vest, and other safety measures ac-

cording to established policies, *to protect patient.*
• Refer patient to psychiatric liaison nurse, social services, community agencies, and such self-help groups as Alcoholics Anonymous. *Resolution of communication problems may require long-term follow-up.*

Evaluations for expected outcomes
• Patient consistently communicates needs to staff, family, or friends.
• Patient's basic needs are met.
• Patient does not show signs of neglect, such as weight loss, dehydration, or constipation.
• Patient does not show evidence of falls, such as bruises, contusions, or cuts.
• Patient states name, place, and time.
• Patient describes relationship between causative factors and impaired communication.
• Patient expresses intent to attend self-help groups.
• Patient identifies resources appropriate to resolving underlying psychological problem.

Documentation
• Patient's concern with level of communication
• Observations of patient's needs, communication attempts, orientation, and safety measures
• Interventions carried out to promote communication
• Contributing factors to poor communication and plans to improve psychological status
• Patient's response to nursing interventions
• Evaluations for each expected outcome.

■ Violence, high risk for: Other-directed

related to excitement or antisocial behavior

Definition
Presence of risk factors for other-directed violence

Assessment
• Age
• Sex
• Recent stressors, coping strategies
• Patient history, including health history, substance abuse history (type, effects on mental status), previous episodes of violence (circumstances, behavior, arrests)
• Reactions of family or significant other to episodes of violence
• Mental status examination (with emphasis on insight and judgment)
• Physical findings, including neurologic examination
• Laboratory studies, including EEG, toxicology screening, blood chemistry

Risk factors
• Boasts regarding past abuse of others
• Clenched fists, angry facial expression, threatening posture, tensed muscles
• Inability to voice feelings
• Increased motor activity, pacing, irritability, agitation
• Possession of gun, knife, or other weapon
• Provocative behavior (argumentative, dissatisfied, overreactive, hypersensitive)
• Purposeful destruction of objects in the environment
• Substance abuse or withdrawal

- Suspicion of others
- Threats

Associated medical diagnoses (selected)
Antisocial personality disorder, bipolar disorder (manic phase), intermittent explosive disorder, impulse control disorder, substance abuse disorders

Expected outcomes
- Patient maintains self-control.
- Patient successfully rechannels hostility into socially acceptable behaviors.
- Patient discusses angry feelings and verbalizes ways to tolerate frustration appropriately.
- Patient expresses the need for long-term treatment by appropriate professional.

Interventions and rationales
- Maintain a low level of stimuli in the patient's environment *to avoid increasing agitation and provoking violent behavior.*
- Remove all objects from the environment that the patient could use to injure others *to provide for the patient's safety and protect potential victims of violence.*
- Instruct staff to maintain and convey a calm attitude toward the patient. *Anxiety is contagious and can be transferred to patient. A calm attitude reinforces a feeling of safety.*
- Explain in a firm, calm voice that patient is expected to remain in control. *Communicating an expectation of self-control encourages the patient to take control of behavior.*
- Set limits on the patient's behavior *to reinforce the expectation that the patient will act in a responsible, controlled manner.*
- Express understanding of the patient's feelings and encourage open discusssion *to provide support, reassurance, and positive reinforcement for desirable behaviors.*
- Administer prescribed medications to help patient control aggressive behavior and remain calm. Monitor for effectiveness. *When used appropriately, medications commonly remove the need for physical restraint.*
- According to hospital policy, restrain or seclude the patient, as necessary, *to prevent serious injury to self or others.* Use seclusion or restraint only after less restrictive measures have failed. Both measures require a doctor's order as well as accurate documentation.
- Establish a daily routine of strenuous exercise and encourage the patient to adhere to it. *Exercise provides an alternative way to handle frustration.*
- Encourage patient to gradually begin discussing hostile feelings *to help patient develop more appropriate ways of dealing with hostility.*
- Refer the patient for appropriate long-term treatment—for example, to a drug or alcohol rehabilitation center, psychiatrist, or psychologist. *Patient may require help from specialized professionals or agencies.*

Evaluations for expected outcomes
- Patient behaves in a nonaggressive manner.
- Patient participates in strenuous physical exercise on a daily basis.
- Patient states what precipitates anger and describes the consequences of failing to control it.
- Patient expresses the need for ongoing treatment.

Documentation
- Patient behaviors that indicate escalating agitation; other observations

about patient's verbal and nonverbal behavior
- Factors that precipitate acts of violence
- Nursing interventions performed to reduce or prevent violent behavior
- Nursing interventions performed to ensure safety of other patients and staff
- Patient's behavior in response to nursing interventions
- Referrals to specialized professionals and agencies
- Evaluations for each expected outcome.

Violence, high risk for: Self-directed

related to suicide attempt

Definition

Presence of risk factors for self-directed violence

Assessment

- Age
- Sex
- Medical history
- Patient's life situation
- Recent stressors; coping behaviors
- Available support systems
- History of suicide attempts, including aggressiveness of suicide attempts, lethality of suicide attempts, prior suicide attempts
- History of substance abuse: type, effects on mental status
- Reaction of family or significant other
- Safety hazards
- Mental status, including abstract thinking, affect, content of thought, general information, insight, judgment, mood, orientation, recent and remote memory, thought processes

Risk factors

- Aggressive suicidal behavior
- Angry facial expression
- Direct or indirect statements indicating desire to kill oneself
- Fear of own impulsivity
- Feelings of helplessness, loneliness, hopelessness
- History of previous suicide attempts
- Possession of destructive implements (such as a gun, knife, razor blade, scissors)
- Putting affairs in order—writing will, giving away possessions
- Real or threatened loss of loved one, memory, prestige, job, health
- Severe depression manifested by feelings of helplessness, loneliness, hopelessness
- Substance abuse or withdrawal
- Tense muscles
- Vulnerable self-esteem

Associated medical diagnoses (selected)

Any illness resulting in long-term disability or incapacity (terminal diseases, degenerative diseases, traumatic injury); dementia; major depressive disorder; personality disorders; schizophrenia; substance use disorders

Expected outcomes

- Patient won't harm self in hospital.
- Patient recovers from suicidal episode.
- Patient discusses feelings that precipitated suicide attempt.
- Patient consults mental health professional.
- Patient describes available resources for crisis prevention and management.
- Patient voices improvement in self-worth.

Interventions and rationales

- Ask patient directly: "Have you thought about killing yourself?" If so, "What do you plan to do?" *Suicide risk increases if patient has a definite plan.*
- Remove from patient's environment anything that could be used to inflict further self-injury (razor blades, belts, glass objects, pills). *This helps to ensure patient's safety.*
- Make short-term contract with patient that he will not harm self during a specific time period. Continue negotiating until there is no evidence of suicidal ideation. *A contract gets subject out in the open, places some responsibility for safety on patient, and conveys acceptance of patient as worthwhile person.*
- Supervise administration of prescribed medications. *Medications may be an appropriate alternative to verbal interventions.* Be aware of drug actions and side-effects. Make sure that patient does not hoard medications.
- Provide supervision (one-on-one observation when possible) for the patient based on hospital policy. *This ensures compliance with legal requirements to protect patient and reassures patient of staff concern.*
- Use warm, caring, nonjudgmental manner *to show unconditional positive regard.*
- Listen carefully to patient and don't challenge him *to communicate caring and support.*
- Demonstrate understanding, but don't reinforce denial of current situation *because roots of suicidal feelings can be masked by denial.*
- Make appropriate referrals to mental health professionals *to help patient work through suicidal feelings and develop healthier alternatives.*
- Help patient set a goal for obtaining long-term psychiatric care. *Ambivalence about psychiatric care or refusal to consult with therapist marks suicidal patient's lack of insight and use of denial.*
- Provide patient with telephone numbers and other information about crisis centers, hot lines, counselors, etc. *Alternatives may ease anxiety about perceived threat of long-term psychotherapy.*

Evaluations for expected outcomes

- Patient's environment is free of potential suicide weapons.
- In the aftermath of initial suicide attempt, patient makes commitment not to act upon suicidal thoughts.
- Patient states reasons for suicide attempt.
- Patient contacts mental health professional.
- Patient identifies crisis prevention resources, such as hotline phone number, local crisis center, or name of therapist.
- Patient expresses positive feelings about self.

Documentation

- Patient's comments about the suicide attempt and current feelings about it
- Observations of patient's behavior
- Interventions to reduce or prevent self-destructive behavior
- Patient's observable responses to interventions
- Evaluations for each expected outcome.

Violence, high risk for: Self-directed or directed at others

related to organic brain dysfunction

Definition

Presence of risk factors for self-directed or other-directed violence

Assessment

- History of head trauma or surgery
- Neurologic status, including cognition, computed tomography scan, electroencephalogram, insight and judgment, level of consciousness, memory (recent and remote), motor ability, orientation, sensory ability
- Psychosocial status, including verbalizations (voice quality and tone, speech content, threats), purposeful actions (pounding fists, throwing things), nonpurposeful actions (tremors, facial expressions), coping skills, drug or alcohol use, family or significant other, personality, socialization, stressors

Risk factors

- Anger
- Clinical evidence of organic brain dysfunction
- Disorientation to time, place, person
- Impairment of memory, judgment, and intellectual functioning
- Inability to voice feelings
- Increased anxiety level
- Increased motor activity, pacing, excitement, irritability, agitation
- Overt and aggressive acts—goal-directed destruction of objects in environment
- Self-destructive behavior and active, aggressive, suicidal acts
- Suspicion of others, paranoid ideation, delusions, hallucinations

Associated medical diagnoses (selected)

Alzheimer's disease, anoxic encephalopathy, Korsakoff's psychosis, organic brain syndrome, senile dementia and psychosis, severe head injury

Expected outcomes

- Patient does not harm self.
- Patient does not harm others.
- Patient voices increased feelings of self-esteem.
- Patient remains calm in a secure environment.
- Patient maintains normal sleep-wake cycle.
- Patient expresses feelings in nonviolent and nondestructive manner.
- Family or significant other explains need for safety and protective measures.
- Family or significant other states intent to use support services.

Interventions and rationales

- Provide close supervision and watch for early signs of agitation or increasing anxiety, such as increased motor activity and unreasonable demands. *Early assessment helps to defuse potentially explosive behavior by giving patient chance to find acceptable ways to deal with aggressive tendencies.*
- Use a calm, unhurried approach when communicating, *to reduce patient's sense of lack of control.* Allow patient to express feelings in nonviolent ways, such as beating a pillow, participating in physical exercise, or working with clay. *Patient can successfully release tension when allowed to do so in presence of caregiver.* Put limits on aggressive and potentially violent behavior, *to reinforce expec-*

tation that patient act in responsible, controlled manner.

- Identify and remove from environment stimuli—persons, objects, or situations—that precipitate potentially destructive behavior. *Such stimuli may precipitate aggressive behavior in patients with cognitive and perceptual deficits.*
- Remove from environment anything patient may use to inflict injury to self or others (belt, razor, glass objects) *to ensure patient's safety.*
- Administer and monitor effectiveness of medications prescribed to control aggressive behavior and help patient remain calm. *Medication is least restrictive intervention and helps reduce patient anxiety and need for physical restraints.*
- Restrain or seclude patient as necessary *to prevent serious injury to self or others.* Be sure to follow hospital policy for these procedures, including obtaining doctor's order and providing accurate documentation, *to ensure compliance with the law.*
- Provide reality orientation if patient is confused and disoriented *to allow for more effective staff-patient interaction and help patient learn to distinguish fantasy from reality.*
- Establish a structured daily routine and help patient follow it. *This helps patient focus on reality, participate in positive goal-directed behaviors, and gradually develop self-control.*
- Assess sleep pattern and establish a regular routine to combat sleep deprivation. *Sleep deprivation is characterized by cognitive, perceptual, behavioral, and performance changes (such as increased irritability, restlessness, confusion, disorientation, agitation, delusions, hallucinations).*
- Discuss reasons for safety and protective measures with family or significant other, *to reduce their anxiety and gain their understanding of need for restrictive interventions.*
- Suggest referral to day-care center or sheltered workshop for continuation of psychosocial treatment. Arrange this through social services or home care program *to facilitate appropriate discharge planning and follow-up care.*

Evaluations for expected outcomes

- Patient does not harm self.
- Patient does not harm others.
- Patient expresses positive feelings about self.
- In environment that is free of potentially harmful stimuli, patient demonstrates appropriate mood and nonaggressive behavior.
- Patient sleeps at least _____ hours nightly and remains awake during daylight hours.
- Patient expresses feelings calmly.
- Family member or significant other communicates understanding of need to protect patient from harming self or others.
- Family member or significant other identifies and contacts available social services and support groups.

Documentation

- Patient's statement of intent to harm self or others
- Observations of behavior, precipitating factors, and methods used to control behavior
- Patient's responses to medical regimen and nursing interventions
- Family's or significant other's statement of understanding of protective safety measures (including seclusion or restraint) and need for follow-up
- Evaluations for each expected outcome.

Violence, high risk for: Self-directed or directed at others

related to panic state

Definition

Presence of risk factors for self-directed or other-directed violence

Assessment

- Medical status
- Patient's life situation
- Recent stressors; coping behaviors
- History of chemical dependency (alcohol, drugs)
- History of suicide attempts (aggressive suicide attempts, lethality of suicide attempts, prior suicide attempts)
- Reaction of family or significant other
- History of violent behavior

Risk factors

- Anger (specifically active, aggressive displays of anger)
- Depression
- Fear of self or others
- History of assaults, weapons possession, or arrests
- Inability to verbalize feelings
- Increasing anxiety level
- Provocative behavior (argumentative, dissatisfied, hypersensitive, overreactive)
- Vulnerable self-esteem

Associated medical diagnoses (selected)

Alcohol withdrawal, brain tumor, drug overdose, drug withdrawal, drug-induced psychosis

Expected outcomes

- Patient maintains self-control.
- Patient reports feelings of losing control.
- Patient expresses the need for help.

Interventions and rationales

- Remove all objects that the patient could use to injure self or others *to ensure safe environment.*
- Use short, declarative sentences when talking to patient. Speak in a firm tone of voice. *Calm, direct, and firm approach demonstrates caregiver's control over situation and reduces patient's own sense of lack of control over aggressive impulses.*
- Call patient by name each time you approach *to demonstrate recognition and respect for patient.*
- Assign patient to a room close to the nurse's station *to allow frequent observation, ensure safety, and reassure patient of staff concern.*
- Do not leave patient alone in the bathroom or the shower *to avoid possible injury.*
- Take patient's feelings seriously. *Patient needs to feel that his feelings are valid and accepted without judgment.*
- Allow distance between yourself and patient. Always keep hands visible to allay fears that you have medication or weapon. *A distance of 8' (2.5 m) is considered nonthreatening and appropriate to maintain caregiver's safety.*
- Explain in a firm, calm voice that patient is expected to remain in control *to encourage patient to take control of behavior.*
- Acknowledge that you are aware of patient's potentially violent behavior. *Doing so reduces patient's need to be defensive.*
- Set limits on patient's behavior. Acknowledge understanding of patient's feelings and invite talking. *Limits reinforce expectation that patient act in a responsible manner. Encouraging talking provides reassurance and reinforces desirable behaviors.*

- Employ physical restraint only if "talking the patient down" is not possible and if appropriate assistance from security officers or other co-workers is immediately available. Follow institutional restraint policies. *If other measures fail, restraints may control violent patients.*
- Administer antianxiety or psychotropic drugs and monitor for effectiveness and side effects. *When used appropriately, medications often remove need for physical restraints.*
- Refer the patient for appropriate assistance from a nurse therapist, psychiatrist, alcohol rehabilitation counselor, drug counselor, or psychologist *to ensure continuity of care.*

Evaluations for expected outcomes

- Patient demonstrates appropriate, nonaggressive behavior.
- Patient contacts staff member and reports potential loss of control before acting on impulses.
- Patient expresses need for help from appropriate support resources.

Documentation

- Patient's statements indicating escalating anxiety levels
- Observations of patient's behavior
- Interventions to ensure safety and control
- Patient's response to interventions
- Referrals
- Evaluations for each expected outcome.

P A R T T W O

ADOLESCENT HEALTH

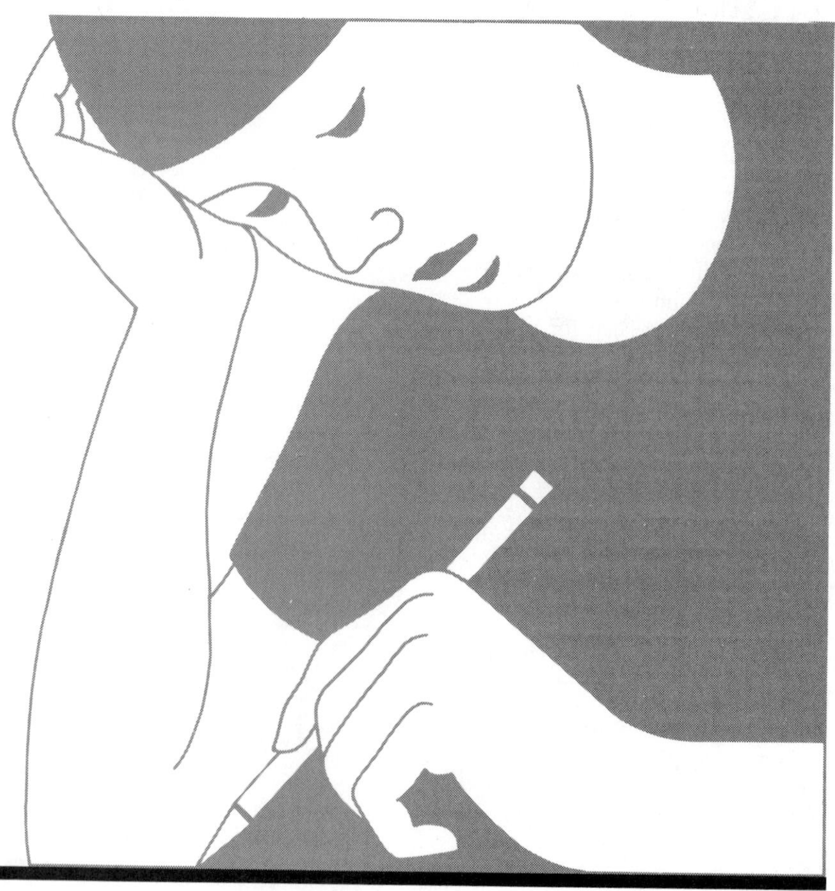

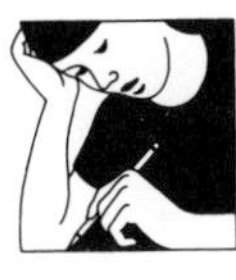

INTRODUCTION

This section focuses on providing nursing care for adolescent patients. The tremendous physiologic and cognitive changes that occur between ages 10 and 18 are commonly accompanied by overpowering emotional turmoil.

The adolescent patient commonly struggles with issues of independence and identity. When taking his history, demonstrate respect for his struggle. Be alert to language; adolescents particularly resent being "talked down to." Let the patient decide the level of parental involvement. While some adolescents prize their independence, others still need parental support during physical examination and history taking. If possible, perform at least part of the nursing assessment in private to allow for open discussion of highly personal issues such as sexuality.

Many adolescents feel invulnerable. This characteristic places them at high risk for such health problems as drug and alcohol abuse, sexually transmitted disease, and trauma. When talking with the patient, explore feelings of personal invulnerability and discuss potential consequences.

When planning interventions, think of ways to foster independence and promote self-esteem while helping the adolescent obtain needed support from parents, health care providers, and others. Refer to plans of care included in the sections on Adult Health and Child Health as well. Use every opportunity to teach the patient about health promotion. Increased knowledge allows the adolescent to assume responsibility for himself.

Adolescence can be a trying time for families as well. In addition to asking direct questions about family relationships, be alert to nonverbal and verbal indications of conflict. Also be aware that parents may be struggling with their child's newfound independence and may need your help as well.

■ Body image disturbance

related to an eating disorder

Definition

Inaccurate self-perception that leads to weight loss in an attempt to conform to an idealized body image

Assessment

- Age, sex
- Health history, including previous eating disorders; dieting; history of physical, emotional, or sexual abuse; episodes of emesis
- Exercise pattern, including type and duration
- Cardiovascular status, including skin color and temperature, heart rate and rhythm, blood pressure, complete blood count
- Nutritional status, including daily food intake, food likes and dislikes, meal preparation, knowledge of dietary requirements; height and weight, weight fluctuations over past year; serum albumin level, lymphocytes, electrolytes
- Psychological status, including expressions of need for control or perceived loss of self-control, behavioral changes, expressions of helplessness, recent emotional crisis, stress, body image
- Perception of ideal feminine form
- Family status, including role performance, perception of role within family
- Use of diuretics and laxatives

Defining characteristics

- Amenorrhea
- Bradycardia
- Change in body structure, body weight, or function
- Decreased blood pressure
- Denial of eating disorder
- Depression, irritability, social isolation
- Dry skin and brittle nails
- Excessive and ritualized exercise
- Excessive need for control of self and environment
- Fear of weight gain
- Hiding body in oversized clothing
- Inability to tolerate cold temperatures
- Lanugo hair
- Lowered body temperature
- Obsession with being organized
- Obsession with food
- Ritualized eating patterns

Associated medical diagnoses (selected)

Amenorrhea, anorexia nervosa, arrhythmias, bulimia nervosa, dehydration, depression, diarrhea, electrolyte imbalance, growth disturbance, malnutrition, tooth enamel erosion

Expected outcomes

- Adolescent complies with prescribed treatment.
- Adolescent expresses feelings associated with food, exercise, weight loss, and medical condition.
- Adolescent expresses understanding of the idea that her eating and exercise patterns are self-destructive.
- Adolescent asks for help in controlling destructive behavior.
- Adolescent participates in decisions about care and treatment.
- Adolescent participates in an eating disorders support group.
- Adolescent expresses insight into the reasons behind her eating patterns and other self-destructive behaviors.
- Adolescent learns and implements new coping behaviors.
- Adolescent expresses positive feelings about self.

• Adolescent expresses satisfaction with parental involvement in care.

Interventions and rationales

• Implement the adolescent's prescribed therapy *to help restore health and body function.*

• Monitor and record the adolescent's vital signs, weight, and electrolytes *to detect abnormal values and prevent complications.*

• Obtain a referral for a dietary consultation *to identify necessary diet modifications and goals for weight-gain and stabilization.*

• Obtain a referral for psychiatric evaluation *to identify problems related to altered body image, poor self-esteem, and difficulty coping.*

• Convey a positive, caring attitude to the adolescent and take steps to ensure continuity of care throughout treatment *to ensure safety and foster a trusting therapeutic relationship.*

• Encourage the adolescent to participate in self-care and, as appropriate, to make decisions about therapy *to foster a sense of control and involvement in restoring health.*

• Tell the adolescent that you accept her as a person and provide reassurance that she can overcome her problems *to validate self-perception and enhance confidence.*

• Maintain communication throughout the adolescent's course of treatment *to assess coping mechanisms and level of self-esteem.*

• Encourage the adolescent to express her feelings about herself, eating, exercise, hospitalization, and medical condition *to correct misconceptions, help the adolescent clarify her thoughts, and reinforce realistic self-appraisal.*

• Reinforce appropriate behaviors *to encourage the adolescent to comply with therapy and to participate in care.* Use behavior modification strategies consistently *to enable the adolescent to predict consequences of behavior.*

• Avoid using coercive techniques to make the adolescent participate in care or adhere to rules. *Use of coercion may encourage the adolescent to view manipulative behavior as acceptable.*

• Monitor food consumption and record intake *to ensure that the prescribed calories are consumed.* Monitor patient in bathroom *to detect episodes of purging.*

• Without conveying an attitude of mistrust, watch for signs of noncompliance. Emphasize that the prescribed caloric intake is necessary to maintain health and won't lead to obesity. *This promotes early detection of self-destructive behavior and may improve the adolescent's sense of control.*

• Inform the adolescent of her progress throughout hospitalization *to increase her awareness of achievements and motivate her to keep trying.*

• Help the adolescent to identify positive aspects of her appearance *to improve self-esteem by correcting her distorted perceptions about her body.*

• Help direct the adolescent's need for control away from body image and eating behaviors by encouraging her participation in appropriate diversional activities *to channel her energies into new areas in which she can take pride.*

• Encourage her participation in group discussions with peers who also have eating disorders *to foster insight and group support.*

• Discuss coping strategies used effectively in the past *to help the adolescent identify appropriate coping strategies.*

• Encourage parents to demonstrate emotional support for the patient throughout her course of treatment *to strengthen the family support system.*
• Encourage parents to participate in a support group with other parents of children with eating disorders *to provide a forum for expressing feelings and obtaining support from individuals who can understand their concerns.*
• Teach parents how to detect signs that their child may be relapsing into self-destructive behaviors *to help them identify the need for early assistance and enhance confidence in their ability to protect their child from harm.*

Evaluations for expected outcomes
• Adolescent complies with prescribed treatment regimen.
• Adolescent expresses feelings associated with food, exercise, weight loss, and medical condition.
• Adolescent describes her perception of personal daily caloric needs.
• Adolescent expresses understanding of the idea that her eating and exercise patterns are self-destructive.
• Adolescent asks for help in controlling destructive behavior.
• Adolescent participates in decisions related to care and treatment.
• Adolescent consumes an appropriate number of calories each day.
• Adolescent participates in an eating disorders support group.
• Adolescent expresses insight into the reasons behind her eating patterns and other self-destructive behaviors.
• Adolescent learns and implements new coping behaviors.
• Adolescent expresses positive feelings about self.
• Adolescent expresses satisfaction with parental involvement in care.

Documentation
• Vital signs
• Weight (recorded daily or weekly according to agency protocol)
• Amount of food consumed at each meal
• Adolescent's description of herself
• Observations of rituals related to food and exercise
• Participation in and response to support group
• Observations of self-destructive behaviors, such as forced emesis or use of laxatives or diuretics
• Observations of manipulative behaviors
• Coping mechanisms
• Exercise patterns
• Behavior modification techniques used by caregivers
• Response to nursing interventions
• Evidence of changes in adolescent's self-perception
• Evaluations for each expected outcome.

■ Caregiver role strain, high risk for

related to developmental state

Definition
Adolescent's inability to meet developmental needs due to responsibilities to act as caregiver

Assessment
• Adolescent caregiver's physical and mental status, including age, sex, and developmental stage; level of cognitive functioning; emotional functioning; self-care abilities
• Care recipient's physical and mental status, including age, sex, illness, self-care limitations, mobility limitations, level of cognitive functioning,

relation to adolescent (parent, sibling, other)
- Available resources, including finances, emotional support system, community services, and health-related services, such as geriatric day care, home health aids
- Home environment, including structural barriers, layout of home, need for medical equipment or devices, availability of transportation
- Cultural, ethnic, and religious background
- Perceived and actual obligations of the adolescent
- Effect of caregiver responsibilities on adolescent
- Adolescent's coping skills, problem-solving abilities, ability to participate in hobbies and preferred activities

Risk factors

Adolescent caregiver:
- caregiver duties that hinder ability to meet personal developmental needs and to perform usual tasks such as schoolwork
- codependence and evidence of dysfunctional coping behaviors within the family
- conflicting role commitments
- drug or alcohol addiction
- lack of preparation for demands of caring for parent or younger sibling
- lack of respite and recreation
- limited financial resources
- poor coping skills

Care recipient:
- cognitive deficits secondary to illness
- drug or alcohol addiction
- home environment poorly adapted to daily needs
- necessity for prolonged care
- severe, unstable, or unpredictable course of illness
- sudden, profound disability

Associated medical diagnoses (selected)

This diagnosis may occur in any chronic illness or disability. Examples include acquired immunodeficiency syndrome (AIDS); Alzheimer's disease; amyotrophic lateral sclerosis; cancer; cerebrovascular accident; cerebral palsy; chronic obstructive pulmonary disease; congestive heart failure; dementia; drug or alcohol addiction; end-stage renal, cardiac, or pulmonary disease; Huntington's disease; macular degeneration; muscular dystrophy; multiple sclerosis; paralysis; Parkinson's disease; and schizophrenia.

Expected outcomes
- Adolescent identifies current stressors.
- Adolescent identifies and implements adaptive coping strategies.
- Adolescent identifies personal developmental needs and tasks.
- Adolescent contacts sources of support to help provide care.
- Adolescent allots time each day for respite, recreation, and personal development activities.
- Adolescent reports a reduction in stress related to performing caregiver duties.

Interventions and rationales
- Assess the developmental stage and needs of the adolescent caregiver *to provide a basis for developing interventions that reduce caregiver role strain. During adolescence, individuals begin establishing their identity by trying various roles without assuming complete responsibility for them. The imposed role of caregiver impedes this developmental task.*
- Help the adolescent identify current stressors. Discuss how her responsibility to act as caregiver places limits

on her lifestyle *to evaluate the degree of caregiver role strain.*
- Encourage the adolescent to discuss coping skills used to manage stress in the past *to reinforce her confidence in her ability to manage the current situation and explore new ways to apply coping strategies.*
- Help the adolescent identify informal sources of support, such as family members, support groups, or church groups, that can help with caregiver tasks *to provide opportunities for respite.*
- Teach the adolescent about formal sources of support, such as home health care agencies, social workers, doctors, clinics, and day care centers, *to allow the adolescent to fulfill other obligations, such as attending school.*
- Urge the adolescent to participate in enjoyable activities, such as sports, hobbies, reading, or social gatherings, *to encourage her to take needed breaks from caregiver responsibilities.*
- Provide the adolescent with information about available support groups and encourage her to participate. *Support groups provide an outlet for expressing feelings and foster a sense of support and belonging.*
- Assess the adolescent's view of her responsibilities as caregiver and correct any misconceptions. *Often, the caregiver's perspective may be clouded by emotional ties to the care recipient, confusion about roles within the family, or codependence. Your input may help her develop a more objective view of the situation.*

Evaluations for expected outcomes
- Adolescent describes her emotional response to stressors in her life.
- Adolescent identifies and uses adaptive coping strategies.
- Adolescent uses available support systems.
- Adolescent schedules respite periods for personal developmental needs and recreation.
- Adolescent distinguishes between actual and perceived caregiver responsibilities.

Documentation
- Care recipient's physical and mental status and adolescent's responsibility for providing care
- Current stressors identified by the adolescent
- Risk factors (developmental, situational, psychological, and pathophysiologic) for caregiver role strain
- Statements by the adolescent indicating her intention to take actions to minimize stress, such as joining support groups, seeking help from support services, scheduling respite
- Observations of the adolescent's response to stress
- Coping strategies identified by the adolescent and nurse
- Referrals provided
- Evaluations for each expected outcome.

Decisional conflict

related to sexual activity

Definition
Uncertainty about whether to engage in sexual activity

Assessment
- Age, sex
- Developmental stage, including physical maturity, cognition, beliefs, values, ethics

- Family system, including nuclear family, extended family, birth order, family roles, evidence of conflict
- History of sexual experiences, including experimentation, trauma
- Psychological status, including level of function, coping mechanisms, support systems, self-image, self-esteem, attitude toward physical appearance
- Sociocultural status, including level of education, ethnic group, religious affiliation
- Sexual orientation

Defining characteristics
- Lack of knowledge or indifference about possible consequences of sexual activity
- Need for peer approval
- Perceived peer pressure to have sex
- Poor self-esteem
- Signs of anxiety, distress, fear, uncertainty (expressed or behavioral)
- Vacillating decisions about sexual behavior

Associated medical diagnoses (selected)
Anorexia, anxiety disorders, bulimia, depression, obesity, personality disorders, pregnancy, psychiatric disorders, sexually transmitted diseases, substance abuse

Expected outcomes
- Adolescent expresses feelings about sexuality and sexual activity.
- Adolescent discusses conflicts between personal values and social pressures to be sexually active.
- Adolescent identifies desirable and undesirable consequences of sexual activity.
- Adolescent describes family conflicts and explores their potential effect on sexual conduct.
- Adolescent accepts help from parents, family, friends, and health professionals.
- Adolescent reports confidence in choosing sexual behavior that's consistent with personal values.

Interventions and rationales
- Visit the adolescent frequently and encourage frequent visits by family members *to promote a trusting therapeutic relationship and ease anxiety and fears.*
- Encourage expression of feelings about social and sexual patterns *to improve recognition of feelings and foster an open discussion.*
- Assess the adolescent's knowledge of sex and sexuality. Discuss sexual behavior and its potential consequences. Provide information about safer sex practices and birth control. Mention abstinence as an option. *Correct information about sexual practices reduces the adolescent's confusion about whether or not to be sexually active.*
- Listen attentively and remain nonjudgmental as the adolescent describes personal fears, values, and desires. *Nonjudgmental, active listening demonstrates your unconditional positive regard for the adolescent.*
- Provide guidance as the adolescent explores options for sexual activity *to promote confidence in decision-making capabilities.*
- Discuss peer pressure. Ask the adolescent if she feels strong social pressure to be sexually active. In what other ways do peers exert an influence? Explore ways of coping with peer pressure. *Peer pressure is a reality that each adolescent must learn to deal with.*
- Discuss family conflicts. Ask the adolescent if she feels troubled family relationships are pushing her to

become sexually active. *Adolescents may seek in sexual relationships the love they can't obtain from family members.*

- Respect the adolescent's right to make choices based upon her personal values, desires, religious beliefs, cultural norms, and sexual preference *to foster autonomy and self-confidence.*
- Help the adolescent identify a support network (friends, family, community services, church or synagogue groups) and encourage her to use this network when making decisions. *An effective support system provides an emotional underpinning and helps the adolescent make decisions and resolve conflicts.*

Evaluations for expected outcomes

- Adolescent expresses feelings related to sexuality and sexual activity.
- Adolescent describes conflicts between her personal values and social pressure to become sexually active.
- Adolescent discusses possible influences, including peer pressure and conflicts with her family, on her decision to be sexually active.
- Adolescent expresses increased understanding of her options regarding sexual activity and their potential consequences.
- Adolescent identifies a support network and uses it to aid decision making.
- Adolescent reports feeling more comfortable with her ability to make decisions regarding sexuality and sexual activity.

Documentation

- Statements indicating the presence of conflict over the decision of whether to be sexually active
- Adolescent's cognitive, emotional, and behavioral levels of functioning
- Adolescent's knowledge of birth control and safer sex practices
- Nursing interventions to help adolescent make choices regarding sexuality and sexual conflict
- Response to interventions
- Evaluations for each expected outcome.

Decisional conflict

related to substance use

Definition

State of uncertainty about a health-related course of action; in this case, whether to use recreational drugs

Assessment

- Age, sex
- Developmental and cognitive state
- Physical maturity
- Sociocultural factors, including level of education, financial status, ethnic group
- Family history, including family roles, coping patterns, family's ability to meet patient's physical and emotional needs, history of substance abuse in family members
- Level of functioning (cognitive, emotional, behavioral)
- Coping mechanisms
- Available support systems
- Evidence of drug use, including drug toxicology screening, urinalysis, personality changes, social withdrawal

Defining characteristics

- Evidence of experimentation with drugs
- Expressed feelings of indestructibility
- Expressions of distress related to uncertainty about drug use

- Expressions of fear related to consequences of drug use
- Indifference toward risks associated with substance abuse
- Need for peer approval and conformity
- Signs of distress, tension, and fear

Associated medical diagnoses (selected)
This diagnosis commonly accompanies any diagnosis related to substance abuse or psychiatric illness and may coincide with many other diagnoses.

Expected outcomes
- Adolescent discusses conflict over drug use.
- Adolescent describes conflict between personal values and options and external value systems (parental, societal, peer, legal).
- Adolescent identifies perceived desirable and undesirable consequences of drug use.
- Adolescent accepts assistance from parents, other family members, friends, and health care providers.
- Adolescent reports increased comfort with making choices that are consistent with personal values.

Interventions and rationales
- Visit the adolescent frequently. Schedule a specific amount of noncare-related time each day for visits *to promote trust and provide a time when the adolescent can discuss his feelings confidentially.*
- Make the adolescent aware that you are willing to discuss all topics, including substance use. Reassure him that all information will be kept confidential *to encourage an honest discussion of concerns.*
- Encourage the adolescent to explore feelings related to drug use, school, family, friends, and other vital topics. Remain nonjudgmental and be willing to listen to his values, beliefs, and concerns *to demonstrate that you regard him as a worthwhile person with valid values and beliefs.*
- Ask the adolescent to describe his family and home life *to assess for family conflict that may be creating emotional distress.* Provide referrals for family counseling if needed.
- Ask the adolescent if he experiences peer pressure to use drugs. Explore ways of coping with peer pressure. *Peer pressure is a reality that all adolescents must learn to cope with.*
- Discuss self-esteem and explore ways of building self-esteem *to strengthen the adolescent's ability to deal with peer pressure.*
- Help the adolescent explore alternative recreational activities, such as sports, art, music, community service, or participation in church or synagogue groups, *to help him develop alternatives to substance use.*
- Teach the adolescent about the health and legal consequences of substance use and abuse. *Accurate information will help him make informed, rational decisions.*
- Encourage the adolescent to identify and use support systems, such as family, friends, clinics, the school nurse, or other health care providers. *A support network and emotional support are important tools in resolving conflicts.*
- Refer the adolescent for long-term counseling if necessary. *Long-standing emotional conflicts may require in-depth intervention.*

Evaluations for expected outcomes
- Adolescent discusses conflict over whether to use drugs.
- Adolescent identifies health and legal consequences of drug use.

- Adolescent discusses peer pressure, family conflict, or other factors that may be influencing him to use drugs.
- Adolescent identifies available sources of emotional support and requests help if needed.
- Adolescent reports increased self-esteem and ability to deal with peer pressure.

Documentation
- Evidence of drug use
- Adolescent's stated feeling about drug use
- Adolescent's level of functioning (cognitive, emotional, behavioral)
- Interventions performed to help adolescent make choices regarding drug use
- Response to interventions
- Evaluations for each expected outcome.

Health maintenance alteration

related to management of insulin-dependent diabetes mellitus

Definition
Lack of knowledge or motivation regarding health practices, in this case adolescent's failure to properly manage insulin-dependent diabetes mellitus

Assessment
- Age, sex
- Developmental stage, including cognitive abilities and physical maturity
- Level of knowledge about insulin-dependent diabetes mellitus, routine health practices, preventive needs and safety measures, treatment and follow-up
- Level of motivation to perform self-care
- Current health status, including height, weight, recent illnesses; adolescent's perception of personal health status
- Social status, including lifestyle, activity level, sports, interests, and socioeconomic status
- Family health history, including history of diabetes mellitus

Defining characteristics
- Disregard for consequences of failing to manage insulin-dependent diabetes mellitus
- Inability or unwillingness to self-administer medication, maintain a proper diet, or identify signs and symptoms of hypoglycemia, hyperglycemia, or ketosis
- Lack of familiarity with available community resources
- Lack of knowledge about importance of diet, exercise, or medication regimen in management of insulin-dependent diabetes mellitus

Associated medical diagnoses (selected)
Insulin-dependent diabetes mellitus

Expected outcomes
- Adolescent describes feelings about self-management of insulin-dependent diabetes mellitus.
- Adolescent describes the disease process.
- Adolescent describes the influence of peer pressure on his health care practices.
- Adolescent describes proper techniques for managing signs and symptoms of hypoglycemia or hyperglycemia and ketosis.
- Adolescent demonstrates ability to perform self-care activities, such as properly administering insulin and choosing appropriate foods.

- Adolescent does not exhibit signs or symptoms of hypoglycemia, hyperglycemia, or ketosis.

Interventions and rationales

- Evaluate the adolescent's understanding of insulin-dependent diabetes mellitus and his attitude about the need to manage it. *This will help you determine which teaching interventions are needed.*
- Correct any misconceptions he may have regarding insulin-dependent diabetes mellitus and the therapeutic regimen. Use teaching materials appropriate for his age *to increase his knowledge of his condition and instill confidence in his ability to manage it.*
- Discuss issues surrounding peer pressure. Ask the adolescent if he feels social pressure causes him to ignore his diet or avoid self-administering insulin. Discuss how and where he carries out his diabetes regimen; explore such issues as timing, privacy, stigma, and adverse effects. Ask if he feels embarrassed about his disorder. Explore ways of coping with peer pressure. *Peer pressure is a reality that each adolescent must learn to deal with.*
- Teach the adolescent how to interpret glycosylated hemoglobin results and correlate these values with the degree of metabolic control *to increase autonomy and decision making skills.*
- Observe the adolescent as he performs self-care activities *to assess his skills and overall progress.*
- Provide the adolescent with written materials that cover each teaching topic. *These materials help reinforce learning now and can refresh the adolescent's memory later.*
- Describe resources available to help the adolescent manage his disorder. Consider arranging a visit with the hospital dietitian or diabetes counselor *to reinforce teaching.*
- Work with the adolescent to develop an exercise plan *to prevent hypoglycemia.* The plan should identify a support person capable of assisting during a hypoglycemic episode and include the following steps:
  - obtaining blood glucose level before and after exercise
  - consuming extra food before exercise (if blood glucose level is between 80 and 180 mg/dl) in the form of carbohydrates
  - abstaining from strenuous exercise if blood glucose level is elevated
  - wearing a medical identification bracelet
  - carrying quick-acting sugar in case hypoglycemia occurs.

These measures ensure the adolescent's safety while allowing him to participate in activity.

- Discuss how to manage diabetes during illness. For example, explain that infections may lead to hyperglycemia or ketosis and that early detection of infection can reduce the severity of these episodes. Also, fever, nausea, vomiting, or diarrhea require modifications in the prescribed diet, such as substituting juice for raw fruits. Teach the adolescent to check over-the-counter medications, such as cold remedies, for sugar content and to avoid products with high levels of sugar. Finally, explain the importance of following the prescribed regimen for increasing insulin dosage in relation to blood glucose test results. *These measures help provide a sense of control, ensure safety, and prevent complications.*
- Teach the adolescent to recognize signs that must be reported to his doctor *to improve management skills and ensure safety.*

• Discuss possible complications, for example, atherosclerosis, which most commonly affects the eyes, kidneys, and lower extremities, and diabetic neuropathy, which may lead to loss of sensation, function, and paraesthesia. *Early understanding of possible major complications may encourage adherence to the prescribed regimen.*
• Encourage adolescent to contact a support group sponsored by the Juvenile Diabetes Association *to provide peer support.*

Evaluations for expected outcomes
• Adolescent demonstrates techniques for managing insulin-dependent diabetes mellitus.
• Adolescent describes signs and symptoms of hypoglycemia, hyperglycemia, and ketosis, and how to manage these conditions.
• Adolescent demonstrates proficiency in self-care activities, including administering insulin and selecting foods.
• Adolescent discusses the influence of peer pressure on his health care practices.
• Adolescent accurately describes the disease process of insulin-dependent diabetes mellitus.
• Adolescent does not exhibit signs or symptoms of hypoglycemia, hyperglycemia, or ketosis.

Documentation
• Adolescent's statements indicating his understanding of insulin-dependent diabetes mellitus, health-promoting activities, management techniques during exercise and illness, and necessary self-care skills
• Adolescent's statements indicating disregard for the consequences of failing to properly manage insulin-dependent diabetes
• Response to interventions
• Literature provided to the adolescent about managing his disorder
• Observations of adolescent's demonstrations of self-care techniques
• Referrals to community resources or hospital services
• Evaluations for each expected outcome.

■ Poisoning, high risk for

related to substance abuse

Definition
Accentuated risk of accidental ingestion of drugs, alcohol, or other potentially hazardous substances in doses sufficient to cause poisoning

Assessment
• Age, sex
• Developmental stage including cognition and physical maturity
• Medication history (prescribed and over-the-counter [OTC] medications)
• Physical status, including evidence or history of renal or hepatic impairment, eating disorders, substance abuse
• Family status, including living arrangement, family dynamics, history or current evidence of substance abuse, financial status
• Social status, including peer group and related social pressures, level of activity
• Knowledge of risks associated with use of drugs, alcohol, or other potentially hazardous substances (such as fumes from glue, nitrous oxide propellants, or lighter fuel gases)
• Psychological status, including evidence of depression or a depressive disorder, feelings of isolation, history

of attempted suicide, level of self-esteem
- Results of laboratory tests

Risk factors
- Access to drugs (prescribed, OTC, or illicit) and alcohol
- Adolescent developmental stage and cognition
- Experimentation with potentially hazardous substances, such as prescribed or illicit drugs, alcohol, glue fumes, or lighter fuel gases
- Expressed feelings of indestructibility
- Family rules (or neglect) that allows the adolescent an inappropriate degree of independence in decision making and activities
- Family system in which most of adolescent's significant relationships are outside the family
- History of psychiatric disorder
- Low self-esteem, confused self-concept
- Multiple stressors caused by dysfunctional family dynamics
- Personal or familial history of substance abuse
- Poor understanding of the potentially lethal effects of drug and alcohol abuse
- Pressure to conform to peer norms (developmental need to be accepted)
- Suicide ideation, threats, or attempts

Associated medical diagnoses (selected)
Depressive disorders, renal or hepatic impairment, substance abuse disorders

Expected outcomes
- Adolescent expresses understanding of the harmful and potentially lethal effects of substance abuse.
- Adolescent remains free from injury during hospital stay.
- Adolescent identifies stressors and feelings that precipitate episodes of substance abuse.
- Adolescent takes only appropriate doses of prescribed medications at designated times.

Interventions and rationales
- Follow the medical regimen to treat toxicity or other injury caused by substance abuse *to ensure the adolescent's safety and promote recovery.*
- Teach the adolescent about the harmful and potentially lethal effects of abusing drugs, alcohol, or other dangerous substances *to enhance his knowledge, which may help him make better informed decisions.* Provide him with appropriate written materials. *Written materials reinforce teaching and can be reviewed after discharge.*
- Help the adolescent identify stressors, such as depression, peer pressure, or family dysfunction, that may precipitate substance abuse *to provide a basis for developing strategies to prevent future episodes of abuse.*
- Describe the resources available in the community to help prevent or treat substance abuse. *Support services and groups can provide the adolescent with safe settings in which to explore feelings and develop methods of coping with them.*
- For adolescents receiving prescribed medication, explain the reason for the medication. Discuss administration techniques, schedule, dosage, cautions, and possible adverse effects *to promote compliance with the medication regimen.*

Evaluations for expected outcomes
- Adolescent describes the harmful and potentially lethal effects of substance abuse.

• Adolescent remains free from toxicity caused by the use of drugs, alcohol, or other hazardous substances.
• Adolescent describes the stressors and feelings that precipitate episodes of substance abuse.
• Adolescent demonstrates two or more constructive techniques for coping with stressors, such as depression, peer pressure, and family dysfunction.
• Adolescent describes his prescribed medication regimen, including dosage and administration schedule, and demonstrates compliance.
• Adolescent describes available community resources and expresses intention to contact appropriate support services.

Documentation
• Interventions to treat toxicity or other injury
• Factors that increase the adolescent's risk of drug toxicity
• Knowledge deficits and learning objectives
• Teaching topics, materials, and methods
• Response to nursing interventions
• Indications that the adolescent is using adaptive techniques to cope with stress, anxiety, peer pressure, dysfunctional family
• Referrals to community resources or professionals for counseling
• Evaluations for each expected outcome.

■ Self-esteem disturbance

related to problematic relationship with parents

Definition
Presence of conflict with parents that disturbs the adolescent's sense of self-esteem.

Assessment
• Age, sex
• Level of education
• Family history, including marital status of parents, financial status, family rules, ability of family to modify rules, consequences when rules are broken, how family members communicate, quality of communication, methods of conflict resolution, family alliances, family stability, ability of family to meet adolescent's physical and emotional needs, disparities between adolescent's needs and family's ability to meet them
• Goals and values, including extent to which family permits adolescent to pursue his own goals and values
• Family genogram
• Parental status, including level of education, knowledge of normal growth and development, ability to agree on appropriate discipline, stability of parental relationship, understanding of adolescent's self-esteem disturbance
• Adolescent's psychological status, including changes in appetite, energy level, motivation, personal hygiene, self-image, self-esteem, sleep patterns; alcohol or drug abuse; reaction to puberty; quality of relationships with authority figures, scholastic performance

Defining characteristics

- Disagreement between adolescent and parents on family rules
- Financial stress or abusive or chaotic family environment
- Frequent fights or arguments between adolescent and parents
- Inability of family members to communicate or to resolve conflicts
- Inability of family members to recognize adolescent's emotional, physical, and social needs or to help him meet them
- Lack of appropriate boundaries between family members
- Lack of flexibility in family rules and rigid consequences when rules are broken
- Parental discord or lack of knowledge of normal growth and development in children

Associated medical diagnoses (selected)

Communication disorders, conduct disorder, learning disabilities, mood disorders, oppositional defiant disorder, post-traumatic stress disorder

Expected outcomes

- Adolescent and parents describe areas of conflict.
- Adolescent begins to openly express feelings to family members.
- Parents encourage and support adolescent's attempt at expression of feelings.
- Adolescent describes his own positive qualities.
- Parents describe positive qualities of their adolescent child and of the family unit.
- Parents and adolescent state plans for continued outpatient family treatment.

Interventions and rationales

- Provide a secure, structured environment for adolescent and parents *to foster open discussion of family conflicts.*
- Educate all family members about the schedule, purpose, and goals of individual and family treatment. *Awareness of the expectations and rationale for treatment will enhance cooperation.*
- Encourage the adolescent to participate in group activities, group therapy, and individual counseling *to provide opportunities for him to develop enhanced self-esteem.*
- Encourage the adolescent to express feelings directly, by using "I" statements, such as "I'm mad because of my curfew." *Such statements help him get in touch with and talk about feelings.*
- Tell the parents that their child is learning to express his feelings directly. *Because family communication patterns are deeply ingrained, the parents may need time to adjust to their child's assertiveness.*
- Assist the parents in understanding the value of talking about feelings *to encourage them to express emotions appropriately and to discourage them from punishing their child for expressing his feelings toward them.*
- Provide a small notebook in which the adolescent can write down positive events as they occur *to encourage him to focus on his strengths and enhance self-esteem.*
- Teach the parents to reward and praise the adolescent for expressing his feelings appropriately *to encourage them to focus on the child's strengths and to strengthen the entire family system.*
- Use role-playing to teach the adolescent different ways to respond to specific family conflicts. *This will help him develop problem-solving and negotiating skills.*

- Communicate with the outpatient clinician *to plan continued treatment for the family.*
- Emphasize to the adolescent and his parents the need for continued support and family therapy after discharge *to enhance compliance.*

Evaluations for expected outcomes
- Adolescent and parents begin to talk about difficulties at home.
- Adolescent and parents identify how they feel during times of conflict.
- Adolescent begins to express feelings directly.
- Parents attend family therapy and educational groups.
- Adolescent participates in group activities and individual and family therapy.
- Adolescent and family agree to participate in outpatient treatment.
- Adolescent uses more positive statements when talking about himself and family.
- Parents make positive statements about adolescent and the family as a whole.

Documentation
- Specific family conflicts as described by adolescent and parents
- Adolescent's and parents' behavior when interacting with each other
- Nursing interventions to facilitate family communication and expression of feelings
- Frequency of family visits and family therapy appointments
- Adolescent's description of his own strengths
- Referrals for continued treatment following discharge
- Evaluations for each expected outcome.

■ Social isolation

related to behavior that fails to conform to social norms

Definition
Negatively perceived loneliness imposed by oneself or others

Assessment
- Age, sex
- Developmental stage
- Level of education
- Reason for hospitalization (physiologic, psychiatric)
- Attitudes of family, friends, teachers, and other important individuals toward the adolescent
- Available support systems
- Factors contributing to social isolation, including delayed physical development, immaturity, altered mental status, changes in behavior or cognition, illness, history of trauma
- Self-esteem
- Coping and problem-solving ability
- Evidence of substance abuse
- Current and past stressors
- Sociocultural factors, including ethnic and religious background

Defining characteristics
- Culturally unacceptable behaviors
- Delayed physical development
- Drug or alcohol addiction or withdrawal
- Dysfunctional family
- Expressions of feeling different, rejected, or alone
- History of physical or sexual abuse
- Inappropriate or immature activities for developmental stage
- Insecurity in public
- Poor interpersonal skills (possibly because of language barriers or auditory or visual impairment)

- Poor self-esteem and self-concept
- Preoccupation with own thoughts (may include narcissism or suicidal ideation)

Associated medical diagnoses (selected)
May accompany any medical diagnoses requiring hospitalization, thereby separating the adolescent from his usual environment. Other associated disorders include attention deficit hyperactivity disorder, drug or alcohol addiction or withdrawal, conduct disorder, depression, panic or anxiety attacks, phobias, and sensory or motor impairment.

Expected outcomes
- Adolescent expresses feelings of social isolation.
- Adolescent identifies causes of social isolation.
- Adolescent participates in planning social activities.
- Adolescent identifies personal behaviors that are considered socially unacceptable.
- Adolescent demonstrates behaviors that are more socially acceptable.
- Adolescent exhibits effective interpersonal communication skills.
- Adolescent interacts with family, staff, and visitors using newly learned behavioral and communication skills.
- Adolescent reports feeling less isolated as social interaction improves.
- Adolescent reports improved sense of self-esteem.

Interventions and rationales
- Assign the adolescent a primary nurse *to enhance continuity of care, establish a trusting relationship, and provide an opportunity to practice developing a one-on-one relationship.*
- Arrange uninterrupted, non-care-related time to talk with the adolescent during each visit. Listen to his concerns and feelings. Provide honest feedback (positive and negative) about his behavior *to encourage appropriate behaviors and reinforce his awareness of inappropriate ones. Feedback is essential to behavior modification.*
- Provide guidance as the adolescent explores possible causes for his sense of social isolation. Help him identify inappropriate behaviors, and teach him ways to improve communication and interpersonal skills *to foster socially acceptable behavior. Once the adolescent becomes aware of the connection between unacceptable behavior patterns and his feelings of isolation, he may be more willing to learn new skills and behaviors.*
- Make a contract with the adolescent that requires him to demonstrate a new behavior within a specific period of time. Reward successful changes in behavior. *Contracts can enhance self-esteem by giving the adolescent responsibility for making changes and allowing adequate time in which to practice new behavior and communication skills without fear of criticism if he falls short. Successful completion of a contract provides positive reinforcement.*
- Demonstrate appropriate communication skills and behaviors in all interactions with the adolescent *to provide him with an example of appropriate behavior and reinforce teaching concepts.*
- Engage the adolescent in role-playing activities that simulate social situations. Provide encouragement and positive reinforcement and avoid criticism *to provide an opportunity to rehearse new skills in a safe environment, which reduces anxiety and boosts self-confidence.*

• Encourage participation in group activities and one-on-one interaction with staff. *Gradual increases in social interaction help reduce the adolescent's feelings of social isolation and instill confidence in newly developed communication and interpersonal skills.*
• Talk to the adolescent about community resources, such as social services or support groups, that can provide ongoing support. Provide names, addresses, and phone numbers whenever possible. *This provides the adolescent with ongoing opportunities for social interaction in a supportive environment.*

Evaluations for expected outcomes
• Adolescent expresses feelings of social isolation and a desire for help.
• Adolescent identifies personal behaviors that are socially unacceptable and acknowledges that changes are necessary.
• Adolescent expresses understanding of the relationship between unacceptable behavior and feelings of social isolation.
• Adolescent demonstrates appropriate behavior and communication skills.
• Adolescent reports increased social interaction and decreased feelings of isolation.
• Adolescent states intention to participate in support group or use community resources to increase social activity.

Documentation
• Observations of adolescent's behavior and communication skills
• Adolescent's description of reasons for impaired social interaction
• Nursing interventions to promote behavior modification and improved socialization
• Adolescent's responses to interventions
• Resources and referrals provided to the adolescent or family members
• Evaluations for each expected outcome.

Trauma, high risk for

related to feelings of personal invulnerability

Definition
Accentuated risk of accidental tissue injury such as burns or fractures

Assessment
• Age, sex
• Level of education
• Developmental factors, including tendency to test independence, tendency to take risks (especially in company of peers), feelings of indestructibility, high level of energy, need for peer approval, access to potential safety hazards (such as complex machinery or tools, farm equipment, car, motorcycle, jet-ski, skimobile)
• Health history, including allergies, sports accidents, auditory or visual impairments, seizure disorders
• Social history, including academic performance, sports, hobbies, social activities, job
• Neurologic status, including level of consciousness, orientation

Risk factors
• Access to alcohol, drugs (prescription, over-the-counter, illicit), poisons, or other toxic substances
• Access to vehicles
• Adolescent developmental stage and level of maturity

- Frequent unsupervised activities with peers
- History of chronic or periodic substance abuse
- Lack of experience operating a car, motorcycle, or other vehicle and poor understanding of safety issues related to operating a vehicle
- Participation in contact sports
- Use of complex power tools or machinery (work, school, or home)

Associated medical diagnoses (selected)
Acute head injury, alcohol or drug overdose, burns, fractures, psychiatric disorders, seizure disorders, spinal cord injury, substance abuse

Expected outcomes
- Adolescent recovers from injury while in hospital.
- Adolescent does not experience additional injury while in hospital.
- Adolescent expresses understanding of appropriate safety precautions (for example, obeying speed limits, following fire prevention precautions, never driving while intoxicated, wearing helmets or seat belts, using protective clothing or equipment).
- Adolescent states intention to adopt appropriate safety precautions.

Interventions and rationales
- Follow the medical regimen to treat the adolescent's injury *to promote recovery.*
- Document risk factors and unsafe practices discovered through observation or through discussions with the adolescent *to plan effective interventions.*
- Select teaching topics that will help the adolescent prevent future injuries and promote personal health, for example, automotive and motorcycle safety, proper use of protective equipment in sports, or alcohol and drug awareness. *Teaching the patient relevant topics increases his knowledge and reinforces the notion that he is responsible for ensuring personal safety.*
- Demonstrate use of appropriate safety equipment, such as protective sports gear, and have the adolescent perform return demonstration *to reinforce learning.*
- Include the adolescent's parents or guardian in teaching sessions. *If properly informed, family and friends can help the adolescent improve safety practices.*

Evaluations for expected outcomes
- Adolescent recovers from existing injuries, if present.
- Adolescent remains free from further injury during hospital stay.
- Adolescent identifies risks and behaviors that should be avoided.
- Adolescent describes appropriate safety precautions.
- Adolescent demonstrates proper use of safety devices and equipment as appropriate (for example, protective sports gear, seat belt, motorcycle helmet).

Documentation
- Adolescent's statements indicating lack of awareness of or disregard for safety practices
- Physical findings
- Observations of unsafe practices
- Medical treatment for existing injuries
- Nursing interventions to reduce the adolescent's risk of future injury
- Response to interventions
- Evaluations for each expected outcome.

■ Violence, high risk for: Self-directed

related to suicidal thoughts, threats, or behavior

Definition

Presence of risk factors for deliberate, self-directed violence

Assessment

- Age, sex
- Developmental stage
- Mood and affect, including persistent depression; feelings of worthlessness, hopelessness, helplessness, isolation, inadequacy, humiliation; feeling of rejection by peers and social group; flat, distant, or remote affect
- Behavioral changes, including loss of interest in personal appearance, loss of interest in hobbies and preferred activities, overeating or eating too little, deterioration in schoolwork, refusal to attend school (cutting class, truancy), acting out (sexual permissiveness, delinquency, running away), low level of energy, sleep disturbances, frequent naps, irritability, frequent somatic complaints, social withdrawal and isolation, antisocial or self-destructive behavior, tendency to be accident prone, acts of self-mutilation
- Availability of weapons
- Preoccupation with death, threats of suicide, history of suicidal or self-destructive behavior
- Reaction to puberty and sexuality
- Recent crisis, trauma, or losses

Risk factors

- Access to a lethal weapon
- Crises concerning sexual development
- Dysfunctional family
- Excessive stress and anxiety
- Expressed or implied statements indicating a desire to commit suicide
- Fear of own impulsiveness
- Feelings of worthlessness, hopelessness, loneliness, helplessness
- History of substance abuse
- History of suicide attempts
- Low self-esteem
- Poor impulse control
- Real or perceived threatened loss of important person or possession
- Recent stressful event, such as parents' divorce or death in family
- Recent suicide of a close friend or relative
- Severe depression
- Substance abuse or withdrawal

Associated medical diagnoses (selected)

Any illness resulting in long-term or permanent disability or incapacity (terminal diseases, degenerative diseases, traumatic injury); major depressive disorders; personality disorders; schizophrenia; substance abuse or withdrawal

Expected outcomes

- Adolescent does not harm himself while in hospital.
- Adolescent recovers from suicidal episode.
- Adolescent discusses feelings that precipitated suicide attempt.
- Adolescent attends therapy sessions with a mental health professional.
- Adolescent describes available resources for crisis prevention and management.
- Adolescent reports improved feelings of self-worth.

Interventions and rationales

- Take all suicide threats seriously. *Early intervention reduces the likelihood of a suicide attempt.*

• Ask the adolescent directly, "Have you thought about killing yourself?" If so, ask, "What do you plan to do?" *The suicide risk increases if the adolescent has a definite plan.*
• Remove any objects in the environment that the adolescent could use to injure himself, for example, razors, belts, glass objects, and pills, *to ensure his safety.*
• Arrange supervision (preferably one-on-one) for the adolescent according to hospital policy. *This ensures compliance with legal requirements to protect the adolescent while demonstrating staff concern.*
• Make a contract with the adolescent that he will not harm himself for a specific period of time. Continue negotiating until there is no evidence of suicidal ideation. *A contract puts the subject of suicide out in the open, places some responsibility for safety on the adolescent, and demonstrates your regard for the adolescent as a worthwhile person.*
• Supervise the administration of all prescribed medications, and be aware of their actions and possible adverse effects. *Medications may be a treatment alternative. By monitoring administration, you prevent the adolescent from hoarding doses, sometimes called "cheeking."*
• Convey a caring and nonjudgmental attitude when talking with the adolescent. *This demonstrates your unconditional positive regard and helps establish a trusting relationship.*
• Listen carefully to the adolescent as he talks without challenging his statements *to communicate caring, support, and understanding and encourage expression of feelings.*
• Be careful not to reinforce adolescent's denial of the current situation. *Denial commonly masks underlying suicidal feelings.*
• Encourage the adolescent to set a goal of cooperating with psychiatric intervention. *Ambivalence about psychiatric care or refusal to attend sessions indicates that the adolescent is still in denial.*
• Provide the adolescent and members of his family with telephone numbers for crisis prevention centers, counselors, and other community support services. *Having many alternatives for support helps reduce the adolescent's anxiety.*

Evaluations for expected outcomes
• Adolescent's environment is free from hazards.
• Adolescent does not harm himself during hospital stay.
• Adolescent enters into contract with nurse not to harm himself for a specific period of time.
• Adolescent discusses feelings and reasons for attempting suicide.
• Adolescent attends counseling sessions with mental health professionals.
• Adolescent describes crisis prevention resources, such as hot-line telephone number, local crisis center, or name of therapist.
• Adolescent expresses an improved sense of self-esteem.

Documentation
• Adolescent's description of his feelings
• Observations of the adolescent's behavior, mood, and affect
• Statements or behavior indicating suicide risk
• Nursing interventions to reduce or prevent self-destructive behavior
• Response to interventions
• Evaluations for each expected outcome.

P A R T   T H R E E

CHILD HEALTH

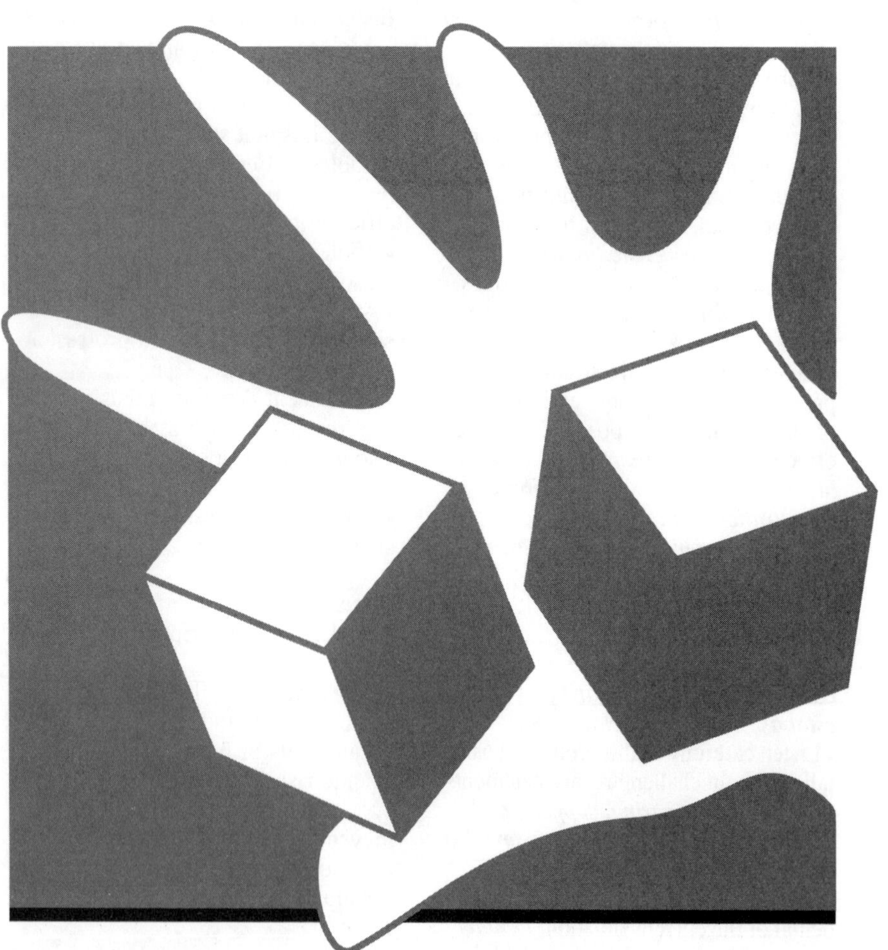

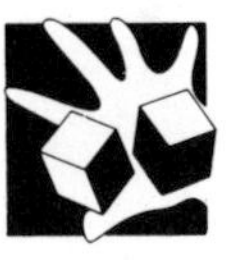

INTRODUCTION

This section focuses on providing care for children, helping them maintain optimal health and achieve their full developmental potential. Your first task is to establish rapport with the child and family under your care. When talking to the child, show understanding and use simple language. If he's frightened, turning portions of your examination into a game may help to calm him. Talk to the child about toys, hobbies, or other subjects of interest and be generous with compliments.

Your plan of care should emphasize working with the entire family. Obtaining accurate assessment information, for example, usually requires the cooperation and trust of family members.

During each stage of growth and development, the child must master specific physical, cognitive, and developmental tasks. Assessment should include an evaluation of the child's growth and developmental level as well as an examination of body systems. Other assessment factors include family roles and relationships, parenting style, stressors, coping patterns, religion, cultural background, living conditions, and financial status. You'll also want to explore how the child and family members perceive the health problem.

After analyzing the assessment data, you'll formulate nursing diagnoses. Your diagnoses should state the child's actual health problems or health problems for which the child is at risk; they may take into account physiologic, psychosocial, or cognitive aspects of the child's well-being. Your nursing plan of care will stem from these diagnoses.

When developing interventions, include steps to encourage the child and family members to participate in care. Some families may need to be encouraged to simply ask questions about the child's status; others may want to become involved in treatment-related decisions. To foster participation, be sensitive to the family's values, ideas, and beliefs. Provide referrals to appropriate social service agencies and other community resources. Keep in mind that your ultimate goal is to make the child and family as self-sufficient as possible in managing the health problem.

Periodically evaluate the child's and family's progress as you implement your plan of care. If you carefully monitor the effectiveness of interventions, necessary revisions to the plan of care will become readily apparent.

Aspiration, high risk for

related to absence of protective mechanisms

Definition

State of being at risk for aspiration of secretions, food, or fluids into tracheobronchial passages

Assessment

- Respiratory status, including rate, depth and pattern of respiration, auscultation of breath sounds, frequency and effectiveness of cough, ability to handle secretions, palpation for fremitus, percussion of lung fields, sputum characteristics (color, consistency, amount, odor)
- Neurologic status, including mental status, level of consciousness
- GI status, including presence or absence of gag and swallowing reflex, gastroesophageal reflux, continuous or intermittent tube feedings
- Diagnostic studies, including arterial blood gas (ABG) levels, chest X-rays, continuous cardiorespiratory monitoring

Risk factors

- Abdominal pain
- Abnormal ABG levels
- Anxiety
- Apprehension
- Bolus tube feeding
- Chest pain
- Choking and gasping for air
- Copious oral secretions (saliva, blood)
- Coughing
- Decreased level of consciousness
- Dehydration
- Depressed cough, gag, or swallowing reflexes
- Dyspnea
- Fever
- GI reflux
- Grunting
- Hiccups
- Increased abdominal girth (with or without vomiting)
- Lack of motor skills (related to developmental delay or age, such as neonate unable to turn head to side)
- Nasal flaring
- Oxygen deficit (mottling, cyanosis, nasal flaring, chest or sternal retractions)
- Pursed lip breathing
- Respiratory infection
- Restlessness
- Sudden drop in heart rate
- Tachypnea
- Use of accessory muscles
- Vomiting (projectile, prolonged, episodic)

Associated medical diagnoses (selected)

Airway obstruction, cardiac arrest, cerebrovascular accident, chest or abdominal surgery, chest trauma, cleft lip or palate, drug intoxication, gastroesophageal reflux, head or neck trauma, hydrocarbon ingestion, neuromuscular diseases or injury, poisoning, postanesthesia recovery, respiratory arrest, tracheoesophageal fistula

Expected outcomes

- Auscultation reveals clear breath sounds.
- Auscultation reveals presence of bowel sounds.
- Child maintains a patent airway.
- Child's pulmonary function remains within normal limits.
- Family members demonstrate measures to prevent aspiration.
- Respiratory rate remains within normal limits for age.
- Family members describe plan for home care, for example, removing

indigestible objects from child's reach.

Interventions and rationales

- Assess child for gag and swallowing reflex. *Impaired reflexes may cause aspiration.*
- Assess respiratory status at least every 4 hours or according to established standards; begin cardiopulmonary monitoring *to detect signs of possible aspiration (increased respiratory rate, cough, sputum production, diminished breath sounds).*
- Auscultate bowel sounds every 4 hours and report changes. *Delayed gastric emptying may cause regurgitation of stomach contents.*
- Elevate head of bed or place child in Fowler's position *to aid breathing.*
- Help child to turn, cough, and deep-breathe every 2 to 4 hours. Perform postural drainage, percussion, and vibration every 4 hours or as ordered. Use suctioning as needed to stimulate cough and clear upper and lower airways. *These measures promote drainage of secretions and full expansion of lungs.*
- Perform chest physiotherapy before feeding child *to decrease risk of emesis leading to aspiration.*
- Hold infant with head elevated during feeding and position in infant seat after feeding. *This position uses gravity to prevent regurgitation of stomach contents and facilitates lung expansion.*
- Recognize progression of airway compromise and report findings *to detect complications early.*
- Encourage fluids within prescribed restrictions. Provide humidification as ordered (such as oxygen tent, nebulizer). *Fluids and humidification liquefy secretions.*
- Place child in lateral or prone position. Change child's position at least every 2 hours *to reduce potential for aspiration by allowing secretions and blood to drain.*
- Instruct child and family members in home care plan. *Child and family members must demonstrate ability to ensure adequate home care before discharge.*

Evaluations for expected outcomes

- Auscultation reveals clear breath sounds.
- Auscultation reveals presence of bowel sounds.
- Family members demonstrate measures to prevent aspiration in child, for example, correct positioning of infant during and after feeding.
- Child breathes easily and does not show signs of respiratory distress.
- Child does not show signs of respiratory infection.
- Respiratory rate remains within normal limits for age.
- Child coughs effectively.
- Child maintains airway patency.

Documentation

- Child's ability to handle oral secretions and feedings
- Observation of respiratory status and response to treatment regimen
- Child's and family members' abilities to carry out home care plan
- Evaluations for each expected outcome.

Body image disturbance

related to alterations in health or invasive medical procedures

Definition

Negative perception of self that interferes with healthful functioning

Assessment
- Physiologic changes in child
- Behavioral changes
- Child's and family members' perceptions of health problem
- Child's developmental stage
- Child's eating pattern, sleeping pattern, usual play activities

Defining characteristics
- Change in child's body structure or functioning
- Immature reasoning with regard to changes in body structure or functioning.
- Loss of body part
- Verbal or nonverbal response to actual or perceived changes in body structure or function

Associated medical diagnoses (selected)
Burns; conditions requiring colostomy, ileostomy, or ileal conduit; congenital anomalies or disease resulting in disfigurement; diabetes mellitus; eating disorders; limb amputation; oncologic disorders; orthopedic disorders including scoliosis and orthopedic conditions requiring casting; trauma

Expected outcomes
- Child acknowledges change in body appearance or function.
- Child expresses positive feelings about self.
- Family members acknowledge change in child's appearance or body functioning and verbalize acceptance of child.

Interventions and rationales
- Hold, rock, or touch child frequently *to give child an awareness of body integrity.*
- Provide opportunity for child to interact with peers who have experienced a similar health problem *to decrease child's feelings of isolation and sense of being different from others.*
- Give child as much freedom as possible. If restraints are called for, use minimum restraint necessary to prevent injury. *Providing the least restrictive environment enhances child's control over surroundings and provides the opportunity to release feelings through physical activity.*
- Explain medical procedures in age-appropriate language. For child under age 7, use dolls and actual medical equipment to describe procedure. *Children in the preoperational stage of development understand best by seeing and manipulating objects.* For older child, use body diagrams to illustrate what changes will and will not appear in body as a result of medical treatment or disease progression. *Illustration is one technique to reinforce learning.*
- For a young child, cover injection sites with adhesive bandages. *A child in the preoperational stage of development may hold the misconception that injections create holes which allow blood to drain out. Adhesive bandages may help reinforce child's sense of body integrity.*
- Encourage young child to participate in play activities *to allow child to act out feelings that he may not have the verbal or cognitive skills to express.*
- Set aside time with older school-age child or adolescent to discuss feelings *to assesss perceptions, clarify misconceptions, and provide an opportunity to ventilate emotions.*
- Ensure privacy during procedures *to accommodate the heightened sense of modesty that children develop beginning in the early school-age years.*
- Encourage family members to express feelings and concerns about changes in child's body appearance

or function. Provide accurate information and answer questions thoroughly. *Encouraging open discussion enables you to provide emotional support and may help ease family members' anxiety.*

Evaluations for expected outcomes
- Child and family members express understanding of changes in the child's body.
- Child expresses positive feelings about self.
- Family members verbalize positive feelings about child and display warmth and affection by holding, comforting, and hugging child as appropriate for child's age.

Documentation
- Child's statements about appearance
- Family members' statements about changes in child's body structure or function
- Account of child's behavior during medical procedures and in play activities
- Observations of family members' behavior toward child and participation in care
- Evaluations for each expected outcome.

■ Body temperature alteration, high risk for

related to dehydration

Definition
State of being at risk for failure to maintain body temperature within normal range

Assessment
- Age
- Vital signs, including pattern of termperature fluctuation
- Hydration status, including mucous membranes, skin turgor, fontanels (in infants)
- Respiratory status, including respiratory rate and depth, dyspnea, use of accessory muscles
- Neurologic health history, including seizures, cerebrospinal fluid infection, abscess, hemorrhage, history of trauma or cranial surgery
- Nutritional status, including decreased intake, vomiting
- Medical history, including effects of drugs or toxins
- Evidence of disturbance in temperature-regulating centers of brain

Risk factors
- Age
- Alteration in metabolic rate
- Dehydration
- Immature temperature-regulating system
- Vigorous activity

Associated medical diagnoses (selected)
Acute viral illnesses; burns; dehydration; cystic fibrosis; eczema; endocrine disorders; GI disorders, such as pyloric stenosis, colitis, or gastroenteritis; head injury; heat stroke; inadequate clotting factors; leukemia; psoriasis; respiratory disease; septic conditions; sunburn; trauma

Expected outcomes
- Child maintains body temperature of 98.6° to 99.5° F (37° C to 37.5° C).
- Child maintains weight within 5% of baseline.
- Child's intake and output are balanced and within normal limits for age.
- Urine specific gravity remains between 1.005 and 1.015.

Interventions and rationales
- Assess child's temperature every 4 hours. Use temperature-taking method appropriate for child's age and size (rectal or axillary for infant or toddler; axillary or oral for preschooler; oral for school-age child or adolescent). *Prolonged elevation of temperature above 104° F (40° C) may produce dehydration and harmful central nervous system effects.*
- Weigh child daily every morning and record results. *A decrease in weight may indicate dehydration.*
- Maintain adequate fluid intake by offering small amounts of flavored fluids at frequent intervals; record intake and output every shift. *A fever increases child's fluid requirements by increasing the metabolic rate. High-calorie liquids, such as colas, fruit juices, and flavored water sweetened with corn syrup, help prevent dehydration.*
- Administer antipyretics as ordered and monitor effectiveness. *Antipyretics act on the hypothalamus to regulate body temperature.*
- Check and record urine specific gravity with each voiding. *Urine specific gravity increases with dehydration. Adequate urine output and urine specific gravity between 1.010 and 1.015 indicates sufficient hydration for children and adolescents.*
- Give tepid sponge bath *to increase vaporization from skin and decrease body temperature.*
- Teach parents to dress child in lightweight clothing when child's body temperature is elevated *to allow perspiration to evaporate, thereby releasing body heat.*

Evaluations for expected outcomes
- Child maintains body temperature of 98.6° to 99.5° F.
- Child maintains baseline weight.
- Child's intake and output are balanced and within normal limits for age.
- Child maintains urine specific gravity of 1.010 to 1.015.

Documentation
- Observation of physical findings
- Nursing interventions, including administration of medications
- Child's body temperature (recorded every 4 hours)
- Child's weight, urine output, and urine specific gravity
- Child's response (behavioral, cognitive, physiologic) to interventions, including administration of antipyretics
- Evaluations for each expected outcome.

Breathing pattern, ineffective

related to decreased energy or fatigue

Definition
Change in rate, depth, or pattern of breathing that alters normal gas exchange

Assessment
- Age
- Allergies
- History of respiratory disorders
- Respiratory status, including rate and depth of respiration, symmetry of chest expansion, use of accessory muscles, nasal flaring, presence of cough, anterior-posterior chest diameter, palpation for fremitus, percussion of lung fields, auscultation of breath sounds, pulmonary function studies, arterial blood gas (ABG) monitoring, pulse oximetry readings

• Cardiovascular status, including history of congenital or acquired heart disease
• Neurologic status, including mental status, level of consciousness
• Emotional well-being
• Knowledge, including understanding of physical condition; physical, mental, and emotional readiness to learn

Defining characteristics
• ABG abnormalities
• Apneic episodes
• Clubbing of fingers and toes
• Cough
• Cyanosis
• Dyspnea
• ECG abnormalities
• Irritability
• Nasal flaring
• Respiratory depth changes
• Restlessness
• Retractions
• Rhinitis
• Tachycardia
• Tachypnea
• Verbal reports of air hunger, fatigue, anxiety

Associated medical diagnoses (selected)
Anemia, asthma, chronic obstructive pulmonary disease, congestive heart failure, congenital heart disease, metabolic acidosis, postoperative conditions, premature birth, rheumatic heart disease, severe burns, viral or bacterial infection

Expected outcomes
• Ausculation reveals no abnormal breath sounds.
• Child's oxygen saturation (SaO_2) level remains above 95%.
• Child's respiratory rate remains within normal limits for age.
• Child demonstrates adequate breathing pattern, with easy, unlabored respirations.
• Child or family member requests oxygen administration, airway suctioning, and other assistance, as needed.
• Child participates in age-appropriate play activities without increased respiratory difficulty.
• Family members develop effective plan of care for child's return home.

Interventions and rationales
• Assess respiratory rate and depth every 2 to 4 hours; monitor for nasal flaring, chest retractions, and cyanosis *to detect early signs of respiratory compromise*.
• Monitor ABG values and pulse oximetry readings *to evaluate oxygenation and ventilation status*.
• Auscultate breath sounds every 2 to 4 hours *to detect decreased or adventitious breath sounds*; report changes.
• Administer oxygen, as ordered, *to help reduce hypoxemia and relieve respiratory distress.*
• Force fluids *to liquefy secretions and prevent dehydration related to increased respiratory rate.*
• Provide nebulizer treatment, vaporizer, or mist tent, as ordered, *to liquefy secretions.*
• Provide postural drainage and chest percussion every 4 hours before meals *to facilitate removal of secretions.*
• Suction the airway, as needed, *to remove secretions*.
• Place the child in Fowler's position, raising the head of the bed. Place an overbed table padded with a pillow in front of the child and have him extend his arms over the table *to promote lung expansion.*

• Remain with the child and offer reassurance during periods of respiratory difficulty *to relieve anxiety.*
• Administer bronchodilators and antibiotics as ordered. *Dilation of the bronchus allows greater passageway for air. Antibiotics treat infection.* Monitor effectiveness and check for adverse reactions *to ensure safety and efficacy of therapy.*
• Prohibit parents and other visitors from smoking in the child's room; explain why. *Smoking depletes a room of its natural oxygen supply and poses a serious fire hazard in a room with oxygen equipment.*
• Schedule necessary care activities to provide frequent rest periods *to prevent fatigue and reduce oxygen demand.* Allow for adequate play time. *For children of all ages, play is an integral part of growth and development.*
• Assist with activities of daily living, as necessary, *to help the child conserve energy and avoid fatigue.*
• Identify the child's developmental level and select appropriate teaching methods. For a preschooler or early school-age child, use stuffed animals, puppets, and drawings. *Preschoolers use sensory experiences to understand information.* For older school-age child, use demonstration and audiovisual materials, such as body outline. *Children in this age-group have the ability to think logically, but not abstractly.* With an adolescent, encourage individual and group discussion and provide written and audiovisual materials. *Adolescents can more readily absorb abstract concepts and learn from a variety of sources.*
• Limit the number of new skills taught each day according to the child's age and ability. Teach preschooler one skill per day; school-age child, two skills per day; adolescent, three or more skills per day. *Limiting daily teaching avoids overloading the child with new information and enhances learning.*
• Teach the child:
  – pursed-lip breathing
  – abdominal breathing
  – relaxation techniques.

These measures allow the child to participate in maintaining health status and to improve ventilation.
• Discuss with the child and family members ways to conserve energy while carrying out daily routine *to prepare the child for discharge from hospital.*
• Help the family plan for care at home. Discuss medication administration, use of assistive equipment, and available community resources. Also discuss signs and symptoms of complications and when to report them. *Increasing family's knowledge improves likelihood of compliance with medical treatment, thereby decreasing risk of recurrence of breathing problem.*

Evaluations for expected outcomes
• Child's respiratory status remains within normal limits for age.
• Pulse oximetry readings reveal SaO_2 above 95%.
• Child and family members express understanding of respiratory problems.
• Child demonstrates correct technique in pursed-lip breathing, abdominal breathing, and relaxation techniques.
• Family members demonstrate correct technique in medication administration, oxygen administration, and suctioning.
• Child's ABG values remain within set limits.

- Child participates in age-appropriate play activities without increased respiratory difficulty.
- Family members describe plan of care to be implemented upon child's return home.

Documentation
- Child's expressions of comfort in breathing
- Child's and family members' understanding of medical diagnosis and readiness to learn
- Child's and family members' responses to teaching
- Physical findings from pulmonary assessment
- Interventions performed and child's and family members' responses to them
- Evaluations for each expected outcome.

Coping, ineffective family

related to prolonged illness

Definition
Destructive behavior on the part of family members during a child's prolonged illness

Assessment
- Child's illness, including severity, duration, and impact on family
- Family process, including number and ages of children, usual patterns of interaction, roles of parents and children, communication patterns, relationship changes (separation, divorce, remarriage), past response to crisis
- Family members' understanding of child's present health status
- Family resources (financial, social, spiritual)
- Parental status, including perception of child's behavior, past responses to stress, child care provisions, history of inappropriate parenting, history of destructive behavior or substance abuse
- Alteration in child's growth and development resulting from illness or dysfunctional parenting
- Transportation limitations, including geographic distances to health resources

Defining characteristics
- Absence of appropriate parenting; parents' inability to provide for basic needs of child
- Behavioral problems or other evidence of children's delayed psychosocial development
- Behavior by family members that indicates lack of concern for one another
- Family members' descriptions or confirmations of incidences of abuse
- Family members' inappropriate responses to stressful situations
- Family members' reports of high number of accidents
- Poor communication among family members
- Role confusion and inconsistency
- Suspiciousness of outsiders

Associated medical diagnoses (selected)
Burns, cancer, chromosomal abnormalities, chronic endocrine disorders, chronic renal disorders, chronic respiratory disorders, congenital anomalies, degenerative disease, developmental disabilities, neuromuscular disorders, trauma

Expected outcomes
- Family members identify factors that trigger stress and inappropriate behavior.

- Family members make use of appropriate sources of support.
- Family members interact appropriately with staff and each other.
- Parents meet the developmental needs of their children.
- Family members express feelings and individual needs.
- Children meet developmental milestones appropriate for age.
- Family members identify measures to meet each others' emotional needs.
- Child's health care needs are met.

Interventions and rationales

- Assess family history *to identify family's strengths and limitations.*
- Determine if family members are prepared to accept help. *Changes in behavior will not take place until family members are ready.*
- Communicate only brief amounts of information at any one time. *Family members under stress often cannot grasp large amounts of information.*
- Help family identify which tasks to tackle now and which can wait until stress level decreases. *Performing easy, familiar activities decreases discomfort during times of stress.*
- Encourage family members to allow open expression of feelings and to avoid passing judgment on one another. *Family members need to be able to communicate openly without putting each other on the defensive.*
- Identify instances of successful communication among family members *to single out and encourage positive behavior.*
- Use play activity to promote self-esteem in children. *Parents frequently forget the developmental needs of children during a crisis. If one child is seriously ill, parents may ignore siblings.*
- Help family members identify situations that trigger inappropriate behavior. *Family members must learn to recognize their tolerance threshold to react appropriately.*
- Help family members identify coping mechanisms used successfully in the past *to enable them to develop appropriate responses without learning new behaviors.*
- Help family members identify options when confronted with difficult decisions. *Members of dysfunctional families commonly believe they lack choices.*
- Teach parents about the health care and developmental needs of their child. *Family-centered care is essential for an ill child.*
- Provide referral to appropriate social service agencies *to help family members find additional resources.*

Evaluations for expected outcomes

- Parents and children state specific factors that lead to inappropriate behavior.
- Family members state their plans for contacting sources of support.
- Family members interact with appropriate verbal and nonverbal behavior.
- Children display appropriate behavior and coping mechanisms.
- Family members meet each others' emotional needs when appropriate.
- Family members meet health care needs of chronically ill child.
- Children show evidence of achieving age-appropriate developmental tasks.
- Family members describe incidents that reveal an increased ability to solve problems independently.

Documentation

- Observation of family members' interactions with each other and with outsiders
- Observations of family members' reactions to stress
- Examples of communication between family members
- Parents' understanding of normal childhood growth and development
- Interventions performed to help improve family members' coping skills
- Family members' level of participation in care of ill child
- Referrals to community resources
- Evaluations for each expected outcome.

Diarrhea

related to malabsorption or inflammation or irritation of bowel

Definition

Alteration of normal elimination pattern characterized by frequent, loose stools

Assessment

- History of bowel disorder or surgery
- GI status, including nausea and vomiting, usual bowel patterns, changes to bowel patterns, stool characteristics (color, amount, consistency, presence of blood or mucous), pain, inspection of abdomen, ausculatation of bowel sounds, palpation for masses and tenderness
- Medication history, including use of antibiotics
- Nutritional status, including dietary intake, appetite, weight, changes to usual diet
- Fluid and electrolyte status, including intake and output, urine specific gravity, skin turgor, mucous membranes, serum potassium and sodium
- Skin integrity

Defining characteristics

- Abdominal pain
- Dehydration
- Fever associated with fluid loss and inflammation
- Increased frequency and mass of stools
- Loose stools
- Redness, irritation, and abnormal skin turgor in perianal area

Associated medical diagnoses (selected)

Crohn's disease, gastroenteritis, lactose intolerance, salmonellosis, shigella, short-bowel syndrome, ulcerative colitis

Expected outcomes

- Child exhibits normal elimination pattern for age.
- Child's intake and output are balanced and within normal limits for age.
- Auscultation reveals normal bowel sounds.
- Child's body temperature remains normal.
- Child's urine specific gravity is between 1.005 and 1.015.
- Child's skin remains intact.
- Caregivers demonstrate appropriate skin care techniques.

Interventions and rationales

- Assess frequency and characteristics of stool, and ausculate bowel sounds every 4 hours, *to monitor effectiveness of treatment.*
- Monitor and record intake and output; urine specific gravity (with each voiding); skin turgor; condition of mucous membranes; presence of tears; and condition of fontanels (in

infants) *to monitor hydration status and need for fluid replacement.*
- Record daily weight before first feeding each morning *to determine if child is suffering from dehydration. Weight loss of 5% or more in the course of a day may indicate dehydration.*
- As ordered, offer oral replacement solution such as Pedialyte or clear liquids in small amounts (5 to 15 ml) every 10 to 15 minutes, waiting 20 to 30 minutes after voiding of a loose stool, *to decrease intestinal irritation and likelihood of further diarrhea.*
- Do not offer fruit juices or carbonated fluids. *The high glucose content and osmolar load associated with these beverages may stimulate further episodes of diarrhea.*
- Offer child BRAT diet (bananas, rice, apple, toast) 4 hours after last loose stool *to help meet child's nutritional needs without exacerbating diarrhea.*
- Check skin in perianal area after each stool. Change diaper frequently and clean skin thoroughly *to prevent skin breakdown.*
- Apply protective ointment to diaper area *to provide a barrier between child's skin and stool.*
- Monitor child's temperature every 2 to 4 hours *to detect fever, which may be associated with fluid loss and inflammation.* Measure temperature using axillary or oral routes *because use of rectal thermometer may stimulate further diarrhea.*
- Teach caregivers importance of frequent diaper changes and meticulous skin care for child. Instruct them not to use powder in diaper area *to avoid caking and subsequent skin breakdown.*

Evaluations for expected outcomes
- Child regains normal elimination pattern.
- Child's intake and output are balanced and within normal limits for age.
- Auscultation reveals normal bowel sounds.
- Child remains afebrile.
- Child's urine specific gravity remains between 1.005 and 1.015.
- Child's skin remains intact, without signs of redness or irritation.
- Caregivers demonstrate appropriate skin care techniques.

Documentation
- Frequency and characteristics of stool
- Appearance of skin
- Intake and output
- Weight (recorded daily)
- Evidence of caregivers' knowledge of dietary management and skin care techniques
- Evaluations for each expected outcome.

Diversional activity deficit

related to long-term hospitalization, isolation, or absence of family

Definition
Restriction or decrease in child's ability to use unoccupied time to advantage or satisfaction

Assessment
- Level of comfort, including mobility, activity tolerance
- Cardiovascular status
- Respiratory status
- Neurologic status, including level of consciousness, orientation, mood, behavior, memory, coordination

- Psychosocial status, including presence of family members, social interaction, cultural and ethnic background, hobbies, interests, changes or adaptations needed to carry out activities
- Environment, including isolation, availability of diversional activities
- Developmental level (physical, cognitive, psychosocial, linguistic), learning needs

Defining characteristics
- Few or no visitors
- Hospital stay beyond acute stage of illness; frequent, lengthy tests or treatments
- Irritability, moodiness, inactivity
- Isolation with limited ability to leave room
- Lack of age-appropriate toys at the bedside
- Physical limitations affecting participation in usual activities
- Statements of boredom or wishing for something to do

Associated medical diagnoses (selected)
This diagnosis can occur in any child hospitalized for a prolonged period. Associated conditions include bronchopulmonary dysplasia requiring mechanical ventilation, burns, cancer requiring chemotherapy or bone marrow transplant, communicable diseases requiring isolation, cystic fibrosis requiring I.V. antibiotic therapy, fractures requiring traction, scoliosis repair.

Expected outcomes
- Child selects and participates in age-appropriate play.
- Child expresses enjoyment in selected play activity.
- Child achieves developmental tasks appropriate to age.

Interventions and rationales
- Provide various toys, supplies, and activities for the child's use. Items should be appropriate to the child's age, developmental level, and environment. *Ready access to diversional activities entices the child to make use of time alone. Age-appropriate items are geared to the child's cognitive, motor, and safety needs.*
- Encourage family members to bring the child's favorite toys, family pictures, or other objects from home. Provide space in the child's room for cards and gifts from family and friends. Encourage parents to tape-record stories for their child, and provide a tape player so the child can listen in the hospital *to maintain sense of attachment to family and provide a sense of security.*
- Encourage the child to visit playroom and participate in individual and group activities. *Participating in play activities will help child meet developmental needs.*
- Discuss the child's diversional activity deficit with the play therapist *to enable the play therapist to better address the child's special needs.*
- Schedule time to personally engage the child in therapeutic or developmental play. Play periods should be scheduled for both day and evening shifts. *This ensures that the child has ample opportunity for diversional activity and prevents the child from being isolated for prolonged periods. Participation in play will also strengthen your relationship with the child.*
- For the child confined to bed, provide creative, challenging games. For example, make a fishing pole with a large safe hook, and challenge the child to pick up items around the room; glue Velcro on soft balls and create a "dart board" on the wall;

make string-and-paper-cup "telephones" to use with other patients in the room. *Creative play encourages age-appropriate behavior, helps make the environment more enjoyable and challenging, and gives the child greater control and independence.*
- Provide the child with opportunities for therapeutic play. For example, encourage the child to play with safe hospital equipment, play nurse or doctor, play house, pound clay, or perform "procedures" on a doll. *Therapeutic play offers the child an opportunity to express fears, fantasies, sadness, and misconceptions; to learn more about the illness and its treatment; and to safely release pent-up feelings. This helps the child develop a better sense of control and enhances the ability to cope with hospitalization and treatment.*
- Provide art and craft supplies for the preschool or school-age child *to enhance the child's creativity, provide an emotional outlet, and encourage development of initative and industry.*
- Provide group activities for an adolescent *to help him learn how his peers are coping with hospitalization and to meet developmental need for peer identity. Participation in group activities may help reduce stress and lessen feelings of isolation and loneliness.*

Evaluations for expected outcomes
- Child voluntarily participates in selected activities.
- Child seeks diversional activities during leisure time.
- Child expresses contentment with activities.
- Child develops increased understanding of treatments.
- Child expresses feelings associated with hospitalization.
- Child achieves age-appropriate developmental milestones.

Documentation
- Child's expression of boredom and desire for activity
- Assessment of child's physical, cognitive, and psychosocial developmental abilities
- Evaluation of child's physical, educational, and psychosocial need for activity
- Nursing interventions directed at providing diversional activity
- Child's response to play
- Evaluations for each expected outcome.

■ Fear

related to unfamiliarity

Definition
Feelings of threat or danger arising from an identifiable source

Assessment
- Age
- Psychosocial factors, including child's understanding of the illness and treatment plan, verbal and nonverbal indicators of fear, availability of family and friends
- Changes in behavior, eating, or sleeping patterns
- Physiologic manifestations of fear, including temperature, pulse rate, blood pressure, respiratory rate, skin color and temperature

Defining characteristics
- Aggressive or angry behavior
- Anticipation of unpleasant events
- Diaphoresis
- Elevated blood pressure
- Excessive crying

- Fatigue, poor sleep patterns
- Increased pulse and respiratory rates
- Loss of bladder or bowel control, enuresis, or encopresis
- Physiologic changes (difficulty swallowing or breathing, muscle tension)
- Rapid, loud speech
- Regression to earlier developmental level
- Restlessness, irritability
- Statements reflecting loss of control
- Verbal acknowledgment of fear
- Vomiting, diarrhea
- Withdrawn behavior

Associated medical diagnoses (selected)
This diagnosis can occur in any hospitalized child.

Expected outcomes
- Child identifies sources of fear.
- Child demonstrates effective use of coping mechanisms.
- Child seeks comfort from parents.
- Child expresses understanding of medical procedures.
- Child's vital signs remain within normal limits for age.
- Child exhibits fewer physiologic or behavioral manifestations of fear.

Interventions and rationales
- Acknowledge the child's fear. *Bringing feelings out into the open allows for discussion and identification of coping strategies.*
- Don't dismiss fear or blithely reassure the child that "everything will be all right." *Refusing to acknowledge fear or giving false reassurance impairs coping.*
- Spend as much time as possible talking with the child. For infants and toddlers, use nonverbal communication such as holding and rocking. *Establishing rapport encourages the child to express feelings and provides comfort.*
- Help the child identify the sources of fear *to enable the child to put emotions into perspective.*
- Provide the child with accurate information about condition and scheduled procedures and treatments. Orient the child to sights and sounds of the hospital. *Accurate information dispels misconceptions that can fuel fear.*
- Encourage parents and family members to stay with the child as much as possible and participate in care, as appropriate, *to enhance the child's ability to cope and decrease fear caused by separation.*

Evaluations for expected outcomes
- Child verbalizes known sources of fear.
- Child's vital signs remain within normal limits for age.
- Child expresses feelings of comfort.
- Child participates in play activities.
- Child exhibits marked decrease in physiologic and behavioral manifestations of fear.

Documentation
- Child's verbal and behavioral expressions of fear
- Physiologic manifestations of fear
- Interventions performed to reduce fear
- Child's response to interventions
- Family's involvement in the child's care
- Child's response to family involvement
- Evaluations for each expected outcome.

Fluid volume deficit

related to active loss

Definition

Excessive loss of fluids and electrolytes caused by diarrhea and vomiting

Assessment

- Age
- Height and weight
- History of diarrhea or vomiting
- GI status, including usual bowel pattern, changes in pattern, stool characteristics (color, amount, size, consistency, frequency), auscultation of bowel sounds, inspection of abdomen
- Stool culture, ova, and parasites
- Nutritional status, including dietary intake, changes from usual pattern, appetite, current weight, recent weight changes
- Fluid and electrolyte status, including intake and output; urine specific gravity; skin turgor; mucous membranes; serum sodium and potassium, blood urea nitrogen, and hematocrit levels
- Medication use, including laxatives, enemas, antibiotics
- Neurologic status, including level of consciousness
- Presence of sick children or adults at home, school, day care
- Respiratory status, including increased respiratory rate
- Child's and family members' knowledge of factors that cause vomiting or diarrhea

Defining characteristics

- Abdominal cramps
- Abdominal distention
- Bloody, mucoid, fatty, or bulky stools
- Changes in stool color
- Evidence of dehydration, including depressed fontanel (in infant), sunken eyes, poor skin turgor, weight loss, dry mucous membranes, decreased urine output
- Hypoactive bowel sounds
- Loose, liquid stools
- Urinary urgency
- Vomiting
- Weight loss

Associated medical diagnoses (selected)

Amebiasis, celiac disease, Crohn's disease, cystic fibrosis, diverticulitis, drug-induced diarrhea, failure to thrive, gastroenteritis, lactose intolerance, salmonellosis, shigella, trichinosis, ulcerative colitis

Expected outcomes

- Child's maintains normal weight.
- Child's intake and output is balanced and within normal limits for age.
- Child's electrolyte values remain within normal limits for age.
- Child maintains urine specific gravity of 1.005 to 1.015.
- Child exhibits moist mucous membranes and good skin turgor.
- Child exhibits normal elimination patterns for age.
- Infant exhibits flat fontanels.
- Child retains feedings and does not experience emesis.

Interventions and rationales

- Record intake and output every shift. Include urine, stool, vomitus, nasogastric or chest tube drainage, and any other output *to obtain fluid status. Increased output and decreased intake indicate fluid deficit.*

• Weigh child each morning before first feeding. *Weight loss of 5% in children indicates a fluid deficit.*
• Assess skin turgor, mucous membranes, and fontanels (in infant) every shift. *Fluid loss occurs first in extracellular spaces, resulting in poor skin turgor, dry mucous membranes, and sunken fontanels.*
• Monitor vital signs every 4 hours or more frequently if needed. *Fever and increased respiratory rate contribute to fluid loss. A weak, thready pulse and a drop in blood pressure indicate dehydration.*
• Check urine specific gravity every voiding. *Increased specific gravity indicates lack of fluids to dilute urine.*
• Monitor laboratory study results (electrolytes, pH, hematocrit). *During fluid loss, electrolytes are excreted. This may lead to electrolyte imbalance.*
• Assess child's behavior and activity level every shift. *Children with dehydration may develop anorexia, decreased activity level, and general malaise.*
• Once diarrhea and vomiting have decreased, offer small amounts (5 to 15 ml) of clear fluids frequently *to replace fluid loss without causing further GI irritation.*
• If the child is to have nothing by mouth, provide mouth care every 4 hours and as needed *to help keep the mucous membranes moist. In infants, oral care and a pacifier help meet the developmental need for sucking.*
• Monitor I.V. fluid infusion every hour. *Because fluid balance is less stable in young children, an infusion rate that's too fast or too slow can lead to fluid imbalance more rapidly than in adults.*
• Secure the I.V. site by wrapping it in Kling bandage *to protect the site and allow the child free movement of extremity.*

Evaluations for expected outcomes

• Child maintains weight.
• Child exhibits balance of intake and output within normal limits for age, good skin turgor, moist mucous membranes, flat fontanels (in infant), and urine specific gravity of 1.005 to 1.015.
• Child's electrolyte levels, pH, and hematocrit remain within age-appropriate ranges.
• Child experiences normal elimination patterns for age.
• Child retains feedings without emesis.

Documentation

• Intake and output
• Weight (recorded daily)
• Skin turgor, mucous membranes, vital signs, and other physical findings
• Urine specific gravity and other laboratory values
• Interventions and child's response
• Evaluations for each expected outcome.

■ Fluid volume deficit, high risk for

related to excessive loss through physiologic routes

Definition

Presence of risk factors that could lead to excessive fluid and electrolyte loss

Assessment

• Age

- History of problems that can cause excessive fluid loss, such as vomiting, diarrhea, hemorrhage, ketoacidosis
- Vital signs
- Level of consciousness
- Fluid and electrolyte status, including intake and output, urine specific gravity, skin turgor, mucous membranes, fontanels (in infant), electrolyte levels, blood urea nitrogen levels
- GI status, including usual bowel pattern, changes in pattern, stool characteristics (color, amount, consistency, frequency), auscultation of bowel sounds, inspection of abdomen
- Nutritional status, including dietary intake, changes from usual pattern, appetite, current weight, recent weight changes
- Psychosocial status, including developmental level, stressors (school, disease process, family discord, separation from family), coping mechanisms
- Respiratory status, including increased respiratory rate
- Child's and family members' knowledge of factors that cause vomiting or diarrhea

Risk factors
- Age (under 12)
- Any disorder that places the child at risk for fluid volume deficit
- Decreased intake
- Excessive diuresis
- Hyperventilation
- Increased fluid output
- Urinary frequency

Associated medical diagnoses (selected)
Acute head injury, diabetes insipidus, diabetes mellitus, Crohn's disease, cystic fibrosis, failure to thrive, gastroenteritis, intractable diarrhea of infancy, viral or bacterial infection, organic brain syndrome, syndrome of inappropriate antidiuretic hormone secretion

Expected outcomes
- Child maintains weight.
- Child's urine specific gravity remains between 1.005 and 1.015.
- Child's intake and output is balanced and within normal limits for age.
- Child exhibits good skin turgor, moist mucous membranes, and flat fontanels (in infant).
- Child exhibits appropriate elimination patterns for age-group.
- Child does not show signs of fluid and electrolyte imbalance.

Interventions and rationales
- Record intake and output every shift. Include urine, stool, vomitus, nasogastric or chest tube drainage, and any other output *to obtain fluid status. Increased output and decreased intake result in fluid deficits.*
- Weigh the child each morning before first feeding. *Weight loss of 5% in children indicates a fluid deficit.*
- Assess skin turgor, mucous membranes, and fontanels (in infant) every shift. *Fluid loss first occurs in extracellular spaces resulting in poor skin turgor, dry mucous membranes, and sunken fontanels.*
- Monitor vital signs at least every 4 hours or more frequently if needed. *Increased temperature and increased respiratory rate contribute to fluid loss. A weak thready pulse and drop in blood pressure indicate dehydration.*
- Check urine specific gravity every voiding. *Increased specific gravity indicates lack of fluids to dilute urine.*
- Monitor laboratory studies (electrolytes, pH, hematocrit). *During fluid loss, electrolytes are excreted, which may lead to electrolyte imbalance.*

• Assess the child's behavior and activity level every shift. *Children with dehydration may develop anorexia, decreased activity level, and general malaise.*
• When diarrhea and vomiting have decreased, offer small amounts (5 to 15 ml) of clear fluids *to replace fluid loss without causing further GI irritation.*
• If the child is to have nothing by mouth, provide mouth care every 4 hours and as needed *to help keep the mucous membranes moist. In infants, oral care and a pacifier help meet the developmental need for sucking.*
• Monitor I.V. fluid infusion every hour. *Because fluid balance is less stable in young children, too rapid or too slow infusion rate can lead to fluid imbalance more quickly than in adults.*
• Secure the I.V. site by wrapping it in Kling bandage *to protect the site and allow the child to move hand or arm freely.*

Evaluations for expected outcomes

• Child maintains weight.
• Child exhibits balanced intake and output within normal limits for age.
• Child exhibits good skin turgor, moist mucous membranes, and flat fontanels (in infant).
• Child's urine specific gravity is between 1.005 and 1.015.
• Child's electrolyte values, pH, and hematocrit remain within age-appropriate ranges.
• Child's elimination patterns are appropriate for age-group.
• Child retains feedings without experiencing emesis.

Documentation

• Intake and output
• Weight (recorded daily)
• Skin turgor, mucous membranes, vital signs, and other physical findings
• Urine specific gravity and other laboratory values
• Interventions and child's response
• Evaluations for each expected outcome.

Grieving, anticipatory

related to potential loss of significant object or person

Definition

Grief response in anticipation of loss of a significant person, ideal, material object, or body part

Assessment

• Child's state of grief and mourning
• Child's developmental level
• Perceived value of the lost object
• Usual patterns of coping with loss
• Behavioral manifestations of grieving
• Somatic problems associated with the grieving process, including appetite, sleep patterns, activity level
• Available support systems

Defining characteristics

• Anger
• Changes in activity level, eating patterns, or sleep patterns
• Communication difficulties
• Denial of potential loss
• Difficulty expressing feelings regarding potential loss
• Expressions of distress or guilt over potential loss
• Sadness
• Withdrawn behavior

Associated medical diagnoses (selected)
This diagnosis may occur in newly diagnosed chronic or terminal diseases, such as acquired immunodeficiency syndrome, cancer, diabetes mellitus, juvenile rheumatoid arthritis, and leukemia and in conditions requiring radical surgery.

Expected outcomes
- Child expresses feelings in a nondestructive manner.
- Child seeks emotional support from family members to help cope with loss.
- Child takes advantage of available resources, such as participation in play therapy, to help cope with loss.
- Family members express understanding of the grieving process.
- Parents participate in care of child and interact positively with child.

Interventions and rationales
- Encourage child to express feelings through drawing, puppetry, or gross motor play *to provide a safe outlet for pent-up emotions. Children do not have verbal and cognitive skills to express feelings and need alternative means of expression. Allow child to express grief in own way; intervene only to prevent physically destructive behavior.*
- Plan to spend time each shift with child. If child doesn't wish to talk, spend the time in silence *to convey concern, understanding, and support.*
- Reassure child that it's all right to be angry or sad. Assess whether child feels responsible for loss, and clear up misconceptions *to help alleviate guilt feelings.*
- Reassure family that grief is a normal reaction to loss; explain the various stages of the grieving process and normal responses. Help parents understand that child's feelings and behavior are normal under the present circumstances. *An understanding of the grieving process will enhance the family's ability to cope.*
- Encourage parents and siblings to participate in care of child. Remind them of child's need for emotional support at this time. *Child may fear he will no longer be loved or cared for after the loss. It is crucial that child receives emotional reassurance.*
- Offer child simple choices related to care issues *to give child a sense of control and to meet developmental needs for initiative and industry.*
- Encourage child and family members to develop coping strategies for dealing with loss, such as participating in diversional activities, reminiscing, or seeking out support groups *to facilitate grieving process.*
- Provide positive feedback for effective coping behavior *to help child and family members regain self-confidence.*

Evaluations for expected outcomes
- Child expresses pent-up feelings in a nondestructive manner.
- Child's verbal expressions and behavior indicate that he does not feel he will be blamed, punished, or abandoned because of loss.
- Family members express understanding of the grieving process.
- Family members express willingness to accept child's behavior.
- Parents participate in care of child.

Documentation
- Child's verbal expressions and behavior
- Child's eating, sleeping, activity patterns
- Observation of emotional responses
- Child's attempts to gain control, such as making decisions, contacting support systems

- Interaction between parents and child
- Nursing interventions and child's response
- Evaluations for each expected outcome.

Growth and development alteration

related to physical disability or environmental deprivation

Definition
State in which a child deviates from developmental norms for age

Assessment
- Child's age, both chronological and developmental
- Nature of physical disability
- Past experience with hospitalization
- Family history, including parents' educational level and knowledge of child development, family member roles and support systems, resources and home environment
- Child's capabilities, including communication skills, motor skills, socialization skills, cognitive abilities

Defining characteristics
- Altered physical growth
- Delay or difficulty in developing skills appropriate to age-group, including motor, language, cognitive and psychosocial skills
- Failure of parents to provide adequate developmental stimulation for child
- Inability to display level of self-control
- Inability to perform self-care activities appropriate for age
- Neurologic impairment

Associated medical diagnoses (selected)
Cardiovascular deficits, cerebral palsy, Down's syndrome, dyslexia, encephalitis, failure to thrive, fetal alcohol syndrome, head trauma, orthopedic disorders, Reye's syndrome, spina bifida, seizure disorder

Expected outcomes
- Child demonstrates skills appropriate for age.
- Child participates in developmental stimulation program to increase skill levels.
- Parents express understanding of norms for growth and development.
- Parents utilize community resources to promote child's development.
- Parents provide play activities to promote child's development.

Interventions and rationales
- Monitor child's height, weight, nutritional intake, and cardiovascular and pulmonary status *to ensure child is healthy enough to participate in activity.*
- Provide appropriate play activities, such as building blocks, dolls, crayons, or games, *to promote development.* Select play activities and related materials according to child's abilities rather than chronological age *to promote use of existing skills as a means of mastering higher skill levels.*
- Teach selected activities to parents and family members and encourage frequent play with child. *To be effetive, learning must be reinforced at home.*
- Monitor developmental progress at regular intervals *to detect changes in level of functioning and, as appropriate, adapt activity program.*
- Provide parents with referrals to appropriate community resources, including sources of financial assis-

tance, child care, and suppliers of adaptive equipment, *to ensure child's right to receive remedial and educational care in accordance with his disability, as guaranteed by federal law.*

Evaluations for expected outcomes

- Child demonstrates skills appropriate for age.
- Child participates in developmentally appropriate play activities.
- Parents express understanding of developmental norms and means to promote child's development.
- Parents participate in program to provide developmental stimulation for child.
- Parents utilize community resources to obtain adaptive equipment and appropriate educational opportunities for child.

Documentation

- Assessment of child's developmental level
- Evidence of parents' knowledge of child's abilities and motivation to promote development
- Interventions performed to stimulate development
- Child's response to nursing interventions
- Evaluations for each expected outcome.

Hyperthermia

related to infection

Definition

Elevation of body temperature above normal range

Assessment

- History of present illness
- History of exposure to communicable disease
- Age, gestational age at birth
- Health history, including chronic disease or disability, pathologic conditions known to cause dehydration, recent traumatic event, exposure to sources of infection (intrauterine or extrauterine), exposure to communicable diseases, other related events
- Medications
- Physiologic manifestations of fever, including vital signs, skin temperature, skin color
- Fluid and electrolyte status, including skin turgor, intake and output, mucous membranes, serum electrolyte levels, urine specific gravity
- Laboratory studies, including white blood cell count, culture and sensitivity findings
- Neurologic status, including level of consciousness, past history of seizures
- Skin integrity, including open lesions, rashes.

Defining characteristics

- Body temperature above 99.5° F (37.5° C)
- Flushed, warm skin
- Increased respiratory and heart rates
- Mild to severe dehydration
- Possible seizures

Associated medical diagnoses (selected)

Bacterial, mycotic, rickettsial, viral, and other infections

Expected outcomes

- Child remains afebrile.
- Child maintains adequate hydration:
  - intake and output are balanced and within normal limit for age
  - urine specific gravity is between 1.005 and 1.015

– Child exhibits moist mucous membranes, good skin turgor, and flat fontanels (in infant).
• Child remains alert and responsive and does not show evidence of seizure activity or decreased level of consciousness.
• Parents identify risk factors for infection and state measures to prevent infection.
• Parents demonstrate correct technique for assessing temperature.
• Parents identify appropriate measures to reduce fever and prevent dehydration.

Interventions and rationales
• Take axillary or oral temperature every 1 to 4 hours (and 1 hour after administration of antipyretics). Record measurements and identify route *to obtain an accurate core temperature.*
• Administer antipyretic medication, as ordered, and record effectiveness. *Antipyretics act on the hypothalamus to regulate temperauture.* Avoid using aspirin. *Administration of aspirin to children with viral symptoms, especially with flulike symptoms or varicella (chicken pox), has been linked to Reye's syndrome.*
• Use nonpharmacologic measures to reduce excessive fever, such as removing sheets, blankets, and most clothing (except diapers and underwear); placing ice bags on axillae and groin; and sponging with tepid water. Explain these measures to child and family members. *Nonpharmacologic measures lower body temperature and promote comfort. Sponging reduces body temperature by increasing evaporation from skin. Tepid water is used because cold water increases shivering, thereby increasing the metabolic rate and causing temperature to rise.*
• Use hypothermia blanket if child's temperature rises above 103° F (39° C). Monitor vital signs every 15 minutes for 1 hour and then as indicated. *Too-rapid reduction of fever can cause vascular collapse in young children.* Turn off blanket if shivering occurs. *Because shivering increases the metabolic rate, it is counterproductive to cooling therapy.*
• Monitor heart rate and rhythm, blood pressure, respiratory rate, level of consciousness and responsiveness, and capillary refill time every 1 to 4 hours *to evaluate the effectiveness of interventions and monitor for complications such as seizures.*
• Determine child's preferences for oral fluids and encourage child to drink as much as possible, unless contraindicated. Monitor and record intake and output, and administer I.V. fluids if indicated. *Because insensible fluid loss increases by 10% for every 1° C increase in temperature, child must increase fluid intake to prevent dehydration.*
• Discuss precipitating factors with parents or primary caregiver. Teach parents:
  – how to take a temperature correctly
  – measures to prevent fever, such as increased fluid intake
  – not to overdress young child.

Effective teaching will help prevent future episodes of hyperthermia.
• Describe complications of fever to parents and explain which symptoms need to be reported to doctor. *Early recognition and treatment of fever reduces risk of complications, such as dehydration and febrile seizures.*

Evaluations for expected outcomes
• Child remains afebrile.
• Child maintains adequate hydration:

– intake and output are balanced and within normal limit for age
– urine specific gravity is between 1.005 and 1.015
– child exhibits moist mucous membranes, good skin turgor, and flat fontanels (in infant).
- Child remains alert and responsive.
- Child does not exhibit evidence of seizure activity.
- Parents identify risk factors for infection and state measures to prevent infection.
- Parents demonstrate correct technique for assessing temperature.
- Parents identify appropriate measures to reduce fever and prevent dehydration.

Documentation
- Observations of physical findings
- Nursing interventions, including administration of medications
- Child's response (behavioral, cognitive, physiologic) to interventions, including administration of antipyretics
- Evaluations for each expected outcome.

Incontinence, total

related to neuropathy, trauma, or disease affecting spinal nerves

Definition
Involuntary, continuous, and unpredictable passage of urine or stool

Assessment
- History of trauma, surgery, congenital anomalies or disease
- History of sensory or neuromuscular impairment
- Vital signs
- Age
- Sex
- Bowel elimination status, including usual bowel pattern, frequency, awareness of need, presence or absence of anal sphincter reflex, bowel sounds
- Genitourinary status, including palpation of bladder, previous bladder elimination procedures, urinalysis, urine characteristics, use of urinary assistive devices, voiding pattern
- Fluid and electrolyte status, including fluid intake and output, mucous membranes, skin turgor, serum electrolyte levels, urine specific gravity
- Neuromuscular status, including degree of neuromuscular function, motor ability to start or stop urine stream, sensory ability to perceive bladder fullness and urge to defecate
- Nutritional status, including usual dietary pattern, appetite, tolerance or intolerance of foods, current weight
- Activity status, including usual play patterns
- Appearance of skin

Defining characteristics
- Constant flow of urine occurring at unpredictable times without distention or uninhibited bladder contractions or spasms
- Involuntary passage of stool
- Lack of awareness of incontinence, perineal fullness, or bladder filling
- Nocturia, enuresis, encopresis

Associated medical diagnoses (selected)
Cerebral tumor; cerebrovascular accident; congenital anomalies, such as spina bifida and myelomeningocele; neuromuscular trauma, such as spinal cord injury; neuromuscular disease, such as spinal cord tumor, cerebral palsy

Expected outcomes

- Child maintains fluid balance, with intake equal to output.
- Child experiences bowel movement when placed on commode or toilet at specified time.
- Child's skin remains clean and intact.
- Parents express understanding of bowel and bladder care.
- Parents express understanding of the need to regulate food and fluid intake to promote continence.
- Parents and child demonstrate correct catheterization technique.

Interventions and rationales

- Monitor and document child's voiding pattern and intake and output. *Careful monitoring allows you to identify problems and individualize interventions.*
- Assist with specific bladder elimination procedures, as ordered, such as:
  - external catheterization. Apply catheter according to established procedure. Maintain patency and avoid constriction. Clean penis or vagina with soap and water at least twice a day. *External catheter keeps skin dry and protected from contact with urine. Clean skin helps prevent skin breakdown and infection.*
  - insertion of indwelling urinary catheter. Insert according to established procedure and monitor patency; keep tubing free of kinks *to avoid drainage pooling and ensure effective drainage.* Keep the drainage bag below bladder level *to prevent urine reflux into the bladder.* Maintain closed drainage *to prevent bacteria from infiltrating into bladder.* Secure the catheter to the leg (in females) or abdomen (in males) *to avoid tension on the bladder and urinary sphincter.*
  - insertion of suprapubic catheter. Monitor patency, change dressing, and perform catheter care according to established protocols *to help prevent skin irritation and breakdown.* Maintain closed drainage *to prevent bacterial infiltration.*
  - use of incontinence aids, including diapers, pads and pants, drip collector, linen protector, or absorbent pouch to cover penis. Use as alternatives to indwelling devices. *Incontinence aids prevent soiling of clothes and linen, reduce embarrassment, and draw urine away from skin. Compared to indwelling devices, incontinence aids allow for greater mobility and carry decreased risk of infection.*
  - intermittent self-catheterization. Assess child's readiness to learn self-catheterization. Instruct child or family member in technique and request return demonstration *to evaluate understanding and ability;* maintain sterile technique in hospital and clean technique at home *to prevent infection.*
- Establish a regular pattern for bowel care; for example, after breakfast each morning, place child on toilet or commode for 1 hour after inserting glycerin suppository; allow child to remain upright for 30 minutes, then cleanse anal area. *Regular bowel care encourages adaptation and routine physiologic function.*
- Teach parents bowel care routine *to foster continuity of care.*
- Teach parents need to regulate child's consumption of foods or

fluids that cause diarrhea or constipation *to promote helpful nutritional patterns.*
• Maintain a diet log *to identify irritant foods that need to be eliminated from child's diet.*
• Teach parents to regulate child's fluid intake according to a specific schedule *to encourage voiding at appropriate time.* Limit fluid intake after dinner *to reduce the need to void at night.*
• Cleanse and dry perianal area after each incontinent episode *to prevent skin breakdown and promote comfort.*

Evaluations for expected outcomes
• Child exhibits normal elimination pattern for age.
• Child's skin remains clean, dry, and intact.
• Parents demonstrate correct technique when implementing bowel and bladder program.
• Parents express understanding of the need to regulate food and fluid intake to maintain continence, and plan appropriate diet for child.
• Child maintains adequate fluid balance, as evidenced by measurements of intake and output and urine specific gravity and assessment of skin turgor.

Documentation
• Observations of incontinence and child's response to treatment regimen
• Nursing interventions performed and child's response
• Instructions given to child and family members and their demonstrated ability to perform bowel and bladder program
• Observations of skin integrity
• Evaluations for each expected outcome.

Injury, high risk for

related to developmental factors

Definition
Risk of tissue injury in a child with physiologic, mental, or emotional disabilities

Assessment
• Age
• Environmental factors, including toxic substances within reach of child, stairs not blocked, unsafe play equipment
• Developmental status, including cognitive abilities (language, reasoning), sensory perception (vision, hearing, touch, taste, smell), response to stimuli (pain, touch, warmth), level of independence, motor skills
• Child's and family members' understanding of safety practices
• Behavior
• Laboratory studies, including toxicology screening

Risk factors
• Age (independence-seeking toddlers and thrill-seeking adolescents especially vulnerable)
• Child's inability to understand safe use of medication or equipment
• Child's lack of knowledge about safety hazards, such as electric sockets or matches
• Decreased level of consciousness
• Decreased or absent sensory perception, including blindness or deafness
• Environmental hazards, such as steep steps, unsteady chairs, clutter, lack of childproofing in home, toxic substances within child's reach

- Family members' lack of knowledge about or indifference toward safety practices
- High bed without side rails
- Hyperactivity

Associated medical diagnoses (selected)
Burns, congenital deformities, depression with suicidal ideation, developmental disorders, learning disabilities

Expected outcomes
- Child remains free of physical injury.
- Family members identify safety hazards in home.
- Family members take action to eliminate household safety hazards.
- Child is adequately protected from environmental hazards while in the hospital.
  - During hospitalization, toxic substances are kept out of child's reach.
  - Play equipment is inspected for safety and unsafe equipment is removed.

Interventions and rationales
- Assess and document any motor, mental, or sensory deficits *to identify specific safety needs.*
- Keep frequently used items within the child's easy reach *to help prevent falls.*
- Encourage the use of necessary assistive devices, such as hearing aids, glasses, and leg braces, *to enhance safety and help prevent injury.*
- Orient child to the immediate environment, as necessary, *to promote mobility and improve safety.*
- Assess amount of supervision needed by child *to ensure safety. Maintaining supervision is especially important if child is hyperactive, disoriented, or unconscious.*
- Keep bed side rails up at all times *to prevent falls.*
- Keep the bed in low position except when providing direct care *to ease getting in and out of bed and to reduce the danger of falling.*
- Use locks on wheelchairs, stretchers, and beds when appropriate, *to immobilize the equipment and enhance safety.*
- Ensure that all equipment, medical supplies, and toys in child's room are appropriate for his developmental age. Make sure an infant's or toddler's room does not contain small objects, sharp instruments, or sharp furniture corners *to reduce the risk of injury.*
- Promote electrical safety. Apply electrical outlet covers to all unused outlets. Inspect all electrical appliances brought from home and have them approved by a safety officer before use. Don't place liquids, jellies, or creams on electrical appliances. Finally, test all electrical equipment before using on child. *Electrical appliances pose potential hazards for both child and staff.*
- Instruct child and family members in standard safety practices, including:
  - wiping up all spills immediately
  - providing nonslip surfaces in hallways, on stairs, and in bathtubs and shower stalls
  - draining all water from bathtubs immediately after completing baths
  - placing toxic substances in locked cabinets or out of reach of child.

Teaching promotes household safety. Including family members in teaching plan is crucial because young children lack cognitive reasoning ability to practice safety on their own.

Evaluations for expected outcomes
- Child remains free of physical injury.
- Child and family members express understanding of safety measures.
- Family eliminates safety hazards from home.

Documentation
- Statements by child or family members that indicate high risk for injury
- Assessment of home environment
- Observation of physical findings
- Child's and family members' knowledge of safety practices
- Nursing interventions to reduce the risk of injury
- Child's and family members' responses to interventions
- Evaluations for each expected outcome.

Knowledge deficit

related to lack of exposure

Definition
Inadequate understanding of information or inability to perform skills needed to practice health-related behaviors

Assessment
- Age
- Developmental status, including learning ability (affective domain, cognitive domain, psychomotor domain), decision-making ability, developmental stage
- Psychosocial status, including family's resources, health beliefs and attitudes, interest in learning, knowledge and skill regarding current health problem, obstacles to learning, support systems (willingness and capability of others to help child), usual coping pattern
- Neurologic status, including level of consciousness, memory, mental status, orientation

Defining characteristics
- Child's or parents' request for information
- Expressions that indicate lack of knowledge
- Lack of prior experience with hospitalization, procedures, and treatments
- Unfamiliarity with diagnosis and nature of illness

Associated medical diagnoses (selected)
This nursing diagnosis can occur in association with any medical diagnosis.

Expected outcomes
- Child and family members communicate a need to gain knowledge.
- Child and family members establish realistic learning goals.
- Child and family members verbalize or demonstrate an understanding of what has been taught.
- Child and family members demonstrate the ability to perform recently learned health-related behaviors.
- Child and family members verbalize their intention to make needed changes in life-style.

Interventions and rationales
- Establish an environment of mutual trust and respect to enhance learning. Communicate openly and honestly with child, and encourage parents and others to visit regularly *to enhance child's feelings of trust in staff and comfort within the hospital environment.*
- Identify child's level of cognitive, physical, linguistic, and perceptual

development *to establish appropriate learning goals.*

- Select teaching methods appropriate to the child's developmental level:
  - For preschooler or early school-age child, use stuffed animals or puppets. *Children in this age-group use their senses and manipulation of objects to learn.*
  - For older school-age child, use demonstration techniques, role-playing, and illustrations. Relate new terms and concepts to child's experiences. For example, to explain a ventricular septal defect you might say "your heart is like a house with four rooms and one of the doors to the room is not working right." *Children at this age think concretely and best understand explanations if related to past experiences.*
  - For adolescent, use individual and group discussion and written and audiovisual materials. *Adolescents can think abstractly and are able to process information from a variety of sources. Because adolescents are concerned with peer identity, group teaching can be especially effective.*
- Limit the number of new skills taught each day according to child's age and ability. A preschooler should learn one skill per day. A school-age child should learn two skills per day. An adolescent may learn three or more skills per day. *Limiting daily teaching helps to avoid overloading child with new information.* Keep in mind that young children who successfully learn single concepts may still have difficulty determining when to apply learned rules.
- Develop a daily schedule for child while in the hospital with plans for rest, meals, play, and performing learned skills. *Establishing routines provides a more controlled, pleasant environment for child and thereby fosters learning. Play is a valuable component of any child's life.*
- Encourage family members to participate in planning child's daily schedule, making it as similar as possible to a typical day in the home environment. *Involving child's family helps reinforce skills necessary for home care after discharge.*
- Regularly discuss progress toward goal achievement with child and family members. Make changes in the plan of care as necessary. *Evaluation helps to reinforce effective learning techniques and identify ineffective techniques. It allows analysis of progress and redirection of activities as necessary.*
- Have child and family members demonstrate learned skills. *Return demonstration allows you to evaluate learning and helps child and family members gain confidence in new skills.*

Evaluations for expected outcomes

- Child and family members express understanding of material being taught.
- Child and family members demonstrate the ability to perform new health-related behaviors correctly.
- Child and family members demonstrate proficiency in specific skills taught.
- Family members express an intent to institute needed changes in child's life-style.

Documentation

- Child's and family members' knowledge and skills
- Child's and family members' statements that indicate knowledge deficit

- Child's and family members' expressions that indicate motivation to learn
- Learning objectives
- Teaching methods used
- Information taught
- Skills demonstrated
- Responses to teaching
- Evaluations for each expected outcome.

Nutrition alteration: Less than body requirements

related to inability to absorb nutrients or insufficient intake

Definition

Insufficient intake or absorption of nutrients that results in changed body weight and inability to meet metabolic needs

Assessment

- Age
- Developmental level
- GI status, including usual bowel pattern, change in bowel habits, stool characteristics (color, amount, size, consistency), pain or discomfort, nausea and vomiting, history of GI disorder or surgery, presence of colic, inspection of abdomen, palpation for masses and tenderness, percussion for tympany and dullness, auscultation of bowel sounds, sucking and swallowing ability of infant
- Medication history, including antibiotic therapy
- Nutritional status, including dietary history, change in type of food tolerated, height, weight, physical growth percentile (pediatic growth grid), meal preparation, sociocultural influences, usual dietary pattern, weight fluctuations in the past year, weight maintenance as height increases
- Change in intrapersonal or interpersonal factors, including desire to eat, rate of food consumption
- Psychosocial status, including body image (perception of observer and self-perception), level of attachment with primary caregiver, financial resources of family
- Laboratory studies, including hemoglobin and hematocrit
- Health status, including heart rate, respiratory status, integumentary status, oral mucosa
- Presence and type of tube feedings
- Activity level, mood

Defining characteristics

- Abdominal pain with or without pathologic condition
- Body weight below 5th percentile for age on pediatric growth grid
- Coated tongue
- Diarrhea, steatorrhea
- Hyperactive bowel sounds
- Impaired sucking or swallowing reflexes
- Loss of body weight with adequate food intake
- Pale conjunctivae and mucous membranes
- Perceived inability to digest food
- Poor muscle tone
- Poor skin turgor
- Pressure ulcers
- Sore, inflamed buccal cavity

Associated medical diagnoses (selected)

Acute gastritis, anorexia nervosa, bleeding esophageal varices, bulimia nervosa, Crohn's disease, congenital anomalies, cystic fibrosis, failure to thrive, gastroesophageal reflux, intestinal obstruction, malabsorption syndrome, paralytic ileus, pyloric stenosis, tumors of GI tract, ulcerative colitis

Expected outcomes

- Child exhibits no further weight loss and, if malnourished, gains 2.2 lb (1 kg)/week.
- Child takes in ____ calories/day.
- Child retains feedings without emesis.
- Child and family members express an understanding of total parenteral nutrition (TPN), if appropriate.
- Child and family members demonstrate an understanding of feeding techniques essential to daily nutritional requirements and a willingness to continue feeding regimen at home.

Interventions and rationales

- Provide diet meeting child's daily caloric requirements. Daily caloric intake is estimated based on age, metabolic status, and activity level. General guidelines include:
  - under age 6 months – 108 kcal/kg/day
  - ages 6 to 12 months – 98 kcal/kg/day
  - ages 1 to 3 – 1,300 kcal/day
  - ages 4 to 6 – 1,800 kcal/day
  - ages 7 to 10 – 2,000 kcal/day
  - ages 11 to 14 – 2,500 kcal/day
  - ages 15 to 18 – 3,000 kcal/day.

A diet meeting child's caloric requirements will help ensure child's maintenance and growth needs are met.

- Provide small, frequent feedings *to reduce fatigue and improve intake.*
- For infants over age 6 months, offer solid foods before formula or milk. Place solid foods in the center of the tongue, using a small spoon to press downward slightly, *to facilitate swallowing. Older infants and young toddlers may resist solid foods, preferring milk or formula.*
- Record and describe food intake. Refer family members to dietitian or nutritional support team for dietary management. *A dietitian or nutritional support team can individualize child's diet within prescribed restrictions.*
- Promote adequate rest *to reduce fatigue and improve child's ability and desire to eat.*
- Obtain and record child's weight each morning before first feeding *to accurately monitor response to therapy.*
- Provide parenteral fluids as ordered *to ensure adequate fluid and electrolyte levels.*
- Monitor electrolyte values and report abnormalities. *Poor nutritional status may cause electrolyte imbalances.*
- Monitor and record the amount, color, consistency, and presence of occult blood of emesis and stools. *Vomitus and stool characteristics provide clues to nutrient absorption.*
- If child is receiving tube feedings:
  - Use a continuous infusion pump, if possible, *to help prevent diarrhea, fatigue, and stimulation of the vagal response. A continuous infusion pump also helps prevent reduction in cough or gag reflex and overstimulation of the stomach.*
  - Provide an infant with opportunities to suck on a pacifier *to satisfy oral needs.*
  - Check feeding tube placement before each feeding *to verify tube placement in the GI tract rather than in the lung.*
  - Begin the regimen with small amounts and diluted concentrations *to decrease diarrhea and improve absorption.* Increase volume and concentration as tolerated.
  - Keep the head of the bed elevated during feedings *to reduce the risk of aspiration.*

– Teach parents correct technique for tube feeding *to ensure compliance with feeding regimen at home.*

- If child is receiving TPN:
  – Carefully monitor delivery of TPN *to promote effective therapy and prevent circulatory overload.*
  – Monitor blood glucose level, urine specific gravity, and urine glucose, protein, and metabolite levels at least every shift *to detect metabolic complications, osmotic diuresis, hypoglycemia, and pulmonary edema.*
  – Provide or assist with oral hygiene *to enhance the child's comfort and improve appetite.*
  – Teach parents correct technique for maintaining TPN infusion at home *to ensure feeding regimen is continued after discharge.*

Evaluations for expected outcomes

- Child's weight stabilizes or increases.
- Child's intake contains adequate calories and essential nutrients.
- Child and family members demonstrate understanding of nutritional principles and requirements, feeding techniques, and special needs.
- Family members express willingness to provide nutritional care at home.

Documentation

- Child's weight, recorded daily
- Child's sucking and swallowing reflexes
- Intake and output
- Incidence of emesis or diarrhea
- Characteristics of emesis or stool
- Presence of complications
- Statements by child and family members that indicate understanding of feeding protocol
- Evaluations for each expected outcome.

■ Pain

related to physical, biological, or chemical agents

Definition

An unpleasant sensation caused by noxious stimulation to sensory nerve endings by physical, chemical, or biological stimuli

Assessment

- Age
- Sex
- Descriptive characteristics of pain, including location, quality, intensity rated on a pictorial assessment scale, temporal factors, sources of relief
- Physiologic variables, including pain tolerance
- Psychological variables, such as body image, personality, previous experience with pain, anxiety, and secondary gain
- Sociocultural variables, including cognitive style, culture or ethnicity, attitude and values, and birth order
- Environmental variables, such as setting and time

Defining characteristics

- Behavioral cues, including grimacing, crying, fist-clenching, restlessness, guarding of body part or area, pulling at ears, withdrawing from social contact, pushing people away, displays of anger, regressive behavior
- Facial mask of pain, characterized by lackluster eyes, a "beaten" look, and fixed or scattered movement
- Physiologic responses to pain, including diaphoresis, pupil dilation, increased muscle tone, and elevated

pulse rate, blood pressure, and respiratory rate
- Statements expressing pain

Associated medical diagnoses (selected)
Pain may be associated with most medical diagnoses.

Expected outcomes
- Child expresses a feeling of improved comfort or demonstrates pain relief through playful, smiling, responsive behavior.
- Child identifies measures effective in relieving pain.
- Parent expresses awareness of child's pain and performs measures to comfort child.

Interventions and rationales
- Assess child's physical symptoms and behavioral cues. If appropriate, encourage child to describe the pain on a pictorial scale depicting a happy face (no pain) and series of grimacing faces gradually increasing to sad face with tears (worst pain possible). *Children lack verbal skills to describe variations in pain sensation. Pain scales and observation of nonverbal behavior provide alternative means to assess pain in young children.*
- Administer analgesics as ordered, and assess and document their effectiveness and adverse effects. *Analgesics depress the central nervous system, thereby reducing pain sensation.*
- Using a pain flow chart, record the time medication was administered and results of pain assessment every hour until the next dose *to closely monitor effectiveness of therapy.*
- Demonstrate acceptance when child reveals pain. *This helps establish a trusting relationship with child and encourages open expression of feelings. Children may deny pain to appear "good."*
- Provide comfort measures, such as massage, repositioning, and instruction in deep breathing and relaxation techniques. *Nonpharmacologic techniques decrease focusing on pain and may enhance effectiveness of analgesics by reducing muscle tension.*
- Apply heat or cold as appropriate to pain site. *Applying heat relaxes muscles and decreases pain. Applying cold results in vasoconstriction, decreasing inflammatory response and reducing pain.*
- Provide diversional activities, such as books, toys, and arts and crafts. *Because of their immature cognitive functioning and short attention span, young children may be distracted from pain by diversional activities. Older children are less easily distracted.*
- Provide honest information to child before potentially painful procedures. Tell child reasons for the pain and how long it should last. *Honest information builds trust and fosters a sense of control over the pain, thereby providing child with an opportunity to increase pain tolerance.*
- Help child obtain uninterrupted periods of rest. *Adequate rest promotes child's well-being and enhances the effectiveness of pain medication.*
- Discuss child's pain with parents or primary caregiver and enlist their help in pain assessment and management. Ascertain parents' usual means of providing comfort to child. *Because parents are most familiar with child's usual behavior, they can offer valuable information to assist pain assessment and management.*
- Try to anticipate the onset of pain. Provide prescribed medication before painful procedures such as dressing changes or activities such as deep breathing. *Careful pain management*

can improve relief and may enable child to cope better with procedures.
• Encourage child to report which pain-relief measures prove most effective *to give child a sense of control, enhance well-being, and allow more effective modifications of therapy.*

Evaluations for expected outcomes
• Child identifies the most effective pain relief measures.
• Parents respond to child's expression of pain and provide comfort to child.
• Child demonstrates reduced pain, as evidenced by verbal reports of pain relief, absence of behavioral signs of pain, and resumption of activities of daily living (age-appropriate diversional activities, social interaction, adequate nutritional intake and rest).

Documentation
• Child's description of pain, feelings about pain, statements about pain relief
• Observations of child's physical and psychological responses to pain
• Comfort measures and medications provided to reduce pain
• Effectiveness of interventions
• Information taught to child and family members about pain and pain relief
• Additional interventions provided to assist child with pain control
• Evaluations for each expected outcome.

■ Parental role conflict

related to child's hospitalization

Definition
State in which one or both parents experience role confusion and conflict in response to crisis

Assessment
• Parental status, including age and maturity; apprehension, fear, guilt; coping mechanisms employed; developmental state of family and other children; knowledge of normal growth and development of children; parents' past response to crises; parents' understanding of child's present condition; previous parent-child relationship; spiritual practices of parents and family; stability of parental relationship; support systems available to parent
• Parent-child interaction, including eye contact, response to appearance (bandages, deformities, hospital equipment), smiling, touching, verbalization
• Child's health status, including severity of illness, health care needs
• Child's level of development

Defining characteristics
• Change in parent-child interaction (speaking and listening, touch, visual contact)
• Ineffective parental coping mechanisms
• Parental relationship breakdown; decreased mutual support and communication
• Parental role changes
• Parents unable or unwilling to participate in child's physical or emotional care

Associated medical diagnoses (selected)
Any disease or condition, short-term or long-term, that results in a child's hospitalization

Expected outcomes
- Parents communicate feelings about present situation.
- Parents participate in daily caretaking of their child.
- Parents express feelings of greater control and ability to contribute more to child's well-being.
- Parents express knowledge of child's developmental needs.
- Parents hold, touch, convey warmth and affection to child.
- Parents use available support systems or agencies to assist in coping.

Interventions and rationales
- Orient parents and primary caregivers to hospital environment, visiting procedures, medical equipment, and staff. *Familiarity with hospital decreases anxiety.*
- Provide family-centered care by obtaining parents input for child's care. *Many of child's needs can best be met by parents rather than staff.* Involve parents in child's case conferences and in physical care of child. *Participation may decrease parents feelings of helplessness.*
- Teach parents normal childhood physical and psychological development *to prepare parents to deal with changes.*
- Encourage parental involvement in appropriate support groups or agencies when necessary or ordered. *Such groups can provide emotional support and help reduce feelings of being overwhelmed.*
- Ask parents if they have questions regarding child's status and provide information as requested *to lessen feelings of helplessness.*
- Provide for needs of parents as appropriate. Offer facilities for showering, sleeping, and eating. Be available to care for child if parents need opportunity to rest. *Helping parents to meet their needs will empower them to meet child care demands.*

Evaluations for expected outcomes
- Parents communicate feelings about present situation.
- Parents participate in daily care of their child.
- Parents express feelings of control in present situation.
- Parents communicate knowledge of child's developmental needs.
- Parents hold, touch, and express warmth and affection to child.
- Parents contact support systems or community agencies to assist in coping.

Documentation
- Observations of parents' ability to cope; their level of involvement in child's hospital care and daily needs
- Interventions performed to assist parents in lowering stress and coping with situation
- Referrals to outside agencies or support groups
- Child's medical and emotional state
- Evaluations for each expected outcome.

Parental role conflict

related to home care of a child with special needs

Definition
State in which one or both parents experience role confusion and crisis in response to the special needs of a child at home

Assessment

- Extent of child's special needs
- Parental status, including age or maturity, developmental state of family, authority within family, employment status, financial needs, marital status, stability of parental relationship, knowledge of normal growth and development, understanding of child's condition and prognosis, expectations regarding child, participation in community, past response to crises, coping mechanisms
- Available support systems, including other family members, friends, visiting nurses, community resources
- Parent-child interaction
- Parent-child relationship before development of special needs, and any changes that have occurred
- Religious practices of parents and family
- Presence of conflict between family's life-style and child's needs
- Home environment

Defining characteristics

- Inadequate physical and psychosocial care provided to child
- Inappropriate, inconsistent discipline
- Lack of physical contact between parents and child
- One or both parents physically, psychologically, or financially unable or unwilling to participate in child's physical or emotional care in the home
- Parents misinformed about child's condition, prognosis, requirements for care
- Parents' expression of apprehension, fear, or inadequacy with regard to caring for child
- Parents' feeling overwhelmed by child's condition and health care needs
- Delays in child's growth and development
- Technology-dependent or chronically ill child requiring multiple daily home treatments or careful monitoring

Associated medical diagnoses (selected)

This diagnosis may be associated with any condition requiring long-term home care. Examples include acquired immunodeficiency syndrome, cystic fibrosis, disorders requiring parenteral nutrition therapy, Down's syndrome and other developmental disabilities, hemophilia, and respiratory disorders requiring mechanical ventilation.

Expected outcomes

- Parents accept external support, education, and assistance in caring for their child at home.
- Parents demonstrate knowledge of child's developmental needs.
- Parents begin to provide physical, emotional, and developmental care to their child at home.
- Parents actively seek outside support in caring for their child at home.
- Parents seek assistance in meeting their own emotional and developmental needs.
- Parents express feelings of greater control and capability in meeting their child's needs.
- Siblings voice their emotional needs.

Interventions and rationales

- Provide family-centered care by involving parents in their child's care. Explain their rights as primary caretakers. Provide information to help them make informed decisions. Give them the opportunity to support child during painful procedures. *Par-*

ents are better able than staff to meet needs of their child. Parents need proper information and to have their own needs met before they are able to meet needs of child.

• Promote emotional well-being of parents by:
  – providing respite care
  – encouraging parents to spend time away from child to enhance their marital relationship
  – providing information about additional sources of support.

Encouraging parents to pay attention to their own emotional needs will enhance their ability to care for their child.

• Listen to parents, child, and siblings openly and without passing judgment *to gain their trust.*

• Help parents develop realistic expectations of their child and formulate achievable short-term goals based on child's needs and abilities *to reduce frustration and feelings of helplessness.*

• Ensure attention to all the child's normal health needs, including dental care, immunizations, safety, and educational and nutritional needs. *A chronically ill child needs total health care, not just illness-related interventions.*

• Pay attention to the needs of siblings at home. Devote time to discussing their feelings about having a brother or sister with special needs. How do their friends react? Contact their school nurse for assistance. Encourage them to help care for their brother or sister, but make sure activities are age-appropriate. *Becoming involved will help siblings achieve greater self-esteem and enhance their sense of control.*

• Advocate normal growth and development for child with special needs. Encourage visits by friends, discourage overprotective behavior *to help child obtain social acceptance. Increased social interaction will encourage parents, siblings, and others to view child as a unique individual instead of a burden. This in turn will help promote child's self-esteem.*

• Act as a liaison between the family and the multidisciplinary health care team, equipment vendors, community agencies, and third-party payers. *An organized approach with one central coordinator decreases stress for family and enhances continuity of care.*

Evaluations for expected outcomes

• Parents express increased knowledge of their child's needs and comfort in caring for child at home.
• Parents make use of community resources to assist in meeting child's physical, psychological, and educational needs.
• Parents seek help to meet their own emotional and developmental needs.
• Siblings come to terms with having a brother or sister with special needs.

Documentation

• Family members' expressions of feelings with regard to their role in caring for child at home
• Observations of parent-child interaction
• Physical and psychological status of child with special needs
• Nursing interventions to resolve parental role conflict in the home
• Parents', child's, and siblings' responses to interventions
• Evaluations for each expected outcome.

■ Parenting alteration

related to lack of knowledge

Definition

Inability of a nurturing figure to promote optimum growth and development in an infant or child

Assessment

- Parental status, including age, apprehension, developmental state; family roles; relationship with spouse or significant other
- Sex, status of other children
- Parents' knowledge of child care, normal growth and development
- Previous bonding history
- Interaction of parent and infant or child, including care practices; eye contact; response to appearance, handicaps, sex of infant; smiling; touching; verbalization; visual and voice responses
- Psychosocial status, including financial stressors, previous experience; support of family, friends, significant other; work demands

Defining characteristics

- Constant verbalization of disappointment in sex or physical characteristics of infant or child
- Delay in growth and development of infant or child
- Evidence of physical and psychological trauma
- Failure to thrive
- Growth and development lag in infant or child
- History of child abuse or abandonment by primary caretaker
- Inappropriate caretaking behaviors (toilet training, sleep and rest schedule, feeding)
- Inappropriate visual, tactile, or auditory stimulation
- Inattention to infant's or child's needs
- Inconsistent or inappropriate discipline
- Lack of parental attachment behaviors
- Negative statements about characteristics of infant or child
- Noncompliance with health appointments for self and infant or child
- Verbalization of inability to control child
- Verbalization of resentment toward infant or child
- Verbalization of role inadequacy

Associated medical diagnoses (selected)

Battered child syndrome, burns, child abuse, failure to thrive, fractures, head trauma, neglect, shaken baby syndrome, soft-tissue injuries

Expected outcomes

- Parents establish eye, physical, and verbal contact with infant or child.
- Parents voice satisfaction with infant or child.
- Parents demonstrate correct feeding, bathing, and dressing techniques.
- Parents express willingness to work to maintain relationship with each other.
- Parents state plans for well-child care.
- Parents express knowledge of developmental norms.
- Parents provide play activities for child.
- Parents identify ways to express anger and frustration that do not harm child.

Interventions and rationales

- Involve parents in care of infant or child immediately *to promote attachment to child.*
- Provide opportunities for caretaking by allowing parents to share room with infant or child or by extending visitation periods. *Participation in care increases parent's feeling of self-esteem and self-worth.*
- Educate parents in:
  - normal growth and development
  - breast- and bottle-feeding techniques
  - infant care, such as bathing and dressing
  - routine well-child care
  - signs and symptoms of illness
  - need for tactile and sensory stimulation.

Knowledge of normal growth and development may decrease unrealistic expectations and increase chances of successful parenting.

- When caring for child in parents' presence, act as a role model for effective parenting skills. *Lack of knowledge of routine child care practices and growth and developmental norms is a significant factor contributing to child abuse. Demonstration is a more effective means of teaching parenting skills than lecturing.*
- Encourage questions about caretaking and provide appropriate information *to allay anxiety and monitor knowledge retention.*
- Praise parents when they display appropriate parenting skills. *Abusive parents are often immature and need positive reinforcement of their abilities.*
- Refer parents to family support group and other community resources such as Parents Anonymous. *Lack of support and sense of being alone is common among battering parents. Participation in support group may help ease isolation.*
- Encourage verbalization of infant's or child's impact on family life. *Ventilation of feelings assists parents to deal more effectively with stress of child care.*
- Be alert for symptoms of child abuse, including neglect, uncleanliness, and frequent accidents or withdrawn, fearful behavior on the part of the child. Report actual or suspected child abuse to appropriate authorities. *Reporting child abuse is your professional duty. Nurses in the United States are legally required to report abuse.*

Evaluations for expected outcomes

- Parents make appropriate physical, verbal, and visual contact when interacting with infant or child.
- Parents make statements indicating satisfaction with infant or child.
- Parents demonstrate correct bathing, dressing, and feeding techniques.
- Parents seek out community resources and participate in support groups for abusive parents.
- Parents express willingness to maintain their relationship with each other.
- Parents bring infant for routine well-child care.
- Parents verbalize knowledge of developmental norms.
- Parents provide play activities for child.
- Parents identify ways to express anger and frustration that do not harm child.
- Child does not experience intentional injuries.

Documentation

- Parents' expressions of feelings about child

• Parents' expression of concern about their performance as parents
• Observation of parental visits, bonding, caretaking, and knowledge level
• Instructions given to parents and parents' understanding of their responsibilities
• Infant's weight
• Evaluations for each expected outcome.

Parenting alteration, high risk for

related to lack of knowledge or ineffective role model

Definition

Presence of risk factors that may interfere with mother's ability to promote optimum growth and development in an infant or child

Assessment

• Ages of mother and child
• Mother's psychosocial status, including developmental state; educational level; family roles; presence or absence of spouse or significant other; financial stressors; previous parenting experience; support of family, friends, or significant other; work demands
• Interaction between mother and infant or child, including care practices; eye contact; response to appearance and sex of infant; smiling; touching; verbalization; visual and voice responses

Risk factors

• Delay in growth and development of infant or child
• Failure to thrive
• Frequent accidents
• Lack of knowledge of appropriate parenting activities
• Lack of parental attachment behaviors
• Mother expresses frustration, anger, sadness, or disappointment over problems in caring for infant or child.
• Mother fails to comply with health appointments for self and infant or child.
• Mother fails to provide appropriate visual, tactile, or auditory stimulation.
• Mother is not attentive to infant's or child's needs.
• Mother is unfamiliar with appropriate caretaking behaviors in areas such as toilet training, sleep, or feeding.

Associated medical diagnoses (selected)

Burns, failure to thrive, fractures, head trauma, neglect, shaken baby syndrome, soft-tissue injuries

Expected outcomes

• Mother establishes eye, physical, and verbal contact with infant or child.
• Mother demonstrates correct feeding, bathing, and dressing techniques.
• Mother states plans to bring infant or child to clinic for routine physical and psychological examinations.
• Mother expresses understanding of developmental norms.
• Mother provides play activities appropriate to child's age.

Interventions and rationales

• Assess the amount of developmental stimulation provided by mother. For example, use Caldwell HOME Inventory Measure on home visit *to assess whether home environment is developmentally stimulating.*

- Instruct the mother in basics of infant and child care, including:
  - breast and bottle-feeding techniques, such as positioning of infant for optimal intake, amount to offer at each feeding, and frequency of feedings based on infant's age
  - bathing and safety precautions during bathing
  - appropriate dressing.

Research shows that the primary source of information about parenting is the mother's own parents. If the mother lacks an effective role model, you may need to supply basic information about parenting.

- When caring for the child in the mother's presence, act as a role model for effective parenting skills. Demonstrate comfort measures, such as rocking the infant, and show the mother how to hold the infant in an en face position *to increase mother's knowledge of routine child care practices.*
- Teach the mother about normal growth and development, and identify ages at which the child should be able to master developmental tasks such as rolling over, crawling, and walking. *This will assist the mother in monitoring the child's growth and development and in practicing appropriate safety precautions, such as blocking stairways, keeping crib side rails secured, and preventing accidents.* Also discuss problem behaviors associated with specific ages, such as colic, temper tantrums, and sleeping difficulties, *to further enhance the mother's understanding of developmental norms.*
- Discuss the child's need for tactile and sensory stimulation. Demonstrate play activities that promote developmental skills, such as shaking a rattle in front of the infant to build eye-and-hand coordination or placing a mobile above the infant to encourage visual tracking and trunk and head control. *Sensory experiences promote cognitive development.*
- Familiarize the mother with techniques for detecting symptoms of illness in an infant or a child, including:
  - taking temperatures and reading thermometers.
  - assessing the child's respiratory status.
  - observing for behavioral cues of illness, such as increased crying, rubbing ears, or drawing legs to abdomen.

Knowledge of how to monitor the child's health status will assist in diagnosis and early treatment of problems.

- Encourage the mother to ask questions about infant and child care. Identify questions parents commonly ask about infant care, such as cord care, feeding techniques, and bathing. Reassure the mother that other parents also need to ask basic questions. *A mother who lacks effective parenting role models may not know what questions to ask or she may hesitate to ask questions because of embarrassment.*
- Praise the mother when she displays appropriate parenting skills *to provide positive reinforcement.*
- Emphasize the importance of making regular visits to a health care professional, even when the child appears healthy. *Routine visits are important for early detection of developmental delays, as well as preventive care such as immunizations.*
- As necessary, refer the mother and family to doctor, nurse practitioner, or social services for follow-up *to ensure continuity of care.*

Evaluations for expected outcomes

- Mother makes appropriate physical, visual, and verbal contact with infant or child.
- Mother demonstrates correct bathing, feeding, and dressing techniques.
- Mother brings infant or child to clinic for routine examinations.
- Mother expresses understanding of developmental norms.
- Mother accurately assesses child's developmental status and needs.
- Mother provides play activities appropriate to child's age.

Documentation

- Evidence of neglect of infant or child
- Observations of mother's caretaking skills and knowledge level
- Presence or absence of mother-child bonding behaviors
- Questions asked by mother about care of infant or child
- Instructions given to mother and mother's response
- Evaluations for each expected outcome.

Self-care deficit: Bathing and hygiene

related to developmental delay

Definition

Inability to carry out aspects of self-care, such as bathing and personal hygiene

Assessment

- Age
- History of neurologic, sensory, or developmental impairment
- Self-care abilities, including knowledge and use of adaptive equipment, preparation of equipment and supplies, technical or mechanical skills
- Musculoskeletal status, including range of motion, muscle tone, gait, muscle size and strength, functional capabilities, mechanical restrictions (splints, casts, traction)
- Neurologic status, including cognition, communication ability, insight or judgment, level of consciousness, memory, motor ability, orientation, sensory ability
- Psychosocial status, including child's affective reaction to imbalances between motor abilities and cognitive reasoning abilities, usual life-style, parents' perception of developmental delay

Defining characteristics

- Depression that interferes with ability to perform self-care
- Immobility or loss of limb
- Inability to gain access to water source
- Inability to regulate water temperature or flow
- Inability to wash body or body parts
- Motor or sensory deficit

Associated medical diagnoses (selected)

This diagnosis can occur with any musculoskeletal, cognitive, or perceptual impairment.

Expected outcomes

- Child's skin remains clean, dry, and intact.
- Child and family members demonstrate appropriate use of assistive devices.
- Child or family member performs self-care program daily.

Interventions and rationales

- Assess child's functional, cognitive, and perceptual level at established periodic intervals. Document and report any changes. *Ongoing assessment allows you to identify changing needs and adjust interventions accordingly.*

- Provide prescribed treatment for child's underlying condition. Monitor and report progress *to provide basis for plan of care.*
- Monitor completion of bathing and hygiene *to evaluate self-care abilities and identify areas of need.* Assist as necessary. Provide help only when child has difficulty.
- Instruct child and family members in bathing and hygiene techniques. Have them perform return demonstrations *to identify problem areas and build self-confidence.*
- Allow ample time to perform self-care. Encourage child to complete each task. Provide constructive feedback. *Rushing creates unnecessary stress and promotes failure. Completing a task without assistance promotes self-confidence. Positive feedback encourages progress.*
- Provide privacy for self-care activities. *Modesty becomes important to a child around age 6.*
- Provide safety equipment *to promote safety.*
- Refer child and family to support groups or community services *to provide continued assistance for efforts to promote self-care independence.*

Evaluations for expected outcomes

- Child and family members voice feelings regarding bathing and hygiene self-care deficit.
- Child displays competence in performing bathing and hygiene through return demonstration.
- Family members display competence in assisting with bathing and hygiene through return demonstration.
- Child's skin remains clean, dry, and intact.

Documentation

- Child's expression of frustration or feelings of inadequacy.
- Family members' expressions of concern regarding child's inability to carry out bathing and hygiene
- Response to treatment for underlying condition
- Child's motor and sensory status
- Observations of child's impaired self-care ability
- Interventions to promote self-care skills and to provide supportive care
- Instructions to child and family members, their understanding of instructions, and their demonstrated ability to carry out bathing and hygiene
- Child's and family members' responses to nursing interventions
- Evaluations for each expected outcome.

■ Self-care deficit: Dressing and grooming

related to developmental delay

Definition

Inability to carry out activities associated with dressing and grooming

Assessment

- Age
- History of neurologic, sensory, or developmental impairment
- Self-care abilities, including knowledge and use of adaptive equipment, preparation of equipment and supplies, technical or mechanical skills

• Musculoskeletal status, including range of motion, muscle tone, gait, muscle size and strength, functional capabilities, mechanical restrictions (splints, casts, traction)
• Neurologic status, including cognition, communication ability, insight or judgment, level of consciousness, memory, motor ability, orientation, sensory ability
• Psychosocial status, including child's affective reaction to imbalances between motor abilities and cognitive reasoning abilities, usual life-style, parents' perception of developmental delay

Defining characteristics
• Impaired ability to dress or undress
• Impaired ability to fasten clothing
• Impaired ability to obtain articles of clothing
• Inability to maintain satisfactory appearance

Associated medical diagnoses (selected)
This diagnosis can occur with any musculoskeletal, cognitive, or perceptual impairment.

Expected outcomes
• Child's is dressed and well groomed each day.
• Child and family members express feelings and concerns regarding child's self-care deficit.
• Child and family members demonstrate correct use of assistive devices, as appropriate.
• Child or family member performs self-care program daily.

Interventions and rationales
• Assess child's functional, cognitive, and perceptual level at periodic intervals. Document and report any changes. *Ongoing assessment allows you to identify changing needs and adjust interventions accordingly.*
• Provide prescribed treatment for the child's underlying condition. Monitor and report progress *to provide basis for plan of care.*
• Monitor completion of dressing and grooming *to evaluate self-care abilities and identify areas of need.* Assist as necessary. Provide help only when child has difficulty. *Appropriate assistance provides an opportunity to teach self-care and promote good habits.*
• Suggest clothing that child can manage easily, such as clothing slightly larger than regular size or pants and shoes with Velcro fasteners *to foster independence and improve self-esteem.*
• Instruct child and family members in dressing and grooming techniques. Have them perform return demonstrations *to identify problem areas and build self-confidence.*
• Allow ample time to perform self-care. Encourage child to complete each task. Provide constructive feedback. *Rushing creates unnecessary stress and promotes failure. Completing a task without assistance promotes self-confidence. Positive feedback encourages progress.*
• Provide privacy for dressing and grooming. *Modesty becomes important to a child around age 6.*
• Refer child and family to support groups or community services *to provide ongoing assistance.*

Evaluations for expected outcomes
• Child and family members voice feelings regarding deficit in grooming and dressing skills.
• Child displays competence in performing dressing and grooming skills through return demonstration.

• Family members display competence in assisting with dressing and grooming through return demonstration.

Documentation

• Child's expression of frustration or feelings of inadequacy
• Family members' expressions of feelings and concerns regarding child's inability to carry out dressing and grooming
• Response to treatment for underlying condition
• Child's motor and sensory status
• Interventions to promote self-care skills and provide supportive care
• Instructions provided to child and family members, their understanding of instructions, and their demonstrated ability to carry out bathing and hygiene
• Child's and family members' responses to nursing interventions
• Evaluations for each expected outcome.

Self-care deficit: Feeding

related to developmental delay

Definition

Inability to carry out feeding routine

Assessment

• Age
• History of injury or disease associated with musculoskeletal impairment
• Self-care abilities, including knowledge and use of adaptive equipment, preparation of equipment and supplies, technical and mechanical skills
• Musculoskeletal status, including coordination, functional ability, muscle tone and strength, range of motion, mechanical restrictions (cast, splint, traction)
• Neurologic status, including cognition, communication ability, level of consciousness, motor ability, sensory status
• Nutritional status, including weight, food preferences
• Psychosocial status, including child's affective reaction to imbalances between motor abilities and cognitive reasoning abilities, usual life-style, parents' perception of developmental delay

Defining characteristics

• Expressions of discouragement or depression
• Inability to bring food from receptacle to mouth
• Loss of upper extremity
• Musculoskeletal impairment

Associated medical diagnoses (selected)

This diagnosis can occur with any musculoskeletal, cognitive, or perceptual impairment.

Expected outcomes

• Child maintains desired weight.
• Child consumes adequate calories.
• Auscultation reveals clear chest sounds.
• Child and family members express feelings and concerns regarding self-care deficit.
• Child and family members demonstrate use of assistive devices.
• Family member assists with feeding program daily.
• Child participates in self-care at optimal level.

Interventions and rationales

• Provide prescribed treatment for the child's underlying condition. Monitor and report progress *to provide basis for plan of care.*

• Weigh child daily and record results *to assess nutritional status.*
• Determine type of food child handles most and tolerates best (formula, finger foods, soft or liquid diet) *to enhance self-feeding ability.*
• Monitor and record breath sounds every 4 hours. Report any evidence of crackles, wheezing, or rhonchi *to detect aspiration.*
• Monitor feeding routine *to evaluate self-care abilities and identify areas of need.* Assist as necessary; for example, cut into bite-size portions. Provide help only when child has difficulty. *Appropriate assistance provides an opportunity to teach self-care and promote good habits.*
• Instruct child and family members in feeding routine. Have them perform return demonstrations *to build self-confidence.*
• Allow ample time to perform self-care activities. *Rushing creates unnecessary stress and promotes failure.* Encourage child to complete each task. *Completing a task without assistance promotes self-confidence.* Provide constructive feedback.
• When feeding child, work slowly. Position child in upright sitting position. Use supportive devices as needed to maintain child's posture. Sit at eye level with child. *These measures will help decrease risk of aspiration. Sitting at eye level will help prevent child from hyperextending his neck, which may increase the risk of aspiration.*
• Teach specific tasks (grasping spoon, opening mouth, closing lips around utensil, swallowing) rather than total feeding skill. Use behavior modification techniques of praise and reward to mark accomplishments. *Children may not have cognitive or motor abilities to complete total skill. Breaking down behavior into smaller units increases likelihood of success.*

Evaluations for expected outcomes
• Child and family members voice feelings regarding feeding routine.
• Child demonstrates correct feeding technique.
• Child maintains weight above 5th percentile on pediatric growth charts.
• Aspiration does not occur as evidenced by clear breath sounds heard during auscultation.

Documentation
• Child's expression of frustration or feelings of inadequacy
• Family members' expression of concerns regarding child's inability to feed self.
• Child's response to treatment for underlying condition
• Child's motor and sensory status
• Interventions performed to promote self-care skills and provide supportive care
• Instructions to child and family members, their understanding of instructions, and their demonstrated ability to carry out feeding routine.
• Child's and family members' responses to nursing interventions
• Evaluations for each expected outcome.

■ Self-care deficit: Toileting

related to developmental delay

Definition
Inability to carry out aspects of self-care associated with bowel and urine elimination

Assessment

- Developmental factors, including age, maturity, smooth muscle control
- History of neurologic, sensory, or developmental impairment
- Self-care abilities, including knowledge and use of adaptive equipment, preparation of equipment and supplies, technical or mechanical skills
- Musculoskeletal status, including range of motion, muscle tone, gait, muscle size and strength, functional capabilities, mechanical restrictions (splints, casts, traction)
- Neurologic status, including cognition, communication ability, insight or judgment, level of consciousness, memory, motor ability, orientation, sensory ability
- Psychosocial status, including child's affective reaction to imbalances between motor abilities and cognitive reasoning abilities, usual life-style, parents' perception of developmental delay

Defining characteristics

- Inability to carry out proper toilet hygiene
- Inability to flush toilet or empty commode
- Inability to get to toilet or commode
- Inability to manipulate clothing for toileting
- Inability to sit on or rise from toilet or commode
- Musculoskeletal, cognitive, or perceptual impairment

Associated medical diagnoses (selected)

This diagnosis can occur with any musculoskeletal, cognitive, or perceptual impairment.

Expected outcomes

- Child maintains normal urine and bowel elimination patterns for age.
- Child and family members voice feelings about impaired toileting ability.
- Child and family members demonstrate correct use of appropriate assistive devices.
- Family member assists with bowel and bladder program as appropriate.
- Child's skin remains clean, dry, and intact.

Interventions and rationales

- Observe the child's functional, cognitive, and perceptual level at established periodic intervals. Document and report any changes. *Ongoing assessment allows you to identify changing needs and adjust interventions accordingly.*
- Provide prescribed treatment for the child's underlying condition. Monitor and report progress *to provide basis for plan of care.*
- Monitor intake and output *to detect fluid and electrolyte imbalances.*
- Assess skin condition, especially in perianal area *to detect evidence of skin breakdown.*
- Assist with toileting when necessary. As much as possible, allow child to perform toilet routine independently *to enhance toileting ability and promote feelings of control and independence.*
- Instruct child and family members in toileting routine. Have child and family members demonstrate toileting routine under supervision. *Return demonstration enables you to evaluate learning and increases child's and family members' confidence.*
- Provide privacy for toileting activities. *Beginning around age 6, modesty becomes important to a child.*
- Assist with specific bladder elimination procedures, such as:
  - intermittent self-catheterization. Assess child's readiness to learn

self-catheterization. Instruct child or family members in technique and request return demonstration *to evaluate understanding and ability;* maintain sterile technique in hospital and clean technique at home *to prevent infection.*
  – use of incontinence aids, including diapers, pads, and pants, as alternatives to indwelling devices. *Incontinence aids prevent soiling of clothes and linen, reduce embarrassment, and draw urine away from skin. Compared with indwelling devices, incontinence aids allow for greater mobility and carry decreased risk of infection.*
- Establish a regular pattern for bowel care; for example, after breakfast each morning, place child on toilet or commode for 1 hour after inserting glycerin suppository; allow child to remain upright for 30 minutes, then clean anal area. *Regular bowel care encourages routine physiologic function.*
- Teach parents bowel care routine *to foster compliance.*
- Maintain a diet log *to identify irritant foods,* and then eliminate such foods from child's diet *to promote regular bowel function.* Teach parents need to regulate child's intake of foods and fluids that cause diarrhea or constipation *to encourage healthful nutritional patterns.*
- Teach parents to regulate child's fluid intake according to a specific schedule and to limit fluid intake after dinner *to encourage voiding at appropriate time.*

Evaluations for expected outcomes
- Child and family members express feelings associated with child's toileting routine.
- Child and family members demonstrate correct toileting activities through return demonstration.
- Child maintains normal elimination patterns for age.
- Child's skin remains intact with no evidence of breakdown.

Documentation
- Child's expression of feelings of inadequacy or depression
- Family members' concerns about child's inability to carry out toileting activities
- Response to treatment for underlying condition
- Child's motor and sensory status
- Interventions to promote self-care skills and to provide supportive care
- Child's and family members' responses to nursing interventions
- Instructions to child and family members, their understanding of instructions, and demonstrated ability to carry out toileting routine
- Evaluations for each expected outcome.

■ Thermoregulation, ineffective

related to illness or trauma

Definition
Potentially extreme fluctuations in body temperature

Assessment
- Age
- History of illness or injury, including related events, such as exposure to sources of infection (intrauterine or extrauterine)
- Perinatal history, including asphyxia

- Health history, including chronic disease or disability
- Medication history
- Vital signs, including temperature, pulse rate, blood pressure, respirations
- Skin color and temperature
- Fluid and electrolyte status, including skin turgor, intake and output, mucous membranes, serum electrolyte levels, urine specific gravity
- Neurologic status, including level of consciousness
- Nutritional status, including willingness and ability to eat, current weight, weight gain pattern (growth chart)

Defining characteristics

- Confusion, lethargy, irritability
- Fluctuations in body temperature above 100° F (37.8° C) or below 96.8° F (36° C)
- Flushed or mottled skin, acrocyanosis
- Skin cool or warm to touch

Associated medical diagnoses (selected)

Brain tumors (especially if located in the hypothalamus, pituitary, or medulla), cerebral edema, chemical toxicity (including reactions to drugs or anesthesia), congestive heart failure, dehydration, infection, near-drowning, smoke inhalation or other anoxic events

Expected outcomes

- Child maintains body temperature at normothermic levels (between 96.8° and 99° F [36° and 37.2° C]).
- Child's fluid intake and output remain balanced and within normal limits for age.
- Child maintains adequate glucose intake and consumes _____ calories per day.
- Child and family members identify risk factors that exacerbate temperature fluctuations.
- Child and family members express understanding of measures to prevent dehydration.
- Family members demonstrate procedure for assessing axillary or oral temperature accurately.

Interventions and rationales

- Take axillary or oral temperature every 1 to 4 hours. Avoid rectal thermometry. Record temperature and route. *Physically and psychologically safer than rectal thermometers, axillary and oral thermometers provide an accurate core temperature.*
- Take the following steps *to reduce excessive fever:*
  - Remove sheets, blankets, and most clothing (except diapers and underwear).
  - Place cool cloths on axilla and groin.
  - Perform tepid sponging procedure.
  - Use hypothermia blanket for temperature above 101.3° F (38.5° C). Discontinue if shivering takes place (*shivering increases the metabolic rate and supports fever*). Set blanket temperature at 41° F (5° C). Use more than one hypothermia blanket if necessary.
  - Monitor vital signs every 15 minutes for 1 hour and as indicated. *Decreasing body temperature too rapidly can cause vascular collapse.*
- Monitor heart rate, rhythm, and respiratory rate. *Careful overall monitoring determines the need for more aggressive intervention.*
- Calculate child's fluid, glucose, and electrolyte requirements. Administer I.V. fluids as indicated. Monitor and

record intake and output *to compensate for the increase in metabolic rate and to prevent dehydration. Insensible fluid losses increase by 10% for every 1° C rise in temperature.*
- Take the following steps *to maintain body temperature:*
  - Use warming blanket for temperature below 96.8° F. Set blanket temperature at 100.4° F (38° C).
  - Keep child wrapped in blankets and cover child's head. *Body surface area, particulary the head, is proportionately larger in young children. Adequate covering will prevent heat loss.*
- Teach parents how to take an accurate temperature and have parents provide a return demonstration *to ensure accurate monitoring after hospital discharge.*
- Determine child's preferences for oral fluids. Push fluids in a manner appropriate to child's age and level of development. *A well-hydrated child's temperature returns to normal range more quickly.*
- Discuss factors that precipitate neurogenic temperature drift with family members *to prevent future episodes.*

Evaluations for expected outcomes
- Child's temperature remains within normal limits.
- Child's fluid intake and output are balanced and within normal limits for age.
- Child expresses an increase in comfort level.
- Family members identify risk factors and describe measures to prevent dehydration.
- Family members demonstrate ability to measure axillary or oral temperature accurately.
- Family members demonstrate measures to care for child with fever, including medication administration, sponging, and maintaining environmental controls

Documentation
- Observations of physical findings
- Nursing interventions performed
- Medications administered
- Child's response to nursing interventions
- Evaluations for each expected outcome.

Verbal communication impairment

related to developmental factors

Definition
Decreased ability to speak, understand, or use words appropriately

Assessment
- Age
- Health history, including past respiratory, neurologic, or musculoskeletal disorders or surgery
- Respiratory status, including dyspnea, use of accessory muscles, respiratory pattern
- Neurologic status, including mental status (level of consciousness, orientation, cognition, memory, insight, and judgment), speech (pattern, signing, and such communication aids as an artificial larynx, computer-assisted speech device, pen and pencil, picture board, and alphabet board)
- Musculoskeletal status, including range of motion, manual dexterity
- Parental status, including understanding of normal speech development, level of frustration with child's speech impairment, coping skills

Defining characteristics
- Inability to communicate verbally because of developmental level or delay in development

Associated medical diagnoses (selected)
This diagnosis may be associated with any disorder that alters the child's ability to speak. Examples include acute respiratory distress, hearing loss or impairment, prematurity, and such birth defects as cleft palate or cleft lip.

Expected outcomes
- Family members express desire to better understand child's communication impairment.
- Family members demonstrate an understanding of verbal development in children and alternative communication techniques.
- Child communicates needs.

Interventions and rationales
- Teach parents measures *to stimulate language development:*
  - Talking, reading, and playing music for child
  - Repeating sound child makes
  - Pointing to objects and naming them
  - Using generative speech ("What would you like to wear today") rather than directive speech ("Do you want to wear the red shirt?"). *Generative speech requires the child to generate words rather than simply responding with yes or no.*
- Describe to family members alternative methods of assessing needs of speech-delayed children. Toddlers and preschoolers may communicate their needs through role-playing with dolls and stuffed animals. Preschoolers and school-age children may communicate through drawing. Parents may use the pictoral (faces) pain scale to assess an ill child's level of discomfort. *These techniques will enable the family to better understand their speech-delayed child.*
- Assess family members' level of understanding of speech development process. Tell them that a toddler has limited receptive language skills and should be given one direction at a time. A preschooler has a limited vocabulary and may communicate through gestures and symbols. Further explain that children develop speech at different rates. If a child has impaired language and cognitive skills, parents may be able to communicate through nonverbal means. *These measures increase family members' understanding of child's speech impairment.*

Evaluations for expected outcomes
- Family members describe the stages of speech development.
- Family members demonstrate three alternative methods of assessing needs of speech-delayed child.
- Child communicates needs.

Documentation
- Family members' understanding of speech development process
- Family members' demonstration of alternative methods of assessing needs of speech-delayed child
- Family members' understanding of alternative methods of communicating with child
- Evaluations for each expected outcome.

PART FOUR

MATERNAL-NEONATAL HEALTH

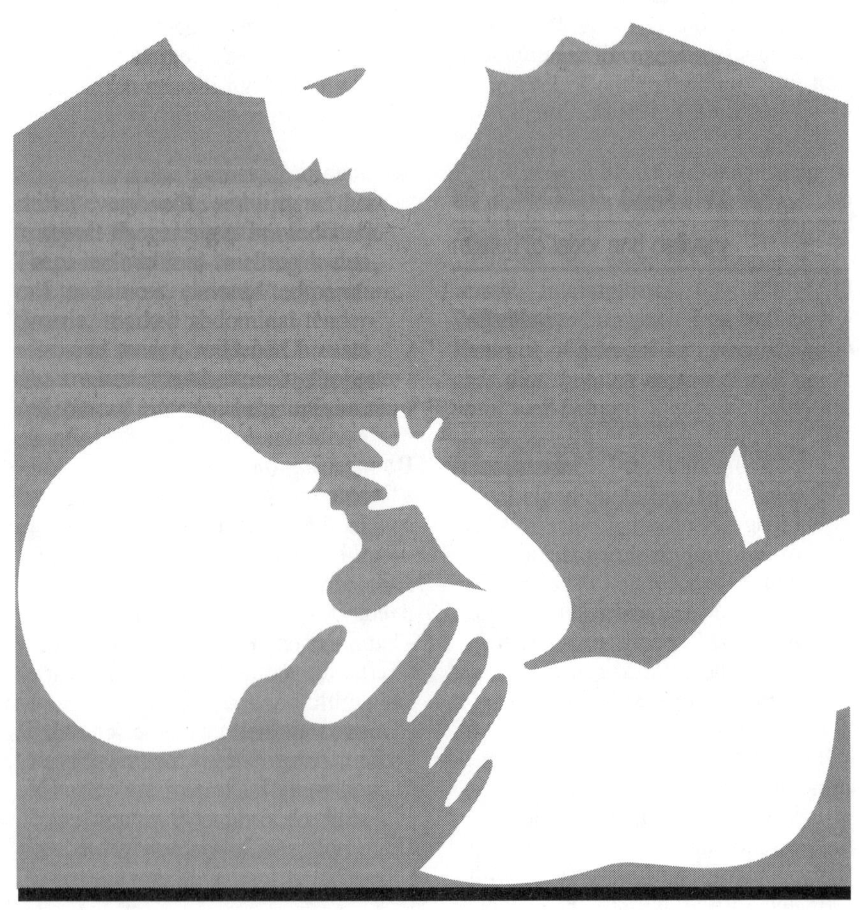

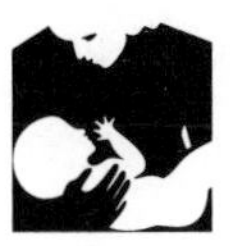

INTRODUCTION

This section discusses maternal, fetal, and neonatal care, with an emphasis on meeting the changing needs of mother, child, and family. Because of the dynamic nature of pregnancy and childbirth, you'll need to be flexible in your care planning. Expect to continually form new nursing diagnoses during the time that you are providing care.

During pregnancy, you'll assess maternal factors, such as age, past experience with pregnancy and delivery, health history, reaction to fetal movement, and nutritional status. Keep in mind that the mother's health status directly affects the fetus's well being.

After birth, you'll assess neonatal factors, such as Apgar scores, gestational age, weight in relation to gestational age, vital signs, feeding patterns, muscle tone, condition of fontanels, and characteristics of the neonate's cry.

Throughout your assessment, maintain a family-centered, holistic approach. Assess family status. Be aware of how pregnancy and the neonate's arrival affect parents, siblings, and the rest of the family. Evaluate how well the mother, father, siblings, and other family members bond with the neonate.

Use information gathered during assessment to develop appropriate nursing diagnoses. In this section, you'll find nursing diagnoses and related etiologies for the prenatal period, labor and delivery, and the postpartum period. Neonatal health is covered as well. These nursing diagnoses state actual or potential health problems of the developing family, focusing on the physiologic and psychosocial needs of its members.

When implementing your plan of care, reinforce your interventions with thorough patient teaching. Encourage family members to become involved in the planning and implementation of care. Stay attuned to their changing educational needs, and remain sensitive to the new mother and supportive of her emotional concerns.

Inform other members of the health care team of your nursing goals, and enlist their support as needed. Keep colleagues informed about the family's progress in attaining goals.

Evaluate the plan of care frequently. This will enable you to promptly determine the need for revisions, thereby ensuring that the plan of care accurately reflects the developing family's current needs.

Anxiety

related to hospitalization and birthing process

Definition

Feeling of threat or danger to self related to pregnancy or birth

Assessment

- History of stress-related signs or symptoms
- Current worries, fears, concerns
- Expectations of labor experience, including knowledge, past experience
- Behavior, including reaction to fetal movement and uterine activity, motor activity, excessive or extraneous movements, interactions with nurse and significant others
- Cognitive status, including ability to concentrate, learn, remember
- Physiologic status
- Usual coping methods
- Mood
- Personality
- Progress of labor

Defining characteristics

- Dilated pupils
- Excessive attention to fetal movement or uterine activity
- Excessive or uncontrolled reaction to labor contractions
- Expressions of concern about pregnancy or birth
- Expressions of feelings of helplessness or incapacity
- Fear, apprehension, wariness
- Focus on self
- Glancing about
- Hypertension
- Inability to concentrate, understand, or remember
- Incoordinate contractions and nonprogressive labor
- Increased muscle tension in body or face
- Perspiration
- Poor eye contact
- Rapid pulse rate
- Restlessness, shakiness, trembling, jittery behavior, extraneous movements
- Vasoconstriction (pale and cool skin)
- Verbalization of fear of unspecified negative outcome

Associated medical diagnoses (selected)

Amniotic fluid embolism, hemorrhagic complications of pregnancy (abruptio placentae, placenta previa, postpartum hemorrhage, disseminated intravascular coagulation), labor (especially transition phase of labor), pregnancy (normal or with complications), shock (anaphylactic reaction to drugs), supine hypotensive syndrome

Expected outcomes

- Patient expresses feelings of anxiety.
- Patient identifies cause of anxiety.
- Patient makes use of available emotional support.
- Patient shows fewer signs of anxiety.
- Patient identifies positive aspects of her efforts to cope during childbirth.
- Patient acquires increased knowledge about childbirth and is better prepared to cope with future births.

Interventions and rationales

- Assess patient's knowledge, experience, and expectations of labor. *Effective intervention requires precise knowledge of source of anxiety.*
- Discuss normal labor progression with patient and explain what to expect during labor *to provide information about the normal progression of*

labor and enable the patient to better understand her own experience.
• Involve patient in making decisions about care *to reduce the sense of powerlessness that some women experience during labor.*
• Share information on labor progression, vital signs, and neonate's condition with the patient *to provide reassurance of normality and increase her sense of participation.*
• Interpret sights and sounds of the environment (electronic fetal monitor strip, fetal monitor sounds, activities in unit) for the patient *to make the environment seem less threatening.*
• Attend to patient's comfort needs *to increase trust and reduce anxiety.*
• Encourage the patient to employ coping skills used successfully in the past *to enhance the patient's sense of control.*
• Teach new coping skills (relaxation, breathing techniques, positioning) *to diminish anxiety by increasing the patient's sense of power and control.* Review skills with patient periodically. *Because anxiety impairs recall, reviewing skills may be necessary.*
• Organize work to spend as much time as possible with patient *to provide a comforting presence and a source of assistance, thereby promoting a sense of security.*
• Allow family members to participate in care *to provide comfort and help the patient cope with labor.*

Evaluations for expected outcomes
• Patient relates feelings of anxiety about pregnancy or birth.
• Patient communicates with nurse or family members to gain reassurance, information, or emotional support.
• Patient's physiologic or behavioral signs return to normal.
• Patient, verbally or nonverbally, indicates that birth was a positive experience.
• Patient expresses satisfaction with her own behavior during birth.
• Patient verbalizes increased confidence in her ability to cope with pregnancy and birth.

Documentation
• Patient's expressions of anxiety
• Patient's description of perceived reasons for anxiety
• Observation of physical or behavioral signs of anxiety
• Interventions to assist patient with coping
• Patient's response to interventions
• Evaluations for each expected outcome.

■ Aspiration, high risk for

related to neonate's immature cough or gag reflex

Definition
Entry of GI secretions, oropharyngeal secretions, or exogenous fluids into neonate's tracheobronchial passages

Assessment
• Gestational age
• Neonate's weight in relation to gestational age
• Maternal sedation before delivery, effects of maternal sedation on labor
• Neonate's health status, including preexisting conditions, anomalies, intrauterine environment, urologic status, cardiovascular status, respiratory status, GI status
• Laboratory studies of neonate, including fluid, electrolyte, and arterial blood gas levels

- Neonate's vital signs
- Neonate's nutritional status, including continuous or intermittent gavage feeding

Risk factors
- Adverse intrauterine environment
- Bolus tube feedings or drug administration
- Decreased GI motility
- Delayed gastric emptying
- Depressed cough or gag reflex
- Endotracheal tube
- Facial, oral, or neck trauma
- GI tubes
- Impaired swallowing
- Increased gastric residual contents
- Increased intragastric pressure
- Polyhydramnios
- Prematurity
- Reduced level of consciousness
- Traumatic intubation
- Vigorous, prolonged suctioning

Associated medical diagnoses (selected)
Asphyxia, aspiration pneumonia, bowel obstruction, cesarean birth, diaphragmatic hernia, duodenal atresia, imperforate anus, intestinal obstruction, intraventricular hemorrhage, prematurity, respiratory depression, respiratory distress syndrome, tracheoesophageal fistula

Expected outcomes
- Neonate is suctioned as needed and maintains a clear airway.
- Neonate does not exhibit gastric distention.
- Neonate demonstrates minimal to moderate quantity of nasopharyngeal and oropharyngeal secretions.
- Neonate tolerates initial feeding.
- Neonate does not demonstrate any color changes during feeding.
- Neonate demonstrates appropriate suck and swallow reflex.
- Neonate has no adventitious breath sounds.
- Neonate does not exhibit signs and symptoms of aspiration.

Interventions and rationales
- Assess neonate's respiratory status on an ongoing basis until stable *to evaluate respiratory system transition to extrauterine life.*
- Monitor vital signs, according to hospital protocol, and report changes *to determine multisystem adjustment to extrauterine existence.*
- Suction as needed to keep upper and lower airways clear. If neonate aspirates meconium, assist doctor with laryngoscopy to suction below vocal cords. In a delivery room, suction oropharynx and nasopharynx with bulb syringe, DeLee catheter, or suction catheter attached to wall suction. *These measures may prevent additional respiratory compromise.*
- Perform head-to-toe physical assessment *to detect abnormalities in other body systems that may impact on respiratory effort.*
- Withhold oral feedings if signs of respiratory distress occur. Provide I.V. fluids as ordered. *Sucking may place additional stress on a neonate in respiratory distress and may lead to aspiration.*
- When offering initial feeding, observe for suck and swallow reflex, gag and cough reflex, and color changes. Have suction equipment available and ready to use. *Early detection of difficulty may prevent neonatal morbidity or mortality.*
- If neonate is receiving gavage feeding:
  - keep head of bed elevated during and after feedings unless contraindicated

- ensure proper positioning of neonate before feeding or administering medication
- monitor residual gastric contents and follow parameters for withholding feedings
- once per shift, measure abdominal girth to check for distention
- stop the gavage feeding immediately if aspiration is suspected. Keep suction apparatus at bedside and suction as needed. Turn neonate on side.

Preventive measures reduce risk of aspiration.

- Review laboratory results and report abnormalities. *Early identification of abnormal laboratory values reduces risk of aspiration.*
- Explain to parents the reasons for interventions. *Gaining parental understanding and cooperation will contribute to a positive outcome.*
- Instruct parents in feeding techniques that will help prevent distended abdomen leading to aspiration. Tell them to avoid overfeeding and to burp neonate at frequent intervals (after intake of ½ to 1 oz). Instruct parents to position neonate on right side with head of bed elevated for 30 to 60 minutes after feeding. *Providing instructions encourages parental understanding and cooperation.*

Evaluations for expected outcomes

- Staff and parents participate in helping neonate to maintain a patent airway.
- Parents become comfortable with techniques for feeding neonate.
- Deviations from normal are noted and responded to promptly to reduce risk of aspiration.

Documentation

- Neonate's tolerance of initial feeding and of gavage feedings
- Residual gastric contents following gavage feeding
- Incidents of vomiting, aspiration, or both
- Breath sounds
- Observations of physical findings
- Interventions performed to prevent aspiration
- Evaluations for each expected outcome.

Breast-feeding, effective

Definition

State in which mother, neonate, or family exhibits proficiency and satisfaction with breast-feeding process

Assessment

- Maternal status, including age and maturity, parity, level of prenatal breast-feeding preparation, past breast-feeding experience, previous postpartum history, physical condition (actual or perceived inadequate milk supply, comfort level), psychosocial factors (apprehension level, body image, stress from family and career, sociocultural views of breast-feeding, emotional support from significant others)
- Neonatal status, including satisfaction and contentment, growth-rate, age-weight relationship, urinary output, quantity and characteristics of stools, ability to latch onto breasts

Defining characteristics

- Neonate appears eager to nurse and is content after feedings
- Neonate eliminates soft stools and a sufficient quantity of unconcentrated urine

- Neonate gains adequate weight
- Mother positions neonate at breast to promote successful latch-on response
- Mother reports satisfaction with breast-feeding process
- Oxytocin release occurs (let-down response or milk-ejection reflex)
- Regular and sustained suckling occurs (every 2 to 3 hours)

Associated medical diagnoses (selected)
Vaginal or cesarean section delivery of term or preterm neonate

Expected outcomes
- Mother breast-feeds neonate successfully and experiences satisfaction with breast-feeding process.
- Neonate feeds successfully on both breasts and appears satisfied.
- Neonate grows and develops in pace with accepted standards.
- Mother continues breast-feeding neonate after early postpartum period.

Interventions and rationales
- Assess mother's knowledge and experience of breast-feeding *to focus teaching on specific learning needs.*
- Educate mother and selected support person about breast-feeding techniques:
  - Clean hands and breasts before nursing.
  - Position neonate for feeding (neonate should be able to grasp most of areola).
  - Change positions to decrease nipple tenderness and use both breasts at each feeding.
  - Remove neonate from breast by breaking suction.
  - Avoid setting time limits in early stage.
  - Practice breast care.

Greater understanding of techniques improves chances for success.
- Teach techniques *to stimulate let-down response.* These include warm showers and compresses, relaxation and guided imagery, infant suckling, holding infant close to breasts, and listening to infant cry.
- Educate mother about her nutritional needs. She requires a well-balanced diet plus an additional 500 calories and two extra glasses of fluid each day *to maintain an adequate milk supply.* She should limit caffeine and avoid foods that make her uncomfortable.
- Teach mother what to expect from breast-feeding neonate *to prepare mother for care of neonate at home.* The neonate should pass 1 to 6 stools and wet 6 to 8 diapers per day. Stools should be soft to liquid and nonodorous. The neonate should feed every 2 to 3 hours and should be quiet after feeding and appear generally well. Explain that the neonate also requires nonnutritive sucking.
- Assist mother and family in planning for home care. The mother needs to rest when neonate sleeps, practice self-care, learn techniques for expression and storage of breast milk, and recognize signs of engorgement and infection. Family members should understand the importance of helping out. *Mothers often stop breast-feeding once they return home and resume work, usually because of fatigue.*
- Provide quiet and privacy *to enhance development of breast-feeding skills.*
- Encourage mother to verbalize concerns about breast-feeding *to reduce anxiety.*
- Offer information about breast-feeding support groups *to help meet emotional and learning needs.*

Evaluations for expected outcomes
- Mother describes breast-feeding procedures, including letting-down, latching-on, breaking suction, and positioning.
- Mother demonstrates successful positioning of neonate, latching-on to nipple, let-down of milk, and removal from breast.
- Neonate feeds on both breasts and in different positions at each feeding.
- Neonate quiets after feeding.
- Neonate's weight and length remain consistent and within 10th and 90th percentiles on a pediatric growth grid.
- Mother expresses satisfaction with breast-feeding.
- Mother breast-feeds neonate as needed.
- Mother continues to breast-feed infant after discharge from hospital.

Documentation
- Mother's expressions about breast-feeding experience
- Observations of breast-feeding techniques and mother-infant interaction during breast-feeding
- Teaching and instructions given
- Neonate's growth and weight
- Referrals to support groups
- Mother's plans for breast-feeding after discharge
- Evaluations for each expected outcome.

Breast-feeding, ineffective

related to dissatisfaction with breast-feeding process

Definition
State in which mother, neonate, or family experience dissatisfaction or difficulty with breast-feeding process

Assessment
- Maternal status, including age and maturity, relationships with significant others, previous bonding history, parity, level of prenatal breast-feeding preparation, knowledge or previous breast-feeding experience, physical condition (actual or perceived inadequate milk supply, nipple shape, comfort level), psychosocial impact (apprehension level, body image and perceptions, such stressors as family and career, actual or perceived sociocultural views of breast-feeding, emotional support from significant others)
- Neonatal status, including satisfaction and contentment, growth rate, age-weight relationship

Defining characteristics
- Abnormal or awkwardly shaped nipple
- Inability of neonate to attach to nipple correctly
- Lack of maternal attachment behavior; reluctance to put neonate to breast as necessary
- Nonsustained suckling at breast
- No observable sign of oxytocin release
- Obvious neonatal hunger with little or no weight gain
- Obvious physical discomfort
- Outward evidence of apprehension, stress, fear (postpartum blues)
- Verbal report of inadequate breast-feeding knowledge

Associated medical diagnoses (selected)
Maternal nipple anomaly, maternal psychological stress, neonatal anomaly, prematurity

Expected outcomes
- Mother expresses physical and psychological comfort with breast-feeding techniques and practice.

• Mother shows decreased anxiety and apprehension.
• Neonate feeds successfully on both breasts and appears satisfied for at least 2 hours after feeding.
• Neonate grows and thrives.
• Mother states at least one resource for breast-feeding support.

Interventions and rationales
• Educate mother in breast care and breast-feeding techniques. *This reduces anxiety and enhances proper nutrition of neonate.*
• Be available yet discreet during breast-feeding. *Assessment of mother's technique can point out problem areas.* Encourage mother's questions, *to increase understanding and reduce anxiety.*
• Teach techniques for let-down response:
  – warm shower
  – breast massage
  – physically caring for neonate
  – holding neonate close to breasts.

These measures reduce anxiety and facilitate let-down response.
• Provide environmental setting conducive to breast-feeding:
  – quiet
  – private
  – comfortable
  – decreased external stressors.

A relaxed environment can promote successful breast-feeding.
• Encourage verbalization of fears and anxieties between mother and significant others. *This reduces anxiety and increases mother's sense of control.*
• Offer written information, a reading list, or information about breast-feeding support groups *to help meet mother's emotional and learning needs.*

Evaluations for expected outcomes
• Mother expresses physical and psychological comfort with breast-feeding techniques and practice.
• Mother displays decreased anxiety and apprehension.
• Neonate feeds successfully on both breasts.
• Neonate appears satisfied for at least 2 hours after feeding.
• Neonate grows and thrives.
• Mother states at least one available resource for breast-feeding support.

Documentation
• Mother's expressions of feelings of comfort with breast-feeding ability
• Observations of bonding and breast-feeding processes
• Teaching and instructions given
• Referrals to support groups
• Neonate growth and weight
• Evaluations for each expected outcome.

■ Breast-feeding, ineffective

related to limited maternal experience

Definition
State in which mother, neonate, or family experiences dissatisfaction or difficulty with breast-feeding process

Assessment
• Maternal status, including age and maturity, relationships with significant others, previous bonding history, parity, level of prenatal breast-feeding preparation, knowledge or previous breast-feeding experience, physical condition (actual or perceived inadequate milk supply, nipple shape, comfort level)
• Psychosocial status, including apprehension level, body image and

perceptions, stressors such as family and career, sociocultural views of breast-feeding, emotional support from significant others
• Neonatal status, including satisfaction and contentment, growth rate, age-weight relationship, neurologic status, respiratory status, sucking reflex, presence of factors that interfere with proper sucking (cleft lip, cleft palate), previous feedings with artificial nipples

Defining characteristics
• Absence of signs of oxytocin release
• Actual or perceived inadequacy of milk supply
• Inability or resistance of neonate to attach to nipple correctly
• Inadequate emptying of breast at feeding
• Inadequate opportunity for suckling at the breast
• Lack of maternal attachment behavior; reluctance to put neonate to breast as necessary
• Mother's expressions of apprehension, stress, fear (postpartum blues)
• Mother's inability to experience comfort with alternate breast-feeding positions
• Neonate's crying and fussing within 1 hour of breast-feeding
• Neonate's failure to sustain suckling at the breast
• Obvious neonatal hunger with little or no weight gain
• Persistence of sore or bleeding nipple beyond first week of breast-feeding
• Physical discomfort of mother
• Signs of inadequate neonatal intake
• Statements indicating inadequate breast-feeding knowledge
• Verbal reports of unsatisfactory breast-feeding

Associated medical diagnoses (selected)
Maternal: Breast engorgement, inverted nipples, mammaplasty, maternal psychological stress. Neonatal: Cleft lip or cleft palate, prematurity.

Expected outcomes
• Mother expresses understanding of breast-feeding techniques and practice.
• Mother displays decreased anxiety and apprehension.
• Mother and neonate experience successful breast-feeding.
• Neonate's initial weight loss is within accepted norms.
• Neonate's nutritional needs are met.

Interventions and rationales
• Assess mother's knowledge *to help direct your interventions.*
• Educate mother in breast care and breast-feeding techniques *to reduce anxiety and help ensure proper nutrition of neonate.*
• Provide appropriate pamphlets and audiovisual aids *to help meet mother's learning needs. Written material can be reviewed at the mother's own pace; audiovisual materials illustrate proper technique.*
• Determine mother's level of anxiety or ambivalence related to breast-feeding. *Anxiety and ambivalence can interfere with the mother's ability to learn and with the let-down reflex.*
• Teach techniques for the let-down reflex:
  – warm shower
  – breast massage
  – relaxation and guided imagery
  – infant suckling
  – holding neonate close to breasts.

These measures reduce anxiety and facilitate let-down reflex.
• Remain with mother and neonate during several feedings *to pinpoint problem areas.* Encourage mother to

ask questions *to increase understanding and reduce anxiety.*
• Evaluate position of neonate's tongue during breast-feeding. *To produce the proper sucking motion, neonate's tongue must be down during breast-feeding, with the nipple directly on top.*
• Instruct mother to offer breast as soon as possible after the neonate awakens; tell her not to wait until neonate is crying vigorously. *Getting an extremely upset neonate to breast-feed effectively is difficult.*
• Evaluate need for nipple shield and instruct mother in its use. *Nipple shields help draw out partially inverted nipples.*
• Make sure neonate is awake and alert when feeding; unwrap as needed. *A tightly wrapped, sleepy neonate will not be alert enough to suckle sufficiently.*
• Sprinkle glucose water on nipples before feeding if needed. *When making preliminary attempts at breast-feeding, neonate may open his mouth upon tasting glucose water. The neonate's open mouth can then be directed and attached to the nipple.*
• Evaluate neonate for presence of anomalies that may interfere with breast-feeding ability *to plan comprehensive treatment and teaching.*
• Instruct mother in proper breast-care techniques, such as wearing supportive bra, using cream, washing, and air drying. *Proper breast care helps prevent nipple drying, cracking, soreness, and bleeding, which can interfere with effective breast-feeding.*
• Instruct mother on ways to alleviate breast engorgement. *Breast engorgement can prevent neonate from effectively attaching to the nipple.*
• Review principles of milk production, and identify factors that can alter production or quality of breast milk, such as emotional upset and intake of alcohol, drugs, and certain foods. *Any substance the mother ingests passes through to breast milk. Mother must be aware of possible dangerous adverse effects.*
• Provide positive reinforcement for mother's efforts *to decrease anxiety and enhance feelings of self-esteem and success.*
• Provide mother with information about breast-feeding support groups. *Participation in a support group after discharge can help meet mother's emotional and learning needs.*

Evaluations for expected outcomes
• Mother demonstrates proper positioning of neonate during breast-feeding.
• Mother demonstrates proper techniques to encourage neonate to attach to nipple correctly.
• Mother expresses continued enthusiasm for breast-feeding.
• Mother demonstrates proper use of supplemental devices if appropriate.
• Mother expresses an understanding of milk production and identifies factors that can alter milk supply.
• Neonate feeds successfully on both breasts and appears satisfied for at least 2 hours after feeding.
• Neonate's initial weight loss remains within accepted norms and his nutritional needs are met.

Documentation
• Mother's level of knowledge related to breast-feeding
• Mother's expressions of dissatisfaction with breast-feeding ability
• Mother's emotional response to breast-feeding
• Mother's breast care practices

- Maternal conditions that may interfere with breast-feeding, such as inverted nipples or mammaplasty
- Mother's and neonate's behavior during and after breast-feeding, including positioning of neonate, neonate's response to being put to breast, neonate's level of satisfaction
- Mother's use of devices such as nipple shield
- Frequency and duration of feedings
- Neonate's growth, weight, output, and any supplemental feedings administered
- Teaching and instructions given and mother's response to instructions
- Goals established by mother
- Referrals to support groups
- Mother's and neonate's responses to nursing interventions
- Evaluations for each expected outcome.

Breast-feeding, interrupted

related to a contraindicating condition

Definition

Break in the continuity of breast-feeding resulting from a maternal or neonatal problem

Assessment

- Maternal status, including age and maturity, employment hours, relationship with significant other, parity, level of prenatal breast-feeding knowledge or experience, physical condition (comfort level, nipple shape, presence of infection, use of medication)
- Neonatal status, including age-weight relationship, growth rate, neurologic status, respiratory status, sucking reflex, presence of factors that interfere with proper sucking (cleft lip, cleft palate)

Defining characteristics

- Failure of the neonate to receive nourishment at breast for some or all feedings
- Mother's continued desire to maintain lactation and provide breast milk for the neonate's nutritional needs
- Mother's lack of knowledge about expressing and storing breast milk
- Separation of mother and infant

Associated medical diagnoses (selected)

Maternal or infant illness, maternal nipple anomaly, maternal psychological stress, neonatal anomaly, neonatal hyperbilirubinemia, prematurity

Expected outcomes

- Mother expresses her understanding of the factors that necessitate interruption in breast-feeding.
- Mother expresses comfort with her decision whether or not to resume breast-feeding.
- Mother expresses and stores breast milk appropriately.
- Mother's milk supply is adequate once breast-feeding is resumed.
- Mother resumes breast-feeding once interfering factors cease.
- Mother obtains relief from discomfort associated with engorgement.

Interventions and rationales

- Assess the mother's understanding of the reasons for interrupting breast-feeding *to evaluate her need for additional instruction.*
- Reassure the mother that the neonate's nutritional needs will be met through other methods *to allay her anxiety.*
- Assess the mother's desire to resume breast-feeding *to help plan interventions.*

• Provide appropriate educational materials, including audiovisual aids and written materials. *Audiovisual aids demonstrate proper expressing and storing techniques; written material allows the mother to review information at her own pace.*
• Instruct the mother in techniques for expressing and storing breast milk *to ensure a proper milk supply.*
• Recommend use of a breast pump according to the following guidelines *to provide maximum stimulation and prolactin production:*
 – Initiate pumping 24 to 48 hours after delivery.
 – Pump a minimum of five times a day.
 – Pump a minimum of 100 minutes a day.
 – Pump long enough to soften breasts each time, regardless of duration.
• Encourage the mother to save her breast milk in a sterile container and store it in a refrigerator or freezer for future feedings. *Preserving breast milk ensures that the neonate receives maternal antibodies and helps to encourage maternal involvement in neonatal care.*
• If prolonged pumping is required, encourage use of a piston-style electric pump. *Using an electric pump produces milk with a higher fat content than does hand pumping.*
• If the mother intends to resume breast-feeding, instruct her in ways to relieve breast engorgement *to prevent discomfort that may keep the neonate from sucking effectively.*
• If appropriate, instruct the mother in use of devices such as a breast shell, *which is designed to alter flat or inverted nipples, a condition that may interfere with successful breast-feeding.*
• Review the mother's daily routine *to advise her how to incorporate breast-feeding into her schedule.*
• Provide the mother with information about breast-feeding support groups. *Participating in a support group can help the mother obtain needed emotional support and continue learning.*
• If the mother doesn't intend to resume breast-feeding, advise her to wear a supportive bra, apply ice, and take a mild analgesic, such as acetaminophen, *to alleviate discomfort associated with engorgement.*

Evaluations for expected outcomes
• Mother describes factors that necessitate interruption in breast-feeding.
• Mother demonstrates proper expression and storage techniques.
• Mother expresses comfort with her decision whether or not to resume breast-feeding.
• Mother resumes breast-feeding when interrupting factors are eliminated.
• Mother's milk supply is adequate when breast-feeding is resumed.
• Mother obtains relief from discomfort associated with engorgement.
• Infant's nutritional needs will be met as evidenced by appropriate weight gain, for example, 1 oz a day for first 6 months of life.

Documentation
• Factors that necessitated interruption in breast-feeding (reassessed periodically to determine status)
• Mother's expression of feelings about the need to interrupt breast-feeding
• Mother's decision whether to continue breast-feeding when possible
• Patient teaching

- Mother's efforts to ensure appropriate milk supply
- Mother's responses to nursing interventions
- Neonate's growth, weight, and output
- Referrals to support groups
- Evaluations for each expected outcome.

Breathing pattern, ineffective

related to adjustment to extrauterine existence

Definition

State in which a neonate's breathing pattern does not provide adequate pulmonary inflation or deflation to promote successful transition to extrauterine life

Assessment

- Gestational age
- Weight in relation to gestational age
- Maternal sedation before delivery
- Preexisting conditions, including anomalies, adverse intrauterine environment, prematurity
- Health assessment, including neurologic status, cardiovascular status, respiratory status, integumentary status, gastrointestinal status, fluid and electrolyte status, laboratory studies

Defining characteristics

- Abnormal arterial blood gas levels
- Altered chest excursion
- Apnea
- Cyanosis
- Grunting
- Nasal flaring
- Retractions
- Tachypnea

Associated medical diagnoses (selected)

Asphyxia, aspiration pneumonia, cesarean birth, choanal atresia, congenital heart disease, diaphragmatic hernia, hyaline membrane disease, hypoplastic lungs, meconium aspiration, persistent fetal circulation, prematurity, respiratory distress syndrome

Expected outcomes

- Neonate establishes normal respiratory rate (40 to 60 breaths/minute) within 1 hour after birth.
- Signs of respiratory distress are absent 1 hour after birth.
- Neonate does not require assisted ventilation.
- Neonate does not require supplemental oxygen.
- Neonate makes a successful transition to extrauterine life with adequate respiratory function.

Interventions and rationales

- Immediately after delivery:
  - Vigorously dry neonate and place under radiant warmer.
  - Suction oropharynx and nasopharynx as needed via a bulb syringe, DeLee catheter, or suction catheter connected to wall suction.
  - Obtain 1-minute and 5-minute Apgar scores.
  - Provide whiffs of oxygen, if indicated.
  - Remove wet blankets and replace with dry ones.
  - Observe for signs of respiratory distress (nasal flaring, tachypnea, retractions, grunting, and accessory muscle breathing).
  - Provide or assist with resuscitative measures, as indicated: bag and mask; naloxone (Narcan) administration, as ordered, if respiratory distress is secondary

to maternal sedation; intubation; and suctioning below vocal cords under direct visualization.

Respiratory difficulties are responsible for most morbidity and mortality during the neonatal period. Accurate assessment and prompt intervention at delivery are critical to sustaining life.

- Transfer neonate to nursery when stable or if more extensive resuscitation measures are needed *to help improve the transition to extrauterine life.*
- Upon admission to nursery:
  - Obtain neonate's vital signs. Observe central and peripheral color. Note signs of respiratory distress.
  - Perform physical assessment, noting anomalies or other abnormal findings.
  - Maintain a neutral thermal environment.
  - Obtain a brief obstetric history, including course of labor and delivery and condition of neonate before arrival in nursery. Note presence of risk factors.
  - Obtain laboratory studies as ordered.
  - Provide resuscitative measures if needed.
  - Continue monitoring vital signs until stable, then routinely or as ordered.

Obtaining baseline data and identifying risk factors will help direct interventions.

- Perform chest physiotherapy as indicated *to clear lungs of fluid.*
- Continually assess need to repeat suctioning in order to maintain patent airway. *Repeated pharyngeal suctioning can prevent aspiration caused by neonate's immature glottal reflex.*

Evaluations for expected outcomes

- Neonate establishes respiratory rate of 40 to 60 breaths/minute within 1 hour after birth and does not require assisted ventilation.
- Neonate does not exhibit signs of respiratory distress 1 hour after birth.
- Apgar score is 8 to 10 at 5 minutes after birth.
- Neonate's central color is pink within 1 hour after birth.
- Retractions, grunting, and nasal flaring cease.

Documentation

- Vital signs
- Physical findings
- Interventions performed to enhance neonate's ability to breathe effectively
- Neonate's responses to nursing interventions
- Evaluations for each expected outcome.

Coping, ineffective family

related to compromised neonatal health

Definition

Inability of family to use adaptive behaviors in response to demands posed by compromised neonate

Assessment

- Family process, including normal pattern of interaction among family members; family's understanding and knowledge of neonate's condition; support systems available (financial, social, spiritual); family's response to past crises, including coping behaviors and problem-solving techniques; recreational activities; communica-

tion patterns used to express anger, affection, confrontation
- Neonate's health status
- Family's perception of present situation
- Degree of difficulty imposed by care of neonate
- Possible impact of neonate on family's future structure and life-style

Defining characteristics
- Change in usual communication patterns
- Chronic fatigue
- Feelings of disappointment about outcome of birth
- General irritability
- Inability to cope, problem-solve, meet role expectations, or ask for help
- Inability to meet neonate's basic needs
- Inappropriate use of defense mechanisms
- Insomnia
- Muscle tension
- Overeating or lack of appetite
- Verbal manipulation

Associated medical diagnoses (selected)
Any disorder that severely compromises a neonate, such as a neurologic disorder, perinatal asphyxia, sequelae of prematurity, single-system or multisystem compromise

Expected outcomes
- Family members communicate feelings regarding neonate's condition.
- Family members engage in healthful coping behaviors.
- Family members become involved in planning and providing neonate's care.
- Family members express feeling of having greater control over their situation.

Interventions and rationales
- Encourage family members to voice feelings about neonate's condition *to decrease tension by clearing up misunderstandings and misconceptions.*
- Identify and reduce unnecessary stimuli in the environment *to enhance family members' ability to focus on caring for neonate.*
- Assess family members' understanding of neonate's condition. Help them view the situation realistically and understand its future implications. *Setting realistic goals helps family plan for the future and avoid unnecessary disappointment.*
- Actively involve family members in learning to care for neonate *to decrease feelings of helplessness and isolation from neonate.*
- Explain to family members the rationale for all treatments and procedures *to help lessen anxiety and enhance cooperation.*
- Involve family members in decision making when possible *to help increase their feelings of involvement and control.*
- Provide positive feedback when family members care for neonate. *This helps increase self-esteem and reinforces ability to care for neonate successfully.*
- Encourage family members to identify and contact support systems and resources, such as family, friends, clergy, and community groups, *to decrease sense of being overwhelmed.*
- Help family members identify and use appropriate coping behaviors *to decrease anxiety and tension.*
- Coordinate referrals to other health care professionals, such as social worker or physical therapist. *This ensures clear communication among health care providers, thus enabling*

the neonate to receive comprehensive care in a timely fashion.
- Provide family members with up-to-date reports on neonate's condition *to ease anxiety and help family plan for future needs.*

Evaluations for expected outcomes
- Family members discuss impact of neonate's condition with health care professionals.
- Family members voice their feelings about neonate's condition.
- Family members identify and use at least two healthy coping behaviors.
- Family members demonstrate ability to meet neonate's special care needs.
- Family members identify and use available support systems.
- Family members set realistic goals for neonate.
- Family members express a feeling of increased control over their lives.

Documentation
- Family members' perceptions of neonate's health and long-term implications
- Observations of family members' behaviors, including interactions with neonate
- Family members' statements indicating their feelings toward neonate
- Teaching and referrals given to family members
- Family members' abilities to meet neonate's physical and emotional needs
- Consultations with other health team members
- Interventions to help family members cope
- Family members' responses to nursing interventions
- Evaluations for each expected outcome.

Coping, ineffective individual

related to labor and delivery

Definition
Inability to use adaptive behaviors in response to labor and delivery

Assessment
- Psychosocial status, including age, developmental stage, health beliefs and attitudes, feelings about pregnancy, decision-making ability, usual coping patterns, support systems, income, ability to learn (cognitive domain, affective domain, psychomotor domain), motivation to learn, obstacles to learning
- Neurologic status, including level of consciousness, orientation, memory, mental status
- Pain threshold, perception of pain, response to analgesia or anesthesia
- Labor, including stage and length of labor, complications, patient's ability to concentrate, patient's ability to use breathing techniques, presence and effectiveness of support person
- Circumstances surrounding delivery, including method of delivery (vaginal [complicated, uncomplicated], cesarean section [elective, nonelective], vaginal birth after previous cesarean section), analgesia or anesthesia, presence and effectiveness of support person, outcome (actual and perceived)
- Previous experience with pregnancy, labor, and delivery; knowledge of birthing process
- Medical history, including preexisting conditions, pregnancy-induced conditions

Defining characteristics

- Altered communication patterns
- Destructive behavior toward self or others
- Inability to concentrate
- Inability to follow instructions, meet basic needs, solve problems, or ask for help
- Inability to meet role expectations
- Inability to tolerate pain
- Manipulation of others
- Muscular tension
- Verbal reports of inability to cope

Associated medical diagnoses (selected)

This diagnosis can occur in any condition associated with labor and delivery. Examples include complicated or uncomplicated vaginal delivery, elective or nonelective cesarean section delivery, and multiple pregnancy.

Expected outcomes

- Patient expresses a need to develop better coping behaviors.
- Patient sets realistic learning goals.
- Patient demonstrates ability to use newly learned coping skills.
- Patient communicates feelings about pregnancy, labor, and delivery.
- Patient maintains appropriate sense of control throughout course of labor and delivery.
- Patient enlists help from support person to obtain physical and psychological comfort.
- Patient demonstrates ability to cope with unexpected change.

Interventions and rationales

- Establish an environment of mutual trust and respect *to enhance patient's learning.*
- Negotiate with patient to develop learning goals *to promote cooperation and help foster a sense of control.*
- Select teaching strategies (discussion, demonstration, role-playing, visual materials) appropriate for patient's individual learning style *to encourage compliance.*
- Teach skills that patient must use during labor and delivery. Have her give return demonstration of each new skill. *Patient must thoroughly understand skills before labor begins because painful contractions will reduce her attention span.*
- During the first (latent) phase of labor (dilation 1 to 4 cm), take the following steps:
  - Encourage patient to ventilate her feelings and to participate in her own care. Offer diversions, such as reading materials. Review breathing techniques to be used during labor. *These measures help allay patient's fears and help her achieve a sense of control.*
  - Involve support person in care and comfort measures *to allay patient's fears.*
  - Provide continuous surveillance *to pinpoint any deviations from normal.*
- During the active phase of labor (dilation 4 to 8 cm), take the following steps:
  - Encourage patient to assume a comfortable position *to promote relaxation between contractions.*
  - Assist patient with breathing techniques *to reduce anxiety and prevent hyperventilation.*
  - Encourage support person to participate in patient care—for example, by changing soiled linen, offering ice chips to suck on, and providing sacral pressure, back support, or back rub—*to provide continuity of care and encourage a therapeutic relationship.*

- Provide encouragement and instruction between contractions *to foster a sense of control.*
- Administer analgesia as ordered *to reduce pain.*
- Provide opportunities for rest between contractions when appropriate. Reassure patient about fetal status. *These measures reinforce patient's ability to cope.*

• During the transitional phase of labor (dilation 8 to 10 cm), take the following steps:

- Assist patient with breathing during contractions. Advise her not to push until complete dilation occurs. Encourage rest between contractions. Identify and reduce unnecessary stimuli in environment. Explain all treatments and procedures, and answer patient's questions. *These measures help allay fear and reduce sensory overload.*

• During delivery, provide these measures:

- Instruct patient in effective pushing techniques *to promote effectiveness of her bearing down efforts.*
- Continue to reassure patient and provide encouragement. Explain physiologic changes and procedures being performed *to prepare patient psychologically for delivery.*
- Escort support person to delivery room. Explain each step of process. Instruct support person in how to effectively coach patient *to provide further support for patient and strengthen her ability to cope.*

• During delivery of the placenta, take these steps:

- Enlist patient's cooperation in maintaining position *to facilitate delivery of placenta.*
- Show neonate to patient and explain care being provided. Reassure patient regarding neonate's condition *to provide emotional support.*
- If permitted, allow patient and support person to hold neonate. If patient desires, allow her to breast-feed neonate *to promote bonding.*

• In a cesarean delivery, allow patient to express feelings. Explain procedure and care being provided. Allow support person to be present before and during delivery, if permitted. *Failure to provide patient with an opportunity to express negative feelings and a source of support may interfere with her ability to cope with impending tasks of motherhood.*

Evaluations for expected outcomes

• Patient becomes more comfortable with expressing feelings.
• Patient participates in establishing care goals.
• Patient successfully uses breathing and relaxation techniques.
• Support person provides effective comfort during labor and delivery.
• Patient seeks support from nurses and support person.

Documentation

• Patient's previous knowledge of labor and delivery
• Patient's expressions indicating her motivation to learn
• Patient's learning objectives
• Methods used to teach patient
• Information taught and skills demonstrated to patient
• Patient's responses to nursing interventions

• Patient's and support person's level of satisfaction with delivery
• Patient's expressions of comfort, discomfort, or both
• Evaluations for each expected outcome.

Family process alteration

related to impending birth

Definition
Altered role functions within the family resulting from pregnancy and pending change in family structure

Assessment
• Age of pregnant woman and partner
• Availability of family members or significant others to help
• Planned versus unplanned pregnancy
• Family status, including number and ages of other children, usual patterns of interaction among family members, family members' assumed or expected roles, communication patterns, support systems, financial resources, past responses to change, spiritual resources, living conditions
• Perceived impact of pregnancy on family unit
• Presence of obstetric or fetal complications or other medical conditions

Defining characteristics
• Anticipated change in family structure
• Family unit unable or unwilling to meet physical or emotional needs of its members
• Pregnancy

Associated medical diagnoses (selected)
This diagnosis can occur in any pregnancy, whether complicated or uncomplicated, planned or unplanned.

Expected outcomes
• Family members take on a portion of the duties carried out by the pregnant woman, such as housecleaning, heavy lifting, and meal preparation.
• Family members voice realistic expectations about pregnancy's impact on their future.
• Family members share their feelings about the pregnancy with each other.
• Family members identify available support systems.
• Family contacts a community agency or support group for continued assistance.
• Family welcomes new member.

Interventions and rationales
• Encourage family members to express their feelings about the pregnancy. Tell them that a wide range of emotions, ranging from fear to excitement, may accompany a diagnosis of pregnancy. *Pent-up feelings can lead to misunderstanding and resentment.*
• Provide emotional support to patient and family members *to help them come to terms with altered roles and responsibilities.*
• Encourage pregnant woman to voice her concerns about pregnancy's potential impact on family structure and finances *to identify unrealistic fears and decrease anxiety.*
• Arrange and participate in family conferences as needed. *Some families may require help to improve interpersonal communication.*
• Refer family members to classes in prepared childbirth or parenting, psychological counseling, or social service and health care agencies, as

appropriate, *to provide additional information and support.*
• Periodically assess woman's acceptance of pregnancy *to determine the need for further interventions. The mother normally grows to accept the pregnancy as the uterus develops and she feels the fetus kick. She may also fantasize about what the neonate will look like and begin preparing for the birth.*

Evaluations for expected outcomes
• Patient and family members voice realistic expectations regarding emotional and financial impact of pregnancy on family structure.
• Patient and family members honestly communicate feelings regarding pregnancy.
• Patient and family members identify potential support groups or organizations.
• Neonate is successfully integrated into family.

Documentation
• Reactions of pregnant woman and partner to diagnosis of pregnancy
• Referrals to outside agencies
• Pregnant woman's adherence to prescribed medical practices
• Observations of pregnant woman's acceptance of and interest in pregnancy as time progresses
• Interventions to assist the pregnant woman and family and their responses to those interventions
• Evaluations for each expected outcome.

■ Family process alteration

related to inclusion of new member

Definition
Disruption in expected role functions within the family structure following the birth of a child

Assessment
• Family status, including assumed or expected roles, communication patterns, developmental stage of family members, number and ages of children, financial resources, past responses to change, available support systems, significant others, spiritual practices
• Family members' perceptions of impact of birth on their assumed roles

Defining characteristics
• Family unable or unwilling to meet physical, emotional, or spiritual needs of its members
• Inability of children to accomplish developmental tasks
• Inability to communicate effectively
• Inability to seek or accept help
• Inability to show respect for individuality and autonomy of family members
• Inappropriate or poorly communicated rules and rituals
• Poor decision making within family
• Rigidity of functions and roles

Associated medical diagnoses (selected)
Childbirth

Expected outcomes
• Family members voice feelings regarding neonate.
• Family members adapt to change in family structure.

• Family members express need to assume new or altered roles within family structure.
• Neonate is successfully assimilated into family structure.

Interventions and rationales
• Encourage family members to express feelings about the arrival of neonate and altered roles and responsibilities *to help clear up misunderstandings and misconceptions.*
• Explore with family members the ways in which neonate will affect family structure and functioning. Topics may include altered finances, changes in living space, caretaking arrangements, and new roles or responsibilities for parents and siblings. *Discussion of legitimate concerns may improve family members' attitudes toward neonate.*
• Discuss with family members the degree of sibling preparation and possibility of sibling rivalry. *Siblings must be reassured that they are still vital members of the family.* Encourage siblings to visit neonate at hospital *to decrease separation anxiety, foster a sense of family, and facilitate bonding.*
• Assess measures taken to prepare home for arrival of neonate. *Lack of preparation may indicate limited financial resources or difficulty accepting neonate.*
• Assess need for help from social services or community agencies and coordinate referrals *to ensure ongoing comprehensive care.*

Evaluations for expected outcomes
• Family members share feelings about neonate with each other.
• Family members assume new or additional responsibilities as needed, such as preparing meals, assisting with transportation, shopping, cleaning, and child care.
• Family members contact community agencies or support group for assistance if needed.
• Family members come to terms with arrival of neonate.

Documentation
• Observations of family members' reactions to neonate
• Statements that indicate family members' attitude toward neonate
• Interventions performed to help family cope with new arrival
• Family members' responses to nursing interventions
• Referrals to outside agencies
• Evaluations for each expected outcome.

■ Fluid volume deficit

related to altered intake during labor

Definition
Excessive loss of body fluids and electrolytes during labor

Assessment
• Vital signs, including temperature, pulse rate, blood pressure, respirations
• Fluid and electrolyte status, including weight, intake and output, urine specific gravity, skin turgor, mucous membranes, electrolyte and blood urea nitrogen levels

Defining characteristics
• Diaphoresis
• Hyperventilation
• Increased or decreased blood pressure
• NPO status
• Peripheral edema

• Presence of any condition that places the patient at risk for fluid volume deficit, such as diarrhea, hemorrhage, pregnancy-induced hypertension (PIH), vomiting
• Proteinuria

Associated medical diagnoses (selected)
Diabetes mellitus, hemorrhage, premature rupture of the membranes, shock, severe PIH

Expected outcomes
• Fluid balance is maintained.
• Patient demonstrates optimal hydration.
• Patient shows no signs of dehydration.

Interventions and rationales
• Monitor vital signs as often as policy dictates. *Decreased blood pressure and increased pulse rate may be a late sign of fluid volume loss. With PIH, the patient may experience increased blood pressure.*
• Assess skin turgor and examine oral mucous membranes for dryness. *Dehydration can cause dry mucous membranes, skin tenting, and cracked, dry lips.*
• Continuously monitor intake and output *to obtain information for maintaining adequate hydration.*
• Monitor electrolyte values and report abnormalities. *Hyponatremia may indicate dehydration, requiring intravenous volume replacement. Hypernatremia may be related to excessive insensible water loss.*
• Provide patient with ice chips or cool, damp, 4″ × 4″ gauze compress *to increase patient comfort and decrease mouth dryness, especially if patient uses mouth breathing techniques.*
• Administer and monitor parenteral fluids. Maintain intake according to doctor's order (usually 125 to 175 ml/hour). Output should approximate intake. *These measures help ensure adequate hydration.*
• Measure amount and character of vomitus *to assess need for antiemetic. When labor begins, blood is rerouted to serve energy needs of contracting uterus and blood flow to the GI tract is decreased. GI motility and absorption are also decreased, and food may remain in the stomach for up to 12 hours. These factors predispose patient to nausea and vomiting, especially during the transition period of labor.*
• As ordered, administer an antiemetic if needed and evaluate its effectiveness *to help control emesis and prevent excessive fluid loss.*
• Keep patient cool and comfortable. Change gown as indicated and apply cool compresses to face and body *to reduce discomfort caused by diaphoresis.*
• Position patient on her left side *to aid kidney perfusion and increase cardiac and urine output.*
• If urine output is reduced, carefully assess patient for peripheral edema, hyperreflexia, increased blood pressure, and presence of urine protein. *Decreased urine output, increased blood pressure, hyperreflexia, and peripheral edema may indicate intrapartal PIH. Proteinuria may result from dehydration, exhaustion, or preeclampsia.*

Evaluations for expected outcomes
• Patient's vital signs are within normal limits.
• Mucous membranes are pink and moist and lips are soft and intact.
• Patient demonstrates optimal skin turgor (brisk return after pinch test, no tenting).

• I.V. intake is maintained at prescribed rate.
• Patient does not develop nausea and vomiting.
• Fluid intake approximates output.
• Patient remains cool and comfortable during the diaphoretic phase of transition.
• Patient maintains urine output of at least 30 ml/hour or 100 ml in 4 hours.

Documentation
• Patient's vital signs
• Observation of patient's fluid volume status
• Intake and output
• Nursing interventions performed to maintain adequate fluid intake
• Patient's response to nursing interventions
• Evaluations for each expected outcome.

■ Fluid volume deficit

related to postpartum hemorrhage

Definition
Excessive fluid and electrolyte loss resulting from excessive postpartum bleeding.

Assessment
• History of problems that can cause fluid loss, such as hemorrhage, vomiting, diarrhea, indwelling catheters
• Vital signs, including temperature, pulse, blood pressure, respirations
• Fluid and electrolyte status, including weight, intake and output, urine specific gravity, skin turgor, mucous membranes, serum electrolyte and blood urea nitrogen levels
• Laboratory studies, including hemoglobin and hematocrit
• Factors that place patient at high risk for postpartum hemorrhage, including grand multipara, overdistended uterus, prolonged labor, previous history of postpartum hemorrhage, traumatic delivery, uterine fibroids, overstimulation with oxytocin, bleeding disorders

Defining characteristics
• Blood loss of 500 ml or more
• Dry or cold, clammy skin
• Low blood pressure (with dizziness or anxiety)
• Pallor
• Rapid, shallow respirations
• Rapid, thready pulse
• Thirst
• Urinary frequency

Associated medical diagnoses (selected)
Postpartum hemorrhage, retained placental fragments

Expected outcomes
• Patient's vital signs remain stable.
• Hematology studies are within normal range.
• Patient's uterus remains firm.
• Signs of possible shock are quickly identified, and treatment is initiated.
• Patient's bladder does not become distended.
• Patient's blood volume returns to normal.

Interventions and rationales
• Immediately after delivery, monitor color, amount, and consistency of lochia every 15 minutes for 1 hour, then every 4 hours for 24 hours, then every shift until discharge. Weigh or count sanitary pads if lochia is excessive. *Hemorrhage is the most common cause of mortality during childbirth.*
• Monitor and record vital signs every 15 minutes for 1 hour, then ev-

ery 4 hours for 24 hours, then every shift until discharge *to detect signs of hemorrhage and shock, such as increased pulse and respiratory rates and decreased blood pressure.*
• Immediately after delivery, palpate fundus every 15 minutes for 1 hour, then every 4 hours for 24 hours, then every shift until discharge. Note location and tone. *Palpation of fundus will enable you to detect uterine atonia (lack of normal uterine muscle tone or strength). Uterine atonia is the most common cause of postpartum hemorrhage.*
• Gently massage boggy fundus; avoid overstimulation. *Stimulation can help the fundus to become firm. Overstimulation, however, can cause relaxation.*
• Explain to patient the process of involution and the need to palpate fundus. Teach patient to assess and gently massage fundus, and to notify you if bogginess persists. *Explaining normal postpartum physiologic adjustments can decrease the patient's anxiety and increase cooperation.*
• Evaluate postpartum hematology studies and report abnormal results. Consider whether typing and cross matching patient for transfusion is necessary. *Comparison of postdelivery hemoglobin and hematocrit with previous results provides information about the amount of blood loss and allows time to plan interventions, such as requesting blood from the blood bank.*
• Administer fluids, blood or blood products, or plasma expanders, as ordered, *to replace lost blood volume.* Monitor for adverse reactions.
• Monitor patient's intake and output every shift. Note bladder distention and catheterize as ordered. *A distended bladder interferes with involution of uterus.*
• Administer oxytocic agents, such as oxytocin (Pitocin), methylergonovine (Methergine), and ergonovine (Ergotrate), as ordered, and evaluate effectiveness. *Oxytocic agents stimulate uterine musculature, controlling postpartum hemorrhage and atonia.*
• Regularly assess patient for signs and symptoms of shock, including rapid, thready pulse; increased respiratory rate; decreased blood pressure and urine output; and cold, clammy, pale skin. *Prompt recognition and treatment of signs of shock helps limit the amount fluid lost and possible impact on other body systems.*

Evaluations for expected outcomes
• Patient's blood loss after delivery is less than 500 ml.
• Patient's uterus remains firm.
• If patient develops shock, it is identified quickly and treated promptly.
• Patient does not develop distended bladder.
• Results of hematology studies are within normal range.
• Patient's fluid volume is replenished.

Documentation
• Estimation of blood loss
• Signs of possible shock
• Location and tone of fundus
• Laboratory results
• Replacement of lost fluid
• Nursing interventions to control active blood loss
• Patient's response to nursing interventions
• Evaluations for each expected outcome.

Growth and development alteration

related to perinatal insult or injury

Definition

State in which neonate deviates from norms for age

Assessment

- Maternal history, including age, use of controlled substances, trauma, anesthesia or analgesia during labor
- Labor and delivery record
- Infant status, including gestational age, Apgar scores, vital signs, feeding patterns, muscle tone, condition of fontanels, characteristics of cry
- Neurologic status, including reflexes, responsiveness, activity level, presence of seizures
- Diagnostic tests, including laboratory studies and ultrasound examinations

Defining characteristics

- Dependence on respiratory support
- Diminished or absent reflexes (Moro's, tonic neck or "fencing", sucking and rooting, grasp, stepping)
- Muscle hypotonia (flaccidity) or hypertonia (rigidity)
- Prematurity
- Small size in relation to gestational age
- Seizure activity

Associated medical diagnoses (selected)

Increased intracranial pressure (ICP), intraventricular hemorrhage, perinatal asphyxia, sepsis, severe prematurity

Expected outcomes

- After evaluation of neonate's alteration in growth and development, supportive measures are initiated.
- Family members express realistic expectations for neonate's growth.
- Family members demonstrate understanding of neonate's special needs.
- Family members accept referrals to available community resources.

Interventions and rationales

- Reposition the hypotonic neonate every 2 hours *to prevent skin breakdown and pulmonary complications of immobility.*
- Measure neonate's head circumference every shift. *Increasing head circumference indicates increased ICP.*
- Evaluate and record activity level every shift. *Altered activity level may be a sign of such conditions as sepsis, hyperbilirubinemia, increased ICP, or intraventricular hemorrhage.*
- Monitor and report changes in neonate's neurologic status *to detect exacerbation or lessening of danger signs.*
- Refer neonate to appropriate health care specialist, such as physical therapist, social worker, developmental specialist, or neurologist. Provide parents or family with information on community resources *to ensure comprehensive care for neonate.*
- Provide emotional support to family members who have difficulty accepting the neonate's condition. Assess their goals for neonate's development. *By offering support and identifying unrealistic goals, you can help family members come to terms with neonate's condition.*
- Involve family members in neonate's daily care and keep them abreast of neonate's condition. *Personal involvement facilitates bonding,*

decreases anxiety, and helps prepare for discharge.
- Assess neonate's ability to suck on an ongoing basis. *A weak sucking reflex may indicate a neurologic defect or a need for nutritional supplementation.*
- Monitor neonate's temperature every 4 hours or as ordered. Maintain a neutral thermal environment *to minimize oxygen consumption, prevent cold stress, and facilitate growth by decreasing unnecessary caloric use.*

Evaluations for expected outcomes
- Neonate's nutritional, physical, and safety needs are met.
- Family members express a realistic understanding of the neonate's present condition and potential for improvement.
- Neonate receives appropriate physical therapy on a regular basis.
- Family members demonstrate ability to meet neonate's physical and emotional needs.
- Family members agree to seek help and support from appropriate community resources.

Documentation
- Observed characteristics of neonate, including seizure activity, characteristics of cry, hypoactive or hyperactive muscle activity, condition of fontanels, presence or absence of reflexes, feeding ability, vital signs
- Use of respiratory support
- Family members' responses to neonate's condition
- Consultations with other health team members
- Referrals to outside agencies
- Nursing interventions and neonate's response
- Evaluations for each expected outcome.

Hypothermia

related to cold, stress, or sepsis

Definition
State in which neonate's body temperature is below normal range

Assessment
- History of present illness
- Gestational age
- Prenatal and intrapartal history
- Presence of maternal risk factors, such as fever, diabetes mellitus, drug use, dystocia, history of perinatal asphyxia
- Neurologic status, including level of consciousness, sensory status
- Cardiovascular status, including core temperature, heart rate and rhythm, blood pressure, capillary refill time
- Respiratory status, including rate, rhythm, and depth; breath sounds; arterial blood gas values
- Integumentary status, including temperature, color (central versus peripheral), turgor
- Nutritional status, including dietary pattern, birth weight, current weight, recent weight changes
- Fluid and electrolyte status, including intake and output, serum glucose and electrolyte levels, urine specific gravity
- Psychosocial status, including behavior, parental stressors, parental coping skills, financial resources

Defining characteristics
- Blood glucose level under 50 mg/dl
- Bradycardia
- Cold, clammy skin
- Core temperature less than 96.8° F (36° C)
- Cyanosis (peripheral or central)

- Decreased absorption of food
- Diminished respirations
- Drowsiness progressing to coma
- Metabolic acidosis
- Pallor
- Shivering
- Slow capillary refill time

Associated medical diagnoses (selected)
Birth trauma, cold stress, congenital chromosomal and genetic syndromes, congenital myxedema, gluconeogenesis depletion, maternal diabetes mellitus, maternal drug overdose, meningitis, perinatal asphyxia, sepsis

Expected outcomes
- Neonate exhibits normal body temperature.
- Neonate's skin is warm and dry and capillary refill time is normal.
- Neonate's cardiovascular status remains normal.
- Neonate does not develop shivering.
- Neonate does not develop signs of hyperthermia related to radiant heat source.
- Neonate is weaned from the Isolette or radiant warmer as tolerated.
- Family members verbalize knowledge of how hypothermia develops and state measures to prevent recurrent hypothermia.
- Family members demonstrate the ability to accurately measure neonate's temperature.

Interventions and rationales
- Monitor body temperature every 1 to 3 hours by axillary or inguinal route (avoid rectal measurement). Record temperature and route. *Monitoring body temperature helps to detect developing complications*. If using an electronic heat source, such as a radiant warmer, monitor the device's temperature reading hourly and compare it with neonate's body temperature *to evaluate the effectiveness of interventions.*
- Monitor and record neurologic status every 1 to 4 hours. *Falling body temperature and slowed metabolic rate may cause decreased level of consciousness.*
- Monitor and record vital signs every 1 to 4 hours. As ordered, initiate and maintain continuous electronic cardiorespiratory monitoring. *These measures help avert metabolic acidosis and respiratory arrest.*
- Provide supportive measures:
  - Maintain a neutral thermal environment. Neutral thermal environment refers to a narrow range of environmental temperature that maintains a stable core (rectal) temperature with minimal caloric and oxygen expenditure. Determination of neutral thermal environment is based on neonate's age and weight.
  - If indicated, place neonate in open crib. For mild hypothermia, dress with undershirt, diaper, and knitted or stockinette cap and cover with double blankets.
  - Avoid overheating neonate.
  - Keep diaper area dry.
  - Cover all metal or plastic surfaces that could come in contact with neonate.
  - Maintain room temperature between 75° and 78° F (23.9° to 25.6° C).
  - Perform all procedures under a radiant warmer, if possible. Postpone bath.

These measures protect neonate from heat loss.
- For severe hypothermia, place neonate in an Isolette or overhead radiant warmer bed.
  - Keep neonate undressed.

– Set mechanism to desired skin temperature (96.8° to 97.8° F [36° to 36.6° C]).
– If neonate is under a radiant warmer, use plastic wrap placed like a blanket to prevent heat and fluid loss. Use sheet large enough to cover only neonate. Border with tape.
– Attach skin probe to right upper quadrant of abdomen. Do not place over bone or rib cage.
– Use heat shield for very unstable neonate inside Isolette.
– Monitor carefully for evaporative loss and insensible fluid loss. Keep in mind that radiant warmer and Isolette therapy increase fluid maintenance needs.

These measures help ensure safe use of radiant warmer or Isolette.

- Follow the prescribed treatment regimen for hypothermia, which may include administering antibiotic in cases of sepsis, administering I.V. fluids, and feeding neonate (small, frequent portions, if appropriate). *Treatment seeks to eliminate infection as well as meet neonate's fluid and nutrient needs.*
- Discuss precipitating factors with family members *to help prevent recurrence.*
- Instruct family members in preventive measures, such as dressing neonate appropriately and providing adequate nutrition for neonate's growth needs. If family requires financial help, refer them to an appropriate social service agency. *These precautions may help protect neonate from future cold stress episodes.*

Evaluations for expected outcomes

- Neonate's temperature returns to normal range.
- Neonate exhibits warm, dry skin and normal capillary refill time.
- Cardiovascular assessment findings are normal.
- Complications of hypothermia do not occur.
- Neonate does not begin shivering.
- Neonate does not demonstrate signs of hyperthermia related to radiant heat source.
- Neonate is successfully weaned from Isolette or radiant warmer bed.
- Family members verbalize understanding of causes of hypothermia and preventive measures.
- Family members demonstrate proper axillary or inguinal temperature measurement technique.
- Family members demonstrate willingness to provide adequate home care for neonate.

Documentation

- Physical findings, including cardiovascular status, temperature, shivering
- Interventions
- Neonate's response to nursing interventions
- Family members' willingness and abilities to provide adequate home care
- Evaluations for each expected outcome.

Infant feeding pattern, ineffective

related to neurologic impairment or developmental delay

Definition

Impaired ability of an infant to suck or coordinate the suck and swallow response

Assessment

- Perinatal history, including gestational age, Apgar score
- Suck and swallow reflex, including condition of lip and palate
- Nutritional status, including intake (type, amount, and frequency of feedings), output (frequency, amount and characteristics of urine), current weight, weight change since birth, skin turgor, signs of dehydration
- Laboratory studies, including glucose, bilirubin levels
- Parental assessment, including age, maturity level, previous experience with infant feeding

Defining characteristics

- Inability to coordinate sucking, swallowing, and breathing
- Inability to initiate or sustain an effective suck

Associated medical diagnoses (selected)

Cleft lip, cleft palate, microcephaly, neonatal anomaly, neurologic impairment, prematurity

Expected outcomes

- Neonate does not lose more than 10% of birth weight within first week of life.
- Neonate gains 4 to 7 oz/week after the first week of life.
- Factors that interfere with the neonate establishing an effective feeding pattern are identified.
- Parents express increased confidence in their ability to perform appropriate feeding techniques.
- Neonate does not experience dehydration.
- Neonate receives adequate supplemental nutrition until able to suckle sufficiently.
- Neonate establishes effective suck and swallow reflexes, which allow for an adequate intake of nutrients.

Interventions and rationales

- Using the same scale, weigh neonate at same time each day *to detect excessive weight loss early.*
- Continuously assess neonate's sucking pattern *to monitor for ineffective patterns.*
- Assess parents' knowledge of feeding techniques *to help identify and clear up misconceptions.*
- Assess parents' level of anxiety with regard to neonate's feeding difficulty. *Anxiety may interfere with parents' ability to learn new techniques.*
- Remain with parents and neonate during feeding *to identify problem areas and direct interventions.*
- Teach parents to place neonate in upright position during feeding *to prevent aspiration.*
- Teach parents to unwrap and position a sleepy neonate before feeding *to ensure that neonate is awake and alert enough to suckle sufficiently.*
- Provide positive reinforcement for parents' efforts to improve feeding technique *to decrease anxiety and enhance feelings of success.*
- For bottle-feeding, record amount ingested at each feeding; for breast-feeding, record number of minutes neonate nurses at each breast and amount of any supplement ingested *to monitor for inadequate caloric and fluid intake.*
- Provide an alternative nipple, such as a preemie nipple. *A preemie nipple has a larger hole and softer texture, which make it easier for neonate to obtain formula.*
- For breast-feeding, ensure neonate's tongue is properly positioned under mother's nipple *to facilitate adequate sucking.*
- Monitor neonate for poor skin turgor, dry mucous membranes, decreased or concentrated urine, and

sunken fontanels and eyeballs *to detect possible dehydration and allow for immediate intervention.*
• Record number of stools and amount of urine voided each shift. *Altered bowel elimination pattern may indicate decreased food intake; decreased amounts of concentrated urine may indicate dehydration.*
• Assess need for gavage feeding. *Neonate may require a temporary, alternative means of obtaining adequate fluids and calories.*
• Alternate oral and gavage feeding *to conserve neonate's energy.*
• If I.V. nourishment is necessary, assess the insertion site, amount infused, and infusion rate every hour *to monitor fluid intake and identify possible complications, such as infiltration and phlebitis.*
• Assess neonate for neurologic deficits or other pathophysiologic causes of ineffective sucking *to identify the need for more extensive evaluation.*

Evaluations for expected outcomes
• Neonate's nutritional needs are met.
• Neonate maintains urine output of 1 ml/kg/day.
• Neonate maintains good skin turgor, moist mucous membranes, and soft, flat fontanels.
• Neonate's urine specific gravity is 1.003 to 1.013.
• Parents demonstrate competence when feeding neonate.
• Neonate retains entire feeding.
• Neonate returns to birth weight by 10 days after delivery.
• Neonate establishes an effective sucking reflex as well as a coordinated suck and swallow response.

Documentation
• Frequency, amount, and type of fluid ingested by neonate
• Effectiveness of suck reflex
• Neonate's daily weight
• Parents' knowledge of feeding techniques, involvement with caretaking, and bonding with neonate
• Frequency of bowel elimination and urination
• Signs of dehydration
• Nursing interventions and neonate's response
• Use of special feeding techniques and equipment
• Parents' and neonate's responses to nursing interventions
• Evidence of neurologic or other physical impairment in neonate
• Evaluations for each expected outcome.

■ Infection, high risk for

related to altered primary defenses during the postpartum period

Definition
Presence of internal or external hazards that threaten physical well-being

Assessment
• Laboratory studies, including white blood cell (WBC) count, clotting factors, platelet count, hemoglobin and hematocrit, serum albumin level, and cultures of blood, body fluid, sputum, urine, and wounds
• Labor and delivery record, including episiotomy; presence of invasive devices, such as I.V. and urinary catheters; premature rupture of membranes
• Presence of medical conditions, such as diabetes mellitus, that may increase incidence of infection
• Signs and symptoms of infection, including pallor, fatigue, malaise, anorexia, chills, foul-smelling lochia, calf tenderness, elevated temperature,

dysuria, marked abdominal tenderness, and tender, reddened breasts that are warm to the touch

Risk factors

- Cesarean delivery
- Indwelling urinary catheter
- Invasive monitoring procedures, such as internal fetal monitoring
- I.V. catheter
- Laceration and tears
- Premature rupture of membranes
- Surgical procedures

Associated medical diagnoses (selected)

Chorioamnionitis, diabetes mellitus, endometritis, gestational diabetes, premature rupture of membranes, pneumonia, urinary tract infection

Expected outcomes

- Vital signs remain within normal range.
- WBC count and differential remain within normal range.
- Cultures do not indicate any pathogens.
- Respiratory secretions are clear and odorless.
- Urine is clear yellow, odorless, and sediment-free.
- Episiotomy and incision sites are free of infection.
- I.V. sites are not inflamed.
- Patient maintains good personal hygiene.
- Patient states risk factors that lead to infection.
- Patient remains free of all signs and symptoms of infection.

Interventions and rationales

- Minimize patient's risk of infection by:
  - washing hands before and after providing care. *Hand washing is the single best way to avoid spreading pathogens.*
  - wearing gloves to maintain asepsis when providing direct care and when in contact with blood or body secretions. *Gloves reduce the possibility of transmitting disease.*
- After delivery, monitor vital signs every 15 minutes for 1 hour, then every 4 hours for 24 hours, then every shift until discharge. Report abnormal readings. *Elevated temperature, pulse or respiratory rates, or blood pressure may indicate infection. A temperature greater than 100.4° F (38° C) on two consecutive readings after the first 24 hours postdelivery may indicate puerperal sepsis, urinary tract infection, endometritis, mastitis, or other infection.*
- Monitor WBC count, as ordered, and promptly report abnormal values. *A total WBC count above 11,000/mm³ indicates increased production of leukocytes by bone marrow, usually in response to the presence of bacterial pathogens.*
- As ordered, culture urine, respiratory secretions, wound drainage, or blood *to identify pathogens and guide antibiotic therapy.*
- Instruct patient in proper personal hygiene, such as use of sitz bath and perineal irrigation bottle, hand washing, and breast care, *to reduce risk of infection.* Explain to the patient that the most common site of localized postpartum infection is the episiotomy site. Tell patient how to apply sanitary pads (front to back) and how to remove them (back to front). Tell her to wipe perineum after elimination and to clean perineum from front to back. *These measures decrease bacterial concentration and help prevent genitourinary infections.*
- Follow hospital infection control policy *to minimize risk of nosocomial infection.*

• Use strict aseptic technique when performing invasive procedures, such as urinary catheterization or I.V. line insertion, *to minimize the risk of introducing pathogens into the body.*
• Assess I.V. site every 4 hours, noting presence of redness or warmth. Change I.V. tubing and site every 72 hours or as dictated by hospital policy. *These measures keep pathogens from entering the body.*
• Instruct postoperative patient to deep-breathe and cough *to help remove secretions and prevent respiratory complications.*
• Ensure adequate nutritional intake. *A diet high in protein, iron, and vitamin C helps promote healing.*
• Assess patient for generalized signs and symptoms of infection (pallor, fatigue, malaise, anorexia, and chills) every shift, and instruct her to report danger signs immediately. These include foul-smelling lochia, calf tenderness, elevated temperature, dysuria, marked abdominal tenderness, and tender, reddened breasts that are warm to the touch. *Prompt detection of infection helps minimize complications.*

Evaluations for expected outcomes
• Patient performs proper personal hygiene on a regular basis.
• Results of laboratory studies do not indicate infection.
• Patient's respiratory secretions and urine do not show evidence of infection.
• Episiotomy and incision sites are free of infection.
• I.V. sites are free of inflammation.
• Patient promptly reports possible signs and symptoms of infection.
• Patient maintains proper nutritional and fluid intake.

Documentation
• Vital signs
• Appearance of episiotomy or incision site
• Date, time, appearance, and sites of cultures
• Date, time, and sites of catheter insertions
• Appearance of invasive catheter and I.V. sites
• Patient teaching about infection control
• Interventions performed to reduce the risk of infection
• Patient's response to nursing interventions
• Evaluations for each expected outcome.

■ Infection, high risk for

related to labor and delivery

Definition
Presence of internal or external hazards that threaten maternal and neonatal well-being

Assessment
• Vital signs, including fetal heart rate
• Health history, including previous infections
• Rupture of membranes, including time of rupture, characteristics of amniotic fluid (amount, color [blood tinged or meconium stained], and odor)
• Laboratory studies, including white blood cell (WBC) count, clotting factors, platelet count, hemoglobin and hematocrit, serum albumin level, cultures (blood or body fluid, sputum, urine, and wounds)
• Signs and symptoms of chorioamnionitis, including maternal pulse

rate over 160 beats/minute, malodorous amniotic fluid, increasing uterine tenderness, fetal tachycardia

Risk factors

- Anemia
- Cervicitis
- Low socioeconomic status
- Obesity
- Poor nutritional status
- Presence of I.V. catheters or invasive monitoring devices
- Previous cervical cerclage
- Rupture of membranes
- Urinary catheterization
- Vaginitis

Associated medical diagnoses (selected)

Chorioamnionitis, pelvic peritonitis, prolonged rupture of membranes, pyelonephritis, septicemia, upper respiratory tract infection, urinary tract infection

Expected outcomes

- Patient maintains good hygiene.
- Patient remains free of signs and symptoms of infection.
- Patient's temperature remains in normal range.

Interventions and rationales

- Monitor and record temperature every 4 hours before rupture of membranes and every 2 hours after rupture. *Temperature elevations are one of the first signs of infection.*
- Use continuous fetal monitoring to assess fetal heart rate and variability. Report rates over 160 beats/minute and variability under 3 to 5 beats/minute to the doctor. *Fetal heart rates over 160 beats/minute and minimal variability may indicate maternal fever.*
- Wash hands thoroughly, using proper technique, before and after providing care *to prevent spread of infection.*
- Maintain universal precautions. Wear gloves if you might come into contact with patient's blood and body secretions. *Universal precautions protect you and the patient from the transfer of microorganisms.*
- Use strict aseptic technique when suctioning the lower airway, applying scalp electrodes, or inserting urinary catheters, pressure catheters, or I.V. lines *to reduces likelihood of nosocomial infections.*
- After spontaneous or artificial rupture of membranes, assess color, amount, and odor of amniotic fluid and presence of blood or meconium. *Alterations in color, amount, and odor of amniotic fluid may indicate infection. Meconium may indicate predisposition to intrauterine infection and fetal distress.*
- After rupture of membranes, keep vaginal examinations to a minimum and always use sterile gloves *to decrease risk of chorioamnionitis or other uterine infection.*
- Maintain good patient hygiene. Clean perineal area from front to back and keep area dry *to reduce risk of infection.*
- Carefully monitor intake and output *to assess for dehydration. Signs and symptoms of infection (tachycardia, dry mucous membranes, poor skin turgor) may resemble those of of dehydration.*

Evaluations for expected outcomes

- Patient's temperature is 97° to 99° F (36.1° to 37.2° C).
- Fetal heart rate ranges from 120 to 160 beats/minute.
- Urine is clear and odorless with no sediment.

- WBC count remains within acceptable limits for labor and delivery (up to 20,000/mm^3).
- Collected cultures show no pathogens.
- Respiratory secretions are clear and odorless.
- Wounds and incisions are clean, pink, and healing.
- Amniotic fluid is clear and odorless.
- I.V. sites show no signs of inflammation.

Documentation
- Maternal vital signs
- Fetal heart rate and variability
- Dates, time, and site of all cultures
- Dates, time, and site of catheter insertions
- Appearance of all invasive catheter and tube sites and wounds
- Nursing interventions performed to reduce the risk of infection
- Patient's response to nursing interventions
- Evaluations for each expected outcome.

Infection, high risk for

related to neonate's immature immune system

Definition
Presence of internal or external hazards that threaten a neonate's physical well-being

Assessment
- Gestational age
- Neonate's temperature and vital signs
- Labor and delivery record, including premature rupture of membranes, characteristics of amniotic fluid (odorous or foul-smelling), maternal temperature
- Maternal infections (recent or current), maternal disease or infection during pregnancy, maternal pathogens passed on during the birth process
- Condition of umbilical cord and skin at base of cord, including redness, odor, discharge
- Signs and symptoms of neonatal infection, including lethargy, poor weight gain, restlessness, jaundice, visible lesions, thrush, temperature elevations or unstable low temperature, hypoglycemia, altered feeding patterns, diarrhea, vomiting, subtle color changes, such as cyanosis, mottling, or grayish skin tones
- Signs of respiratory distress, including grunting, retractions, nasal flaring, cyanosis
- Evidence of chronic intrauterine infections, including growth retardation, microcephaly, hepatosplenomegaly

Risk factors
- Amnionitis
- Chlamydia
- Chronic intrauterine infection
- Gonorrhea
- Infection with group B streptococci or TORCH group of viruses (toxoplasmosis, rubella, cytomegalovirus, and herpes simplex)
- Premature rupture of membranes
- Prematurity
- Syphilis

Associated medical diagnoses (selected)
This diagnosis may be associated with maternal disease during pregnancy or maternal pathogens passed on to the neonate during the birth process. Examples include acquired immunodeficiency syndrome, amnionitis, chlamydia, chronic intra-

uterine infection, gonorrhea, syphilis, or infection with herpesvirus, gonococci, group B streptococci, or TORCH group of viruses.

Expected outcomes

- Neonate's vital signs remain in normal range.
- Neonate is free of signs and symptoms of infection.
- Umbilical cord and circumcision site are healing and free of infection.
- Family members demonstrate good hand-washing technique before handling neonate.

Interventions and rationales

- Review maternal chart and delivery record *to detect risk factors that predispose neonate to infection.*
- Assess neonate's gestational age. *Passive immunity of neonate via placenta increases significantly in the last trimester, making a premature neonate much more susceptible to infection.*
- Observe principles of asepsis. Remove all rings, bracelets, and wrist watches before handling neonate. Scrub hands and arms with antimicrobial preparation before entering nursery and after contact with contaminated material. Wash hands again after handling neonate. Instruct parents and siblings in hand-washing techniques and procedures. *These measures help prevent spread of pathogens.*
- Monitor all hospital personnel, parents, and visitors for potential infection *to prevent spreading infection to neonate.*
- Organize nursery. Make sure aisles are 3′ (1 m) wide and cribs are 18″ (45 cm) apart. Keep individual supplies separate for each neonate. *These measures help prevent cross-contamination.*
- Provide cover gowns for nonnursing personnel who enter nursery *to prevent spread of pathogens.*
- Provide eye prophylaxis as hospital policy dictates *to prevent ophthalmia neonatorum or infections from gonococci or chlamydia.*
- Perform umbilical cord care with each diaper change, as hospital policy dictates, *to promote healing, remove urine and stool, and facilitate desiccation process.*
- Assess respirations, pulse, and blood pressure every 15 minutes for 1 hour, then every hour for 4 hours, then once a shift or more frequently as indicated. Assess temperature every 4 hours for 24 hours, then every 8 hours or as indicated. *Unstable vital signs, persistent elevations in temperature, or hypothermia may indicate neonatal infection.*
- Observe neonate for signs and symptoms of infection. Notify doctor immediately if signs and symptoms of infection appear *to ensure rapid identification and early treatment.*
- Observe universal precautions. Wear gloves before neonate's first bath and when in contact with blood and body secretions. *Following universal precautions prevents cross-contamination and transmission of pathogens, including human immunodeficiency virus.*
- Encourage mother to begin breastfeeding early if indicated. *Colostrum and breast milk contain high amounts of immunoglobulin A, which provides passive immunity to neonate and helps reduce infection.*
- As ordered, monitor laboratory studies, including white blood cell (WBC) count, serum levels of immunoglobulin M (IgM), and blood cultures. Culture any lesions, pustules, or drainage. *Decreased WBC count commonly indicates infection in neo-*

nate; elevated IgM levels indicate that an infectious process has occurred in utero. Cultures are used to identify pathogens and guide antibiotic therapy.

- Administer topical, oral, and parenteral antibiotics, as ordered, *to eradicate pathogenic organisms.*
- Observe circumcision site for color, healing, and presence of drainage. *A fresh, healing circumcision site is a port of entry for bacteria.*

Evaluations for expected outcomes

- Neonate's skin color is pink, with no subtle color changes.
- Neonate is alert and active.
- Weight loss during first 5 days after birth does not exceed 10% of birth weight.
- Neonate does not have diarrhea.
- Umbilical cord is clean, dry, and healing.
- Oral mucous membranes are moist and pink.
- Eyes are clean, sclera is white, with no signs or symptoms of drainage.
- Family members demonstrate proper hand-washing technique before handling neonate.

Documentation

- Vital signs
- Appearance of umbilical cord
- Dates, times, and sites of all cultures
- Feeding patterns and weight gain
- Bowel elimination patterns
- Condition of oral mucosa
- Skin color and rashes
- Activity pattern
- Interventions performed to reduce risk of infection
- Neonate's response to nursing interventions
- Evaluations for each expected outcome.

Injury, high risk for

related to induction or augmentation of labor

Definition

Increased risk to well-being of mother or fetus resulting from oxytocin stimulation

Assessment

- Previous pregnancies
- Prenatal history, including prenatal laboratory studies, pelvic measurements, allergies, weight gain, last menstrual period, and estimated date of confinement
- Physical examination, including maternal vital signs, Leopold's maneuvers (to determine fetal position), palpation of uterus (to assess frequency, intensity, and duration of contractions), sterile vaginal examination (to assess ripeness of cervix [Bishop score], presentation, estimation of maternal pelvis, fetal heart rate
- Diagnostic studies, including ultrasound test to determine gestational age and fetal size; non-stress test or contraction stress test to assess fetal-placental function
- Laboratory studies, including complete blood count, blood type and Rh factor, platelets, nitrazine test (to confirm rupture of membranes), urine protein and glucose levels
- Contraindications to oxytocin stimulation, such as absolute cephalopelvic disproportion; fetal distress; grand multipara; overdistention of the uterus from multiple gestation or polyhydramnios; vaginal bleeding; unfavorable fetal presentation or position

Risk factors

- Dysfunctional labor
- Hypotonic contractions
- Patient who lives far from hospital
- Postmaturity
- Previous precipitous delivery
- Prolonged rupture of the membranes

Associated medical diagnoses (selected)

Abortion (stimulation of uterus to pass conceptus), chorioamnionitis, chronic hypertension, cyanotic maternal cardiac disease, dystocia, fetal demise, diabetes, renal disease

Expected outcomes

- Uterine contractions occur every 2 to 3 minutes, with intensity of 40 to 60 mm Hg (by internal monitoring).
- Fetal heart rate maintains a variability of 6 to 10 beats/minute, with a reassuring pattern, as demonstrated by continuous fetal monitoring.
- Mother achieves a good labor pattern and neonate is delivered without complications.
- Adverse responses to oxytocin stimulation are identified and appropriate interventions initiated.
- Fluid balance is maintained.
- Optimal maternal-fetal well-being is maintained.

Interventions and rationales

- Explain oxytocin protocol to patient and her support person. Describe how oxytocin-induced contractions may peak more quickly and last longer than spontaneous contractions *to allay apprehension and encourage patient participation.*
- Before applying fetal monitor or administering oxytocin, encourage patient to void. Palpate bladder every 2 hours for distention. *A full bladder causes discomfort, especially when equipment is placed on patient's abdomen.*
- Monitor intake and output and measure urine specific gravity. *Decreased output with increased specific gravity may indicate urine retention, which may impede fetal descent.*
- Place patient in as comfortable a position as possible. A left lateral tilt relieves pressure of the gravid uterus on the inferior vena cava and facilitates blood flow to the placenta. *Correct positioning enhances patient comfort and may help you obtain a clearer fetal monitoring strip.*
- Apply fetal monitor and obtain a 15- to 20-minute baseline strip *to ensure adequate assessment of the fetal heart rate pattern and contractile status.*
- Use an 18G or 20G catheter when starting the main I.V. line *to prepare for possible emergency interventions, such as a cesarean section or blood administration.*
- Prepare oxytocin as ordered. Add drug to dextrose 5% injection or normal saline solution (initially, 10 units to 1,000 ml of solution). Label bottle with patient's name, amount of oxytocin, date and time prepared, and your name. Note that a doctor must be present in the hospital during oxytocin infusion. *Strict procedure ensures uniform administration and accurate assessment of uterine response.*
- Piggyback oxytocin solution to main I.V. line at the site most proximal to patient. Use an I.V. infusion pump to control flow rate. *Insertion at most proximal site to patient prevents a bolus infusion if oxytocin is stopped and primary I.V. rate is increased. An infusion pump guarantees exact dose administration.*
- Begin infusion at a rate of 0.5 to 1 milliunit/minute. Remain with pa-

tient during the first 20 minutes. *Initiating oxytocin at this rate enables you to evaluate patient's individual response to stimulation.*

- Increase oxytocin infusion by increments of 1 to 2 milliunits/minute, as ordered, every 30 to 60 minutes until desired contraction pattern is achieved and cervical dilation is 5 to 6 cm. Monitor blood pressure before and after each advancement of drug. *Advancing oxytocin slowly avoids hyperstimulation, which can cause fetal distress and uterine hypoxia.*
- If you advance to an infusion rate of 20 milliunits/minute without patient achieving desired contractile pattern, notify the doctor. *Increments above 20 milliunits/minute increase the risk of hyperstimulation and water intoxication.*
- Monitor maternal vital signs every 15 to 30 minutes, as indicated by hospital policy, *to assess for oxytocin-induced hypertension.*
- Monitor contractile pattern and fetal heart rate every 15 minutes. Assess contractions by palpation or intrauterine pressure catheter. At least every 30 minutes, document heart rate, variability, and fetal monitor strip changes. *Assessment of fetal heart rate and variability will enable you to detect nonreassuring fetal heart patterns. Palpation of contractions or intrauterine catheter monitoring will enable you to monitor uterine activity.*
- If patient responds poorly to oxytocin infusion, take the following steps:
  - Check I.V. mixture.
  - Check lines for patency.
  - Increase oxytocin flow rate, according to hospital policy.
  - Palpate uterine fundus for quality, duration, and relaxation of contractions.

Errors in oxytocin mixture and I.V. administration can cause a poor uterine response. An unripe cervix or uterus will also diminish the desired response. If patient's response does not improve, the infusion may have to be discontinued after 8 to 12 hours and restarted the next day.

- Observe for hypertonicity—contractions longer than 90 seconds' duration and less than 2 minutes apart. When using an intrauterine pressure catheter, a reading greater than 75 mm Hg indicates hypertonicity. *Because hypertonicity is unpredictable, it must be monitored carefully.*
- If you detect hypertonicity, discontinue infusion immediately. Check maternal vital signs and notify doctor. Increase primary I.V. fluids and position patient on left side. *These measures will help arrest hypertonicity.*
- Monitor continuously for loss of variability, late decelerations, or persistent bradycardia *to detect fetal distress. Fetal distress may result from impaired uteroplacental perfusion caused by increased tonicity of contractions.*
- If you detect signs of fetal distress, take the following steps:
  - Discontinue oxytocin infusion.
  - Administer 8 to 12 liters of oxygen via tight rebreathing mask *to increase oxygen supply to the fetus.*
  - Increase flow rate of primary I.V. line.
  - Reposition patient on left or opposite side *to increase placental blood flow.*
  - Notify the doctor *to expedite medical evaluation of maternal and fetal status.*
  - Assess maternal vital signs.
  - Perform or assist with sterile vaginal examination *to rule out*

the possibility of umbilical cord prolapse.
– Make sure patient is not left unattended.

• Assess patient's intake and output and monitor amount of oxytocin administered over the course of stimulation. Total fluid intake should not exceed 125 ml/hour. *Over a period of time, the antidiuretic effects of oxytocin combined with the administration of large volumes of electrolyte-free solutions can lead to water intoxication.*

Evaluations for expected outcomes

• Patient expresses understanding of how oxytocin may help induce or augment labor and consents to the use of oxytocin.
• Patient is assessed for contraindications to oxytocin stimulation.
• Patient is placed in a left lateral recumbent position with the head of the bed elevated.
• Patient's doctor or his designate is in attendance in the hospital during oxytocin administration.
• A baseline fetal monitoring strip is obtained before oxytocin stimulation, showing fetal heart rate within the normal range of 120 to 160 beats/minute, with average long-term variability.
• Oxytocin infusion is piggybacked to primary tubing close to catheter site.
• Induction is started at 0.5 to 1 milliunit/minute, with titration of 1 to 2 milliunits/minute every 20 to 30 minutes.
• Vital signs, contractile pattern, and fetal heart rate characteristics are recorded every 30 minutes or according to hospital policy.
• Contractions occur every 2 to 3 minutes, last 30 to 60 seconds, and are of moderate intensity with adequate resting tonus.
• Patient is monitored constantly.
• Signs of hypertonicity, fetal distress, late decelerations, or bradycardia are absent.
• I.V. intake should not exceed 125 ml/hour.
• Patient responds adequately to the stress of oxytocin stimulation with the assistance of nurse and support person.

Documentation

• Patient's vital signs on admission and every 15 to 30 minutes, according to hospital policy
• Baseline assessment of uterine activity before oxytocin stimulation and every 30 minutes thereafter via continuous electronic fetal monitoring (frequency, intensity, interval, duration, and tonus)
• Assessment of fetal heart rate, including baseline rate, long-term variability, short-term variability (with internal monitoring), accelerations and periodic changes
• Patient's physical and emotional response to induction or augmentation of labor, or both
• Nursing interventions to reduce risk of injury to patient or fetus from oxytocin stimulation
• Patient's response to nursing interventions
• Evaluations for each expected outcome.

■ Injury, high risk for

related to internal and external neonatal risk factors

Definition

Accentuated risk of accidental tissue damage

Assessment
- Ability of individuals caring for neonate
- Apgar scores
- Developmental stage (neonate and parents or caregivers)
- Environment, including air temperature, water temperature, stability of equipment
- Labor and delivery record
- Laboratory studies, including blood glucose and bilirubin levels, white blood cell count, clotting factors, platelet count, hemoglobin and hematocrit, maternal and neonatal blood types
- Neonatal health history, including traumatic delivery, blood dyscrasia, hypothermia, hyperthermia
- Neurologic status (neonate and parents or caregivers)
- Prenatal history

Risk factors
- Extremes in environmental temperature
- Hyperbilirubinemia
- Improperly functioning radiant warmer and temperature probe
- Improper padding of cold surfaces
- Litter or liquid spills on floor
- Malfunctioning equipment
- Parents or caregiver experience cognitive, emotional, or motor difficulties
- Parents' or caregiver's lack of familiarity with information resources
- Placement of neonate near drafts
- Requests for information by parents or family members
- Unsafe handling of neonate
- Water temperature at improper setting for washing neonate

Associated medical diagnoses (selected)
Birth injury, childbirth, hyperbilirubinemia, meconium aspiration, perinatal asphyxia

Expected outcomes
- Neonate's physical and safety needs are met.
- Family members provide safe environment for neonate following discharge.
- Family members recognize and report dangerous or potentially dangerous situations.
- Neonate does not experience any injury.

Interventions and rationales
- Assess family members' baseline knowledge of neonate safety. Instruct them as needed. *Education in safety techniques minimizes risk of injury.* Consider which teaching methods (pamphlets, videotapes, demonstrations) best suit each family member's individual learning style *to facilitate the learning process.*
- Immediately report malfunctioning equipment to the appropriate individual for replacement or repair *to help prevent accidents.*
- Keep one hand 1" to 2" (2.5 to 5 cm) above neonate when measuring weight *to prevent neonate from accidentally slipping off scale.*
- When transporting neonates from nursery, take one bassinet at a time, if possible, *to improve safety.*
- Discourage family members from walking in hall while holding neonate *to avoid falls caused by wet or slippery floors.*
- Discourage mother from sleeping in bed with neonate. *While sleeping, she may accidentally turn over onto, or lose her grip on, neonate.*
- Monitor neonate's skin color for signs of jaundice every shift. *Hyperbilirubinemia occurs in approximately 50% of all neonates. Elevated bilirubin levels can lead to neurologic and developmental difficulties.*

• Test water temperature before washing neonate. Temperature should not exceed 100° F (37.8° C). *Neonates' fragile skin cannot tolerate high temperatures.*
• Do not allow ill staff members or visitors to approach neonate *to prevent transfer of pathogens.*
• Assess neonate's potential for injury based on prenatal and labor and delivery records. *Early detection and treatment can minimize injury from intrauterine or perinatal insults.*
• Never leave neonate unattended in unprotected area. *Neonates are totally dependent on others for their physical, emotional, and safety needs.*
• Monitor respiratory and neurologic status as well as laboratory test results. Promptly report abnormal findings *to ensure immediate intervention and prevent complications.*
• Avoid heat loss to neonate from evaporation. *Cold stress leads to increased metabolic rate, which can result in oxygen consumption and hypoglycemia.*
• Review with family members state regulations regarding car seats before discharge *to decrease the risk of automobile injury or fatality.*

Evaluations for expected outcomes
• Family members express an understanding of techniques to ensure neonate's safety.
• Family members practice safety techniques during neonate's stay in hospital.
• Laboratory studies are within normal limits. If not, abnormal results are promptly reported to doctor.
• Family members express their intention to provide safe environment for neonate after discharge.
• Neonate does not experience injury.

Documentation
• Neonate's skin color
• Temperature of radiant warmer and presence of functioning temperature probe
• Laboratory results
• Observations of physical findings
• Observations or knowledge of unsafe practices
• Teaching and instructions given to family members, and their responses
• Interventions performed to prevent injury
• Neonate's response to nursing interventions
• Evaluations for each expected outcome.

■ Knowledge deficit

related to lack of information about birth process

Definition
Inadequate understanding of, or inability to perform, skills needed to cope effectively with the process of labor

Assessment
• Age
• Psychosocial status, including developmental stage; previous experience with childbearing; expectations of the birth process; current level of knowledge about pregnancy, birth, and recovery; interest in learning
• Ability to learn, including cognitive domain, intellectual and conceptual skills, attention span
• Support systems, including presence of support person, support persons's interest and ability to participate in helping patient

Defining characteristics

- Nulliparous state
- Patient's expressions indicating difficulty coping with pregnancy and birth
- Patient's expressions indicating lack of knowledge about birth process
- Patient's requests for information
- Patient's statements indicating anxiety related to lack of knowledge or skills
- Patient's statements indicating unrealistic expectations about birth process (may be unrealistically positive or unnecessarily pessimistic)

Associated medical diagnoses (selected)

Pregnancy, with or without associated complications

Expected outcomes

- Patient recognizes that increased knowledge and skill will help her cope better with the process.
- Patient demonstrates understanding of what she is taught.
- Patient demonstrates ability to perform skills needed for coping with labor.
- Patient expresses realistic expectations about the birth process.
- Patient's level of anxiety about giving birth is realistic.
- Patient expresses satisfaction with her increased knowledge.

Interventions and rationales

- Find a quiet, private environment for teaching patient and support person. *Freed of distractions, the patient and support person will learn more effectively.*
- Establish a trusting relationship with the patient. Develop mutual goals for learning. *These measures will enhance learning.*
- Select teaching strategies appropriate to the material to be taught and learning style of the patient (lecture, discussion, demonstration, practice, audiovisual materials). *Careful selection of teaching strategies will enable you to better meet the patient's needs.*
- Teach information and skills needed for understanding and coping during birth *to decrease patient's anxiety and increase her sense of competence.* Evaluate patient's level of understanding and ability to use knowledge during the birth process.

Evaluations for expected outcomes

- Patient expresses intention to put knowledge to use during labor.
- Patient describes birth process in her own words.
- Patient correctly performs labor skills.
- Patient expresses realistic expectations of labor.
- Patient responds to labor without undue anxiety.
- Patient uses breathing, relaxation, and position changes to cope during birth.
- Patient voices satisfaction with newly acquired knowledge and skills.

Documentation

- Patient's current understanding about birth process
- Patient's expression of need for better understanding or skills
- Learning goals established in cooperation with patient
- Information and skills taught to patient
- Teaching method used
- Patient response to teaching
- Patient mastery of information, including demonstration of new skills
- Evaluations for each expected outcome.

Knowledge deficit

related to neonatal care

Definition

Inadequate understanding of, or inability to perform, skills needed to provide neonatal care

Assessment

- Psychosocial status, including age, learning ability (affective domain, cognitive domain, psychomotor domain), decision-making ability, developmental stage, financial resources, health beliefs and attitudes, interest in learning, knowledge and skills regarding neonatal care, obstacles to learning, support systems (willingness and capability of others to help), usual coping pattern
- Neurologic status, including level of consciousness, memory, mental status, orientation

Defining characteristics

- Inability to demonstrate skills related to care of neonate.
- Lack of familiarity with informational resources
- Request for information
- Statements indicating insufficient recall, poor understanding, or misinterpretation of information

Associated medical diagnoses (selected)

Childbirth

Expected outcomes

- Patient voices need to improve her understanding of neonatal care.
- Patient sets realistic learning goals for developing competence in caring for neonate.
- Patient expresses understanding of neonatal care.
- Patient demonstrates ability to care for neonate independently or with minimal assistance.
- Patient identifies specific learning goals and target dates for mastering new skills.
- Patient expresses intention to adjust life-style to accommodate arrival of neonate.
- Patient or family member contacts community resources when necessary.
- Family members take active role in caring for neonate.

Interventions and rationales

- Establish an environment of mutual trust and respect *to enhance learning. Achieving rapport is especially important in light of the maternity patient's short length of stay.*
- Assess the patient's level of knowledge. Does she have other children? Has she had recent experience caring for a neonate? *Answering these questions will determine whether the patient requires basic information or a reinforcement of previous learning.*
- Negotiate with patient to develop goals for learning. *Allowing the patient to participate in decision making enhances learning.*
- Select teaching strategies appropriate for patient's individual learning style, such as one-on-one discussion and demonstration, attending a unit-based neonatal care class, or viewing audiovisual materials. *Choosing the approach that will serve the patient best increases the chance for successful learning.*
- Teach skills that patient must incorporate into daily life-style *to ensure relevance of learning experience.* Have patient give return demonstration of each new skill, such as feed-

ing, diapering, and bathing neonate, *to increase comfort level and identify areas of misunderstanding.*
- Have patient incorporate learned skills into daily routine during hospital stay. Encourage patient to care for neonate in hospital and allow for rooming-in if possible. *Practicing skills leads to proficiency.* Acknowledge positive efforts *to increase patient's self-esteem.*
- Provide patient with names and telephone numbers of resources (such as local breast-feeding association, child welfare service) to contact with questions. *The patient may benefit from additional sources of support during her hospital stay as well as after discharge.*
- Encourage family members to become involved in care of neonate *to promote family unity and bonding with neonate.*

Evaluations for expected outcomes
- Patient is comfortable holding and playing with neonate.
- Patient demonstrates ability to bottle-feed neonate and burps neonate at appropriate intervals.
- When applicable, patient demonstrates ability to breast-feed neonate.
- When applicable, patient demonstrates ability to care for circumcised neonate.
- Patient demonstrates ability to provide cord care.
- Patient demonstrates ability to bathe neonate and provide scalp care.
- Patient is comfortable with diapering neonate.
- Patient or family members express willingness to follow up on referrals to community resources.
- Family members demonstrate willingness to take active role in neonatal care.

Documentation
- Patient's current level of knowledge and skills
- Patient's expressions indicating her motivation to learn
- Patient's learning objectives
- Methods used to teach patient
- Teaching and instructions given
- Skills demonstrated
- Patient's response to teaching
- Evaluations for each expected outcome.

Knowledge deficit

related to postpartum self-care

Definition

Inadequate understanding of postpartum self-care activities or inability to perform skills needed to practice health-related behaviors

Assessment
- Psychosocial status, including age, learning ability (affective domain, cognitive domain, psychomotor domain), decision-making ability, developmental stage, financial resources, health beliefs and attitudes, interest in learning, knowledge and skill regarding current health problem, obstacles to learning, support systems (willingness and capability of others to help patient), usual coping pattern
- Neurologic status, including level of consciousness, memory, mental status, orientation
- Physical ability to perform self-care activities

Defining characteristics
- Expression of problem
- Inability to perform self-care tasks

• Lack of familiarity with sources of information
• Requests for information

Associated medical diagnoses (selected)
Pregnancy (vaginal delivery, with or without complications; cesarean section)

Expected outcomes
• Patient communicates desire to learn how to care for herself after delivery.
• Patient establishes realistic learning goals.
• Patient verbalizes or demonstrates understanding of what she has learned about self-care.
• Patient incorporates newly learned skills into daily routine.
• Patient states intention to make changes in postpartum routine, including seeking the assistance of a health care professional if necessary.

Interventions and rationales
• Establish an environment of mutual trust and respect *to enhance patient's learning. Establishing rapport is especially important in light of the maternity patient's short length of stay.*
• Assess patient's level of understanding of postpartum self-care activities *to establish a baseline for learning and provide direction for goal development.*
• Negotiate with patient target dates for mastering postpartum self-care skills. *Having the patient participate in decision making will facilitate learning.*
• Select teaching strategies (discussion, demonstration, role-playing, visual materials) best suited for patient's individual learning style *to enhance the learning process.*
• Teach skills that the patient must incorporate into daily postpartum routine, including: perineal care; use of sitz bath; use of witch hazel compresses; application and removal of perineal pads; and breast care. *Relevant topics will enhance the patient's motivation to learn.*
• Have patient give return demonstration of each new skill *to reinforce learning.*
• Teach patient about the process of involution *to help her understand postpartum occurrences.*
• Teach patient the importance of adequate nutrition and hydration *to ensure proper urinary and bowel elimination.*
• Discuss the importance of adequate rest *to promote emotional and physical stability.*
• Have patient incorporate learned skills into daily routine during hospitalization. Acknowledge her efforts. *Practicing learned skills will help the patient gain proficiency.*
• Provide patient with names and telephone numbers of appropriate resource people and community service agencies *to provide further resources to help with problem solving, both during the patient's hospital stay and after discharge.*

Evaluations for expected outcomes
• Patient expresses motivation to learn and establishes realistic goals for herself.
• Patient understands process of involution and recognizes and reports deviations from normal.
• Patient performs breast and perineal care.
• Patient resumes normal bowel and bladder elimination.
• Patient incorporates rest and sleep periods within daily routine.
• Patient demonstrates ability to use sitz bath.

- Patient displays knowledge of hemorrhoidal care.
- Patient says she will make changes in daily routine and seek the assistance of a health care professional if necessary.

Documentation
- Patient's understanding of and skill in postpartum self-care (including insight into her own abilities)
- Patient's expressions that indicate her motivation to learn
- Learning objectives
- Methods used to teach patient
- Information imparted to patient
- Skills demonstrated to patient
- Patient's responses to teaching
- Evaluations for each expected outcome.

Knowledge deficit

related to premature labor

Definition
Inadequate understanding of, or inability to perform, skills needed to cope with premature labor

Assessment
- Age
- Psychosocial status, including decision-making ability, developmental stage, financial resources, health beliefs and attitudes, interest in learning, knowledge and skill regarding pregnancy and birth process, learning ability (affective domain, cognitive domain, psychomotor domain), obstacles to learning, previous experience with premature labor, support systems (willingness and capability of others to help patient), usual coping pattern
- Neurologic status, including level of consciousness, memory, mental status, orientation

Defining characteristics
- Anxiety over premature labor
- Expressions of confusion over signs and symptoms of premature labor
- Expressions of desire for more information
- Expressions of difficulty understanding and coping with premature labor
- History of premature labor

Associated medical diagnoses (selected)
Premature labor

Expected outcomes
- Patient communicates desire to learn about premature labor.
- Patient sets realistic learning goals.
- Patient expresses understanding of causes and management of premature labor.
- Patient recognizes signs and symptoms of premature labor.
- Patient identifies and immediately reports danger signals during and after hospitalization.
- Patient voices emotional response to premature labor.
- Patient uses available support systems.
- Patient copes successfully with premature labor as demonstrated by verbal and nonverbal behaviors.
- Pregnancy results in a positive outcome.

Interventions and rationales
- Introduce yourself to patient and support person and orient them to surroundings. Explain all procedures beforehand. *These measures lessen the patient's anxiety.*
- Establish an environment of mutual trust and respect *to calm patient, de-*

creasing uterine stimulation from stress, and to provide an atmosphere conducive to learning.
• Work with patient to develop realistic goals for learning. *Unrealistic goals will frustrate you and the patient. Failure to achieve goals may reduce patient's interest in learning.*
• Select teaching strategy most appropriate for patient and support person *to enhance learning.*
• Assess patient's understanding of pregnancy and premature labor *to establish basis for nursing care plan and help guide future interventions.*
• Explain the causes, signs, and treatment of premature labor to patient and support person *to prepare them to actively participate in care.* Avoid information overload. *Anxiety may limit the patient's ability to assimilate information.*
• Project a warm, caring attitude and convey a willingness to listen *to encourage the patient to ask questions and voice feelings.*
• Don't place unrealistic demands on the patient *to avoid exacerbating feelings of inadequacy and anxiety.*
• Remain with the patient for uninterrupted periods of time. Assure patient and support person that they can rely on staff for emotional support *to ease anxiety and establish a therapeutic relationship.*
• Include patient in decision-making process when possible *to give her a feeling of participation and control.*
• Provide positive feedback to patient *to strengthen her self-esteem.*
• Provide patient with information related to her health status and condition of fetus. Inform support person as well. *Continued knowledge of maternal and fetal health status helps relieve anxiety.*
• Teach patient danger signs to report immediately, such as: contractions occurring every 10 minutes or less for 1 hour; fluid leaking from vagina; lack of or altered fetal movement. *Prompt identification and reporting of danger signs helps avoid premature labor.*
• If patient is discharged to home before delivery, review discharge instructions. Emphasize taking prescribed medications, limiting activities as instructed, and reporting danger signs. *If the patient understands her needs and limitations, she may be able to avoid recurrence of premature labor.*

Evaluations for expected outcomes
• Patient identifies possible causes of, signs of, and treatments for premature labor.
• Patient and support person are kept current on maternal and fetal condition.
• Patient promptly reports danger signs, and appropriate interventions are initiated.
• Patient states realistic expectations concerning pregnancy.

Documentation
• Patient's statements indicating her understanding of premature labor
• Patient's expressions indicating her motivation to learn
• Learning objectives
• Methods used to teach patient and support person
• Information discussed with patient and support person
• Patient's and support person's responses to teaching
• Maternal and fetal physical status
• Evaluations for each expected outcome.

Knowledge deficit

related to self-care activities during pregnancy

Definition

Inadequate understanding of information needed to practice health-related behaviors during pregnancy

Assessment

- Age
- Psychosocial status, including decision-making ability, developmental stage, financial resources, health beliefs and attitudes, interest in learning, knowledge and skill regarding pregnancy, learning ability (affective domain, cognitive domain, psychomotor domain), obstacles to learning, previous obstetric history, support systems (willingness and capability of others to help patient), usual coping pattern
- Neurologic status, including level of consciousness, memory, mental status, orientation

Defining characteristics

- Patient's expressions that indicate lack of knowledge about self-care during pregnancy
- Patient's requests for information
- Patient's statements indicating lack of familiarity with information resources

Associated medical diagnoses (selected)

Pregnancy

Expected outcomes

- Patient communicates a need for more information about self-care.
- Patient sets realistic learning goals.
- Patient demonstrates understanding of material taught.
- Patient performs health-care activities during pregnancy.
- Patient demonstrates ability to perform new health-related behaviors she has learned (specify skills and target dates).
- Patient continues to practice health-care behaviors after pregnancy.

Interventions and rationales

- Establish an environment of mutual trust and respect *to help patient relax and be receptive to learning.*
- Negotiate realistic learning goals with patient. *Unrealistic goals will frustrate you and patient. Failure to achieve goals may reduce patient's interest in learning.*
- Using open-ended questions, assess patient's knowledge of pregnancy-related health practices *to establish basis for nursing care plan and help guide future interventions.*
- Adapt teaching strategies to patient's individual learning style. Different strategies include discussion, demonstration, role-playing, and use of visual materials. *Tailoring teaching and content to patient's learning style helps enhance learning.*
- Refer patient to appropriate resource people, agencies, or organizations *to ensure comprehensive care.*
- Discuss appropriate dental care and instruct patient to visit a dentist early in pregnancy. *Poor oral hygiene and caries may result from nausea, vomiting, heartburn, and gum hyperemia associated with pregnancy.*
- Review possible effects of caffeine, alcohol, addicting drugs, and tobacco on the developing fetus *to help ensure fetal well-being*. Tell patient that any substance she ingests during pregnancy can affect the fetus. Intake of alcohol may cause developmental anomalies. Use of marijuana and tobacco may cause intrauterine

growth retardation and prematurity. Cocaine use may cause abruptio placentae in the mother and prematurity, poor feeding patterns, irritability, and increased respiratory and cardiac rates in the neonate. Effects of excessive caffeine intake are being investigated.

• Urge patient to consult her doctor or nurse-midwife before taking any medications *to avoid possible teratogenic effects on the fetus.*

• Review exercise routines designed for pregnant women and, if appropriate, refer patient to organized exercise group. *A regular exercise program during pregnancy enhances well-being and helps improve muscle tone in preparation for childbirth.*

• Review dietary intake for 1 week and instruct patient in proper nutrition during pregnancy. Explain to patient that she needs an extra 300 calories each day, for a total of 2,100 to 2,400 calories per day. Refer patient to dietitian if appropriate. *Increased caloric intake is required for optimal utilization of protein, fetal and maternal tissue synthesis, and increased basal metabolic needs.*

• Discourage patient from wearing constrictive clothing, tight shoes, or high-heeled shoes. *High-heeled shoes increase the likelihood of developing low back strain, backache, and poor balance. Constrictive clothing and shoes can alter venous circulation.*

• Discuss exposure to possible sources of toxic chemicals or gases *to avoid possible teratogenic effects on the developing fetus.*

• Review patient's daily routine at home and at work. *The patient may need to alter her routine during pregnancy. For example, if she holds a sedentary job, she should walk about periodically to increase circulation to the legs. If she stands for long periods, she may need to adopt a less physically demanding posture.*

• Instruct patient to contact doctor or nurse-midwife immediately if she experiences any danger signs or symptoms, including severe vomiting, frequent and severe headaches, epigastric pain, visual disturbances, swelling of fingers or face, altered or absent fetal movements after quickening, signs of vaginal or urinary tract infection, unusual or severe abdominal pain, or fluid discharge from vagina. *Prompt identification of danger signs reduces risk of abnormal pregnancy.*

Evaluations for expected outcomes

• Patient communicates a need for more information about self-care and establishes realistic learning goals.

• Patient's dietary intake, reviewed for 1 week, reflects an understanding of appropriate diet during pregnancy.

• Patient limits or stops smoking, if applicable.

• Patient does not consume alcohol during pregnancy.

• Patient limits daily caffeine intake.

• Patient explains how she can adapt her daily schedule to allow for rest periods throughout pregnancy.

• Patient expresses an understanding of the effects of illicit drugs on the developing fetus.

• Patient checks with her doctor or nurse-midwife before taking any medication.

• Patient avoids areas where toxic chemicals or gases may be present.

• Patient consistently follows an appropriate exercise regimen throughout pregnancy.

• Patient does not wear constrictive clothing and shoes or high-heeled shoes.

• Patient promptly reports danger signals to the doctor or nurse-midwife.

• Patient visits a dentist early in pregnancy.
• Patient takes prenatal vitamins as prescribed.

Documentation

• Patient's knowledge of self-care activities during pregnancy
• Expressions indicating patient's motivation to learn
• Learning objectives
• Teaching methods
• Subject matter discussed in teaching session
• Record of dietary intake for 1 week
• Demonstration and return demonstration of skills
• Patient's response to teaching
• Written and audiovisual materials given to patient
• Evaluations for each expected outcome.

Nutrition alteration: Less than body requirements

related to ineffective suck reflex

Definition

Inability to ingest sufficient fluids and nutrients resulting from an ineffective sucking reflex

Assessment

• Gestational age
• Perinatal history
• Apgar score
• Suck and swallow reflex, including intactness of lips and palate
• GI assessment, including vomiting and regurgitation, stool characteristics (color, amount, consistency, frequency), inspection of abdomen, auscultation of bowel sounds, palpation for masses, percussion for tympany or dullness
• Nutritional status, including intake and output, current weight, weight change since delivery, skin turgor, urine characteristics (frequency, amount), signs of dehydration, feedings (type, amount, frequency)
• Laboratory studies, including urine glucose levels, urine bilirubin levels, urine specific gravity
• Maternal assessment, including anesthetic used during labor and delivery, parity, knowledge level, breast-feeding (condition of nipples, positioning of neonate)

Defining characteristics

• Altered bowel elimination pattern
• Daily intake less than 130 ml/kg
• Decreased muscle tone
• Diarrhea or steatorrhea
• Dry mucous membranes
• Inelastic skin turgor
• Loss of more than 10% of birth weight within 5 days after delivery
• Sunken eyeballs
• Sunken fontanels
• Urine specific gravity greater than 1.015

Associated medical diagnoses (selected)

Cleft lip or cleft palate, hyperbilirubinemia, hypoglycemia, hypoxia, Pierre Robin syndrome, prematurity, tracheoesophageal fistula

Expected outcomes

• Mother demonstrates effective feeding techniques.
• Neonate does not lose more than 10% of birth weight.
• Neonate retains entire feeding without vomiting or regurgitating.
• Neonate ingests 95 to 145 calories/kg and 130 to 200 oz/kg each day.
• Neonate establishes effective suck and swallow reflexes, allowing for an adequate intake of nutrients.

- Infant gains at least 1 oz each day for first 6 months following birth.

Interventions and rationales

- Obtain neonate's weight at the same time each day, using the same scale, *to ensure early recognition of excessive weight loss.*
- If bottle-feeding, record amount ingested at each feeding. If breast-feeding, record number of minutes neonate nurses at each feeding, as well as ingestion of any supplement, *to aid in early recognition of inadequate caloric and fluid intake.*
- Assess parents' knowledge of feeding techniques, and provide instruction in positioning neonate during and after feeding; burping neonate; preparing formula; and proper amount and frequency of feedings. *Early detection of knowledge deficits and appropriate instruction help eliminate misconceptions.*
- Assess neonate's sucking pattern on an ongoing basis. Try to correct ineffective sucking patterns *to help eliminate ongoing difficulties.*
- Provide a preemie nipple or breast shield, as appropriate. *A preemie nipple's larger hole and softer texture make it easier for the neonate to obtain formula. A breast shield helps draw out an inverted nipple.*
- Make sure neonate's tongue is properly positioned under the nipple *to enable neonate to suck adequately* .
- Make sure neonate is awake before feeding. Unwrap blanket and tap soles of feet. *A tightly wrapped, drowsy neonate is less likely to be interested in feeding. The neonate must be fully awake and stimulated to suck effectively.*
- Record the number of stools and amount of urine voided each shift. *Decreased amounts of concentrated urine may indicate dehydration; altered bowel elimination pattern may indicate decreased food intake.*
- Monitor neonate for signs of dehydration, such as poor (inelastic) skin turgor, dry mucous membranes, decreased or concentrated urine, and sunken fontanels and eyeballs, *to establish need for immediate medical intervention.*
- Assess neonate for neurologic or other physical causes of ineffective sucking *to identify the need for more extensive evaluation.*
- Assess need for gavage feeding. *Neonate may require an alternative means of obtaining adequate fluids and calories temporarily.*

Evaluations for expected outcomes

- Neonate maintains good (elastic) skin turgor, moist mucous membranes, and flat, soft fontanels.
- Neonate's urine specific gravity is between 1.005 and 1.015.
- Mother demonstrates competence when feeding neonate.
- Neonate ingests 95 to 145 calories/kg and 130 to 200 oz/kg each day.
- Neonate retains entire feeding.
- Neonate returns to birth weight by 10 days after delivery.

Documentation

- Frequency, amount, and type of fluid ingested
- Incidence of vomiting and regurgitation
- Effectiveness of suck reflex
- Neonate's daily weight
- Parent's knowledge, level of caretaking, and bonding with neonate
- Frequency of bowel elimination and urination
- Signs of dehydration

- Nursing interventions and neonate's response
- Use of special nipple (such as preemie nipple)
- Results of laboratory studies
- Presence of physical or neurologic impairment
- Evaluations for each expected outcome.

Pain

related to physiologic changes of pregnancy

Definition

Subjective sensation of discomfort resulting from multiple sensory nerve interactions generated by physical, chemical, biological, or psychological stimuli

Assessment

- Characteristics of pain, including location, quality, intensity on a scale of 1 to 10; temporal factors; sources of relief
- Physiologic variables, such as age and pain tolerance
- Psychological variables, such as body image, personality, previous experience with pain, anxiety, and secondary gain from symptoms
- Sociocultural variables, such as cognitive style, culture or ethnicity, and attitude and values
- Environmental variables, such as setting and time
- Understanding of pregnancy and birth process

Defining characteristics

- Alteration in muscle tone (may range from flaccid to rigid)
- Altered time perception, withdrawal from social contact, and impaired thought process
- Autonomic responses, including diaphoresis, pupillary dilation, increased or decreased respiratory rate, blood pressure and pulse rate changes (these responses do not occur in chronic stable pain)
- Behavior that indicates pain
- Facial mask of pain, characterized by lackluster eyes, a "beaten" look, fixed or scattered movement, or grimacing
- Guarding or protective behavior, such as favoring a body part
- Moaning and crying
- Seeking distractions, such as conversation or activities
- Self-focusing
- Verbal reports of pain

Associated medical diagnoses (selected)

Abdominal infections, appendicitis, backache, Braxton Hicks contractions, breast masses or infection, cervical disk abnormality, cholecystitis, constipation, eclampsia, gastric ulcer, headache, gallbladder disease, hyperemesis gravidarum, heartburn, hemorrhoids, hiatal hernia, hydatidiform mole, intestinal flu, labor, leg cramps, pleurisy, preeclamptic headache, pulmonary emboli, round ligament pain, thrombosed veins, thrombophlebitis, urinary frequency, urinary tract infection, varicosities

Expected outcomes

- Patient identifies characteristics of pain.
- Patient articulates factors that intensify pain and modifies behavior accordingly.
- Patient carries out appropriate interventions for pain relief.

Interventions and rationales

- Provide care for patient experiencing nausea and vomiting.
  - Assess and document extent of nausea and vomiting *to create a data base for nursing interventions and patient teaching.*
  - Reassure patient that nausea will usually subside by the fourth month *to reduce patient's anxiety level and enhance compliance with nursing interventions.*
  - Instruct patient to eat dry, unsalted crackers before rising in the morning *to prevent nausea resulting from empty stomach.*
  - Tell patient to avoid greasy or spicy foods. *Spicy foods irritate stomach. Fats with meals depress gastric motility and digestive enzyme secretion, and slow intestinal peristalsis. These effects may lead to gastroesophageal reflux.*
  - Tell patient to avoid cooking odors that predispose her to nausea and to use a fan while cooking *to help avoid nausea. Air circulation dilutes odors.*
  - Advise patient to eat six small meals a day instead of three large ones *to avoid overloading stomach.*
  - Advise patient to eat foods high in carbohydrates. *Such foods are easier to digest.*
  - Tell patient to take iron pills and vitamins after meals *to avoid irritating stomach.*
  - Advise patient to take frequent walks outdoors. *Walking in fresh air reduces nausea and helps reinforce a positive outlook.*
  - Tell patient to separate food and fluid intake by ½ hour. *Drinking excessive fluids with meals distends the stomach, predisposing the patient to nausea. Taking fluids between meals also prevents dehydration.*
  - Advise patient to avoid very cold fluids and foods at mealtimes. *Cold fluids and foods may cause nausea and abdominal cramping.*
  - Caution patient to consult doctor before taking over-the-counter medications to treat nausea and vomiting *to avoid harmful effects on the fetus.*
- Provide care for the patient experiencing urinary frequency.
  - Assess patient for frequency and dysuria *to rule out possible urinary tract infection.*
  - Reassure patient that urinary frequency is normal in the early and late stages of pregnancy because an enlarging uterus places pressure on the bladder. *Reassurance may reduce patient's confusion and anxiety.*
  - Tell patient to avoid drinking large amounts of liquids within 2 to 3 hours of bedtime *to prevent frequent nocturnal urination and sleep loss.*
  - Instruct patient to ingest required amount of liquids early in the day *to reduce need for evening liquids.*
  - Instruct patient to void when the urge occurs *to prevent bladder distention and urinary stasis, which may predispose patient to urinary tract infection.*
  - Instruct patient in the signs and symptoms of urinary tract infection. Urge her to promptly report signs and symptoms to the doctor. *Early detection of urinary tract infection allows early treatment and helps to prevent complications, such as pyelonephritis and premature labor.*

- If the patient experiences breast fullness and tingling, take the following measures.
  - –Assess patient's breast discomfort *to obtain a data base for further interventions.*
  - –Assure patient that breast changes and discomfort are natural. Tell her that fullness will last entire pregnancy but that tenderness will resolve after first trimester. *Reassurance decreases patient's anxiety level and promotes compliance.*
  - –Advise patient to wear supportive bra with wide, adjustable straps and smooth lining *to decrease irritation and provide support for enlarging breasts.*
  - –Instruct patient to avoid tight bras and clothing that may confine breasts. *Pressure increases tenderness, tingling sensations, and discomfort.*
  - –Teach patient anatomy and physiology of breast changes during pregnancy. If indicated, begin preparation for breastfeeding at end of third trimester *to enhance the nursing experience.*
- Provide care for the pregnant patient who develops a headache.
  - –Assess type and location of headache, and associated signs and symptoms. *Assessment provides information for selection of interventions and clues to patient's discomfort. The presence of associated factors, such as proteinuria, weight gain, edema, elevated blood pressure, and hyperreflexia, may indicate occurrence of pregnancy-induced hypertension.*
  - –Advise patient to sleep 8 hours a night and to nap or rest for 2 hours in the afternoon *to alleviate fatigue.*
  - –Advise patient to drink 6 to 8 glasses (1,500 to 2,000 ml) of fluid per day *to prevent or alleviate headache resulting from dehydration. Increasing fluids may eliminate headache by increasing vascular space and dilating cerebral veins.*
  - –Instruct patient to apply cool, wet compresses to forehead and back of neck and to massage neck, shoulders, face, and scalp. *Cool compresses may eliminate headaches resulting from emotional tension and spasms of sternocleidomastoid muscles of neck and back.*
  - –Instruct patient to take two tablets of acetaminophen every 4 to 6 hours, as ordered. Tell her to avoid aspirin because of its anticoagulant action. Remind her to consult her doctor before taking over-the-counter medications. *Acetaminophen effectively relieves minor headaches of pregnancy.*
- Provide care to the patient experiencing heartburn.
  - –Assess patient's nutritional habits *to obtain clues to patient's discomfort and information for selection of interventions.*
  - –Reassure patient that normal pregnancy changes can cause heartburn, *to decrease her anxiety and increase her compliance with nursing interventions.*
  - –Advise patient to eliminate greasy and spicy foods from her diet and to avoid fats. *Such foods decrease stomach motility and increase secretion of stomach acids and gastric acidity.*

- Instruct patient to reduce fluid intake with meals. *Liquids tend to inhibit gastric juices.*
- Instruct patient to avoid very cold foods. *Very cold foods promote gastric reflux.*
- Instruct patient to drink cultured milk, such as buttermilk, rather than regular whole milk. *Cultured milk has less fat than regular milk.*
- Instruct patient in good posture. *Good posture gives the stomach more room to function.*
- Instruct patient to take small, frequent meals *to avoid overloading the stomach* and to remain upright for 3 to 4 hours after a meal *to decrease possibility of reflux.*
- Advise patient to use antacids that are low in sodium *to lessen the risk of tissue edema* and that contain both aluminum and magnesium (Maalox, Riopan). *Aluminum-based antacids (such as Amphojel) may cause constipation. Magnesium-based antacids (such as Milk of Magnesia) have a laxative effect. Aluminum-magnesium combinations tend to balance these effects.* Tell patient to avoid antacids that contain sodium bicarbonate.

• Provide care for the patient with round ligament pain.
- Assess onset and site of round ligament discomfort and associated uterine activity *to rule out the possibility of premature labor activity.*
- Reassure patient that round ligament pain is a normal occurrence during pregnancy, caused by the stretching of the ligaments that support the expanding uterus. *Reassurance will decrease anxiety and promote cooperation.*
- Instruct patient to avoid sudden jerky movement, to rise slowly from recumbent positions, and to avoid excessive exercise, standing, or walking. *Sudden, jerky movements or twisting of the torso pulls on the round ligaments, causing unilateral or bilateral pain. Excessive exercise, standing, or walking can also strain the abdominal muscles.*

• Provide care to the patient who experiences backache.
- Assess patient's posture, lifting techniques, and footwear *to pinpoint causes of pain.*
- Instruct patient to wear low-heeled shoes, maintain good posture, and hold shoulders back *to increase spinal curvature, which may reduce backache.*
- Instruct patient in proper body mechanics *to help her avoid stress to the lower back.*
- Tell patient to rest in recumbent position or with her legs bent and elevated on a bed or chair *to relieve strain on lower back.*
- Instruct patient to perform moderate daily exercise *to tone and maintain muscle strength in lower back.*
- Discuss benefits of massaging and applying warm, moist heat to the lower back. *These measures will help relax and soothe tight muscles.*

• Provide care for the patient with hemorrhoids.
- Assess patient's diet for fiber, fluids, and iron intake *to plan appropriate diet that will enhance bowel function.*
- Assess prepregnancy bowel habits and history of hemorrhoids

to provide a data base for planning interventions.
- Instruct patient to avoid constipation through increasing intake of dietary fiber, bran cereals, and fluids. She should also drink warm water when she arises in the morning. *Avoiding constipation helps prevent straining at stool and lessens risk of hemorrhoids. Dietary fiber, bran cereals, and fluids increase intestinal peristalsis and facilitate bowel function.*
- Encourage patient to take sitz baths and to use witch hazel and Epsom salt compresses. *Warm sitz baths cause tissue dilation, increased blood flow, and healing. Witch-hazel pads (such as Tucks) and Epsom salt compresses are used to reduce tissue swelling.*
- According to the doctor's recommendation, encourage use of analgesic ointments and topical preparations *to reduce pain.*
- Administer stool softeners, as ordered, *to allow normal evacuation without straining.*

• Provide care for the pregnant patient with varicosities.
- Assess for degree of pain, family history, level of exercise, extent of varicosities, and history of varicosities before pregnancy. *Assessing pain helps rule out thrombophlebitis. Assessing extent of varicosities and patient's level of exercise helps plan for nursing interventions.*
- Reassure patient about the cause and usual duration of her discomfort *to decrease anxiety and promote compliance.*
- Tell patient to rest in recumbent position, with her legs elevated above the level of the body, twice a day *to promote venous return and avoid stagnation and pooling of venous blood.*
- Instruct patient to put on supportive hose before arising in the morning and to raise her legs when putting them on. *Supportive hose facilitate venous return and promote comfort.*
- Tell patient to avoid garters and tight knee-high stockings and not to cross her legs *to lessen risk of venous pooling and thrombus formation.*
- Advise patient to perform regular exercise, take frequent walks, and avoid sitting for long periods *to increase blood flow and retard stasis and pooling.*

• Provide care for the patient suffering from leg cramps.
- Assess patient's diet for excessive soft drink intake or inadequate dairy protein. *Inadequate dairy protein or excessive intake of soft drinks, which contain large amounts of phosphorus, can disrupt the body's calcium-phosphorus ratio, thereby leading to leg cramps.*
- Instruct patient to limit intake of soft drinks *to reduce consumption of phosphorus.*
- Reassure patient that leg cramps are normal during pregnancy *to reduce anxiety and promote compliance.*
- Tell patient to consult with doctor about supplementing milk intake with aluminum hydroxide (Amphojel). *Taken with milk, aluminum hydroxide helps to remove dietary phosphorus from the intestinal tract.*
- Instruct patient to elevate legs periodically and to avoid lying prone with toes pointed. *Lying prone with toes pointed predis-*

poses the patient to blood vessel occlusion and subsequent cramping.
- Tell patient to exercise and use good body mechanics *to prevent leg cramping by increasing general circulation.*
- Advise patient to take warm baths at bedtime *to relax muscle fibers and increase blood flow circulation to the muscles.*
- If cramping occurs, straighten the affected leg and dorsiflex the foot. *These measures pull the contracted muscle taut, thus relieving a cramp caused by contraction.*
- Caution patient not to rub the affected calf *to avoid risk of dislodging an undetected thrombus.*

• Provide care for the patient who experiences Braxton Hicks contractions.
- Assess patient for frequency, strength, and regularity of contractions *to rule out preterm or true labor.*
- Reassure the patient that Braxton Hicks contractions are normal in pregnancy, *to reduce anxiety.*
- Instruct patient to walk. *Walking may cause Braxton Hicks contractions to cease and can be effective in distinguishing them from true labor.*
- Advise patient to assume left lateral position when at rest *to increase blood flow to the uterus, which may decrease the intensity and frequency of the contractions.*

Evaluations for expected outcomes

• Patient identifies characteristics of pain, lists factors that intensify pain, and modifies behavior accordingly.
• Patient is free of vomiting and effectively reduces her level and frequency of nausea.
• Patient consumes adequate fluids during the day and limits intake in the evening.
• Patient wears a supportive bra.
• Patient reports proper care and preparation of her breasts for nursing.
• Patient is free of headaches.
• Patient is free of heartburn.
• Patient reports a decrease in the frequency and duration of round ligament pain.
• Patient demonstrates proper posture, body mechanics, and footwear.
• Patient reports reduced back pain.
• Patient increases her intake of fiber, bran cereals, and fluids.
• Patient reports a decrease or absence of hemorrhoidal pain.
• Patient is free of constipation.
• Patient is free of of varicosities.
• Patient reports a decrease or absence of leg cramps.
• Patient reports a decrease in frequency and intensity of Braxton Hicks contractions.

Documentation

• Patient's description of pain and expression of feelings about pain
• Observations about the patient's physical, psychological, and sociocultural responses to pain
• Comfort measures and medications provided to reduce pain and the effectiveness of these interventions
• Patient teaching about pain and pain relief
• Additional nursing interventions performed by the nurse to assist the patient with pain control
• Evaluations for each expected outcome.

Pain

related to physiologic response to labor

Definition

Subjective sensation of discomfort resulting from multiple sensory nerve interactions generated by physical, chemical, biological, or psychological stimuli

Assessment

- Descriptive characteristics of pain, including location, quality, intensity on a scale of 1 to 10; temporal factors; sources of relief
- Physiologic variables, including age and pain tolerance
- Psychological variables, including body image, personality, previous experience with pain, anxiety, and secondary gain from symptoms
- Sociocultural variables, including cognitive style, culture or ethnicity, and attitude and values
- Environmental variables, including setting and time
- Understanding and expectations of labor and delivery

Defining characteristics

- Alteration in muscle tone (may range from flaccid to rigid)
- Altered time perception, withdrawal from social contact, and impaired thought process
- Autonomic responses, including diaphoresis, pupillary dilation, increased or decreased respiratory rate, blood pressure and pulse rate changes (these responses do not occur in chronic stable pain)
- Behavior that indicates pain
- Facial mask of pain, characterized by lackluster eyes, a "beaten" look, fixed or scattered movement, or grimacing
- Guarding or protective behavior, such as favoring a body part
- Moaning and crying
- Seeking distractions, such as conversation or activities
- Self-focusing
- Verbal reports of pain

Associated medical diagnoses (selected)

Impending eclampsia, abruptio placentae, uterine rupture, labor

Expected outcomes

- Patient identifies characteristics of pain.
- Patient articulates factors that intensify pain and modifies behavior accordingly.
- Patient expresses a decrease in the intensity of her discomfort.
- Patient experiences satisfaction with her performance during labor and delivery.

Interventions and rationales

- Orient patient on admission to labor and delivery suite. Show the patient her individual room and explain operations of her bed and call light. Explain admission protocol and the labor process. *These measures will allay the patient's initial anxiety.*
- Assess patient's knowledge of labor process and her current anxiety level *to plan supportive strategies.*
- Explain available analgesics and anesthesia to the patient and support person. *Awareness that medications are available reduces anxiety.*
- Encourage support person to remain with patient in labor. *A woman in labor will respond more readily to supportive measures if offered by a familiar, caring person.*

• Instruct the patient and support person in techniques to decrease the discomfort of labor.
 – Discuss techniques of conscious relaxation. *During labor, relaxation enables the patient to use coping techniques.*
 – Tell patient to concentrate on an internal or external focal point. *A focal point allows controlled thought while breathing.*
 – Instruct patient in basic deep chest breathing, which is similar to normal breathing, but slower and deeper. *Deep chest breathing creates a sense of relaxation during contractions.*
 – Instruct patient in shallow chest breathing. Tell her to take slow, panting-like breaths. Breathing should be slow to avoid hyperventilation. *Shallow chest breathing lifts the diaphragm from the uterus during contractions, thereby decreasing the intensity of contractions.*
 – Instruct patient in effleurage — light, rhythmic, circular stroking of the abdomen with the fingertips. Tell her to use both hands, to begin at the pubes, and to stroke upward and outward. *Effleurage soothes the patient, enhances relaxation, and may complement use of learned breathing techniques.*

• In early labor, provide the patient with diversional activities, such as watching TV, *to decrease anxiety.*
• As labor progresses, modify environment to reduce distractions (close door, turn off TV, close curtains). *These measure help patient to concentrate during active phase of labor.*
• Apply sacral pressure to patient if needed *to decrease back pain.*
• Help patient to change positions and use pillows to make herself more comfortable. Make sure all body parts are supported, with joints slightly flexed. *Frequent position changes reduce stiffness, prevent pressure sores, and promote comfort.*
• Assess bladder for distention, and encourage patient to void every 2 hours. *A distended bladder increases patient's discomfort during contractions and interferes with fetal descent.*
• Provide frequent mouth care. According to protocol, provide ice chips, water-based jelly, or a wet 4″ × 4″ gauze swab for dry lips *to relieve dry mouth and lips caused by breathing techniques and NPO status.*
• Apply a cool, damp cloth to patient's forehead *to relieve diaphoresis.*
• Change patient's gown and bed linens as needed. *Diaphoresis and vaginal discharge can dampen the gown and bed and cause discomfort.*
• Encourage patient to rest and relax between contractions *to decrease fatigue. Fatigue worsens pain perception and decreases patient's ability to cope with contractions.*
• Discuss with patient and support person which pain medications are available if alternate pain control methods prove inadequate. *The patient may need prescribed analgesics to cope with the labor process.*

Evaluations for expected outcomes

• Patient effectively uses learned breathing techniques to cope with stresses of labor.
• Patient copes with labor in a relaxed manner.
• Patient articulates a need for analgesia.
• Patient articulates a decrease in the intensity of her discomfort.
• Patient assumes a comfortable position.
• Patient's personal hygiene needs are met.

• Patient expresses satisfaction with her performance during childbirth.

Documentation
• Patient's childbirth preparation and plans for giving birth
• Patient's description of pain
• Observation of patient's response to labor
• Nursing interventions to decrease discomfort
• Patient's response to nursing interventions
• Evaluations for each expected outcome.

Pain

related to postpartum physiologic changes

Definition
Subjective sensation of discomfort derived from multiple sensory nerve interactions generated by physical, chemical, biological, or psychological stimuli

Assessment
• Descriptive characteristics of pain, including location, quality, intensity on a scale of 1 to 10, temporal factors, sources of relief
• Physiologic variables, such as age and pain tolerance
• Psychological variables, such as body image, personality, previous experience with pain, anxiety, and secondary gain
• Sociocultural variables, including cognitive style, culture or ethnicity, attitude and values, and birth order
• Environmental variables, such as the setting and time
• Physical factors, including perineal pain, sulcus tears, hemorrhoids, hematomas, uterine discomfort, breast fullness and engorgement, nipple soreness or cracking, episiotomy (type, extension, redness, edema, ecchymosis, discharge, approximation)

Defining characteristics
• Alterations in muscle tone (may span from flaccid to rigid)
• Altered time perception, withdrawal from social contact, impaired thought processes
• Autonomic responses, including diaphoresis, pupillary dilation, increased or decreased respiratory rate, blood pressure and pulse rate changes (these responses do not occur in chronic stable pain)
• Expressions of pain
• Facial mask of pain, characterized by lackluster eyes, "beaten" look, fixed or scattered movement, grimace
• Guarding or protective behavior, such as posturing or favoring a body part
• Moaning, crying
• Seeking distractions, such as conversation or activities
• Self-focusing

Associated medical diagnoses (selected)
Mastitis, pelvic thrombophlebitis, perineal lacerations and extensions, puerperal infections, septicemia, vulvar or vaginal hematoma

Expected outcomes
• Patient identifies characteristics of pain.
• Patient articulates factors that intensify pain and modifies behavior accordingly.
• Patient expresses a feeling of comfort and relief from pain.
• Patient understands and carries out appropriate interventions for pain relief.

Interventions and rationales

- Assess patient's pain symptoms *to obtain information and plan appropriate nursing interventions.*
- As ordered, administer pain medications *to provide pain relief.*
- Discuss with patient reasons for her discomfort and its expected duration *to decrease anxiety and increase compliance.*
- Examine episiotomy site for redness, edema, ecchymosis, drainage, and approximation *to detect trauma to the perineal tissues or developing complications.*
- Inspect the rectum for hemorrhoids. Provide instruction on hemorrhoidal care, as appropriate. Tell patient to apply ice for 20 minutes every 4 hours; apply witch hazel compress; and use sitz baths. *Hemorrhoidal care will help decrease patient discomfort. Ice aids in the regression of hemorrhoids and vulvar irritation by promoting localized vasoconstriction.*
- Apply ice packs to the episiotomy site for the first 24 hours *to increase vasoconstriction and reduce edema and discomfort.*
- Encourage the use of sitz baths. Baths should be cool to cold for the first day, and warm (100° to 105° F [37.8° to 40.6° C]) thereafter. Patient should take sitz baths three or four times a day, with each lasting about 20 minutes. *Sitz baths with cold water decrease edema and promote comfort. After 24 hours, moist heat increases circulation to the perineum, reduces edema, promotes healing, and enhances oxygenation and nutrition of tissues.*
- As ordered, instruct patient in the proper use of sprays, creams, and ointments for the perineal area. *Creams, sprays, and ointments penetrate sensory nerve endings, providing a depressant effect on the peripheral nerves, thereby reducing the response to sensory stimulation. Astringents, such as witch hazel, shrink tissues and reduce swelling.*
- Assess for uterine tenderness and presence and frequency of after-birth pains every hour for the first 24 hours, then every shift as indicated. *In the first 12 hours after birth, uterine contractions are strong and regular. Factors that may intensify contractions include multiparity, breast-feeding, and oxytocin administration.*
- Encourage patient to tighten buttocks before sitting and to sit on a flat, padded surface. She should avoid foam donuts or soft pillows. *Tightening gluteal muscles before sitting reduces stress and direct pressure on the perineum. Because foam donuts separate the buttocks, they may decrease venous blood flow to the affected area, thereby increasing discomfort.*
- Inspect breast and nipple tissue for engorgement or cracked nipples *to ensure selection of appropriate nursing interventions.*
- Encourage breast-feeding mother to wear supportive bra *to increase comfort* and to position neonate properly during feedings. She should not use the same position all the time. *This will help prevent sore nipples.*
- If breast-feeding patient is engorged, instruct her to use warm compresses or take a warm shower before breast-feeding and to breast-feed more often *to relieve discomfort. Warm compresses and showers help stimulate the flow of milk and may help relieve stasis and engorgement.*
- If the breast-feeding mother's nipples become sore, instruct her to air-dry nipples for 20 to 30 minutes after feedings *to help toughen nipples* and to apply breast creams as or-

dered *to soften nipples and relieve irritation.* If only one nipple is sore or cracked, instruct her to offer the nontender nipple first for several feedings *to reduce potential trauma on the sore nipple.*
• Tell the non-breast-feeding patient to wear a tight supportive bra or breast binder and apply ice packs as needed *to prevent or reduce lactation.*
• Assess for bladder distention. Implement measures to facilitate voiding and provide appropriate patient teaching. *Bladder fullness can be a source of discomfort.*
• After epidural or spinal anesthesia, assess patient for spinal headache. Pain is primarily located behind the eyes but may radiate to the temples and occipital area. Pain is relieved when patient assumes the supine position but increases when she sits or stands. Avoid pain medications before medical evaluation of the source of the headache. Increase oral fluids, and notify doctor or anesthesiologist, as indicated. *Epidural or spinal anesthesia may lead to leakage of cerebrospinal fluid (CSF) and subsequent headache. Increasing oral fluids helps to compensate for loss of CSF.*
• After a cesarean section, provide an abdominal pillow and teach patient to splint the incision when moving or coughing *to provide support for the abdominal muscles.*

Evaluations for expected outcomes
• Episiotomy site is clean, intact, and heals well. Signs of redness, edema, ecchymosis, discharge, and approximation are absent.
• Patient demonstrates perineal care measures, such as taking a sitz bath, to aid in comfort and promote hygiene.
• Patient successfully uses prescribed creams, sprays, and ointments.
• Patient ambulates freely without excessive discomfort.
• In the nonlactating patient, the breasts are soft and nontender.
• In the breast-feeding patient, the breasts are emptied regularly and not engorged, with soft, nonirritated nipples.
• Patient voids adequately without pressure or dysuria.
• Uterine afterbirth pains are minimal and relieved with prescribed medications.

Documentation
• Patient's description of physical pain, pain relief, and feelings about pain
• Nurse's observations about patient's physical, psychological, and sociocultural responses to pain
• Comfort measures and medications provided to reduce pain (including effectiveness of each intervention)
• Information provided to the patient about pain and pain relief
• Additional nursing interventions performed to assist the patient with controlling pain
• Evaluations for each expected outcome.

Parenting alteration

related to inadequate attachment to high-risk neonate

Definition
Inability of a nurturing figure to promote optimum growth and development of a high-risk neonate

Assessment
• Parental status, including age and maturity; apprehension; parental role models during childhood; knowledge

of child care and normal growth and development; previous bonding history; available support systems; coping mechanisms; feelings about pregnancy and neonate
• Family status, including age, sex, status, and developmental stage of other children; parents' relationship with each other and with other children
• Mother's medical condition
• Neonatal status, including medical condition, separation from parents, presence of medical equipment
• Psychosocial status, including financial stressors, work demands

Defining characteristics
• Expression of disappointment in neonate's physical characteristics
• Expression of negative feelings toward neonate's bodily functions
• Expression of resentment toward neonate
• Expression of role inadequacy
• Expressions of apprehension, fear, guilt
• Inability of parents to accept neonate's medical condition
• Inability or unwillingness to participate in neonate's physical or emotional care
• Inappropriate verbal, tactile, and auditory stimulation of neonate
• Inattention to neonate's needs
• Infrequent phone calls to nursery
• Infrequent visits to see neonate
• Lack of parental attachment behavior
• Neonate separated from parents soon after birth because of medical complications and placed in the neonatal intensive care unit (NICU)

Associated medical diagnoses (selected)
Any disease or illness associated with high-risk neonates

Expected outcomes
• Parents establish contact with neonate.
• Parents communicate feelings and anxieties regarding neonate's condition and their parenting skills.
• Parents express willingness to care for neonate and demonstrate competent parenting skills.
• Parents demonstrate knowledge of neonate's developmental needs.
• Parents become involved in planning and providing neonate's care.
• Parents use available support systems to assist with care of neonate.

Interventions and rationales
• Before parents' first visit to NICU, explain appearance of neonate and presence of supportive devices *to prepare parents for sights and sounds that may otherwise upset them.*
• Encourage mother to visit NICU. Assess whether mother is physically able to go to nursery and offer assistance if necessary. *Mother may be hesitant to ask for help or may be unsure of physical surroundings.*
• Provide parents with picture of neonate *to help them accept the reality of the birth.*
• If transfer to another institution is necessary, arrange for parents to meet transfer team and visit with neonate beforehand. *Seeing neonate and meeting transfer team will increase parents' feelings of involvement and help them to come to terms with neonate's condition.*
• Encourage father or other family member to visit neonate soon after admittance to NICU or transfer to other institution, especially if mother can't visit. *First-hand reports from a family member regarding neonate's condition and physical surroundings will help allay fears of mother and other family members.*

• Assess parents' level of understanding of neonate's condition and their expectations for the future *to clear up misunderstandings, allow for prompt intervention, and promote realistic planning.*
• Encourage parents to express anxieties related to neonate's condition and their parenting skills *to identify and clarify misconceptions.*
• Make sure parents are informed of neonate's ongoing condition *to help decrease their anxiety and help them plan for the future.*
• Encourage parents to touch and talk to neonate and call neonate by name. Reassure them that touching infant will not cause any harm. *This will stimulate bonding between parents and infant.*
• Allow time for parents to care for neonate within the security of the hospital. Provide positive feedback for parent's efforts to care for neonate *to increase parents' self-confidence.*
• Provide parents with NICU telephone number and encourage phone calls at any time *to make information about neonate readily available.*
• Refer parents to social services, as needed, *to help ensure comprehensive care.*
• Encourage parents to bring in personal items for neonate, such as small stuffed animals or pictures of family members, *to encourage emotional bonding with neonate.*

Evaluations for expected outcomes
• Parents initiate regular contact with neonate.
• Parents are kept informed of neonate's condition.
• Parents voice their anxieties about neonate's condition and their ability to provide care.
• Parents express understanding of available sources of support.
• Parents demonstrate ability to meet neonate's basic needs and, if appropriate, special care needs.
• Parents display appropriate attachment behaviors, including providing neonate with appropriate verbal, tactile, and auditory stimulation.
• Parents set realistic goals for neonate.

Documentation
• Observations of parents' behavior
• Parents' statements concerning the neonate
• Information provided to parents and their level of understanding
• Parents' interactions with neonate
• Parents' willingness to meet neonate's physical and emotional needs
• Consultations with health team members
• Parents' and neonate's responses to nursing interventions
• Evaluations for each expected outcome.

■ Self-esteem disturbance

related to behavior during labor and delivery

Definition
Negative perception of behavior that disturbs healthy functioning

Assessment
• Availability of support
• Patient's and support person's perception of labor and delivery
• Patient history, including past labor and delivery experience, ethnic and cultural background, and usual pattern of coping with stress

- Physiologic and behavioral changes during labor and delivery

Defining characteristics
- Difficulty accepting positive reinforcement
- Inability to use coping strategies
- Lack of eye contact
- Low self-esteem

Associated medical diagnoses (selected)
Vaginal or cesarean section delivery of term, postterm, or preterm infant

Expected outcomes
- Patient expresses feelings about labor and delivery.
- Patient sets realistic goals for her behavior during labor and delivery.
- Patient receives adequate emotional and physical support during labor and delivery.
- Patient projects a positive self-concept through behavior and verbal expression.

Interventions and rationales
- Encourage patient and support person to articulate their expectations of the labor and delivery experience *to identify and correct misconceptions early in the couple's experience.*
- Provide positive feedback concerning patient's behavior on an ongoing basis *to clear up misconceptions and increase feelings of self-esteem.*
- Emphasize realistic goals for behavior during labor and delivery. *Placing unrealistic demands on the patient can lead to feelings of inadequacy and poor self-esteem.*
- Encourage support person to express feelings regarding labor and delivery. *The patient may misunderstand how the support person viewed her behavior during labor.*
- Encourage patient to take an active role in self-care activities after delivery *to reinforce patient's ability to care for self and increase self-esteem.*

Evaluations for expected outcomes
- Patient expresses feelings about labor and delivery.
- Patient expresses realistic understanding of what to expect from her own behavior during labor and delivery.
- Patient expresses satisfaction with emotional and physical support received during labor and delivery.
- Patient's behavior and remarks reflect a positive self-image.

Documentation
- Patient's behaviors and expressions that indicate lowered self-esteem
- Nurse's perceptions of patient's readiness for decision making
- Nursing interventions to improve patient's self-concept
- Patient's response to nursing interventions
- Patient's willingness to perform self-care activities
- Patient's expressions of well-being
- Evaluations for each expected outcome.

■ Skin integrity impairment

related to episiotomy or abdominal incision

Definition
Interruption in skin integrity after delivery

Assessment
- Age
- Vital signs
- Integumentary status, including color, elasticity, hygiene, lesions, moisture, quantity and distribution of

hair, sensation, skin temperature, texture, and turgor
- Musculoskeletal status, including area affected by anesthetic procedure, joint mobility, muscle strength and mass, paralysis, and range of motion
- Health history, including past skin problems, trauma, surgery, chronic debilitating disease, and immobility
- Nutritional status, including appetite, dietary intake, hydration, present weight, change from normal
- Laboratory studies, including hemoglobin and hematocrit, serum albumin levels
- Psychosocial status, including coping patterns, family or significant other, mental status, occupation, self-concept, and body image
- Knowledge, including patient's current understanding of her physical condition; physical, mental, and emotional readiness to learn
- Presence of medical condition that may interfere with healing
- Extent of interruption in skin integrity due to delivery

Defining characteristics
- Destruction of skin layers surrounding episiotomy or abdominal incision
- Disruption of skin surfaces
- Invasion by pathogens
- Presence of external factors adversely affecting skin integrity (chemical agents, cold, heat, pressure)

Associated medical diagnoses (selected)
Cesarean delivery, lacerations (first-, second-, third-, and fourth-degree), tubal ligation, vaginal delivery

Expected outcomes
- Patient demonstrates understanding of self-care activities.
- Patient performs skin care routine.
- Patient regains skin integrity.
- Incision heals without infection.
- Patient expresses feelings about possible change in body image.

Interventions and rationales
- Inspect incision every shift following REEDA (redness, edema, ecchymosis, discharge, and approximation) method. Document findings. *Frequent assessment can detect signs and symptoms of possible infection.*
- Perform prescribed treatment regimen. Monitor progress and report favorable and adverse responses. *Periodic cleaning decreases bacterial concentrations, thus aiding the healing process. Monitoring response to treatment can help identify possible need for alternative interventions.*
- Instruct and assist patient with general hygiene, including hand washing and toileting practices. *Proper hand washing is the most effective method of disease prevention. Bacteria from hands can easily contaminate other areas.*
- Instruct and assist patient in use of sitz baths (three to four times daily) and perineal irrigation bottle (after each elimination). *Sitz baths aid the healing process by increasing circulation to the perineum and decreasing edema. Perineal irrigation bottles maintain cleanliness, thus decreasing bacterial concentration.*
- Teach patient how to apply and remove maternity perineal pad. Tell her to apply a clean pad from front to back and to remove a soiled sanitary pad from back to front *to decrease risk of contaminating the vaginal area with stool.*
- Maintain infection control standards *to help minimize the risk of nosocomial infections.*
- Provide splinting pillow for patient with abdominal incision. *Splinting*

provides support to the area, minimizing discomfort and encouraging patient to move and cough.
- Help patient assume a comfortable position *to minimize incidence of pain-induced immobility.*
- Inform patient of purpose of self-care practices *to increase compliance.*
- Encourage patient and partner to discuss impact of altered skin integrity. The patient's self-esteem may be lowered because of scar from abdominal incision. The patient or partner may be concerned about effect episiotomy will have on sexual relations. *Open communication increases understanding between partners.*
- Instruct patient and partner in possible danger signs and symptoms that should be reported to doctor immediately. These include:
  - temperature above 100.4° F (38° C) on two consecutive readings
  - incisional drainage
  - increased discomfort at episiotomy or incision site
  - reddened or warm skin surrounding episiotomy or incision site.

Prompt reporting of danger signs and symptoms may help prevent major complications.

Evaluations for expected outcomes
- Patient demonstrates correct self-care practices.
- Redness, edema, ecchymosis, and discharge do not occur at incision site. Edges are approximated.
- Patient identifies possible danger signs and reports them immediately to doctor.
- Patient and partner communicate feelings about possibly altered body image or sexuality.

Documentation
- Patient's concerns about change in skin integrity
- Patient's willingness and ability to perform self-care practices
- Observations of incision site and response to treatment regimen
- Presence and type of skin closure method
- Instructions regarding treatment regimen and patient's understanding of instructions
- Prescribed treatment
- Interventions to provide supportive care
- Patient's response to nursing interventions
- Self-care practices performed by patient
- Evaluations for each expected outcome.

Thermoregulation, ineffective

related to immaturity

Definition
Fluctuations in body temperature caused by thermoregulatory disturbances in neonate

Assessment
- Gestational age
- Weight in relation to gestational age
- Neurologic status, including level of consciousness, motor status, sensory status
- Cardiovascular status, including blood pressure, capillary refill time, electrocardiogram, heart rate and rhythm, pulses (apical and peripheral), temperature
- Respiratory status, including arterial blood gas measurements; breath

sounds; rate, depth, and character of respirations
- Integumentary status, including color, temperature, turgor
- Fluid and electrolyte status, including blood urea nitrogen levels, intake and output, serum electrolyte levels, urine specific gravity
- Laboratory studies, including clotting factors, hemoglobin and hematocrit, platelet count, white blood cell count
- Environmental factors that contribute to heat loss, including radiation (loss of heat to objects not in direct contact with neonate), conduction (loss of heat through direct contact with cooler objects), convection (loss of heat from body surface to cooler surrounding air), evaporation (changing of a liquid to a vapor)
- Coexisting conditions and diagnoses
- Maternal sedation before delivery

Defining characteristics
- Fluctuations in body temperature above or below the normal range
- Flushed or mottled skin
- Increased or decreased respiratory and heart rate
- Mild to severe dehydration
- Neonate large or small in relation to gestational age
- Seizures or convulsions
- Skin warm or cool to touch

Associated medical diagnoses (selected)
Apnea, congenital heart disease, intrauterine growth retardation, intraventricular hemorrhage, neonatal sepsis, postmaturity, prematurity, respiratory distress syndrome (hyaline membrane disease)

Expected outcomes
- Neonate maintains body temperature at normothermic levels.
- Neonate has warm, dry skin.
- Neonate maintains heart rate, respiratory rate, and blood pressure within normal range.
- Neonate does not exhibit signs of compromised neurologic status.
- Staff and parents or family members recognize and avoid possible sources of heat loss.
- Family members express an understanding of neonate's thermoregulatory disturbance and the principles of thermoregulation.

Interventions and rationales
- Monitor neonate's body temperature on admission to hospital *to obtain a baseline.* According to hospital protocol, continue routine monitoring of neonate's body temperature until discharge *to determine need for intervention and effectiveness of therapy. Timely intervention is necessary to prevent complications related to prolonged cold stress.*
- Monitor and record heart rate, respiratory rate, and blood pressure on admission and routinely thereafter until discharge *to help ensure prompt diagnosis and treatment of conditions that may affect thermoregulation.*
- Monitor results of laboratory studies for indications of sepsis or of metabolic or respiratory disorders. *Difficulty maintaining normal body temperature may indicate an underlying disorder. Conditions resulting from cold stress may further interfere with effective thermoregulation. For example, hypoxia, central nervous system trauma, or hypoglycemia may impair neonate's ability to maintain normal body temperature.*
- Place neonate under radiant warmer device, with temperature probe, on admission. When temperature is stable, transfer healthy neonate to regular open crib. Transfer sick neonate to servo-controlled open warmer bed

or incubator. *These measures will help minimize oxygen consumption and metabolic rate, will cause sweat gland activity to cease, and will maintain deep body temperature at an appropriate level.*

- Closely monitor neonate's temperature and compare with temperature of warming device. Be aware of potential hazards:
  - Make sure temperature probe does not become detached from neonate's skin *to prevent hyperthermia. Overheating increases metabolic rate and, subsequently, oxygen consumption and may lead to apneic spells, particularly in a premature neonate.*
  - Do not place temperature probe between neonate and mattress. *This can result in a falsely high reading, causing the warming device to decrease heat output, thus leading to hypothermia.*
  - Maintain accurate record of environmental and core temperatures. Observe for variations in heater output. *Consistent variations in heater output may be symptomatic of sepsis.*
  - Monitor neonate for signs of dehydration, including inelastic skin turgor, increased urine specific gravity, and dry mucous membranes. *Warming devices may contribute to insensible water loss.*
- Provide fluids based on neonate's age, size, and condition. Monitor intake and output, and administer parenteral fluids as ordered. *An increase in fluids may be needed to compensate for water loss caused by an increase in metabolic rate.*
- Maintain environmental temperature at a comfortable setting.
  - Dry neonate thoroughly after delivery.
  - Provide bath only when neonate's temperature is stable. After bath, return neonate to incubator or warmer device until temperature returns to normal range.
  - Monitor nursery temperature and humidity.
  - Provide heated, nebulized oxygen when ordered.
  - Use an overhead warmer during procedures and extensive examinations.
  - Keep incubator or radiant warmer away from windows and cold walls.
  - Ensure that linen and clothing are clean and dry.
  - Warm hands before examinations and procedures.
  - Warm examination table and instruments, such as scales and stethoscope, when possible, before exposure to neonate.

Maintaining temperature of external environment reduces effects of heat loss from body surface to environment.

- Instruct family members regarding:
  - signs and symptoms of altered body temperature, such as cool extremities
  - factors in the home that contribute to neonatal heat loss and ways to minimize heat loss
  - signs of prolonged heat loss, including poor weight gain
  - the importance of contacting the health care provider when problems related to temperature regulation arise.

Careful teaching allows family members to take active role in maintaining neonate's health.

Evaluations for expected outcomes

- Neonate's temperature is stable at 96.8° to 98.6° F (36° to 37° C) within 4 hours of birth.
- Neonate is kept in neutral thermal environment throughout hospitalization.
- Potential for heat loss in home environment is minimized or eliminated.
- Mother, other family member, or caregiver incorporates precautions against ineffective thermoregulation into routine care of neonate.

Documentation

- Physical findings
- Intake and output
- Laboratory results
- Vital signs, including blood pressure
- Environmental temperature
- Teaching provided to mother or other family member regarding thermoregulation
- Mother's or other family member's expressions indicating understanding of problems related to thermoregulation
- Nursing interventions
- Neonate's response to interventions
- Evaluations for each expected outcome.

Urinary elimination pattern alteration

related to sensory impairment during labor

Definition

Alteration or impairment in urinary function

Assessment

- Vital signs
- History of sensory or neuromuscular impairment, urinary tract trauma, surgery, or infection
- Genitourinary status, including palpation of the bladder, voiding pattern, urine characteristics, presence of pain or discomfort
- Labor and delivery, including anesthesia (regional, local), oxytocin induction or augmentation
- Fluid and electrolyte status, including skin turgor, intake and output, urine specific gravity, inspection of mucous membranes
- Neuromuscular status, including ability to perceive bladder fullness

Defining characteristics

- Bladder distention
- Clinical evidence of neuromuscular or sensory impairment
- Hesitancy
- Retention
- Urgency

Associated medical diagnoses (selected)

Hemorrhage, severe intrapartal pregnancy-induced hypertension, episiotomy, vaginal laceration

Expected outcomes

- Patient empties bladder regularly, as confirmed by abdominal palpation.
- Patient's intake and output remain roughly equivalent.
- Urinary function remains normal and free of complications.

Interventions and rationales

- Review patient's intake and output before and during labor. Note amount of urine, color, concentration, and specific gravity. *Decreased output may indicate dehydration, hemorrhage, pregnancy-induced hypertension, and excessive oxytocin stimulation. Specific gravity reflects the kidneys' ability to concentrate urine and the patient's hydration status.*

• Assess for dehydration (poor skin turgor; flushed, dry skin; confusion; dry mucous membranes; fever; and rapid, thready pulse). *Dehydration leads to decreased circulatory blood volume and decreased urine output.*
• Palpate the abdomen above the symphysis pubis every 2 hours *to detect bladder distention and degree of fullness.*
• Encourage patient to void every 2 hours *to promote optimum bladder tone, prevent distention, and assist in promoting fetal descent.*
• To facilitate voiding, help patient to relax by:
 – having her sit in an upright position. Assist her to the bathroom, if appropriate. *An upright or squatting position promotes contraction of the pelvis and intra-abdominal muscles, thereby assisting in sphincter control and bladder contraction.*
 – providing privacy *to promote relaxation.*
 – pouring warm water over the perineum *to stimulate the urge to void.*
 – providing audible sound of slow running water. *This technique helps many patients void through the power of suggestion.*
• As ordered, catheterize patient if she cannot void independently. *An overdistended bladder can cause atony and impede fetal descent or can become traumatized by the presenting part of the fetus during delivery.*

Evaluations for expected outcomes
• Patient's vital signs remain within normal range.
• Patient's urinary function remains normal and free of complications.
• Patient does not exhibit signs or symptoms of dehydration.
• Patient empties her bladder adequately at least every 2 hours.

Documentation
• Intake and output
• Vital signs
• Results of bladder assessment
• Nursing interventions performed to promote voiding
• Patient's response to nursing interventions
• Evaluations for each expected outcome.

PART FIVE

GERIATRIC HEALTH

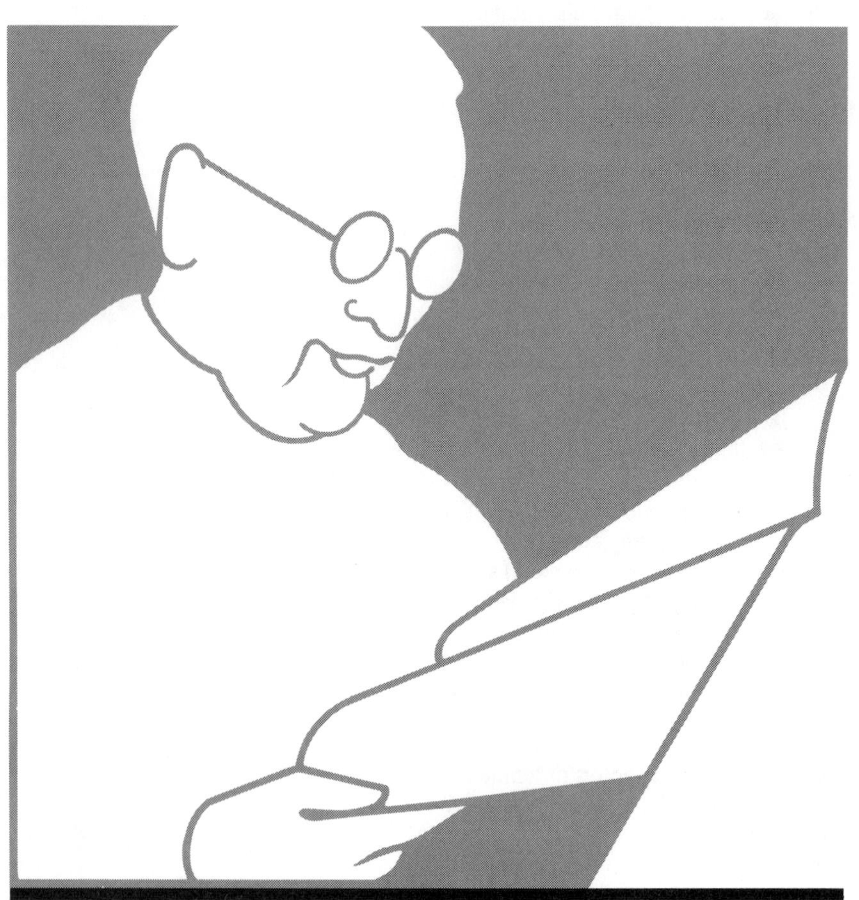

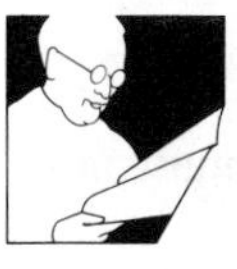

INTRODUCTION

This section focuses on nursing diagnoses and plans of care for patients age 65 and older—an age-group that already makes up approximately 12.8% of the North American population and that is growing twice as fast as younger age-groups.

Traditionally, our culture has valued youth over old age. In keeping with this cultural prejudice, our health care system emphasizes cure over care, acute intervention over long-term rehabilitation, and highly specialized technology over nurturing and support. Not surprisingly, such a system frequently fails to adequately meet the needs of elderly patients. With the elderly population growing so rapidly, nurses and other health care providers are challenged to find new and better approaches to geriatric care. Nursing diagnoses and associated plans of care offer an important alternative framework for meeting the needs of elderly patients.

Holistic geriatric care involves not only helping the patient cope with the effects of aging and chronic illness but also supporting his efforts to maintain self-reliance and autonomy. Your assessment should therefore take into account the patient's psychosocial functioning as well as physiologic status. Don't neglect to consider such factors as the amount and quality of contact with family and friends, the opportunity to perform meaningful life roles, access to transportation, and available financial resources. Such factors can have a tremendous influence on the older patient's well-being.

Because older people now lead longer and more productive lives, geriatric care is increasingly focused on health promotion. Your interventions may include encouraging the patient to make life-style changes, such as seeking and maintaining social support, moving to a more healthful environment, or exercising and eating properly. If the patient becomes ill, your task may be to help restore optimal functioning. If recovery is unlikely, your task may be to help the patient adjust to his condition and make sure he receives necessary assistance.

Keep in mind always that interventions must be tailored to the individual patient's needs. Although aging is common to all, each person ages differently. Factors that influence aging include genetics, culture, nutrition, environment, stress, and life-style, among others. Modifying your plan of care to meet the patient's individual needs not only leads to better nursing practice but also demonstrates respect for the patient's rich life experiences.

■ Activity intolerance

related to functional changes accompanying the aging process

Definition

Insufficient physiologic or psychological energy to endure or complete required or desired daily activities.

Assessment

- Usual activity level, including self-care (dressing self, feeding self, toileting), transfer, walking, stair climbing, aids for ambulation
- Pain
- Cardiovascular status, including blood pressure, heart rate and rhythm (at rest and with activity), skin temperature and color, edema, chest pain or discomfort
- Respiratory status, including arterial blood gases; auscultation of breath sounds; rate, rhythm, depth and pattern of respiration at rest and with activity
- Musculoskeletal status, including range of motion, muscle size, strength, tone, and functional mobility as follows:
  - 0 = Completely independent
  - 1 = Requires use of equipment or device
  - 2 = Requires help, supervision, or teaching from another person
  - 3 = Requires help from another person and equipment or device
  - 4 = Dependent, does not participate in activity
- Laboratory studies, including complete blood count
- Environmental factors, including safety hazards
- History of chronic illnesses (cardiopulmonary, cardiovascular, musculoskeletal, neuromuscular)
- Sensory deficits, including hearing, vision, tactile
- Psychosocial status, including cognitive and mental status, mood, affect, behavior, family support, coping style
- Economic status
- Medication history, including prescribed and over-the-counter medications

Defining characteristics

- Cognitive impairment
- Decreased mobility, caused by chronic illness, contractures or stiffness of muscles or joints, pain on movement, or an unsafe environment
- Depression
- Feelings of isolation
- Inability to manage one or more activities of daily living, such as shopping, housekeeping, laundry, and cooking
- Inability to perform one or more self-care activities

Associated medical diagnoses (selected)

Advanced cardiopulmonary illness, advanced dementia, cataracts, chronic obstructive pulmonary disease, glaucoma, macular degeneration, osteoarthritis, parkinsonism, rheumatoid arthritis

Expected outcomes

- Patient's pulse, respirations, and blood pressure remain within established parameters.
- Patient uses assistive devices to carry out activities.

- Patient modifies activities to adjust to decreased activity tolerance.
- Patient seeks help in performing activities of daily living as needed.
- Patient demonstrates willingness to perform activities needed to follow prescribed plan of care.
- Patient verbalizes acceptance of decreased activity level.
- Patient experiences less discomfort when ambulating, transferring, or performing other activities.
- Patient states plan to use support services.

Interventions and rationales

- Establish realistic goals for improving patient's activity level, taking into account patient's physical limitations and energy level, *to help improve patient's quality of life. Keep in mind that, in some older patients with chronic conditions, even minimal improvements in activity level are noteworthy.*
- Demonstrate use of assistive devices, such as cane or walker, shopping cart on wheels, or trapeze, *to teach methods of conserving energy and maintaining independence.*
- Establish progressive goals to increase ambulation, for example:
  - Ambulate 20′ (6 m) three times a day for 1 week.
  - Ambulate 40′ (12 m) three times a day for 1 week.
  - Ambulate 60′ (18 m) three times a day for 1 week.

Older patients may fatigue easily; therefore, activity level should be increased gradually. Monitor vital signs before and after ambulation *to detect cardiovascular insufficiency.*

- Provide encouragement if patient achieves even small improvements in activity level, *to help restore self-confidence.*
- Coordinate the activities of the interdisciplinary team when developing an activity regimen for patient. For example, the doctor can prescribe treatment for the medical condition, the physical therapist can design an exercise program, the dietitian can design a nutrition plan, and the social worker can locate community resources, such as Meals on Wheels or home health services, *to address patient's physical and psychosocial needs.*
- Refer depressed patient to mental health practitioner *to address psychosocial problems that may be causing impairment in activity.*
- Encourage patient to express feelings about decreased energy levels that may accompany advanced age *to enhance acceptance.*
- Teach patient about good nutrition and the importance of getting adequate rest *to improve poor health practices.*
- Monitor patient's medication regimen on a regular basis *to identify drugs that may cause gait, posture, or ambulatory problems.*
- Assist patient in identifying activities that are personally meaningful and developing a realistic plan to incorporate meaningful activities into daily routine *to heighten satisfaction with energy expenditure.*
- Encourage patient to become involved in exercise and social activities as tolerated *to increase stamina and decrease social isolation.*
- Modify environment *to maximize independent activity.* For example, place bed on first floor of home with easy access to bathroom and instruct patient to obtain and use energy-sav-

ing devices, such as elevated toilet seat, trapeze bar on bed, and chair with arms and seat that raises patient to standing position, *to promote independence.*
• Perform periodic health assessments and monitor for complaints of weakness or fatigue *to assess whether acute illness or exacerbation of chronic condition is causing activity intolerance.*
• Refer to home health agency for follow-up care. Discuss impact of incorporating help from attendants or use of assistive devices on self-esteem. Encourage patient to interview and select home health personnel *to maintain a sense of independence.*

Evaluations for expected outcomes
• Patient's pulse, respirations, and blood pressure are within established parameters.
• Patient uses assistive devices to carry out activities.
• Patient demonstrates necessary skills for modifying activity level to adjust to activity intolerance.
• Patient requests help to complete activities of daily living when necessary.
• Patient demonstrates willingness to perform activities needed to follow plan of care, including maintaining a balanced diet, getting adequate rest, and participating in a modified exercise program.
• Patient's verbal statements indicate that he is learning to accept decreased energy level and to come to terms with the fact that he may not regain former level of activity.
• Patient reports experiencing less discomfort and pain when ambulating, transferring, and performing activities of daily living.
• Patient states that acceptance of support services will not damage self-esteem or alter independent living efforts.

Documentation
• Observations of patient's activity level, both deficits and improvements
• Patient's compliance with treatment regimen and response to multidisciplinary approach
• Teaching provided to patient and family members and their responses
• Modification of home or institutional environment to ease patient's activity level
• Evaluations for each expected outcome.

■ Body image disturbance

related to negative self-image

Definition
Disruption in self-perception that results from normal physical changes associated with aging

Assessment
• Sensory acuity, including vision, hearing
• Skin changes, including discoloration (for example, aging spots); thinning; sagging; dryness associated with diminished sebaceous gland production; wrinkling associated with diminished underlying connective structures
• Hair, including thinning, loss of color
• Musculature, including diminished muscle mass, alterations in body shape, sagging skin
• Mental status, including denial, depression, discouragement, fear, grief

Defining characteristics

- Excessive or inappropriate use of cosmetics to cover signs of aging
- Excessive or inappropriate use of hair-coloring products
- Frequent, disparaging remarks concerning aging and its physical manifestations
- Hypersensitivity to remarks about advancing age
- Inappropriate dress in light of safety and comfort needs
- Indulgence in dangerous physical activities with the intent of demonstrating youthful capabilities
- Personal rigidity or unwillingness to change
- Reluctance or refusal to wear corrective lenses
- Reluctance or refusal to wear hearing aids
- Use of cosmetic surgery to reverse signs of aging
- Unwillingness to admit to physical changes associated with aging
- Unwillingness or inability to view aging in a positive light

Associated medical diagnoses (selected)

Cataract, depression, hearing and visual deficits, impotence, osteoarthritis, osteoporosis, psoriasis, rheumatoid arthritis, sexual dysfunction

Expected outcomes

- Patient alters skin care routine to reflect age-related changes.
- Patient identifies physical changes caused by aging in a nondisparaging manner.
- Patient identifies at least one positive aspect of aging.
- Patient uses visual and auditory aids appropriately.
- Patient dresses appropriately with regard to safety, comfort, and personal taste.
- Patient cleans and styles hair appropriately, without excessive coloring.
- Patient uses makeup apppropriately.
- Patient demonstrates increased flexibility and willingness to consider life-style changes.
- Patient exercises and engages in other physical activity at a level consistent with desire, ability, and safety.

Interventions and rationales

- Encourage patient to express feelings about physical changes associated with aging. *Active listening conveys a caring and accepting attitude.*
- Provide information on appropriate self-care activities:
  - maintaining proper diet
  - bathing less frequently
  - using skin lotions to combat dryness
  - exercising appropriately to maintain muscle mass, bone strength, and cardiorespiratory health
  - avoiding fractures related to osteoporosis.

Providing accurate self-care information helps patient establish realistic goals.

- Encourage patient to consider new grooming styles or to seek advice from barber or cosmetologist on "updating" hair and makeup styles. *Attractive, tasteful grooming may help the older patient achieve a sense of control over the aging process.*
- Provide patient with referrals for corrective lenses and auditory aids *to address sensory deficits.*
- Provide patient with positive role models. For example, offer to share literature that emphasizes the accomplishments, capabilities, and contributions of older adults *to promote formation of positive self-image and a*

more positive view of the elderly population.
• During conversations with the patient, focus on patient's strengths and what the patient can do; emphasize positive aspects of aging *to increase patient's self-esteem.*
• Encourage patient to engage in social activities with people from all age-groups *to foster opportunities for increased human interaction, positive feedback, and development of new interests.*

Evaluations for expected outcomes
• Patient's skin appears clean and well cared for; cosmetics are used appropriately.
• Patient identifies an age-related physical change and comments on it positively.
• Patient identifies at least one personal advantage to growing older.
• Patient identifies one aspect of his life or his personality that is better than it was 10 years ago.
• Patient uses visual and auditory aids comfortably.
• Patient dresses appropriately.
• Patient's hair appears clean and well groomed.
• Patient participates in at least one social activity or group regularly.
• Patient makes a positive statement about a new interest, idea, or activity.
• Patient makes a positive statement about another older adult.
• Patient identifies at least one thing that he does well.
• Patient engages in regular, appropriate exercise activity.

Documentation
• Patient's statements about appearance, ability, and age
• Mental status assessment (baseline and ongoing)
• Physical assessment
• Interventions directed toward improving the patient's body image
• Patient's response to nursing interventions
• Evaluations for each expected outcome.

■ Body temperature alteration, high risk for

related to decreased sensitivity of thermoreceptors

Definition
State of being at risk for failure to maintain body temperature within normal range

Assessment
• Age
• History of present illness
• Medical history, especially endocrine or nervous system illness
• Environmental temperature
• Medication history
• Neurologic status, including level of consciousness, sensory status, motor status, mental status, knowledge level
• Cardiovascular status, including heart rate and rhythm, blood pressure, pulses, capillary refill time, electrocardiogram
• Respiratory status, including breath sounds; arterial blood gases; respiratory, rate, depth, and character
• Integumentary status, including temperature, color, turgor
• GI status, including evidence of enema or laxative abuse, inspection of abdomen, auscultation of bowel sounds
• Support systems, including family, friends, volunteer organizations, clergy

Risk factors
- Advanced age
- Altered metabolic rate
- Dehydration
- Exposure to various environmental temperatures
- Inactivity
- Inappropriate clothing for temperature
- Obesity or underweight
- Sedation
- Vasoconstrictor or vasodilator drug therapy
- Vigorous activity

Associated medical diagnoses (selected)
Thermoreceptors in the elderly patient may be impaired by any disease, injury, or degenerative change.

Expected outcomes
- Body temperature remains normal.
- Skin remains warm and dry.
- Patient states feelings of comfort.
- Patient does not exhibit signs of hypothermia or hyperthermia.
- Patient or family member identifies warning signs of hypothermia and hyperthermia.
- Patient or family member expresses understanding of factors that cause hypothermia and hyperthermia.
- Patient or family member describes ways to prevent altered body temperature.

Interventions and rationales
- Monitor patient's body temperature every 8 hours or more frequently, as indicated, *to ensure temperature doesn't vary more than 1° F from average normal (98.6° F [37° C] oral)*. If it does, monitor more frequently.
- Assess patient's knowledge and lifestyle before teaching about hypothermia and hyperthermia *to gear teaching plan to patient's needs.*
- Using large black type, provide patient with a list of signs and symptoms of altered body temperature.
  - Hypothermia: shallow respirations; slow, weak pulse; low blood pressure; and pallor
  - Hyperthermia: shivering, shaking chill; feeling hot; thirst; elevated temperature; and high blood pressure

Listing signs and symptoms helps patient to learn and identify warning signals of altered body temperature. Using large black type makes it easier for older patient to read information.
- Encourage patient to remain active when in cool environment *to keep warm and maintain normal metabolism.*
- Explain to patient or family member why warm clothing is needed in cool climates, even indoors. Suggest socks, nonslip house shoes, and leg warmers *to provide warmth to vulnerable lower extremities, where vascular changes may cause decreased temperature sensation.*
- Instruct patient or family member to label home thermostats with large numbers using black or bright contrasting colors to indicate appropriate temperature settings. *Easy-to-read labels will help patient maintain room temperature.*
- Teach patient or family member about the dangers of too much direct sunlight on warm days *to prevent overheating in older patient with faulty thermoreceptors.*
- Discuss appropriate clothing for warm and cool climates. Suggest wearing clothes in layers, which can be removed or added as needed, *to accommodate increased susceptibility to temperature variations caused by aging vasculature.*

• Suggest that a friend, family member, or volunteer from a local community organization visit the patient on a daily basis *to help ensure patient's safety.*

Evaluations for expected outcomes

• Patient's body temperature remains within normal limits.
• Patient's skin remains warm and dry.
• Patient reports absence of pain.
• Patient does not exhibit or report signs or symptoms of hypothermia or hyperthermia.
• Patient or family member correctly identifies factors that may cause hypothermia or hyperthermia.
• Patient or family member describes changes to life-style that will prevent recurrence of altered body temperature.

Documentation

• Patient's or family member's perception of the problem, including reports of excessive cold or heat
• Patient's temperature
• Observations of risk factors for altered body temperature
• Instructions regarding preventive measures
• Patient's or family member's understanding of instructions
• Evaluations for each expected outcome.

Cardiac output, decreased

related to reduced myocardial perfusion

Definition

Cardiovascular or respiratory symptoms resulting from insufficient blood being pumped by the heart

Assessment

• Mental status, especially sudden mental deterioration accompanied by confusion, agitation, restlessness
• Cardiovascular status, including history of arrhythmias and syncope; skin color, temperature, and turgor; jugular vein distention; hepatojugular reflux; heart rate and rhythm; heart sounds; blood pressure; peripheral pulses; electrocardiogram (ECG); echocardiogram; phonocardiogram; serum digitalis level; aspartate aminotransferase (formerly SGOT), lactate dehydrogenase, and creatine phosphokinase isoenzyme levels
• Respiratory status, including respiratory rate and depth, breath sounds, chest X-ray, arterial blood gases
• Renal status, including weight, intake and output, urine specific gravity, serum electrolyte levels

Defining characteristics

• Abnormal cardiac enzyme levels
• Arrhythmias, ECG changes
• Cold, clammy skin
• Confusion
• Cyanosis
• Decreased blood pressure
• Decreased peripheral pulses
• Dizziness
• Dyspnea
• Enlarged liver
• Fatigue and weakness
• Irregular pulse
• Jugular vein distention
• Light-headedness
• Nausea, vomiting
• Orthopnea
• Pallor of skin and nails
• Paroxysmal nocturnal dyspnea
• Restlessness, anxiety
• Retrosternal pain
• Shortness of breath
• Syncope
• Tachypnea, palpitations

Associated medical diagnoses (selected)
Adams-Stokes syndrome, advanced liver disease, anemia, arrhythmias, carotid sinus syndrome, chronic heart block, congestive heart failure, cor pulmonale, diabetes mellitus, digitalis toxicity, hypertension, hyperthyroidism, myocardial infarction (MI), rheumatic heart disease, sick sinus syndrome, syncope

Expected outcomes

- Patient does not experience tachypnea, restlessness, anxiety, dyspnea, confusion, fainting, dizzy spells, light-headedness, nausea, fatigue, or weakness.
- Patient tolerates exercise and activities at usual level, taking into account any cardiac damage.
- Patient maintains respiratory status within established parameters.
- Patient's cardiac status stabilizes, with no evidence of arrhythmias.

Interventions and rationales

- Administer medications as ordered, monitor intake and output, and observe for adverse reactions. *In older patients, decreased renal and liver function may lead to rapid development of toxicity.*
- Monitor for dyspnea or breathlessness every 2 to 4 hours, and report changes from baseline. *Older patients with silent or painless MI frequently develop dyspnea related to left ventricular failure.*
- Monitor mental status every 2 to 4 hours and report deviations from baseline. *Dizziness, confusion, light-headedness, and restlessness may indicate decreased cerebral blood flow caused by a slow carotid sinus reflex.*
- Administer diuretics cautiously to patient. Monitor closely for cardiac overload by taking frequent vital signs and documenting intake and output accurately. Report symptoms of cardiac overload, such as elevated central venous pressure, fluid intake above output, and increased pulmonary artery pressure. *When fluid in lungs and lower extremities is mobilized and returns to the circulation, it may overtax the patient's weakened myocardium.*
- Assess apical and radial pulses every 2 to 4 hours, and report deviations from baseline, *to monitor for arrhythmias, impending cardiac arrest, hypertension, or shock.*
- Administer oxygen to patient as ordered, especially after patient eats or during heightened activity, *to increase oxygenation of the brain and heart.*
- Make sure patient gets adequate rest and does not exceed activity tolerance level *to ease dyspnea, decrease oxygen demand on the myocardium, and prevent hydrostatic pneumonia, venous thrombosis, and cardiovascular deconditioning.*
- Teach patient or family member signs and symptoms of possible cardiac problems:
  - dizziness
  - indigestion
  - nausea
  - retrosternal pain
  - dyspnea or shortness of breath
  - unusual fatigue and weakness.

Knowledge of signs and symptoms of decreased cardiac functioning helps patient to feel greater control of situation and encourages compliance with treatment plan.

- Reduce stressful elements, such as excessive noise or light, from patient's environment *to help decrease arrhythmias, anxiety, and restlessness.*
- Encourage patient to increase fluid intake and dietary fiber and to take natural stool softeners *to avoid Val-*

salva's maneuver during defecation, which can increase heart rate and blood pressure, cause reflex bradycardia, and decrease cardiac output.

Evaluations for expected outcomes

- Patient experiences fewer dyspneic episodes, with no syncope or dizzy spells.
- Physical examination reveals that arrhythmias are absent.
- Patient returns to normal activity and exercise levels (taking into account extent of cardiac damage).
- Patient and family member understand and comply with prescribed therapeutic regimen.

Documentation

- Patient's chief complaint
- Signs or symptoms of decreased cardiac output
- Therapeutic interventions and patient's responses
- Activity and exercise tolerance
- Diet and sleep patterns
- Teaching provided to patient and family member
- Evaluations for each expected outcome.

Constipation

related to diet, fluid intake, activity level, and personal bowel habits

Definition

Change in normal bowel habits characterized by decrease in frequency and passage of dry, hard stool

Assessment

- History of bowel disorder or surgery
- GI status, including nausea and vomiting, usual bowel habits, tenesmus, distention, flatulence, laxative or enema use, medications
- Oral status, including inspection of oral cavity (gums, tongue, and dentition), pain or discomfort, salivation
- Activity status, including type, duration, and frequency of exercise; life-style; access to toilet facilities during work and recreation
- Nutritional status, including appetite, dietary intake, amount and type of dietary fiber, fluid intake, food likes and dislikes, meal pattern, access to food supply and storage facilities, access to shopping and transportation, financial resources available for food
- Drug history, including use of constipating agents, such as aluminum-based antacids, anticholinergics, antidepressants, iron supplements, laxatives, narcotics; history of laxative abuse

Defining characteristics

- Abdominal mass
- Decreased amount of stool
- Decreased appetite
- Immobility
- Lack of response to urge to defecate
- Less than usual bowel frequency
- Rectal fullness or pressure
- Straining at stool
- Sedentary life-style

Associated medical diagnoses (selected)

Anxiety, atonic colon, cerebrovascular accident, dehydration, depression, diabetes mellitus, diverticulitis, GI tumors, hemorrhoids, hypokalemia, hypothyroidism, irritable bowel syndrome, multiple polyposis

Expected outcomes

- Patient participates in development of bowel program.
- Patient reports urge to defecate, as appropriate.

- Patient increases fluid and fiber intake.
- Patient reports easy and complete evacuation of stool.
- Patient increases activity level.
- Patient's elimination pattern is within normal limits.
- Patient describes changes in personal habits that will help maintain normal elimination.

Interventions and rationales

- Monitor frequency and characteristics of patient's stool. *Careful monitoring forms the basis of an effective treatment plan.*
- Monitor and record patient's fluid intake and output. *Inadequate fluid intake contributes to dry feces and constipation. Monitoring fluid balance ensures adequate fluid intake and promotes elimination.*
- Provide privacy for elimination *to promote physiologic functioning.*
- Encourage patient to use bedside commode or walk to toilet facilities. Avoid use of bedpan. *Using a bedpan may inhibit normal positioning for evacuation, thereby exacerbating constipation.*
- Work with patient in planning and implementing an individualized bowel regimen *to establish regular elimination schedule.*
- Emphasize to patient the importance of responding to the urge to defecate. Be alert for any mental status changes that may impair patient's ability to recognize or attend to the need to defecate or to report the need to a caregiver. *Timely response to the urge to defecate is necessary to maintain normal physiologic functioning and to avoid pressure and discomfort in lower GI tract.*
- Teach patient to locate public restrooms and to wear easily removable clothing on outings *to promote normal bowel functioning.*
- Teach patient to massage his abdomen once a day. Show him how to locate and gently massage along the transverse and descending colon. *In an older patient, neural centers in lower intestinal wall may be impaired, making it more difficult for the body to evacuate feces. Massage may help stimulate peristalsis and the urge to defecate.*
- If abdominal pressure is inadequate to complete defecation, encourage patient to perform rocking motion of upper body *to aid in elimination.*
- Plan and implement exercise routine, such as walking, leg raising, abdominal muscle strengthening, and Kegel exercises. *Exercise promotes abdominal and pelvic muscle tone necessary for normal elimination.*
- Encourage intake of high-fiber foods. *Many older patients have reduced intestinal muscle tone and decreased strength in abdominal muscles, resulting in slower peristalsis, dry feces, and decreased ability to exert pressure for evacuation. High-fiber foods supply bulk for normal elimination and improve intestinal muscle tone.*
- Unless contraindicated, encourage fluid intake of 6 to 8 glasses daily *to maintain normal metabolic processes and prevent excessive reabsorption of fluid from GI contents.*
- Teach patient the sensible use of laxatives and enemas *to avoid laxative dependency. Overuse of laxatives and enemas may cause fluid and electrolyte loss and damage to intestinal mucosa.*
- Help patient understand diet modification plan. If appropriate, have patient consult with dietitian *to discourage patient from departing from prescribed diet.*

Evaluations for expected outcomes
- Patient participates in planning and implementing bowel program.
- Patient achieves routine bowel function without excessive use of laxatives, enemas, straining, or discomfort.
- Patient's diet includes daily intake of high-fiber foods and adequate fluids.
- Patient makes adaptations to life-style to ensure maintenance of bowel function, including increasing activity level.

Documentation
- Patient's expressions of concern regarding constipation, dietary changes, laxative use, and bowel pattern
- Physical findings
- Intake and output
- Observations of diet, characteristics of stool, and activity level
- Teaching provided and patient's response
- Patient's expressions indicating understanding of bowel program
- Evaluations for each expected outcome.

■ Coping, ineffective family

related to caring for dependent, aging family member

Definition
State in which a normally functioning family experiences a dysfunction

Assessment
- Patient status, including age, medical history, self-concept, physical disabilities or limitations, present living arrangements, role in family
- Family assessment, including communication style, family coping style, perceptions of the aging process (myths vs. realities), health problems of other members, financial status, available support systems, additional stressors
- Patient's current health crisis (emotional or physical)

Defining characteristics
- Anger
- Excessive involvement with patient
- Guilt
- Inadequate involvement with patient
- Incorrect knowledge regarding aging process
- Ineffective communication patterns among family members
- Lack of respect for patient
- Patient exhibits mental confusion or disorientation
- Patient is socially isolated

Associated medical diagnoses (selected)
Any condition that results in temporary or permanent dependence on family members, such as Alzheimer's disease, cancer, cerebrovascular accident, cirrhosis, depression, hip fracture, Parkinson's disease, rheumatoid arthritis

Expected outcomes
- Family members express feelings about responsibilities of caring for an older relative.
- Patient and family members express understanding of maturational and developmental issues that contributed to crisis.
- Patient and family members locate and make use of appropriate community services.
- Patient and family members demonstrate improved capacity for making decisions on health-related matters and planning care for older relative.

Interventions and rationales

- Identify primary caregiver within the family and assess the roles of other family members *to establish family hierarchy and plan interventions.*
- Educate patient and family members about aging process. Discuss how changes in patient have affected the family *to assess the needs of patient and family members.*
- Avoid becoming involved in a power struggle among family members. *The patient may no longer be able to fulfill his role within the family. The sudden shift in roles may lead to a power struggle among family members. The patient or family members may try to manipulate you as part of this power struggle. Maintaining a neutral, objective approach will help family members to adjust to role changes.*
- As appropriate, arrange and conduct a conference for family members; include patient when possible. *Long-established communication patterns may interfere with family members' ability to resolve conflicts and make decisions. Your presence may help family members to express feelings, identify needs and resources, and develop more healthy ways of interacting.*
- Encourage family members to express their feelings about caring for an older family member. *A nonjudgmental attitude promotes effective communication.*
- Encourage family members to identify strengths and weaknesses within the family system. Help them explore values, beliefs, perceived changes, and actual role changes related to older patient's altered physical or emotional condition *to enhance insight.*
- Assist patient and family members in developing short- and long-term goals and contingency plans *to provide patient and family members with a sense of control and direction for future.*
- Assist patient and family members in deciding whether to seek help and in identifying appropriate community services, such as adult day care, respite care, and geriatric outreach services, *to provide access to additional sources of support.*
- Help family members explore coping strategies used effectively during past crises and discuss how to apply these strategies to the present situation *to make family members aware of their demonstrated ability to adapt to change.*
- Provide emotional support for primary caregiver. *A family member who takes on the most responsibility for the patient has the double burden of caring for an older adult and adjusting to a new role within the family.*
- Maintain a nonjudgmental attitude while working with family members. Some families may be hesitant to accept outside help. Other families may be unwilling to make even small sacrifices to care for an older relative. Remember that, if family members have not been supportive or close to patient in the past, you are unlikely to change their attitude. *Ultimately, a nonjudgmental outlook benefits both patient and family members. Learning to accept your limitations will help to avoid burnout.*
- Remain supportive and understanding if patient or family members are reluctant to use needed community resources, such as adult day care, respite care, and home health services. *The older patient may feel that using outside resources means sacrificing independence; family members may feel that asking for help indicates a lack of caring.*

Evaluations for expected outcomes

- As appropriate, family members assume responsibilities formerly performed by patient.
- Patient and family members share feelings about current crisis.
- Patient or family members acknowledge need for outside help to cope with crisis.
- Patient or family members identify and contact community resources.
- Patient and family members demonstrate improved capacity for short- and long-term planning.
- Patient and family members express satisfaction with their improved ability to cope with the current crisis.

Documentation

- Patient's and family members' understanding of aging process and current health crisis
- Observations of patient's and family members' reactions to crisis
- Family members' willingness to become involved in patient care
- Nursing interventions performed and patient's and family members' responses
- Teaching provided and patient's and family members' responses
- Referrals to community agencies
- Evaluations for each expected outcome.

Coping, ineffective individual

related to inability to solve problems or adapt to demands of daily living

Definition

Inability to use adaptive behaviors in response to difficult life situations

Assessment

- Age
- Life-style changes necessitated by disease or illness
- Role changes caused by retirement or relocation; death of spouse, family members, or friends
- Changes associated with normal aging, such as decreased vision, hearing, and physical endurance
- Perceived coping ability
- Usual coping mechanisms
- Support systems, including family, friends, church, community organizations

Defining characteristics

- Disheveled appearance
- Disorganized behavior that may be mistaken for senility
- Frequent accidents or illness
- Heightened sense of fear and anxiety
- Hypersensitivity to normal aging changes
- Inability to meet basic needs
- Inability to meet role expectations
- Inability to solve problems
- Isolation
- Poor personal hygiene
- Verbal expressions that indicate inability to cope with present demands

Associated medical diagnoses (selected)

Alcoholism; Alzheimer's disease; amyotrophic lateral sclerosis; cancer; cataracts; cor pulmonale; depression; diabetes mellitus; end-stage renal, pulmonary, or cardiac disease; paralysis; Parkinson's disease; rheumatoid arthritis

Expected outcomes

- Patient verbalizes a sense of enhanced ability to cope.
- Patient expands support network to meet social and emotional needs.
- Patient locates and uses appropriate resources for help in problem solving.

• Patient reports increased success in meeting demands of daily living.
• Patient makes changes to environment to ensure enhanced coping or moves into a long-term care facility as needed.

Interventions and rationales

• Refer patient to social service agencies, such as geriatric assessment centers, adult day-care programs, and home health care agencies, as appropriate *to expand his support network and help him cope with physical, psychosocial, and economic stressors.*
• Assist patient in becoming involved with informal community programs, such as volunteer, foster grandparent, church, or synagogue groups. *Increased community involvement will provide peer and social contact, thereby decreasing older patient's sense of loneliness and isolation.*
• Encourage patient to reminisce about past *to help him recall past challenges and successful coping strategies.*
• Provide patient with information about the aging process, how to cope with stress, and techniques used by other older adults to meet the demands of daily living *to assist patient in implementing coping strategies.*
• If patient must enter a long-term care facility or undergo a lengthy home-based convalescence, help him put the situation in perspective. Explain to patient that extreme stress can overwhelm anyone, even well-adapted individuals with strong support systems. When stress becomes overwhelming, rehabilitation in a secure environment may be the best option. Entering a long-term care facility is not "the beginning of the end," as many people think, but rather an additional mechanism for ensuring optimal recovery. *Taking the time to provide a carefully worded explanation may help patient come to terms with his situation.*
• If treatment in a long-term care facility is required, provide the least restrictive environment possible *to reduce patient's fear and anxiety, help him retain a sense of control, and encourage him to use his abilities to the maximum.*
• Discuss with patient the possibility of making life-style changes *to improve ability to cope*—for example, moving closer to relatives, moving to a retirement community, or hiring someone to help with housework.

Evaluations for expected outcomes

• Patient states understanding of strategies to improve coping ability.
• Patient lists resources available to help with problem-solving.
• Patient reports success in developing support network to meet social and emotional needs.
• Patient reports being able to meet demands of daily living.
• Patient identifies life-style changes that will improve his ability to cope.
• Patient states that he understands and accepts need to move to a long-term care facility or retirement community.

Documentation

• Patient's expression of feelings about present life situation and difficulty coping
• Formal and informal sources of support identified by patient or family members
• Observations of patient's behavior in response to stressful situations
• Teaching provided and patient's response
• Use of outside support services
• Evaluations for each expected outcome.

Denial

related to fear or anxiety about aging

Definition

Attempt to disavow knowledge or meaning of an event to reduce fear of growing older

Assessment

- Age
- Appearance
- Activity patterns, including sudden interest or participation in activities that may be dangerous
- Self-concept, including self-esteem, body image, perception of self in the life continuum
- Coping behaviors
- Mental status, including affect, communication, memory, mood, orientation, perception, abstract thinking, judgment, insight

Defining characteristics

- Inappropriate dress that suggests misguided attempt to project youthful appearance
- Indulgence in physically hazardous activities with intent of demonstrating youthful capabilities
- Frequent negative comments about aging and the elderly
- Lying about age
- Refusal to acknowledge significance of signs and symptoms of aging or chronic illness
- Refusal to frequent places or participate in activities enjoyed by peers
- Refusal to talk about growing older

Associated medical diagnoses (selected)

This diagnosis may be associated with any disorder that causes physical disability or limitations. Examples include angina pectoris, arteriosclerosis, atherosclerosis, chronic obstructive pulmonary disease, chronic renal failure, fractured hip, hypertension, osteoporosis, presbycusis, presbyopia, renal calculi, rheumatoid arthritis.

Expected outcomes

- Patient discusses aging process and impact of aging on ability to participate in hobbies and other activities.
- Patient expresses interest in becoming involved in age-appropriate community activities.
- Patient states intention to set aside time for reminiscing as part of daily routine.
- Patient expresses a more positive view of growing older.

Interventions and rationales

- Discuss the challenge of being an older adult in today's youth-oriented society *to encourage patient to express feelings and help him recognize that he does not have to accept society's prejudices with regard to aging.*
- Discuss with patient and family members changes that normally occur as part of the aging process *to correct misconceptions.* Discuss how to adapt activities and hobbies to accommodate physiologic changes that occur with aging *to avoid excess physical stress.*
- Discuss advantages of growing older, for example, having increased time to pursue hobbies and other interests, *to help patient develop a positive view of aging.*
- Emphasize the variety of activities that the patient can continue to do well *to enhance self-esteem.*
- Encourage patient to set aside time for reminiscing as part of daily routine. *Reminiscing helps patient to affirm past and promotes self-esteem.*

- Provide information about senior volunteer groups and part-time work or volunteer opportunities *to help patient maintain physical and mental functioning and promote social interaction.*
- Invite an active member of a senior citizens club, social group, senior sports league, or advocacy group to visit patient *to provide a positive role model.*

Evaluations for expected outcomes
- Patient states intention to attend an age-appropriate community activity.
- Patient expresses positive and negative feelings about aging.
- Patient expresses willingness to set aside time for reminiscing.
- Patient adapts activities to avoid unnecessary physical stress on body.

Documentation
- Evidence of patient's difficulty adjusting to the aging process
- Nursing interventions
- Referrals provided
- Patient's response to nursing interventions
- Patient's statements, which indicate a more positive attitude toward growing older
- Evaluations for each expected outcome.

■ Gas exchange impairment

related to carbon dioxide retention or excess mucus production

Definition
Interference in cellular respiration caused by inadequate exchange or transport of oxygen and carbon dioxide

Assessment
- Age
- Sex
- Smoking history
- Occupational or environmental risk factors, such as exposure to asbestos, smog, pollutants
- Respiratory status, including history of respiratory disorders, breath sounds, sputum characteristics, accessory muscle use, cyanosis, arterial blood gas levels
- Cardiovascular status, including skin color and temperature, heart rate and rhythm, heart sounds, blood pressure, hemoglobin and hematocrit, red blood cell count, white blood cell count, platelet count, prothrombin time, partial thromboplastin time, serum iron concentrations
- Psychosocial status, including mental status, knowledge level, life-style, support systems
- Activity status, including ability to perform activities of daily living

Defining characteristics
- Confusion
- Decreased exercise tolerance
- Dyspnea
- Fatigue
- Hypercapnia
- Hypoxia
- Immobility
- Inability to mobilize secretions
- Irritability
- Somnolence

Associated medical diagnoses (selected)
Adult-onset asthma, cerebrovascular accident, chronic obstructive pulmonary disease, congestive heart failure (CHF), lung cancer, pneumonia, pulmonary embolism, tuberculosis

Expected outcomes
- Patient increases endurance and exercise tolerance.

- Patient performs activities of daily living without experiencing dyspnea or excess fatigue.
- Patient maintains adequate fluid intake.
- Patient maintains clear breath sounds.

Interventions and rationales

- Establish baseline values for respiratory assessment. *Older adults take shorter breaths. This decreases maximum breathing capacity, vital capacity, residual volume, and functional capacity. A baseline assessment helps to distinguish age-related changes that may mimic disease states.*
- Auscultate lungs every 4 hours, taking into account anatomic changes that may occur in older patients, such as kyphosis, deviated trachea, and dowager's hump, *to detect abnormal breath sounds.* Report abnormalities.
- Administer and monitor oxygen therapy, as ordered, *to enhance oxygenation and detect signs of decompensation. Older patients have a high incidence of chronic cardiac and chronic pulmonary disorders. Detecting early changes in condition allows for early intervention.*
- Teach patient relaxation techniques and ask for return demonstrations. *Using relaxation techniques may help reduce tissue oxygen demand.*
- Incorporate patient's past experiences into teaching plan when conveying information about disease, medications, and life-style changes. *Information becomes more meaningful when related to previous experiences.*
- Help patient schedule activities of daily living to allow for rest periods. *In older patients, alveoli are more fibrous and less elastic and contain fewer functional capillaries, which decreases exertional capacity. Rest periods are necessary to conserve patient's respiratory effort.*
- Help patient identify positions that maximize ventilatory capacity, such as leaning over bedside table when sitting or using large wedge pillow under shoulders. *In an older patient, accessory muscles of the pharynx and larynx atrophy, making it necessary for patient to assume breathing positions that maximize ventilation, perfusion, and thoracic expansion.*
- Encourage adequate fluid intake. *Older adults may have a diminished sense of thirst, which may lead to dry mucous membranes. Dry mucous membranes in turn may impede removal of secretions and promote respiratory infection. Consuming adequate fluids helps to liquify secretions, thereby reducing the energy required to mobilize them.* Record intake and output *to monitor fluid status.*
- Perform bronchial hygiene, such as positioning, coughing, deep breathing, percussion, postural drainage, and suctioning, *to promote and maintain patent airway.*
- Evaluate home environment and recommend changes, such as moving patient's bedroom to first floor, *to reduce need for exertion.*

Evaluations for expected outcomes

- Patient performs activities of daily living with minimum fatigue and increased endurance.
- Patient maintains adequate ventilation.
- Patient or family members state understanding of causes for impaired gas exchange and related preventive behaviors.
- Auscultation reveals clear breath sounds.

Documentation

- Patient's complaints of dyspnea or fatigue
- Observations of patient's condition
- Patient's response to nursing interventions
- Teaching provided and patient's response
- Patient's expressions indicating understanding of plan of care
- Evaluations for each expected outcome.

Grieving, anticipatory

related to perceived potential loss of life

Definition

Grief response in anticipation of perceived loss of life

Assessment

- Age
- Developmental stage
- Presence of living will, durable power of attorney for health care, other advance directives
- History of chronic illness or terminal diagnosis
- Mental status, including level of consciousness, orientation
- Emotional status, including evidence of anger, apathy, depression, hostility
- Support systems, including family members, significant other, friends, clergy
- Spiritual practices, including religious affiliation, use of spiritual support systems
- Customs and beliefs related to illness, death, suffering

Defining characteristics

- Altered communication patterns
- Anger
- Anxiety
- Difficulty in expressing loss
- Expressions of distress over potential loss of life
- Guilt
- Physical deterioration
- Sorrow
- Weight loss

Associated medical diagnoses (selected)

This diagnosis may be associated with exacerbation of any chronic or terminal illness, for example, bronchopneumonia; cancer; end-stage pulmonary, cardiac, or renal disease; influenza A.

Expected outcomes

- Patient expresses feelings about anticipated death.
- Patient progresses through the stages of the grieving process in his own way.
- Patient practices religious rituals and uses other coping mechanisms appropriate to the end of life.
- Family members or significant other participate in providing supportive care and comfort to patient.

Interventions and rationales

- Provide time for patient to express feelings about death or terminal illness. *Active listening helps patient to lessen feelings of loneliness and isolation.* Do not approach patient with a busy, hurried attitude, *which can block communication.*
- Establish a relationship that encourages patient to express concerns about death. *Basic nursing care combined with genuine interest in patient fosters trust and understanding.*
- Guide patient in life review. Encourage him to write or tape life history as a lasting gift to family members. *Life review allows patient to survey events from*

his past and give them a meaningful interpretation.

• Involve interdisciplinary team (including psychologist, nurse, patient, nutritionist, doctor, physical therapist, chaplain) in providing care for dying patient. *Each team member offers unique expertise for meeting dying patient's needs.*

• Encourage family members to become involved in care of dying patient. Communicate with patient and family members honestly and compassionately. *Giving family members a role in patient care helps to relieve anxiety and lessen feelings of regret and guilt. Honest communication is important because family members need opportunity to acknowledge loss and to say farewell.*

• Demonstrate acceptance of patient's response to anticipated death, whatever that response may be: Crying, sadness, anger, fear, or denial. *Each patient responds to dying in his own way. Helping him express his feelings freely will enhance his ability to cope.*

• Help patient progress through the psychological stages associated with anticipated death. *Dr. Elisabeth Kübler-Ross has identified five stages of grief for the patient with a terminal illness: shock and denial, anger, bargaining, depression, and acceptance. Knowing these stages will help you anticipate the dying patient's psychological needs. Keep in mind, however, that not all dying patients will go through each stage.*

• Support patient's spiritual coping behaviors. For example, arrange for patient to have at the bedside objects that provide spiritual comfort (such as Bible, prayer shawl, pictures, statues, rosary beads). *Even patients for whom religious practice has not been a dominant part of their lives frequently turn to religion when confronted by death or serious illness.*

• Inform patient about hospice services. Hospice services emphasize symptomatic relief and caring, with the aim of improving patient and family comfort until death occurs, instead of prolonging life for its own sake. *Hospice care is an appropriate alternative for a patient with an incurable illness.*

• Provide referrals for home health assistance if patient will be cared for at home *to support patient's decision to remain at home.*

Evaluations for expected outcomes

• Patient expresses feelings about anticipated death.

• Patient accepts feelings and behaviors brought about by the possibility of death.

• Patient progresses through stages of grief in his own way.

• Patient participates in religious rituals and uses other appropriate coping mechanisms.

• Patient receives adequate support during end of life from family members, friends, and members of the health care team.

Documentation

• Patient's verbal expressions indicating feelings about anticipated death.

• Observations of emotional responses, such as crying, anger, and withdrawal

• Interventions performed to help patient cope with anticipated death

• Patient's requests for assistance in achieving spiritual comfort (spiritual objects; visits from minister, priest, or rabbi)

• Patient's responses to interventions

• Evaluations for each expected outcome.

Home maintenance management impairment

related to impaired cognitive, emotional, or psychomotor functioning

Definition

Disruption in the patient's ability to meet household maintenance needs adequately

Assessment

- Age
- Sex
- Home environment
- Financial resources
- Patient's psychosocial status, including perception of reality, communication patterns, role responsibilities, degree of awareness and concern, history of psychiatric-related illness, support systems, and cognitive, memory, and motor abilities
- Caregiver's psychosocial status, including stressors, support systems, understanding of patient care requirements

Defining characteristics

- Caregiver expresses uncertainty regarding patient's competence
- Changes in patient's mental capacity
- Consistent inattention to personal and environmental needs
- Lack of sufficient material resources to meet needs
- Presence of emotional or physical difficulties that hinder the patient's ability to maintain activities of daily living within the home

Associated medical diagnoses (selected)

This diagnosis may occur in any acute or chronic alteration in the patient's health status, for example, arthritis, cancer, chronic obstructive pulmonary disease, coronary artery disease, Parkinson's disease.

Expected outcomes

- Patient and caregiver express concern about poor home maintenance.
- Patient and caregiver verbalize plans to correct identified health and safety hazards in the home.
- Patient and caregiver identify community organizations that can help ease the transition from hospital to home or long-term care facility.
- Patient and caregiver develop schedule for doing household tasks.

Interventions and rationales

- Help patient and caregiver identify strengths and weaknesses in current home maintenance practices *to provide a focus for interventions.*
- Discuss with patient and caregiver any obstacles to meeting home maintenance needs *to provide basis for program to meet health and safety requirements.*
- Determine patient's capability and motivation to achieve a higher level of home maintenance. *Self-motivation is necessary to ensure change.*
- Help patient and caregiver explore resources available in the community, such as Meals on Wheels, senior centers, home health care agencies, homemaker services, cleaning services, self-help groups, church programs, and retired senior volunteer programs, *to ease the transition from hospital to home.*
- Allow caregiver to express feelings about having responsibility for patient's health care regimen and household upkeep. When appropriate, discuss opportunities for caregiver to assign responsibility to other family members or make use of community resources. Encourage caregiver to ask questions, seek help,

and make decisions *to enhance communication and help caregiver and family members formulate realistic expectations.*

• Conduct a home visit or evaluate patient's description of home, *to assess safety needs and make recommendations for structural alterations. For example, the patient may benefit from installing ramps or enlarged doorways or moving second floor bedroom to first floor family room.*

• Discuss alternative housing opportunities with patient and caregiver, such as moving patient to life-care community, *to provide necessary information to make appropriate decisions regarding patient's future.*

• Based on assessment of patient's health and home environment, determine the need for assistive devices, including the following:
  - hearing aids
  - hand-held or table-stand magnifying glasses
  - hospital bed
  - large print items
  - telephones for the hearing-impaired
  - telephone dial covers with large numbers
  - telephones with programmed dialing
  - wheelchair
  - amplifiers for phone receivers
  - clocks that chime or recite the time
  - canes
  - walkers
  - handrails
  - safety bars for toilet and bath
  - automatic chair lifts
  - commode chairs
  - shower chairs
  - orthotics.

Using assistive devices helps patient remain independent and contributes to self-confidence and self-esteem.

• Help patient develop written daily and weekly schedules for performing household tasks *to provide structure and consistency and set standards for measuring progress.*

• Involve patient in the decision-making process by providing choice of where, when, and how to carry out appropriate home maintenance activities. *Participation in decision-making increases patient's feelings of independence and self-esteem.*

• If patient cannot perform certain tasks without assistance, educate caregiver or other appropriate personnel on how to provide help *to ensure patient's needs are met.*

Evaluations for expected outcomes

• Patient and caregiver express an understanding of the changes needed to promote maximum health and safety within the home.

• Patient and caregiver list community resources available to assist with identified home maintenance deficits.

• Patient and caregiver establish and follow daily and weekly schedules for home maintenance activities.

Documentation

• Patient's perception of problems in home maintenance

• Observations regarding the magnitude of home maintenance deficits

• Interventions performed to alleviate home maintenance deficits

• Responses of caregiver and others asked to assist patient with home maintenance

• Evaluations for each expected outcome.

Incontinence, stress (female)

Definition
Involuntary passage of urine, which occurs when intravesical pressure exceeds the maximum ureteral pressure in the absence of detrusor activity

Assessment
- History of incontinence symptoms, including onset, pattern
- Physical observations, including personal and perineal hygiene, complete bladder assessment
- Mental status, including cognition, affect
- Mobility status
- Emotional status, including evidence of social withdrawal
- Current medication regimen

Defining characteristics
- Frequent "accidents" due to inability to reach toilet in time
- Urinary frequency and urgency
- Urine odor
- Withdrawal from social activities and reluctance to leave home

Associated medical diagnoses (selected)
Alzheimer's disease, atrophic senile vaginitis, atrophic urethritis secondary to estrogen deficiency, cerebrovascular accident, cirrhosis, depression, diabetes mellitus, obesity, urethrocele, urinary tract infections, uterine prolapse

Expected outcomes
- Patient understands the causes of stress incontinence.
- Patient establishes a plan compatible with life-style to manage symptoms.
- Patient resumes normal social activities.
- Patient maintains continence with the aid of pads or frequent toileting.

Interventions and rationales
- Discuss stress incontinence and associated social stigma with patient in a nonjudgmental manner. Tell patient incontinence is a problem many people share. *The patient may be reluctant to discuss incontinence, which can have a negative effect on self-image. A nonjudgmental approach may help to ease embarrassment and encourage open discussion of the problem.*
- Assist patient in obtaining appropriate evaluation and care for underlying causes of stress incontinence *to ensure prompt diagnosis and treatment.*
- Review current medication regimen for drugs that can contribute to stress incontinence, including diuretics, CNS depressants, and anticholinergics. Discuss with doctor the possibility of changing the medications or the medication schedule *to relieve symptoms.*
- If appropriate, develop an individualized toileting schedule, increasing intervals by 30 minutes until a 2- to 3-hour pattern is achieved. *Bladder retraining may help alleviate symptoms.*
- Teach patient to do Kegel exercises to strengthen pelvic floor muscles. Instruct patient to tighten the muscles of the pelvic floor to stop the flow of urine while urinating and then to release muscles to restart the flow. *Kegel exercises may help to strengthen the urinary sphincter muscle and restore control.*
- Discuss the benefits and costs of padding with patient. *Padding, while costly, is nonintrusive, easy to manage, and easily removed.*
- Encourage patient to take short trips outside the home when her symptoms are under control *to help*

enhance patient's confidence and reduce social embarrassment associated with stress incontinence.
• When mobility is a problem, help patient obtain a bedside commode *to reduce the need for adult incontinence pads, which can adversely affect patient's self-image.*

Evaluations for expected outcomes
• Patient expresses, without embarrassment, an understanding of causes of stress incontinence.
• Patient states she is managing her symptoms successfully.
• Patient states she has begun to resume social activity.
• Patient maintains continence with the aid of pads or frequent toileting.
• Patient performs Kegel exercises.

Documentation
• Patient's symptoms of stress incontinence, including onset and pattern
• Patient teaching, including Kegel exercises, padding, and other control strategies
• Patient's responses to nursing interventions
• Evaluations for each expected outcome.

Injury, high risk for

related to elder abuse

Definition
Accentuated risk for neglect or abuse of older adult by a family member

Assessment
• Age
• Sex
• Patient's health status, including presence of acute or chronic illness, changes or deterioration in mental or physical functioning
• Family status, including communication patterns, presence or absence of extended family
• Family's willingness and ability to provide physical and emotional support to patient
• Evidence of physical abuse, including malnutrition, imprint of hand or fingers, marks from restraints, unexplained bruises, burns, welts, cuts, dislocations, or abrasions
• Evidence of emotional abuse, including observation or reports of insults, ridicule, or humiliation
• Evidence of financial abuse, including unexplained changes in bank accounts, transfer of funds to caregivers
• Evidence of neglect, including inappropriate clothing, unsanitary living conditions, inadequate food supplies, lack of medication, absence of needed eyeglasses, hearing aids, cane, or walker

Risk factors
• Caregiver expresses frustration over responsibilities of caring for older family member
• Family has limited education or inadequate financial resources
• Family is isolated from community, without relatives living nearby
• Patient is forced to be dependent on family members for daily care
• Patient reports lack of social contacts outside family
• Patient suffers from deteriorating health, frailty, or impaired mobility

Associated medical diagnoses (selected)
Alzheimer's disease, arteriosclerosis, atherosclerosis, cerebrovascular accident, chronic obstructive pulmonary disease, coronary artery disease, dementia, depression, end-stage cardiac

disease, hip fracture, hypertension, osteoarthritis, rheumatoid arthritis

Expected outcomes

- Patient remains free of injury and states that incidents of abuse no longer occur.
- Patient expresses understanding of right to be free from abuse.
- Patient reports increased social contact outside the family.
- Patient establishes a mutual "buddy system," whereby he and a friend visit or telephone each other at regularly scheduled intervals.
- Patient maintains control over mail, telephone, and other personal effects.
- Caregiver states intention to contact respite care services, support groups, and other community resources.
- Patient and caregiver report improved communication patterns.

Interventions and rationales

- Monitor patient closely at each visit for evidence of physical or mental abuse or neglect. Observe for bruises or abrasions, body odor, or dirty, unkempt appearance *to ensure his safety and well-being.* Question him privately about findings *to encourage trust and promote open communication.*
- Encourage patient to discuss incidents of abuse or threats of abuse. Be willing to listen and be careful to convey a nonjudgmental attitude. *Older patients may be reluctant to discuss abuse or threats of abuse because of fear of retaliation, embarrassment, or reluctance to report family members to authorities. By communicating that you care and are willing to listen, you may help patient overcome these barriers.*
- Educate patient regarding his right to be free from abuse. Discuss the responsibility of law enforcement agencies to investigate incidents of abuse. Provide a list of social service agencies that are available to provide counseling. *Education may help empower patient to resist or prevent episodes of abuse.*
- Encourage patient to maintain use of personal telephone and open his own mail *to promote sense of control and self-worth and maintain contact with people outside the home.*
- Encourage patient to participate in community activities, such as church groups and retired senior volunteer organizations, *to establish social contacts necessary for a strong support network.*
- Suggest use of Meals-On-Wheels or community geriatric outreach for homebound patient *to prevent isolation and provide respite for family caregiver.*
- Encourage friends to visit patient at home. Suggest that patient and friend develop a "buddy system," whereby each takes turns telephoning or visiting the other at regular intervals *to provide social contact, respite for caregiver, and an additional safeguard against abuse.*
- If appropriate, encourage patient and family members to periodically hold conferences. Help patient and family members identify productive topics for discussion, such as strategies for dealing with patient's self-care deficits or scheduling respite care, *to foster open communication, diffuse tension, and develop solutions to the practical problems of caring for an older family member.*
- Inform caregiver about state and county services for the elderly, respite services, adult day-care, support groups for children of aging parents, and other community resources *to enhance caregiver's ability to cope and thereby diminish the likelihood of abuse.*

• Report actual or suspected elder abuse to local authorities and provide follow-up or emergency care, if needed. *Nearly every state has laws mandating that suspected elder abuse be reported to the authorities.*

Evaluations for expected outcomes

• Patient does not exhibit injuries and states that incidents of abuse have stopped.
• Patient expresses understanding of right to be protected from abuse.
• Patient reports satisfaction with ability to maintain or increase social contacts outside family.
• Patient establishes "buddy system" with a friend outside the home.
• Patient maintains control over mail, telephone, and other personal effects.
• Caregiver regularly attends a community support group and contacts appropriate social service agencies and other sources of support.
• Caregiver reports increased ability to cope with responsibilities of caring for an older family member.
• Patient and caregiver report improved communication.

Documentation

• Evidence of emotional, physical, or financial neglect or abuse.
• Patient's statements, which indicate risk for abuse
• Caregiver's statements indicating feelings about caring for an older family member
• Caregiver's statements indicating willingness to attend support groups or use community resources
• Patient's and caregiver's expressions indicating understanding of teaching provided by nurse
• Patient's response to nursing interventions
• Evaluations for each expected outcome.

Knowledge deficit

related to difficulty understanding disease process and its effect on self-care

Definition

Lack of knowledge regarding any aspect of health care, including disease process, medications, treatment plan, community resources, or coping strategies

Assessment

• Current knowledge level
• Interest and motivation to learn
• Preferred learning style
• Comprehension ability, reading level
• Other factors that may affect learning, such as cultural influences; religious practices and beliefs; sensory, cognitive, or physical impairment; support systems; economic status; feelings of anger, depression, or hopelessness

Defining characteristics

• Acknowledgment (overt and subtle) of inability to comprehend the disease process, medications, or treatment
• Difficulty following instructions
• Inability to describe what actions are needed to alleviate self-care deficits
• Inability to explain basic facts about disease process, medications, or treatment
• Overreaction to disease process, medications, or treatment
• Poor understanding of how to incorporate the management of disease process into activities of daily living

Associated medical diagnoses (selected)

Alzheimer's disease, arthritis, cancer, cerebrovascular accident, chronic obstructive pulmonary disease, cirrhosis, congestive heart failure, coronary artery disease, diabetes mellitus, hypertension, Parkinson's disease

Expected outcomes

- Patient expresses understanding of disease process, medication regimen, and treatment plan.
- Patient makes informed choices when addressing health care problems and self-care deficits.
- Patient demonstrates ability to accurately implement chosen health care strategy.

Interventions and rationales

- Incorporate older patient's life experiences when developing teaching plan. *New information is easier to assimilate if it is built upon existing knowledge.*
- Provide a quiet and calm environment for learning *to enable patient to process information without being distracted by background noise or stress.*
- Limit the length of each teaching session *to avoid information overload.*
- Ask patient if he wants to learn new or additional information. If not, discuss why. *Open discussion helps to identify barriers to learning and determine if these barriers may be eliminated. Discussion also promotes acceptance of patient's right to choose his own level of participation.*
- Encourage patient to use memory aids, such as preset alarms on watch, calendar for noting scheduled appointments, and small notepad for recording questions or symptoms, *to help compensate for memory lapses.*
- Write instructions in large letters, using black ink or contrasting colors. *The older patient sees black best and may have difficulty distinguishing pastels or monotone color schemes.*
- Modify teaching style to accommodate normal aging changes:
  - Face the patient when speaking.
  - Use a well-modulated voice.
  - Allow ample time for teaching sessions.

Understanding normal age-related changes enhances teaching effectiveness.

- Set aside time during each session for answering questions and clarifying information. *The older patient may simply need affirmation that the knowledge he possesses is current and correct. Discussion may also stimulate the exchange of ideas and further learning.*
- Encourage patient to join a support group, such as a club for stroke survivors or a support group for cancer patients, *to reinforce education and promote contact with others in same situation.*
- Involve caregiver in teaching sessions when appropriate *to reinforce information and ensure continuity of care at home.*

Evaluations for expected outcomes

- Patient expresses increased understanding of disease process, treatment plan, and medications.
- Patient describes at least three basic concepts relevant to the disease process and its impact on activities of daily living.
- Patient states at least four strategies to improve self-care.
- Patient expresses understanding of how implementing chosen strategies will provide relief from the disease process and improve his ability to perform activities of daily living.
- Patient demonstrates ability to implement chosen strategies on an ongoing basis.

Documentation
- Patient's verbal statements and behavior, which indicate knowledge deficit
- Teaching provided and patient's or caregiver's response
- Questions and comments made by patient during teaching sessions
- Patient's description of chosen intervention strategies
- Patient's actual implementation of strategies, as evidenced by verbal statements and behavior
- Evaluations for each expected outcome.

Nutrition alteration: More than body requirements

related to a decline in basal metabolic rate and physical activity

Definition
Change in normal eating pattern or activity level that results in increased body weight

Assessment
- Activity level
- Health history, including evidence of impaired mobility, chronic illness, use of appetite-stimulating medications, lack of exercise, family history of obesity
- Nutritional status, including height and weight, usual dietary pattern, stated food preferences, weight fluctuations
- Psychosocial factors, including life-style, ethnic background, socioeconomic status, level of education, available transportation, internal and external cues that trigger desire to eat, motivation to lose weight, rate of food consumption
- Home environment, including presence of family members or significant other, responsibility for grocery shopping and meal preparation, presence of food storage and food preparation facilities, access to transportation

Defining characteristics
- Consistent snacking on low-nutrient foods
- Difficulty understanding what constitutes a proper diet
- Eating as a method for coping with boredom
- Eating triggered by emotions, such as anger or depression
- Lack of motivation to prepare balanced meals because of solitary life-style
- Sedentary life-style
- Taking majority of caloric intake at the end of the day
- Weight 20% over ideal for frame and height

Associated medical diagnoses (selected)
Atherosclerotic renal vascular disease, cerebrovascular accident, chronic obstructive pulmonary disease, cirrhosis, congestive heart failure, coronary artery disease, degenerative joint disease, depression, diabetes mellitus, diverticulitis, hyperglycemia, hyperosmolar nonketotic syndrome, hypertension, myocardial infarction, osteoarthritis

Expected outcomes
- Patient expresses understanding of why obesity is a problem.
- Patient develops realistic goals for weight reduction and a plan to achieve these goals.
- Patient loses ___ lb per week.
- Patient carries out exercise and activity plan.

Interventions and rationales

- Assess patient's perception of weight problem. Determine whether patient understands that obesity affects life-style and creates certain health risks *to evaluate patient's motivation to lose weight and determine appropriate plan of action.*
- Encourage patient to keep a food diary *to accurately track dietary intake.*
- Teach patient about changes in nutrient and vitamin needs that occur with aging *to promote well-informed food choices. Dietary requirements diminish with age; the older patient's caloric requirements decrease by 10% to 25%.*
- If patient lacks the motivation or resources for preparing balanced meals, provide information on appropriate community services, such as Meals on Wheels or federally sponsored nutrition programs, *to help patient obtain healthier meals.*
- Encourage patient to make gradual improvements in eating habits; for example, slowly introduce low-calorie, nutritious foods into diet. Keep in mind that older patient has developed current habits over many years. *Planning for gradual changes increases chances of success.*
- Set a realistic goal for weight loss; For older patients, a weekly loss of ½ to 1 lb (0.2 to 0.45 kg) is adequate. *Realistic goals ensure success of the weight-control program and help patient to become motivated.*
- If appropriate, have a registered dietitian discuss meal planning and food preparation with patient. *The dietitian may be able to provide appropriate nutritional guidance, taking into account physical, psychological, socioeconomic, and cultural factors.*
- Develop a modified exercise plan, such as regular walking. *Besides burning calories, promoting endurance, and maintaining musculoskeletal strength, regular exercise enhances patient's motivation and self-concept.*
- Provide ongoing support and recognition of patient's progress *to reinforce changes in eating habits and to help patient accurately assess progress.*
- Provide patient with information on social events and artistic, cultural, and educational programs *to stimulate patient to become more active.*

Evaluations for expected outcomes

- Patient expresses understanding of the consequences of continued obesity.
- Patient actively participates in developing weight-reduction goals.
- Patient implements goal-directed changes in eating patterns.

Documentation

- Patient's weight
- Patient's expression of feelings about obesity
- Observations of patient's eating patterns
- Weight-reduction plan implemented
- Teaching provided and patient's response
- Evaluations for each expected outcome.

■ Poisoning, high risk for

related to drug toxicity or polypharmacy

Definition

Accentuated risk of ingestion of drugs or dangerous products in doses sufficient to cause poisoning

Assessment

- Age
- Sex

• Drug history, including prescribed and over-the-counter medications
• Use of alcoholic beverages
• Health history, including evidence of hepatic or renal impairment
• Nutritional status, including weight changes, protein intake, and fluid status
• Psychosocial history, including activity level, knowledge level, financial status, mental status, living arrangements
• Laboratory studies, including toxicology screening; serum digitalis, serum electrolyte, blood urea nitrogen, serum creatinine, and bilirubin levels; liver enzymes, such as aspartate aminotransferase (formerly SGOT), alanine aminotransferase (formerly SGPT), and alkaline phosphatase; total serum protein, albumin to globulin ratio

Risk factors

• Cognitive or emotional difficulties, including forgetfulness or confusion
• Drugs stored near bedside
• History of drug abuse or alcoholism
• Impaired vision
• Inability to read medication labels
• Living alone
• Multiple health care providers, multiple drug prescriptions, and multiple pharmacies
• Poor bowel habits, including chronic use of enemas or laxative abuse
• Poor understanding of drug interactions
• Poor understanding of drug usage
• Poor understanding of precautions necessary for safe drug therapy

Associated medical diagnoses (selected)

Alzheimer's disease, arteriosclerotic heart disease, cataracts, cerebrovascular accident, chronic obstructive pulmonary disease, congestive heart failure, degenerative joint disease, depression, diabetes mellitus, diverticulitis, glaucoma, hepatic disease, myocardial infarction, hypertension, pneumonia, renal disease, rheumatoid arthritis, urinary tract infections

Expected outcomes

• Patient expresses understanding of medication regimen.
• Patient does not experience episodes of toxicity.
• Patient's medical conditions remain under control.
• Patient takes only prescribed medications in appropriate quantities at appropriate times.

Interventions and rationales

• Instruct patient or family member in drug regimen, including reasons for taking drugs, safety precautions, and how to monitor effectiveness of drugs *to increase compliance.*
• Review and document patient's entire medication regimen on a regular basis *to monitor use of medications, to assess whether certain medications should be discontinued, and to monitor for drug interactions.*
• Instruct patient or family member to store drugs in secure area away from the bedside *to prevent accidental ingestion. Often, older patients will keep medications at their bedside to decrease the need to arise during the night.*
• If color-coding medications, use only bright contrasting colors. *Older patients can't distinguish pastel colors well.*
• Help patient or family member identify behaviors that may contribute to risk of toxicity, for example, obtaining prescriptions from various health care providers or using differ-

ent pharmacies, *to raise awareness of potential hazards.*
- Encourage patient or family member to retain a primary doctor who can coordinate care. *Older patients with multiple health problems may receive care from various providers who are unaware of each other's treatment plans and drug regimens.*
- Provide instructions for use of medications, including size, frequency, and number of doses, *to enhance understanding of medication regimen and increase compliance.* Make sure instructions are clearly written in black or blue ink. *Older patients can read black or blue type more easily.*
- Be sure all medication labels are inscribed in large print and include dosage instructions *to avoid medication errors.*
- Help patient maintain an accurate and effective system for following medication regimen, such as a check-off calendar system or separate pill boxes labeled for each day of the week, *to reduce errors.* Encourage patient to work with pharmacist when developing this system.
- Monitor patient's urine and serum toxicity levels when indicated. *Age-related changes in bodily function may lead to decreased renal, liver, and GI clearance of drugs, thereby increasing the patient's risk of toxicity. In addition, the variety of drugs commonly used by the older patient increases the risk of toxicity from drug interactions.*
- Discuss with the doctor the possibility of using alternative drugs, such as long-acting preparations or drugs that require only one dose per day, *to simplify the drug regimen and thereby decrease the risk of toxicity.*

Evaluation for expected outcomes
- Patient expresses understanding of medication regimen.
- Patient does not experience episodes of toxicity.
- Patient's existing medical conditions remain under control.
- Patient takes only prescribed drugs in appropriate quantities at appropriate times.

Documentation
- Evidence of patient's or family member's lack of understanding of or poor compliance with medication regimen
- Additional factors that increase patient's risk of drug toxicity
- Physical findings
- Instructions provided about safe drug practices and patient's or family member's response to instructions
- Patient's responses to nursing interventions
- Evaluations for each expected outcome.

■ Powerlessness

related to perceived loss of control over life situation

Definition
Feeling of helplessness, hopelessness, and lack of control

Assessment
- Environmental factors, including institutional setting, if appropriate
- Impact of therapeutic regimens on life-style, including use of cane or walker, changes in diet, medication regimen
- Economic status, including retirement income, medical expenses such as ongoing home care or placement

in a nursing home, Medicare or other insurance coverage
- Emotional status, including recent loss of spouse, history of dependence on others
- Physical impairments, including arthritic conditions, loss of limb use, diminished vision, lengthy or chronic illness

Defining characteristics
- Angry outbursts
- Disinterest in improving or modifying own care
- Emotional withdrawal
- Expressions of hopelessness
- Expressions of loss of control over life situation
- Extreme, unwarranted dependency on others
- Hopelessness
- Lack of participation in activities of daily living, including personal hygiene and nutrition
- Perceived lack of control over life situation

Associated medical diagnoses (selected)
Anxiety disorders, cancer, cerebrovascular accident, chronic obstructive pulmonary disease, cirrhosis, congestive heart failure, degenerative joint disease, dementia, depression, diabetes mellitus, macular degeneration, maladaptive coping, osteoporosis, Parkinson's disease, rheumatoid arthritis

Expected outcomes
- Patient identifies aspects of life still under his control.
- Patient participates in development of schedule for self-care activities.
- Patient participates in decisions about own care and life-style.

Interventions and rationales
- Guide patient through life review. Encourage patient to reflect on past achievements *to foster a sense of satisfaction and promote acceptance of current status.* Assist patient in establishing realistic expectations and goals. *Having realistic expectations will help avoid failures, which might exacerbate feelings of powerlessness.*
- Help patient identify aspects of his life that are still under his control. For example, offer patient the opportunity to request changes to the arrangement of furniture in the room. Recognize patient's right to express feelings. *Empowering the older patient in any way possible may prevent feelings of powerlessness from becoming overwhelming.*
- Encourage patient to make his own choices in scheduling daily routine, including personal hygiene, dressing and grooming, meals, and physical therapy. Emphasize that the patient, not the staff, has the authority to make scheduling decisions. *This helps patient reassert control.*
- Ask patient open-ended questions, rather than questions that can be answered "yes" or "no." *Open-ended questions encourage patient to assert his opinions and, thereby, regain a feeling of control.*
- Encourage staff members to express interest in patient's progress and set aside time to listen attentively to patient *to acknowledge and reinforce efforts to regain control.*
- Encourage patient to take an active role in choosing among available social and recreational activities *to enhance patient's life-style and further diminish feelings of powerlessness.*

Evaluation for expected outcomes

- Patient describes actions that can be taken to improve or modify his routine.
- Patient displays an appropriate sense of responsibility in scheduling self-care activities.
- Patient expresses more realistic expectations and increased satisfaction with current situation.
- Patient selects appropriate social and recreational activities.

Documentation

- Patient's verbal and behavioral expressions of powerlessness
- Patient's level of involvement in self-care activities
- Patient's level of participation in the therapeutic and social milieu
- Patient's responses to nursing interventions
- Patient's statements indicating increased feelings of control
- Evaluations for each expected outcome.

■ Role performance alteration

Definition

Disruption in ability to perform social, vocational, and family roles

Assessment

- Age
- Sex
- Patient's perception of social, vocational, and family roles
- Neurologic status, including level of consciousness, memory, mental status, orientation, cognitive and perceptual functioning
- Physical disabilities or limitations
- Coping behaviors
- Developmental status, including evaluation of age-appropriate task resolution, for example, accepting changes in mental and physical capacities, relinquishing past roles, creating new social relationships, substituting new activities and interests for those that can no longer be pursued, and revising goals, values, and self-concept to accommodate life-style changes
- Family status, including roles of family members, effect of illness on patient's family, family's understanding of patient's illness
- Family members' perceptions of patient's ability to perform social, vocational, and family roles

Defining characteristics

- Patient describes experiencing change in ability to perform social, vocational, and family roles
- Patient experiences changes in mental capacity that affect ability to perform social, vocational, and family roles
- Patient experiences changes in physical capacity that affect ability to perform social, vocational, and family roles

Associated medical diagnoses (selected)

Any chronic medical condition or age-related change that may affect an older patient's role performance. Examples include Alzheimer's disease; angina pectoris; arteriosclerosis; blindness; bursitis; chronic obstructive pulmonary disease; congestive heart failure; dementia; diabetes mellitus; deafness; end-stage renal, cardiac, or pulmonary disease; hip fracture; Parkinson's disease; rheumatoid arthritis

Expected outcomes

- Patient discusses plans to reevaluate social, family, and vocational roles and adapt them to present physical and mental status.
- Family members express willingness to take over responsibilities previously performed by patient.
- Patient expresses feelings about limitations imposed by aging.
- Patient continues to perform usual social, family, and vocational roles to extent possible.
- Family members express willingness to provide emotional support as patient adjusts to altered role performance.

Interventions and rationales

- Discuss with patient factors that make it difficult to fulfill his usual vocational role. For example, has the patient recently been forced to retire? How does the patient cope with free time? How does the patient feel about no longer being the family breadwinner? *Discussion helps patient gain insight and rationally define problems and potential solutions.*
- Explore ways in which patient can continue to contribute to society, such as participation in a retired senior volunteer program, *to develop an activity program for patient that will help restore sense of purpose.*
- Discuss factors that make it difficult for patient to fulfill usual social roles. For example, have many of patient's close friends died? Is it difficult for patient to obtain transportation to social events? *This will help patient identify the causes of diminished social interaction.*
- Investigate available support groups, senior citizen centers, and other community resources *to help patient find new outlets for forming social relationships.*
- Discuss with family members ways they can help patient cope with altered role performance. Family members can help by visiting frequently, providing emotional support, and requesting patient's input into family decisions *to help maintain patient's self-esteem.*
- Encourage patient to continue to fulfill life roles within constraints imposed by aging *to maintain sense of purpose and preserve connection with others.*
- Encourage family members to express feelings about patient's altered role performance. Discuss alternative ways for family members to partially or fully assume roles once performed by patient *to enhance family coping.*
- Provide patient and family members with information about developmental tasks of aging. *As with other age-groups, elderly patients must perform certain developmental tasks to successfully master the process of aging. These tasks may include accepting changes in mental and physical capacities, relinquishing past roles, creating new social relationships, substituting new activities and interests for those that can no longer be pursued, and revising goals, values, and self-concept to accommodate life-style changes. Helping patient and family members understand that these tasks are a normal part of the aging process may enhance coping.*

Evaluations for expected outcomes

- Patient describes plans to adapt to changes related to aging and chronic illness.
- Patient expresses desire to continue to fulfill family, social, and vocational responsibilities to extent possible.

• Family members express willingness to take on responsibilities formerly held by patient.
• Family members express willingness to provide emotional support for patient as he adjusts to altered role performance.
• Patient describes new activities he will undertake to maintain sense of purpose in life.

Documentation
• Patient's expression of feelings and concern associated with altered role performance
• Nursing interventions performed to assist patient to understand and accept changes in role performance
• Patient's response to nursing interventions
• Statements by family members indicating their attitude toward patient's altered role performance
• Referrals to support services for patient and family members
• Evaluations for each expected outcome.

Self-esteem, situational low

related to hospitalization and forced dependence on health care team

Definition
Negative self-evaluation or feelings that develop in response to increased dependence on others

Assessment
• Changes in physical appearance, including wrinkles, sagging skin, gray hair, aging spots, scoliosis, dowager's hump, increased truncal fat
• Changes in social status, including recent retirement (forced or voluntary)
• Changes in sleep patterns, including trouble falling asleep, frequent awakenings, restless sleep
• Family status, including recent loss of spouse or significant other
• Reason for current hospitalization
• Medical history, including chronic illnesses
• Mental status, including evidence of depression, hopelessness, discouragement, preoccupation with bodily functions, unrealistic fear of developing a serious disease

Defining characteristics
• Difficulty making decisions
• Patient expresses feeling helpless or useless
• Patient expresses frustration, sadness, or regret over inability to handle life events
• Patient expresses negative view of self in response to life events

Associated medical diagnoses (selected)
Acute exacerbation of any chronic illness, such as arthritis, cardiovascular disease, cataracts, hypertension, obesity, varicose veins

Expected outcomes
• Patient participates in care.
• Patient maintains eye contact and initiates conversations.
• Patient maintains an upright and open posture.
• Patient's body language and speech content are congruent.
• Patient talks about impact of changes caused by chronic illness or aging on life-style.
• Patient expresses (verbally or through behavior) increased acceptance of changes caused by chronic illness or aging.
• Patient expresses increased self-esteem.

Interventions and rationales

- Ask permission to enter the patient's personal space. This may include areas around the bed, bedside tables, and closet. *As patient's self-esteem decreases, significance of personal space increases. Asking permission to enter personal space provides patient with a sense of control and raises self-esteem.*
- Encourage patient to wear own pajamas or gowns and robes *to contribute to a positive self-identity.*
- Arrange patient's personal items on the bedside stand so that they are within easy reach *to maintain patient's independence.*
- Incorporate appropriate exercise activities into patient's daily care *to enhance strength, endurance, and coordination, all of which affect self-esteem.*
- Encourage patient to reminisce *to help focus patient's attention on past accomplishments.*
- If patient's mobility is limited, install an over-the-bed trapeze *to promote feelings of independence.*
- Incorporate tactile stimulation into daily activities through such techniques as back rubs, foot massages, or touching of hand or arm. *Frequent touching enhances the patient's sense of self-worth.*
- Encourage patient to express feelings about chronic illness or aging process. Also encourage patient to discuss fears about loss of independence and diminished ability to participate in work and leisure activities. *This allows patient to gain insight and to rationally define problems and potential solutions.*
- Provide information about appropriate support groups. *Interacting with individuals who have successfully adapted to illness or limitations may increase patient's coping skills.*

Evaluation for expected outcomes

- Patient carries out activities of daily living while in the hospital.
- Patient initiates conversations and maintains eye contact.
- Patient is open and receptive to others.
- Patient's speech and body language are congruent.
- Patient states at least two ways hospitalization will impact upon his lifestyle.
- Patient discusses feelings associated with aging, chronic illness, loss of independence, and diminished ability to participate in work and leisure activities.
- At least once each day, patient makes statements reflecting greater self-esteem.

Documentation

- Patient's expressions of lowered self-esteem
- Mental status assessment (baseline and ongoing)
- Interventions directed toward improved self-esteem
- Patient's response to nursing interventions
- Evaluations for each expected outcome.

■ Sensory or perceptual alteration (auditory)

related to altered sensory reception, transmission, or integration

Definition

Changes in the sense of hearing

Assessment

- Mental status, including mood, affect, comprehension level, recent stressors

• Occupational hazards
• Auditory status, including physical examination of ears (cerumen build-up, excessive hair in canal), previous ear trauma or surgery, use of hearing aid
• Audiometric evaluation, including Rinne, Weber's, Schwabach, and speech and noise tests
• Adaptive or maladaptive communication-related behaviors, such as lip reading, gestures, withdrawal, isolation
• Medication history, including drugs that may cause hearing loss, such as aspirin, streptomycin, kanamycin, neomycin

Defining characteristics
• Anxiety
• Auditory deficits and misperceptions
• Change in behavior pattern
• Decreased social interaction
• Depression
• Diminished sense of trust
• Excessive dependence on others
• Passivity or apathy
• Reported or measured change in hearing

Associated medical diagnoses (selected)
Acoustic tumors, diabetes mellitus, drug-related deafness, otosclerosis, recurrent otitis media, trauma, tinnitus, tumors of the nasopharynx, vascular lesions, viral infections

Expected outcomes
• Patient expresses understanding of normal hearing changes that occur with age.
• Patient expresses feelings with regard to hearing deficits and impact deficits have on life-style.
• Patient demonstrates correct use of hearing aids.
• Patient incorporates alternative communication techniques, such as lip reading, gestures, and written information, into daily activities.
• Patient expresses interest in attending community support groups.
• Patient takes steps to enhance communication where possible, such as decreasing background noise and looking at the speaker's mouth while listening.

Interventions and rationales
• Provide information about progressive hearing loss that occurs with age (presbycusis) *to enhance patient's understanding of hearing deficits.*
• Encourage patient to express feelings about hearing loss. *Because of the stigma attached to hearing loss, the older patient may be reluctant to discuss this problem. Offering support and encouragement may help overcome patient's self-consciousness.*
• Incorporate written communication methods (such as flash cards and word lists) and visual speech (such as sign language, gestures, and facial expressions) into daily care *to provide patient with an alternative means of communication and to enhance his sense of control.*
• When speaking to the patient, eliminate background noises, such as television, air conditioning, fans, chatter, and radios, *to help patient concentrate on what you're saying.*
• Speaking slowly and carefully, orient patient to the topic of conversation *to reduce feelings of paranoia that may cause the patient to withdraw from social interaction.*
• Speak to the patient in a moderate, low-pitched voice, maintaining an even volume throughout each sentence. *Speaking louder will not assist patient's hearing because presbycusis first causes a loss in high-pitched sound recognition.*

• Face patient when speaking and enunciate words carefully, especially consonant sounds, *to help patient read lips.*
• If patient has difficulty understanding a sentence, rephrase it *to overcome possible barriers in language comprehension.*
• Encourage patient to participate in activities, such as cards or checkers, which do not require a high level of verbal communication, *to promote social activity.*
• Describe to patient the types of adaptive hearing devices available and their care *to help patient make informed choices and maintain independence.*
• Provide information about support groups, such as the nationally affiliated hearing-impaired support group "Self Help for Hard of Hearing People (SHHH)," *to promote continuity of care through community support.*
• Make sure other staff members are aware of patient's hearing deficit. Tell staff members that "selective hearing" may be related to patient's decreased ability to hear high frequencies and that fatigue or environmental distractions may contribute to hearing deficits. *Teaching colleagues about presbycusis will help ensure quality care.*

Evaluation for expected outcomes
• Patient expresses understanding of hearing loss that occurs with aging.
• Patient verbalizes feelings regarding hearing deficits.
• Patient discusses how to modify life-style to adapt to hearing deficits.
• Patient demonstrates correct care of adaptive hearing devices.
• Patient uses alternative communication techniques to express needs or wants.
• Patient expresses interest in attending appropriate community support groups.
• Patient takes appropriate steps to enhance communication where possible, such as decreasing background noise.

Documentation
• Patient's statements that indicate feelings about hearing deficits
• Patient's behavioral response to hearing loss
• Nursing interventions to help patient cope with hearing deficits
• Patient teaching, including explanation of hearing loss, instructions on how to care for hearing aids, and instructions on alternative communication techniques
• Patient's responses to nursing interventions
• Evaluations for each expected outcome.

Sensory or perceptual alteration (visual)

related to altered sensory reception, transmission, or integration

Definition
Changes in the sense of sight

Assessment
• Age
• Visual status, including visual fields, corneal reflexes, extraocular movements, visual acuity, intraocular pressure, previous eye trauma, infection, or surgery, accommodation, night blindness, physical examination of the eye including ophthalmoscopy, use of glasses
• State of remaining senses

- Patient's life-style and physical environment
- Mental status, including behavior, mood, affect, coping mechanisms
- Family history of visual problems

Defining characteristics
- Altered conceptualization
- Anger
- Anxiety
- Apathy or passivity
- Change in behavioral pattern
- Changes in response to visual stimuli
- Clinical evidence of decreased visual ability
- Depression
- Distorted visual perception
- Restlessness

Associated medical diagnoses (selected)
Cataracts, diabetic retinopathy, ectropion, entropion, glaucoma, macular degeneration, retinal detachment, retinitis pigmentosa

Expected outcomes
- Patient discusses impact of vision loss on life-style.
- Patient expresses a feeling of safety, comfort, and security.
- Patient shows interest in external environment.
- Patient uses adaptive devices to compensate for vision loss.

Interventions and rationales
- Teach patient about the normal age-related changes of the eye (presbyopia) *to increase patient's understanding of visual changes he is experiencing.*
- Encourage patient to undergo annual eye examinations *to monitor for progressive vision loss. Decreased vision can exacerbate acute confusion.*
- Install night lights in patient's room. Strategically arrange lighting to avoid abrupt changes in light. *The aged eye takes longer to accommodate to changes in lighting levels.*
- Provide adequate light for performing activities of daily living. *A patient over age 60 needs twice the illumination for close tasks that a patient age 20 does.*
- Adjust lighting to reduce glare from shiny surfaces, such as magazine paper and walls. *Aging eyes are more sensitive to glare.*
- If color-coding medications, use only bright contrasting colors. *Pastel colors, such as light blues and greens, look alike to the aging eye.*
- When teaching patient, use large black print, *which is easier to see and read.*
- Provide large-print objects, such as clocks, calendars, and telephone dials, *to promote a sense of independence.*
- Confer with patient before moving furniture or other items in a room *to help patient maintain independence in activities of daily living.*
- Provide a brightly colored strip on the edge of the bedside tray and table *to prevent objects from falling on the bed or floor as a result of depth perception problems.*
- Touch patient *to communicate that you are listening.*
- Provide patient with low-vision aids, such as large-print books and magnifying glasses, *to help increase patient's independence level.*

Evaluation for expected outcomes
- Patient describes effects of vision loss on life-style.
- Patient regains vision to the extent possible and begins to come to terms with any potentially permanent vision loss.
- Patient expresses interest in external environment.

- Patient uses adaptive devices to compensate for vision loss.

Documentation
- Patient's expression of feelings about visual deficits
- Patient's behavioral response to visual deficits
- Use of adaptive equipment or devices
- Teaching provided to patient and patient's response
- Patient's response to nursing interventions
- Evaluations for each expected outcome.

Sexuality pattern alteration (female patient)

related to illness, medical treatment, or age-related changes

Definition
State in which a person expresses concern about personal sexuality

Assessment
- Changes in female reproductive organs related to aging
- Hormone replacement therapy (postmenopause or postoophorectomy), including estrogen, progesterone, or both
- Relationship with spouse or significant other
- Psychosocial status, including self-perception, ability to cope with aging process, usual sexual activity pattern, social interaction patterns
- Chronic illnesses
- Impaired mobility
- Perceived changes in sexual activity resulting from surgery or illness

Defining characteristics
- Anger
- Constricted affect
- Depressed mood
- Noncompliance with prescribed therapies
- Reported changes, difficulties, or limitations in sexual activity
- Withdrawal from social interaction

Associated medical diagnoses (selected)
Diabetes mellitus, hysterectomy, menopause, multiple sclerosis, musculoskeletal disorders of pelvis and lower back, osteoporosis, parkinsonism, rheumatoid arthritis, therapy with antihypertensives, therapy with estrogen or progesterone, thyroid deficiency, vaginal atrophy

Expected outcomes
- Patient expresses feelings associated with sexuality and self-concept.
- Patient discusses variety of options involved in maintaining intimacy throughout her life span.
- Patient expresses understanding of normal physiologic changes that occur with aging.
- Patient expresses understanding of options available to relieve discomfort associated with menopause or hysterectomy.

Interventions and rationales
- Provide information regarding hysterectomy and menopause. *After menopause or hysterectomy, older women need reassurance that sexual activity can still be enjoyable.*
- Teach patient about the impact of normal physiologic changes on sexuality. For example, the vagina becomes smaller and less elastic, the vaginal walls become thin and smooth, and the external genitalia may be softer. Also, vaginal lubrication may take longer. The patient may also have abdominal pain or

irritability of the bladder during intercourse. *Explaining how the aging process affects sexuality may help patient to accept these physiologic changes.*

- Encourage patient to express feelings about sexuality *to reassure patient that you are willing to discuss her concerns.*
- Discuss variety of options involved in intimacy, for example, hugging, touching, and closeness, *to reaffirm patient's identity as a sexual being.*
- Provide information concerning alternative techniques and adaptations that can assist sexual satisfaction *to encourage patient to explore and accept her sexuality.* Topics may include:
  - lubrication
  - Kegel exercises (for vaginal muscle tone)
  - self-stimulation
  - alternative sexual positions and activities.
- Discuss the impact that chronic illness or adverse drug reactions can have on patient's sexuality *to explore ways of eliminating barriers to sexual enjoyment.* Discuss with doctor the possibility of providing alternative medications.
- Teach patient the benefits and risks associated with hormone replacement therapy, for example:
  - reduced postmenopausal osteoporosis
  - decreased risk of cardiovascular disease
  - increased risk of endometrial cancer (with estrogen therapy alone)
  - presence of monthly period with combined estrogen and progestin therapy.

Education will help patient make the most informed decision possible.

- Discuss psychosocial issues that may affect patient's sexuality, such as financial concerns about remarriage or family member's objections to her relationship with a male companion, *to help patient focus on specific concerns and avoid misunderstandings.*
- If patient lives in a long-term care facility or life-care community, encourage her to participate in social activities *to enhance opportunities for sexual expression.*

Evaluations for expected outcomes

- Patient discusses feelings related to sexuality and self-concept.
- Patient discusses options for maintaining intimacy throughout her life.
- Patient describes physiologic changes in the reproductive organs that occur with aging.
- Patient describes risks and benefits of hormone replacement therapy.

Documentation

- Patient's expression of feelings about sexuality and aging
- Teaching provided and patient's response
- Observations of patient's behavioral responses to care
- Expressions indicating patient's improved ability to achieve sexual enjoyment and intimacy
- Evaluations for each expected outcome.

■ Skin integrity impairment, high risk for

related to the aging process and impaired mobility

Definition

Presence of risk factors for interruption in skin integrity

Assessment

- Age

- Physical examination, including inspection of lower limbs, sensation testing of lower limbs, palpation of peripheral pulses, presence of edema
- Integumentary status, including color, elasticity, hygiene, lesions, moisture, quantity and distribution of hair, sensation, temperature and blood pressure, texture, turgor, condition of nails
- Psychosocial status, including coping patterns, life-style, presence of family members or significant other, mental status, self-concept and body image
- Mobility status, including activity level, joint range of motion, contractures, muscle mass and tone
- Mental status
- Evidence of incontinence
- Recent changes in medication regimen
- History of skin problems, including pressure ulcers, dermatitis, trauma
- Ability to perform skin-care regimen

Risk factors

- External (environmental) factors, including pressure, friction, shearing forces, restraints, physical immobilization, confinement to bed or chair, excretions and secretions, moisture, hypothermia, or hyperthermia
- Internal (somatic) factors, including altered nutritional status (cachexia or debilitation), decreased serum albumin level, dehydration, dependence on others for self-care, skin maceration, bladder or bowel incontinence, comatose state, paralysis, skeletal prominences, decreased circulation, obesity, localized infection in pressure-supporting areas, loss of subcutaneous tissue or muscle mass, altered metabolic state, or vitamin deficiency

Associated medical diagnoses (selected)

Anemia, Buerger's disease, cerebrovascular accident, chronic renal disease, cirrhosis, degenerative joint disease, diabetes mellitus, hip fracture, hyperparathyroidism, malnutrition, obesity, peripheral vascular disease, Raynaud's disease, surgical procedures with associated wound or incision healing, thrombophlebitis, venous stasis ulcers

Expected outcomes

- Patient maintains intact skin.
- Patient or caretaker describes normal aging changes in the skin and risk factors for potential disturbance in skin integrity.
- Patient or caretaker implements strategies to prevent skin breakdown.
- Patient or caretaker carries out skin-care regimen.

Interventions and rationales

- Educate patient or caretaker in changes to skin caused by aging *to motivate patient or caretaker to implement a skin-care regimen. Physiologic changes associated with aging increase the risk of skin breakdown. For example, older patients, especially those immobilized with chronic health problems, are at a high risk for pressure ulcers. Physiologic changes also leave older patients vulnerable to problems associated with dry skin.*
- Help patient to obtain appropriate evaluation and treatment of underlying skin condition *to promote healing and minimize complications.*
- Assist patient or caretaker in implementing a pressure-relief movement and massage program to prevent pressure ulcers. Patient's position should be changed at least every 2 hours. *Frequent turning and massage*

promotes adequate tissue perfusion and prevents necrosis.

- Use preventive skin-care devices as needed, such as a foam mattress, an alternating pressure mattress, sheepskin, pillows, or padding, *to avoid discomfort and skin breakdown. These measures do not replace need for turning.*
- Instruct patient in need for good nutrition, including the importance of meeting caloric requirements and the benefits of adequate vitamin and protein intake. *Good nutrition helps to maintain adequate tissue nourishment, perfusion, and oxygenation.*
- Assist patient or caretaker in developing and implementing a daily routine of skin inspection and care. Discuss the need to:
  - maintain good personal hygiene.
  - use nonirritating (nonalkaline) soap.
  - pat rather than rub skin dry.
  - inspect skin on a regular basis.
  - avoid prolonged exposure to water, sun, cold, wind.
  - recognize beginning of skin breakdown (redness, blisters, discoloration) and report symptoms.

A daily program of skin inspection and maintenance will protect older patient's skin integrity.

- Encourage patient or caretaker to seek immediate attention in the event of skin injury or trauma *to help prevent further insult and conditions requiring extensive treatment.*
- Monitor any wounds or incisions for infection and follow prescribed treatment regimen *to prevent infection, which may delay healing.*

Evaluations for expected outcomes

- Patient's skin remains intact.
- Patient or caretaker describes skin changes that result from aging and lists risk factors for impaired skin integrity.
- Patient or caretaker implements a daily program of skin inspection and care, including frequent turning and movement.

Documentation

- Observations of patient's skin
- Presence of risk factors for impaired skin integrity
- Patient teaching provided and patient's response
- Patient's response to nursing interventions
- Evaluations for each expected outcome.

Social isolation

related to physiologic, environmental, or emotional barriers

Definition

Self-imposed or environmentally imposed lack of contact with others

Assessment

- Age
- Psychosical status, including available support systems, financial resources, coping and problem-solving ability, cultural background, activities or hobbies
- Health status, including visual or hearing deficits, chronic illness, incontinence, pain
- Self-care abilities, including knowledge and use of adaptive equipment and supplies, technical and mechanical skills
- Living conditions, including home environment, site of activities and resources, available transportation
- Mental status, including behavior, mood, affect

• Musculoskeletal status, including coordination; functional ability; gait; muscle tone, size, and strength; range of motion; presence of tremor or paralysis

Defining characteristics

• Absence of family and friends
• Behavioral and emotional problems, including withdrawal; insecurity in public; lack of eye contact; preoccupation with own thoughts; sad, dull affect
• Environmental barriers to social activity, such as unsafe neighborhood, lack of transportation, living alone, confinement to long-term care facility
• Failure to join organized social groups or participate in group activities
• Loss of social roles or relationships
• Physiologic limitations, including hearing deficits, impaired mobility, impaired vision, impaired speech, chronic illness, decreased muscle strength and endurance, incontinence, pain
• Problems in social interaction, such as difficulty asking for help, initiating a conversation, or responding to a question
• Refusal to participate in organized activities offered by long-term care facility or retirement community
• Verbal expression of feeling different from others
• Verbal expressions indicating feelings of being rejected by others
• Verbal expression of lacking purpose in life

Associated medical diagnoses (selected)

Alcoholism, Alzheimer's disease, amyotrophic lateral sclerosis, arthritis, cerebrovascular accident, cirrhosis, degenerative joint disease, diabetes mellitus, malnutrition, osteoporosis, Parkinson's disease, schizophrenia or other psychiatric disorders

Expected outcomes

• Patient expresses feelings associated with social isolation.
• Patient seeks assistance or information from staff to overcome social isolation.
• Patient makes use of available community resources.
• Patient describes an increased number of social contacts.
• Patient expresses satisfaction with level of social contacts.

Interventions and rationales

• Assign a primary nurse or case manager to patient *to provide consistency and promote trust.*
• Discuss with patient causes and contributing factors of social isolation. Find out what factors patient believes interfere most with his ability to develop relationships with others *to determine patient's wants and needs.*
• Find out if patient is willing to make changes in life-style or daily routine to increase contact with others. *Patient needs to be motivated to change for nursing interventions to be successful.*
• If appropriate, address any physical limitations that are interfering with patient's ability to form social relationships. For example, if patient has a hearing deficit, make a referral to the audiologist for a hearing aid; if patient has a mobility impairment, make a referral to the physical therapist for an exercise program or for recommendations for assistive devices. *Physical limitations may need to be addressed before patient can overcome social isolation.*
• Assess the influence of the home environment on patient's social life. For example, is patient afraid to go

outside because of the high crime rate in the neighborhood? If so, consider investigating options, such as moving to a retirement community or residential care facility, that might offer better social opportunities. *The patient may not be aware of alternative living options.*
- Investigate available activity groups, support groups, senior citizens centers, health education programs, and other community resources *to develop an activity program for patient.*
- Investigate availability and cost of public transportation. Familiarize patient with route to planned activities. *Overcoming barriers to transportation is essential to gaining access to the outside world.*
- Involve patient in planning activities that will enhance his social life and assist him in identifying resources *to individualize care planning and reduce feelings of dependency and helplessness.*

Evaluations for expected outcomes
- Patient expresses feelings associated with social isolation.
- Patient expresses desire to increase social relationships.
- Patient expresses desire for assistance in increasing participation in social activities.
- Patient makes use of available resources, such as social services, senior citizens centers, American Association of Retired Persons, or religious organizations.
- Patient indicates that social contacts have increased and feelings of social isolation have diminished.

Documentation
- Factors that have caused or contributed to patient's social isolation
- Statements that indicate patient's dissatisfaction with social situation
- Community resources identified for patient
- Planning done by patient, family member, primary nurse, and case manager.
- Patient's use of community resources
- Evaluations for each expected outcome.

Verbal communication impairment

related to physiologic or psychosocial changes

Definition
Decreased ability to appropriately speak, understand, or use words that is caused by organic and environmental factors

Assessment
- History of neurologic disease
- Speech characteristics, including pattern (rate of speech, phrase length, effort, fluency, prosody, repetition, information content), vocabulary, level of comprehension, presence of aphasia (Broca's, Wernicke's, transcortical, receptive, global) or dysarthria
- Ability to use alternative forms of communication (eye blinks, gestures, pictures, nods, written notes)
- Auditory status, including use of hearing aid, history of hearing deficits, presence of cerumen
- Visual status, including use of eyeglasses, history of visual deficits, visual acuity (near and distant), visual fields
- Neurologic status, including level of consciousness, orientation, cognition,

memory (recent, remote), insight, judgment, cranial nerves (IX, X, XII), primitive reflexes (snout, suck, palm-chin), diagnostic studies (arteriogram, EEG, computed tomography scan, magnetic resonance imaging scan)
- Psychosocial status, including family; friends; other support systems; recent relocation; recent losses; efforts to express sadness, frustration, anxiety, or other emotions associated with verbal communication impairment
- Medication status, including use of prescribed and over-the-counter medications

Defining characteristics
- Decreased ability to comprehend language
- Decreased ability to use meaningful language
- Difficulty with producing speech sounds (phonation)
- Disorientation
- Dyspnea
- Garbled or incomprehensible speech
- Impaired articulation
- Inability to identify objects
- Inability to modulate speech
- Inability to speak in sentences
- Incessant, incoherent speech
- Perseveration
- Stuttering or slurring

Associated medical diagnoses (selected)
Alcoholic cerebellar degeneration, Alzheimer's disease, amyotrophic lateral sclerosis, cerebrovascular accident, dementia, Huntington's disease, intracranial tumors, myasthenia gravis, normal pressure hydrocephalus, Parkinson's disease, septic meningitis, subacute spongiform encephalopathy (Creutzfeldt-Jakob disease)

Expected outcomes
- Patient improves communication skills to the extent possible.
- Patient attends sessions with speech therapist.
- Visitors and staff demonstrate appropriate respect when speaking with patient.
- Patient communicates needs without excessive frustration.
- Patient or family member identifies and contacts appropriate support services.
- Patient indicates through gestures, behavior, writing, or speaking that he is coming to terms with his impaired ability to communicate.

Interventions and rationales
- When initiating communication, face patient, maintain eye contact, speak slowly, and enunciate clearly *to make it easier for patient to receive and process your message.*
- Take steps to enhance communication while providing care:
  - Communicate one idea at a time.
  - Use "yes" and "no" questions.
  - Avoid abstract thoughts and controversial topics.
  - Use plain, everyday vocabulary.
  - Allow longer response time.
  - Guess at meaning of incorrect words.
  - Reduce distractions.
  - Eliminate unnecessary noise.
  - Encourage patient to use gestures or other alternative means of communication.

Facilitating communication efforts will help decrease patient's frustration.
- If patient's communication problems are exacerbated by hearing deficits, use appropriate techniques to overcome hearing problems:

- Minimize glare in patient's room *to make it easier for patient to read your lips.*
- Use normal voice when speaking. *Shouting makes your voice frequency higher and does not assist hearing.*
- Check for proper use of adaptive hearing devices. If patient wears a hearing aid, be sure the battery is working and the hearing aid is in place correctly *to enhance hearing ability.*
- Use paper and pencil if hearing is severely impaired *to provide an alternative means of communication.*

• If patient does not follow your conversation, rephrase ideas using simpler wording *to overcome differences in language or culture that may block communication.*

• Do not rush patient when he is struggling to express his thoughts. Demonstrate tact and a willingness to listen. Even if you can't understand patient, let him know you accept his efforts to communicate and you empathize with his frustration. *The patient with impaired verbal communication experiences isolation, despair, and frustration. Demonstrating compassion and fostering a therapeutic relationship is the single most important step for improving communication.*

• Avoid conversing with patient when he is tired. *Patient's attention span may deteriorate when he is fatigued, thereby making efforts to communicate even more frustrating.*

• Encourage patient to engage in social activities, such as attending therapy sessions and eating with other patients at group tables, *to reduce feelings of isolation.*

• If appropriate, help patient reintegrate into family life; for example, arrange for patient to attend family gatherings. *The patient with impaired verbal communication usually can no longer perform his role within the family. When possible, providing an opportunity to reintegrate patient into family life may help diminish loneliness and anxiety.*

• Encourage patient to reminisce. Use photographs, gestures, and visits from family members and friends to stimulate patient's desire to express himself. *Recalling meaningful experiences from the past may motivate patient to try to communicate and may enhance feelings of self-worth.*

• Encourage family members and colleagues to use speech appropriate for adults when talking to patient and not to talk about him within his range of hearing *to convey respect.*

• Obtain referral to speech therapist. Educate family members and colleagues about methods prescribed by therapist to enhance communication *to ensure continuity of care.*

• Refer patient and family members to appropriate community resources, such as a club for stroke survivors or a support group for relatives of Alzheimer's patients, *to help them cope with communication impairment after discharge.*

Evaluation for expected outcomes

• Patient improves communication skills to the extent possible.

• Patient attends sessions with speech therapist _______ times/week.

• Visitors and staff demonstrate appropriate respect when speaking with patient by using adult speech and not talking about him within his hearing range.

• Patient communicates needs, using gestures, behavior, writing, or speech, without excessive frustration.

• Patient takes steps to decrease isolation from friends and family members.
• Patient or family member identifies and contacts appropriate support services.
• Patient indicates, through gestures, behavior, writing, or speech, that he is coming to terms with his impaired ability to communicate.

Documentation
• Observations of impaired speaking ability, use of communication aids, and expressions of frustration
• Interventions implemented to decrease barriers to effective communication
• Efforts to communicate on behalf of patient using gestures, behavior, writing, or speech
• Patient teaching and patient's response to teaching efforts
• Referrals to speech therapist and other support services
• Evaluations for each expected outcome.

■ Violence, high risk for: Self-directed

related to suicide attempt

Definition
Presence of risk factors for self-directed violence

Assessment
• Age
• Sex
• Race
• Religion
• Marital status (widowed, divorced, married, single)
• Life situation, including recent retirement, unemployment, or move to a new area, isolation (lives in urban area, lives alone)
• Mental health history, including coping behaviors, statements of low self-esteem, family dynamics, communication patterns
• Recent stressors, including divorce or death of spouse, relocation
• Mental status, including orientation, level of consciousness, thought processes
• Available support systems

Risk factors
• Changes in mood or affect
• Changes in physical or mental status
• Confusion
• Direct or indirect statements of intent to commit suicide
• Experience of multiple losses, such as loss of spouse, loss of income, loss of friends
• Expression of feelings of hopelessness, helplessness, or depression
• Getting affairs in order, for example, changing or making a will
• Giving away money or valuables
• Hoarding medications
• Purchasing gun or other weapon
• Visiting doctor about somatic complaints

Associated medical diagnoses (selected)
Any mental or physical illness that decompensates patient and in which prognosis is poor, such as cancer, dementia, major depression, substance abuse, terminal illness, traumatic injury

Expected outcomes
• Patient is free from self-harm and remains in controlled environment.
• Patient willingly participates in therapeutic milieu.
• Patient verbalizes feelings associated with suicide attempt.
• Patient expresses desire to live.
• Patient expresses improved self-concept.

- Patient discusses appropriate coping skills to avoid future suicidal episodes.

Interventions and rationales

- Remove items that could be used in suicide attempt *to ensure patient's safety.*
- Set aside time for listening to patient *to communicate that you care.*
- Approach patient with understanding and concern *to alleviate angry or embarrassed feelings related to emotional breakdown or previous unsuccessful suicide attempt.*
- Commmunicate a nonjudgmental attitude *to build trust and rapport.*
- Recognize patient's feelings of inadequacy and take steps to bolster self-esteem. Encourage patient to participate in life review, revisit places where significant past events took place, put together a scrapbook, research family genealogy, or attend family, class, or church reunions. *These activities help patient experience emotions, which ultimately promotes better integration of self and improved self-esteem.*
- Discuss problems that led patient to crisis state. *Talking about specific events may help patient achieve catharsis and guide patient in developing appropriate coping skills.*
- Avoid comparing patient with others *to reduce stereotyping and allow for individuality.*
- Ask patient directly: "Have you thought about killing yourself?" If so, ask, "What do you plan to do?" *to assess for suicidal ideation.*
- Supervise and educate patient or family member in the use of prescribed antidepressants. Explain that geriatric doses differ from those for a younger patient. *Knowledge of medications and careful monitoring help to guard against adverse effects.*
- Help patient identify community resources *to obtain continued therapy and support after hospitalization.*

Evaluations for expected outcomes

- Patient's environment is safe.
- Patient participates in therapeutic milieu.
- Patient verbalizes feelings and thoughts in a way that promotes the healing process.
- Patient's states that he feels better about himself.
- Patient states that he experiences fewer suicidal thoughts.
- Patient expresses understanding of the importance of increased social support and improved coping skills in avoiding future suicidal episodes.

Documentation

- Patient's exact description of suicidal thoughts and recent suicide attempt
- Observations of patient's behavior
- Interventions performed to prevent suicide
- Patient's responses to therapeutic milieu
- Evaluations for each expected outcome.

APPENDICES AND INDEX

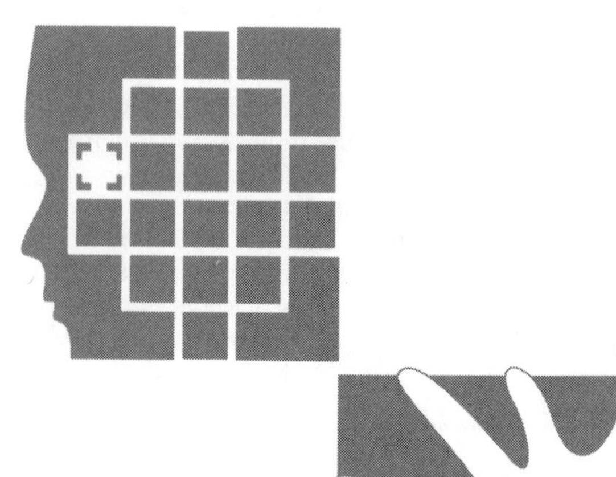

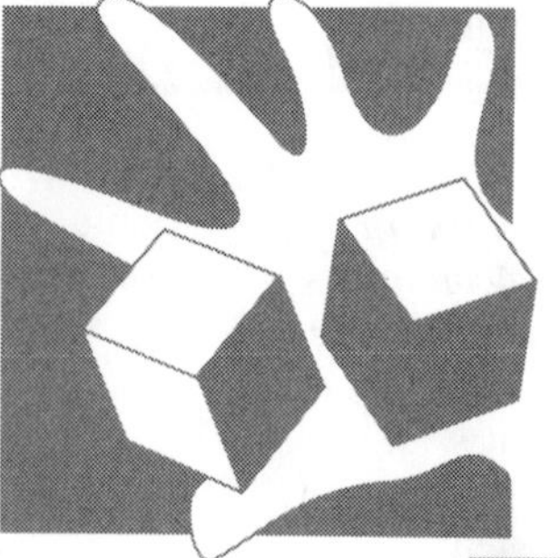

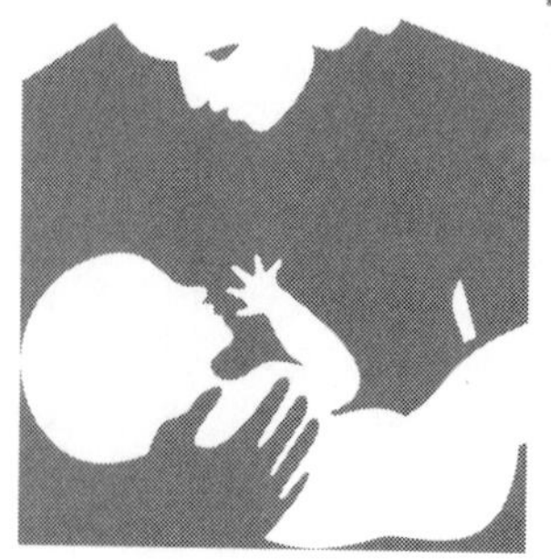

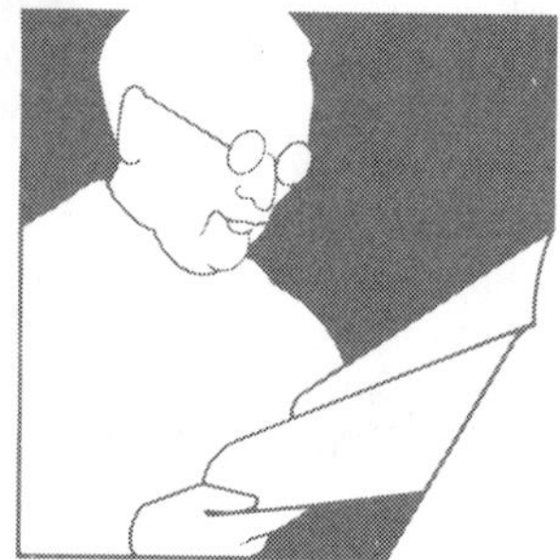

NURSING DIAGNOSIS CROSS-REFERENCES

NURSING DIAGNOSES BY MEDICAL DIAGNOSES

Cardiovascular disorders

Adams-Stokes syndrome
- Anxiety
- Cardiac output, decreased
- Tissue perfusion alteration

Anaphylactic shock
- Anxiety
- Cardiac output, decreased
- Tissue perfusion alteration (cardiopulmonary, renal)

Angina pectoris
- Anxiety
- Cardiac output, decreased
- Denial
- Pain
- Role performance alteration

Aortic aneurysm
- Anxiety
- Breathing pattern, ineffective
- Pain
- Tissue perfusion alteration (peripheral, renal)

Aortic stenosis or insufficiency
- Cardiac output, decreased
- Mobility impairment
- Tissue perfusion alteration (cardiopulmonary)

Arterial insufficiency
- Anxiety
- Cardiac output, decreased
- Pain
- Tissue integrity impairment
- Tissue perfusion alteration (peripheral)

Arterial occlusion
- Pain
- Sensory or perceptual alteration (olfactory, tactile)
- Skin integrity impairment
- Tissue perfusion alteration (peripheral)

Arteriosclerosis
- Denial
- Health-seeking behaviors
- Incontinence, reflex
- Poisoning, high risk for
- Role performance alteration
- Sensory or perceptual alteration (tactile)
- Tissue perfusion alteration (cardiopulmonary)
- Verbal communication impairment

Arteriovenous malformation
- Mobility impairment
- Tissue perfusion alteration (cerebral)
- Verbal communication impairment

Buerger's disease
- Sensory or perceptual alteration (tactile)
- Skin integrity impairment, high risk for
- Thermoregulation, ineffective
- Tissue integrity impairment
- Tissue perfusion alteration (peripheral)

Cardiac arrest
- Anxiety
- Aspiration, high risk for
- Breathing pattern, ineffective
- Cardiac output, decreased

Cardiac arrhythmias
- Cardiac output, decreased
- Fluid volume deficit, high risk for
- Tissue perfusion alteration (peripheral)

Cardiac disease: End-stage
- Activity intolerance
- Cardiac output, decreased

- Caregiver role strain
- Caregiver role strain, high risk for
- Coping, defensive
- Coping, ineffective individual
- Decisional conflict
- Denial
- Grieving, anticipatory
- Grieving, dysfunctional
- Hopelessness
- Injury, high risk for
- Self-esteem, situational low

Cardiac tamponade
- Activity intolerance
- Cardiac output, decreased
- Pain
- Tissue perfusion alteration (cardiopulmonary)

Cardiogenic shock
- Anxiety
- Cardiac output, decreased
- Gas exchange impairment
- Tissue perfusion alteration (cardiopulmonary, renal)

Carotid sinus syndrome
- Cardiac output, decreased

Congestive heart failure
- Activity intolerance
- Activity intolerance, high risk for
- Airway clearance, ineffective
- Breathing pattern, ineffective
- Cardiac output, decreased
- Caregiver role strain
- Caregiver role strain, high risk for
- Fatigue
- Fluid volume excess
- Gas exchange impairment
- Home maintenance management impairment
- Hopelessness
- Infection, high risk for
- Injury, high risk for
- Knowledge deficit
- Nutrition alteration: More than body requirements
- Pain
- Poisoning, high risk for
- Powerlessness
- Role performance alteration
- Thermoregulation, ineffective
- Tissue perfusion alteration (cardiopulmonary)
- Tissue perfusion alteration (peripheral)

Coronary artery disease
- Activity intolerance
- Anxiety
- Cardiac output, decreased
- Gas exchange impairment
- Health-seeking behaviors
- Home maintenance management impairment
- Knowledge deficit
- Management of therapeutic regimen, ineffective
- Nutrition alteration: More than body requirements
- Pain
- Role performance alteration
- Sexuality pattern alteration
- Tissue perfusion alteration (cardiopulmonary)

Endocarditis
- Activity intolerance
- Cardiac output, decreased
- Diversional activity deficit
- Fluid volume excess
- Knowledge deficit
- Nutrition alteration: Less than body requirements
- Thought process alteration
- Tissue perfusion alteration (peripheral)

Hypertension
- Cardiac output, decreased
- Fluid volume excess
- Health maintenance alteration
- Injury, high risk for
- Knowledge deficit
- Management of therapeutic regimen, ineffective
- Noncompliance
- Nutrition alteration: More than body requirements
- Pain
- Poisoning, high risk for
- Powerlessness
- Self-esteem, situational low
- Sexuality pattern alteration

Hypervolemia
- Tissue perfusion alteration
- Ventilation, spontaneous: Inability to sustain

Hypovolemia
- Fluid volume deficit
- Tissue perfusion alteration (renal)
- Ventilation, spontaneous: Inability to sustain

Hypovolemic shock
- Cardiac output, decreased
- Oral mucous membrane alteration
- Tissue perfusion alteration (cardiopulmonary, renal)

Leriche's syndrome
- Pain
- Sexual dysfunction
- Skin integrity impairment
- Tissue perfusion alteration (peripheral)

Mitral stenosis or insufficiency
- Activity intolerance
- Cardiac output, decreased
- Fatigue
- Thought process alteration
- Tissue perfusion alteration (cardiopulmonary)

Myocardial infarction
- Activity intolerance
- Adjustment impairment
- Anxiety
- Aspiration, high risk for
- Cardiac output, decreased
- Coping, ineffective individual
- Denial
- Hypothermia
- Nutrition alteration: More than body requirements
- Pain
- Poisoning, high risk for
- Self-esteem, situational low
- Sexual dysfunction
- Sexuality pattern alteration
- Sleep pattern disturbance
- Tissue perfusion alteration (peripheral, renal)

Neurogenic shock
- Cardiac output, decreased
- Tissue perfusion alteration (cardiopulmonary, renal)

Pericarditis
- Anxiety
- Breathing pattern, ineffective
- Cardiac output, decreased
- Fluid volume excess
- Pain
- Tissue perfusion alteration (cardiopulmonary)

Peripheral circulatory failure
- Peripheral neurovascular dysfunction, high risk for

Peripheral vascular disorder
- Activity intolerance
- Disuse syndrome, high risk for
- Diversional activity deficit
- Infection, high risk for
- Mobility impairment
- Peripheral neurovascular dysfunction, high risk for
- Skin integrity impairment
- Skin integrity impairment, high risk for
- Tissue integrity impairment
- Urinary elimination pattern alteration

Pulmonary artery infarct
- Tissue perfusion alteration (cardiopulmonary)

Raynaud's disease
- Sensory or perceptual alteration (tactile)
- Skin integrity impairment, high risk for
- Thermoregulation, ineffective
- Tissue integrity impairment
- Tissue perfusion alteration (peripheral)

Rheumatic heart disease
- Activity intolerance
- Cardiac output, decreased
- Pain
- Skin integrity impairment

Tetralogy of Fallot
- Activity intolerance
- Cardiac output, decreased
- Growth and development alteration

Thrombophlebitis
- Pain
- Skin integrity impairment
- Skin integrity impairment, high risk for
- Tissue perfusion alteration

Varicose veins
- Pain
- Self-esteem, situational low
- Tissue perfusion alteration

Vascular insufficiency
- Peripheral neurovascular dysfunction, high risk for

Vascular occlusion
- Peripheral neurovascular dysfunction, high risk for

Venous ulcers
- Skin integrity impairment
- Skin integrity impairment, high risk for

Endocrine disorders

Adrenal insufficiency (Addison's disease)
- Body image disturbance
- Body temperature alteration, high risk for
- Coping, ineffective family
- Fluid volume deficit
- Hopelessness
- Hypothermia
- Infection, high risk for
- Self-esteem, chronic low
- Sexual dysfunction
- Sleep pattern disturbance
- Tissue perfusion alteration (peripheral)

Cushing's syndrome
- Activity intolerance
- Body image disturbance
- Body temperature alteration, high risk for
- Coping, ineffective family
- Coping, ineffective individual
- Fluid volume excess
- Grieving, dysfunctional
- Hopelessness
- Nutrition alteration: Less than body requirements
- Self-esteem, chronic low
- Sexual dysfunction
- Skin integrity impairment

Diabetes insipidus
- Body temperature alteration, high risk for
- Coping, ineffective family
- Fluid volume deficit, high risk for
- Hopelessness
- Oral mucous membrane alteration

Diabetes mellitus
- Adjustment impairment
- Body image disturbance
- Body temperature alteration, high risk for
- Cardiac output, decreased
- Constipation
- Coping, ineffective family
- Coping, ineffective individual
- Fluid volume deficit, high risk for
- Grieving, anticipatory
- Hopelessness
- Hyperthermia
- Hypothermia
- Incontinence, stress
- Incontinence, total
- Infection, high risk for
- Injury, high risk for
- Knowledge deficit
- Management of therapeutic regimen, ineffective
- Noncompliance
- Nutrition alteration: More than body requirements
- Nutrition alteration, high risk for: More than body requirements
- Oral mucous membrane alteration
- Poisoning, high risk for
- Powerlessness
- Role performance alteration
- Self-esteem, chronic low

- Sensory or perceptual alteration (auditory, olfactory, visual, tactile)
- Sexual dysfunction
- Sexuality pattern alteration
- Skin integrity impairment
- Skin integrity impairment, high risk for
- Social isolation
- Tissue integrity impairment
- Tissue perfusion alteration (peripheral, renal)
- Urinary elimination pattern alteration

Diabetic ketoacidosis
- Body temperature alteration, high risk for
- Social interaction impairment
- Thought process alteration

Diabetic neuropathy
- Body temperature alteration, high risk for
- Coping, ineffective family
- Incontinence, bowel
- Pain, chronic
- Urinary retention

Hyperglycemia
- Nutrition alteration: More than body requirements

Hyperosmolar nonketotic syndrome
- Fluid volume deficit
- Nutrition alteration: More than body requirements

Hyperparathyroidism
- Anxiety
- Body temperature alteration, high risk for
- Breathing pattern, ineffective
- Coping, ineffective family
- Coping, ineffective individual
- Fluid volume deficit, high risk for
- Hopelessness
- Nutrition alteration: Less than body requirements
- Self-esteem, chronic low
- Sexual dysfunction
- Skin integrity impairment, high risk for
- Thought process alteration

Hyperpituitarism (acromegaly)
- Activity intolerance
- Body image disturbance
- Body temperature alteration, high risk for
- Coping, ineffective family
- Coping, ineffective individual
- Hopelessness
- Pain
- Self-esteem, chronic low
- Sexual dysfunction

Hyperthyroidism (Graves' disease, thyrotoxicosis)
- Body image disturbance
- Body temperature alteration, high risk for
- Cardiac output, decreased
- Coping, ineffective family
- Diarrhea
- Fluid volume deficit, high risk for

Hypoparathyroidism
- Body temperature alteration, high risk for
- Breathing pattern, ineffective
- Cardiac output, decreased
- Constipation
- Coping, ineffective family
- Coping, ineffective individual
- Hopelessness
- Nutrition alteration: More than body requirements
- Self-esteem, chronic low
- Skin integrity impairment
- Thought process alteration

Hypothyroidism (myxedema)
- Body image disturbance
- Body temperature alteration, high risk for
- Constipation, colonic
- Coping, family: Potential for growth
- Coping, ineffective family
- Coping, ineffective individual
- Fluid volume excess
- Hopelessness
- Hypothermia
- Incontinence, functional
- Mobility impairment
- Self-esteem, chronic low
- Sexuality pattern alteration

Eye, ear, nose, and throat disorders

Blindness
- Body image disturbance
- Diversional activity deficit
- Fear
- Injury, high risk for
- Mobility impairment
- Powerlessness
- Role performance alteration
- Sensory or perceptual alteration (visual)

Cataracts
- Activity intolerance
- Body image disturbance
- Coping, ineffective individual
- Grieving, anticipatory
- Health maintenance alteration
- Injury, high risk for
- Pain
- Poisoning, high risk for
- Self-esteem, situational low
- Sensory or perceptual alteration (visual)

Deafness
- Body image disturbance
- Diversional activity deficit
- Fear
- Injury, high risk for
- Role performance alteration
- Sensory or perceptual alteration (auditory)
- Verbal communication impairment

Detached retina
- Body image disturbance
- Diversional activity deficit
- Mobility impairment
- Pain
- Sensory or perceptual alteration (visual)

Diabetic retinopathy
- Sensory or perceptual alteration (visual)

Glaucoma
- Activity intolerance
- Body image disturbance
- Diversional activity deficit
- Pain
- Poisoning, high risk for
- Sensory or perceptual alteration (visual)

Laryngitis
- Oral mucous membrane alteration
- Pain
- Verbal communication impairment

Macular degeneration
- Activity intolerance
- Body image disturbance
- Powerlessness
- Sensory or perceptual alteration (visual)

Ménière's disease
- Mobility impairment
- Sensory or perceptual alteration (auditory)
- Trauma, high risk for

Nasal polyps
- Sensory or perceptual alteration (olfactory)

Nasopharyngitis
- Sensory or perceptual alteration (olfactory)

Otitis media
- Body image disturbance
- Infection, high risk for
- Sensory or perceptual alteration (auditory)
- Verbal communication impairment

Otosclerosis
- Body image disturbance
- Pain
- Sensory or perceptual alteration (auditory)
- Sleep pattern disturbance

Presbycusis
- Body image disturbance
- Denial
- Sensory or perceptual alteration (auditory)

Presbyopia
- Body image disturbance
- Denial
- Sensory or perceptual alteration (visual)

Retinitis pigmentosa
- Injury, high risk for
- Sensory or perceptual alteration (visual)

Rhinitis or sinusitis
- Sensory or perceptual alteration (olfactory)

Tinnitus
- Injury, high risk for
- Sensory or perceptual alteration (auditory)

Gastrointestinal disorders

Appendicitis
- Infection, high risk for
- Nutrition alteration: Less than body requirements
- Pain
- Skin integrity impairment

Atonic colon
- Constipation
- Nutrition alteration: Less than body requirements
- Pain

Celiac disease
- Diarrhea
- Fluid volume deficit
- Nutrition alteration: Less than body requirements

Colitis
- Adjustment impairment
- Body image disturbance
- Constipation, colonic
- Diarrhea
- Fluid volume deficit
- Nutrition alteration: Less than body requirements
- Pain
- Tissue perfusion alteration (gastrointestinal)

Constipation
- Constipation
- Constipation, colonic
- Constipation, perceived
- Pain

Crohn's disease
- Body image disturbance
- Coping, ineffective family
- Coping, ineffective individual
- Diarrhea
- Fluid volume deficit
- Fluid volume deficit, high risk for
- Hopelessness
- Nutrition alteration: Less than body requirements
- Pain
- Self-esteem, chronic low
- Self-esteem, situational low
- Sexual dysfunction
- Skin integrity impairment
- Tissue perfusion alteration (gastrointestinal)

Diverticulitis
- Constipation
- Diarrhea
- Fluid volume deficit
- Nutrition alteration: Less than body requirements
- Nutrition alteration: More than body requirements
- Poisoning, high risk for

Dumping syndrome
- Anxiety
- Diarrhea
- Nutrition alteration: Less than body requirements

Duodenal ulcer
- Fluid volume deficit
- Tissue perfusion alteration (gastrointestinal)

Esophageal or tracheal anomalies
- Ventilatory weaning response, dysfunctional

Esophageal varices
- Diarrhea
- Fluid volume deficit
- Fluid volume deficit, high risk for

- Nutrition alteration: Less than body requirements
- Skin integrity impairment
- Thought process alteration
- Tissue perfusion alteration (gastrointestinal)

Gastritis
- Fluid volume deficit, high risk for
- Nutrition alteration: Less than body requirements
- Pain

Gastroenteritis (food poisoning, intestinal flu)
- Diarrhea
- Fluid volume deficit
- Pain

Gastroesophageal reflux
- Airway clearance, ineffective
- Aspiration, high risk for
- Nutrition alteration: Less than body requirements

Gingivitis, glossitis, periodontitis, and stomatitis
- Nutrition alteration: Less than body requirements
- Oral mucous membrane alteration
- Pain

Hemorrhoids
- Constipation
- Knowledge deficit
- Pain

Hernia
- Activity intolerance
- Aspiration, high risk for
- Breathing pattern, ineffective
- Constipation
- Pain

Intestinal obstruction
- Aspiration, high risk for
- Constipation
- Fluid volume deficit, high risk for
- Fluid volume excess
- Incontinence, urge
- Nutrition alteration: Less than body requirements
- Pain
- Tissue perfusion alteration (gastrointestinal)
- Urinary retention

Intussusception
- Constipation
- Diarrhea
- Pain

Irritable bowel syndrome
- Body image disturbance
- Constipation
- Diarrhea

Malabsorption syndrome
- Diarrhea
- Nutrition alteration: Less than body requirements
- Thought process alteration

Pancreatitis
- Fluid volume deficit
- Hopelessness
- Hypothermia
- Nutrition alteration: Less than body requirements
- Pain
- Tissue perfusion alteration (gastrointestinal)

Paralytic ileus
- Constipation
- Fluid volume deficit, high risk for
- Nutrition alteration: Less than body requirements
- Tissue perfusion alteration (gastrointestinal)

Peptic ulcer
- Fluid volume deficit
- Noncompliance
- Nutrition alteration: Less than body requirements
- Pain
- Tissue perfusion alteration

Peritonitis
- Constipation
- Infection, high risk for
- Nutrition alteration: Less than body requirements
- Tissue perfusion alteration

Tracheoesophageal fistula
- Aspiration, high risk for
- Nutrition alteration: Less than body requirements

Genetic disorders

Albinism
- Body image disturbance
- Coping, ineffective family
- Coping, ineffective individual
- Sensory or perceptual alteration (visual)
- Skin integrity impairment, high risk for

Cleft lip or palate
- Aspiration, high risk for
- Breast-feeding, ineffective
- Coping, family: Potential for growth
- Infant feeding pattern, ineffective
- Nutrition alteration: Less than body requirements
- Verbal communication impairment

Congenital heart disease
- Breathing pattern, ineffective
- Cardiac output, decreased
- Hypothermia
- Thermoregulation, ineffective

Cystic fibrosis
- Airway clearance, ineffective
- Body temperature alteration, high risk for
- Breathing pattern, ineffective
- Coping, family: Potential for growth
- Diversional activity deficit
- Fluid volume deficit
- Hypothermia
- Parental role conflict

Down's syndrome
- Coping, ineffective family
- Growth and development alteration
- Hypothermia
- Parental role conflict

Hemophilia
- Altered protection
- Body temperature alteration, high risk for
- Coping, family: Potential for growth
- Gas exchange impairment
- Hypothermia
- Parental role conflict
- Self-esteem, chronic low
- Tissue perfusion alteration
- Trauma, high risk for

Sickle cell anemia or sickle-cell crisis
- Gas exchange impairment
- Mobility impairment
- Pain
- Tissue perfusion alteration (renal, venous)

Genitourinary disorders

Atrophic urethritis
- Incontinence, stress

Benign prostatic hypertrophy
- Sexual dysfunction
- Sexuality pattern alteration
- Urinary elimination pattern alteration
- Urinary retention

Cystitis
- Coping, ineffective individual
- Incontinence, urge
- Pain
- Sexual dysfunction
- Sexuality pattern alteration
- Sleep pattern disturbance
- Urinary elimination pattern alteration

Ectopic ureter, epispadias, and bladder exstrophy
- Incontinence, total
- Sexual dysfunction
- Sexuality pattern alteration
- Urinary elimination pattern alteration

Urinary tract infection
- Incontinence, stress
- Incontinence, urge
- Infection, high risk for
- Pain
- Poisoning, high risk for
- Urinary elimination pattern alteration

Hematologic disorders

Anemia
- Activity intolerance
- Altered protection
- Body temperature alteration, high risk for
- Breathing pattern, ineffective
- Cardiac output, decreased
- Fatigue
- Gas exchange impairment
- Infection, high risk for
- Injury, high risk for
- Sensory or perceptual alteration (olfactory)
- Skin integrity impairment
- Skin integrity impairment, high risk for
- Tissue integrity impairment
- Tissue perfusion alteration (cardiopulmonary)

Disseminated intravascular coagulation
- Altered protection
- Anxiety
- Body temperature alteration, high risk for
- Injury, high risk for
- Tissue perfusion alteration (renal)

Polycythemia vera
- Fatigue
- Gas exchange impairment
- Sensory or perceptual alteration (visual)

Thalassemia
- Anxiety
- Gas exchange impairment
- Growth and development alteration

Thrombocytopenia
- Altered protection
- Gas exchange impairment
- Infection, high risk for
- Injury, high risk for
- Tissue perfusion alteration (venous)
- Trauma, high risk for

Hepatobiliary disorders

Cirrhosis
- Breathing pattern, ineffective
- Coping, ineffective family
- Fluid volume excess
- Hopelessness
- Hypothermia
- Incontinence, stress
- Infection, high risk for
- Knowledge deficit
- Nutrition alteration: Less than body requirements
- Nutrition alteration: More than body requirements
- Powerlessness
- Self-care deficit
- Skin integrity impairment
- Skin integrity impairment, high risk for
- Social isolation
- Thought process alteration
- Tissue integrity impairment
- Tissue perfusion alteration (venous)

Gallbladder disorders
- Gas exchange impairment
- Nutrition alteration: Less than body requirements
- Pain

Hepatic disease or hepatic failure
- Cardiac output, decreased
- Hopelessness
- Incontinence, functional
- Poisoning, high risk for
- Tissue perfusion alteration (gastrointestinal, venous)

Hepatitis
- Hopelessness
- Infection, high risk for
- Nutrition alteration: Less than body requirements
- Sensory or perceptual alteration (gustatory)
- Skin integrity impairment, high risk for
- Social isolation

Laënnec's cirrhosis
- Fluid volume excess
- Health maintenance alteration
- Hopelessness
- Mobility impairment
- Self-care deficit
- Skin integrity impairment

Immune disorders

Acquired immunodeficiency syndrome (AIDS)
- Altered protection
- Caregiver role strain
- Caregiver role strain, high risk for
- Coping, defensive
- Denial
- Grieving, anticipatory
- Hopelessness
- Incontinence, urge
- Infection, high risk for
- Management of therapeutic regimen, ineffective
- Parental role conflict
- Powerlessness
- Sexuality pattern alteration
- Social isolation
- Tissue integrity impairment

Anaphylaxis
- Anxiety
- Cardiac output, decreased
- Diarrhea

Ankylosing spondylitis
- Activity intolerance
- Fatigue
- Mobility impairment
- Pain

Dermatomyositis and polymyositis
- Activity intolerance
- Disuse syndrome, high risk for
- Growth and development alteration
- Health maintenance alteration
- Mobility impairment
- Skin integrity impairment

Graft-versus-host disease
- Altered protection
- Infection, high risk for
- Powerlessness

Juvenile rheumatoid arthritis
- Grieving, anticipatory
- Growth and development alteration
- Mobility impairment
- Sensory or perceptual alteration (tactile)

Lupus erythematosus
- Airway clearance, ineffective
- Fluid volume excess
- Grieving, anticipatory
- Hopelessness
- Infection, high risk for
- Mobility impairment
- Tissue perfusion alteration (peripheral)

Muscular dystrophy
- Caregiver role strain
- Caregiver role strain, high risk for
- Coping, family: Potential for growth
- Fatigue
- Health maintenance alteration
- Hopelessness
- Injury, high risk for
- Mobility impairment
- Self-care deficit
- Sensory or perceptual alteration (kinesthetic)

Rheumatoid arthritis
- Activity intolerance
- Altered protection
- Body image disturbance
- Coping, ineffective family
- Coping, ineffective individual
- Denial
- Disuse syndrome, high risk for
- Fatigue
- Grieving, anticipatory
- Health maintenance alteration
- Home maintenance management impairment
- Hopelessness
- Infection, high risk for
- Injury, high risk for
- Knowledge deficit
- Management of therapeutic regimen, ineffective
- Mobility impairment
- Pain
- Pain, chronic
- Poisoning, high risk for

- Powerlessness
- Role performance alteration
- Self-care deficit
- Self-esteem, situational low
- Sensory or perceptual alteration (tactile)
- Sexual dysfunction
- Sexuality pattern alteration
- Social isolation
- Tissue perfusion alteration (peripheral)

Sjögren's syndrome
- Oral mucus membrane alteration
- Pain
- Sensory or perceptual alteration (gustatory)

Infection

- Activity intolerance
- Breathing pattern, ineffective
- Fluid volume deficit, high risk for
- Hyperthermia
- Incontinence, functional
- Incontinence, urge
- Pain
- Thermoregulation, ineffective
- Thought process alteration
- Tissue integrity impairment

Amebiasis and *Campylobacter* dysentery
- Diarrhea
- Fluid volume deficit
- Fluid volume deficit, high risk for

Candidiasis
- Oral mucous membrane alteration
- Skin integrity impairment
- Swallowing impairment

Chronic fatigue and immune dysfunction syndrome
- Activity intolerance
- Fatigue
- Management of therapeutic regimen, ineffective

Common cold
- Fatigue
- Sensory or perceptual alteration (gustatory, olfactory)

Herpes zoster
- Sensory or perceptual alteration (tactile)

Influenza
- Activity intolerance
- Hyperthermia
- Sensory or perceptual alteration (gustatory)

Poliomyelitis
- Fatigue
- Health maintenance alteration
- Mobility impairment

Rabies
- Anxiety
- Fluid volume deficit, high risk for
- Sensory or perceptual alteration (tactile)

Rubella (German measles)
- Hyperthermia
- Infection, high risk for
- Skin integrity impairment

Salmonellosis and shigellosis
- Diarrhea
- Fluid volume deficit
- Fluid volume deficit, high risk for
- Urinary retention

Septic shock
- Body temperature alteration
- Cardiac output, decreased
- Tissue perfusion alteration (cardiopulmonary, renal)

Streptococcal infection
- Infection, high risk for
- Ventilation, spontaneous: Inability to sustain

Tetanus
- Disuse syndrome, high risk for
- Health maintenance alteration
- Injury, high risk for
- Mobility impairment

Trichinosis
- Diarrhea
- Fluid volume deficit

Integumentary disorders

Cellulitis
- Mobility impairment
- Pain
- Skin integrity impairment

Dermatitis (eczema)
- Body temperature alteration, high risk for
- Skin integrity impairment
- Tissue integrity impairment

Open wounds and lesions
- Infection, high risk for
- Skin integrity impairment
- Skin integrity impairment, high risk for
- Tissue integrity impairment

Pressure sores
- Altered protection
- Diversional activity deficit
- Infection, high risk for
- Skin integrity impairment

Psoriasis
- Body image disturbance
- Body temperature alteration, high risk for
- Powerlessness
- Skin integrity impairment
- Social isolation

Mental and emotional disorders

Affective disorders (cyclothymic, dysthymic, organic)
- Anxiety
- Coping, ineffective individual
- Powerlessness
- Role performance alteration
- Sensory or perceptual alteration
- Sexual dysfunction
- Thought process alteration

Alcoholism
- Altered protection
- Caregiver role strain
- Caregiver role strain, high risk for
- Coping, defensive
- Coping, ineffective individual
- Denial
- Incontinence, functional
- Mobility impairment
- Oral mucous membrane alteration
- Powerlessness
- Self-care deficit
- Sensory or perceptual alteration (tactile)
- Sexual dysfunction
- Sleep pattern disturbance
- Social isolation
- Tissue integrity impairment
- Violence, high risk for

Anorexia nervosa and bulimia
- Anxiety
- Body image disturbance
- Constipation
- Denial
- Family process alteration
- Fluid volume deficit
- Hyperthermia
- Nutrition alteration: Less than body requirements
- Oral mucous membrane alteration
- Parenting alteration
- Powerlessness
- Self-esteem, chronic low
- Sleep pattern disturbance
- Social isolation

Anxiety disorders (obsessive-compulsive disorder, panic disorder, posttraumatic stress disorder)
- Anxiety
- Constipation, colonic
- Coping, defensive
- Denial
- Diarrhea
- Home maintenance management impairment
- Incontinence, functional
- Nutrition alteration: More than body requirements

- Nutrition alteration, high risk for: More than body requirements
- Powerlessness
- Self-esteem, chronic low
- Self-esteem disturbance
- Sensory or perceptual alteration
- Thought process alteration
- Verbal communication impairment

Autism
- Health maintenance alteration
- Self-care deficit
- Self-mutilation, high risk for

Bipolar disorder: Depressive phase
- Constipation
- Coping, ineffective individual
- Denial
- Health maintenance alteration
- Home maintenance management impairment
- Hopelessness
- Mobility impairment
- Nutrition alteration: Less than body requirements
- Powerlessness
- Self-care deficit
- Self-esteem, chronic low
- Sensory or perceptual alteration
- Sexual dysfunction
- Sleep pattern disturbance
- Social isolation
- Thought process alteration
- Urinary elimination pattern alteration
- Verbal communication impairment
- Violence, high risk for: Self-directed

Bipolar disorder: Manic phase
- Coping, ineffective individual
- Denial
- Health maintenance alteration
- Home maintenance management impairment
- Mobility impairment
- Nutrition alteration: Less than body requirements
- Self-care deficit
- Self-esteem, chronic low
- Sensory or perceptual alteration
- Sexual dysfunction
- Sleep pattern disturbance
- Social isolation
- Thought process alteration
- Verbal communication impairment
- Violence, high risk for: Other-directed

Delusional disorders (organic, paranoid)
- Home maintenance management impairment
- Powerlessness
- Sensory or perceptual alteration
- Thought process alteration

Dementia
- Activity intolerance
- Caregiver role strain
- Caregiver role strain, high risk for
- Family process alteration
- Incontinence, functional
- Incontinence, urge
- Injury, high risk for
- Powerlessness
- Role performance alteration
- Sensory or perceptual alteration
- Verbal communication impairment
- Violence, high risk for: Self-directed

Depression
- Constipation
- Constipation, colonic
- Coping, ineffective family
- Coping, ineffective individual
- Denial
- Diversional activity deficit
- Fatigue
- Home maintenance management impairment
- Hopelessness
- Hyperthermia
- Incontinence, functional
- Incontinence, stress
- Injury, high risk for
- Nutrition alteration: Less than body requirements
- Nutrition alteration: More than body requirements
- Nutrition alteration, high risk for: More than body requirements
- Oral mucous membrane alteration
- Pain
- Parenting alteration
- Poisoning, high risk for
- Powerlessness
- Self-esteem, chronic low
- Self-esteem disturbance
- Sensory or perceptual alteration

- Sexual dysfunction
- Sleep pattern disturbance
- Social isolation
- Violence, high risk for: Self-directed

Drug addiction
- Caregiver role strain
- Caregiver role strain, high risk for
- Coping, defensive
- Coping, ineffective individual
- Denial
- Health maintenance alteration
- Powerlessness
- Sexual dysfunction
- Sleep pattern disturbance

Drug or alcohol withdrawal
- Coping, ineffective individual
- Powerlessness
- Sensory or perceptual alteration
- Social interaction impairment
- Thought process alteration
- Violence, high risk for

Dyslexia
- Growth and development alteration
- Self-esteem disturbance

Factitious disorder
- Coping, ineffective individual
- Self-mutilation, high risk for

Hypochondriasis
- Anxiety
- Coping, ineffective individual
- Health maintenance alteration
- Powerlessness
- Thought process alteration

Korsakoff's psychosis
- Sleep pattern disturbance
- Thought process alteration
- Violence, high risk for

Malingering
- Coping, ineffective individual
- Self-mutilation, high risk for

Maternal psychological stress
- Anxiety
- Breast-feeding, ineffective
- Breast-feeding, interrupted
- Powerlessness

Mental retardation
- Coping, family: Potential for growth
- Growth and development alteration
- Health maintenence alteration
- Incontinence, functional
- Injury, high risk for
- Knowledge deficit
- Poisoning, high risk for
- Powerlessness
- Self-care deficit
- Self-mutilation, high risk for

Multiple personality disorder
- Home maintenance management impairment
- Personal identity disturbance
- Self-mutilation, high risk for

Personality disorders (antisocial, borderline, dependent, impulse control, narcissistic)
- Coping, ineffective individual
- Home maintenance management impairment
- Powerlessness
- Role performance alteration
- Self-esteem, chronic low
- Self-esteem disturbance
- Self-mutilation, high risk for
- Sensory or perceptual alteration
- Sexual dysfunction
- Violence, high risk for

Phobic disorders
- Anxiety
- Home maintenance management impairment
- Powerlessness
- Fear

Psychoses
- Health maintenance alteration
- Self-care deficit
- Sexual dysfunction
- Thought process alteration
- Verbal communication impairment
- Violence, high risk for

Psychosexual disorders (paraphilias)
- Anxiety
- Coping, defensive
- Denial
- Personal identity disturbance

- Role performance alteration
- Self-esteem, chronic low
- Self-mutilation, high risk for
- Sexual dysfunction
- Social interaction impairment
- Violence, high risk for

Schizophrenia
- Anxiety
- Caregiver role strain
- Caregiver role strain, high risk for
- Coping, ineffective individual
- Fluid volume deficit
- Home maintenance management impairment
- Hopelessness
- Incontinence, functional
- Nutrition alteration: Less than body requirements
- Poisoning, high risk for
- Powerlessness
- Role performance alteration
- Self-care deficit
- Sensory or perceptual alteration
- Sexual dysfunction
- Sleep pattern disturbance
- Social isolation
- Thought process alteration
- Violence, high risk for: Self-directed

Self-destructive or suicidal behavior
- Anxiety
- Denial
- Injury, high risk for
- Poisoning, high risk for
- Self-esteem, chronic low
- Self-mutilation, high risk for
- Violence, high risk for: Self-directed

Spouse abuse
- Posttrauma response
- Rape-trauma syndrome
- Violence, high risk for: Other-directed

Substance abuse
- Anxiety
- Coping, ineffective individual
- Home maintenance management impairment
- Incontinence, functional
- Infection, high risk for
- Parenting alteration
- Powerlessness
- Role performance alteration
- Self-esteem, chronic low
- Self-esteem disturbance
- Thought process alteration
- Violence, high risk for

Metabolic and nutritional disorders

Homeostatic imbalance (hypocalcemia, hypokalemia)
- Cardiac output, decreased
- Constipation, colonic
- Sensory or perceptual alteration (tactile)
- Thermoregulation, ineffective

Hypoglycemia
- Hypothermia
- Incontinence, functional
- Nutrition alteration: Less than body requirements
- Self-esteem, chronic low
- Thought process alteration

Lactose intolerance
- Diarrhea
- Fluid volume deficit

Malnutrition
- Altered protection
- Fluid volume excess
- Infection, high risk for
- Nutrition alteration: Less than body requirements
- Oral mucous membrane alteration
- Skin integrity impairment
- Skin integrity impairment, high risk for
- Social isolation
- Thought process alteration

Metabolic acidosis
- Breathing pattern, ineffective
- Fluid volume deficit
- Self-esteem, chronic low
- Thought process alteration

Metabolic alkalosis
- Breathing pattern, ineffective
- Fluid volume deficit, high risk for
- Sensory or perceptual alteration

Obesity
- Incontinence, stress
- Nutrition alteration: More than body requirements
- Nutrition alteration, high risk for: More than body requirements
- Self-esteem, situational low
- Skin integrity impairment, high risk for
- Tissue integrity impairment
- Ventilatory weaning response, dysfunctional

Pellagra
- Mobility impairment
- Nutrition alteration: Less than body requirements
- Skin integrity impairment

Scurvy
- Infection, high risk for
- Nutrition alteration: Less than body requirements
- Oral mucous membrane alteration

Vitamin deficiencies
- Mobility impairment
- Sensory or perceptual alteration (gustatory, tactile)
- Urinary retention

Musculoskeletal disorders

Backache
- Activity intolerance
- Activity intolerance, high risk for
- Adjustment impairment
- Fatigue
- Injury, high risk for
- Pain
- Pain, chronic
- Sexuality pattern alteration

Bursitis and tendinitis
- Activity intolerance
- Disuse syndrome, high risk for
- Fatigue
- Injury, high risk for
- Mobility impairment
- Role performance alteration

Carpal tunnel syndrome
- Mobility impairment
- Pain
- Peripheral neurovascular dysfunction, high risk for

Compartment syndrome
- Peripheral neurovascular dysfunction, high risk for

Degenerative joint disease
- Nutrition alteration: More than body requirements
- Poisoning, high risk for
- Powerlessness
- Skin integrity impairment, high risk for
- Social isolation

Gout and osteoarthritis
- Activity intolerance
- Body image disturbance
- Home maintenance management impairment
- Injury, high risk for
- Knowledge deficit
- Mobility impairment
- Nutrition alteration: More than body requirements
- Pain
- Self-care deficit
- Sensory or perceptual alteration (tactile)

Herniated disk
- Mobility impairment
- Pain
- Sensory or perceptual alteration (tactile)
- Sexuality pattern alteration
- Urinary retention

Osteomyelitis
- Body image disturbance
- Coping, ineffective individual
- Injury, high risk for
- Mobility impairment
- Pain
- Skin integrity impairment
- Tissue perfusion alteration

Osteoporosis
- Body image disturbance
- Denial
- Injury, high risk for
- Powerlessness
- Sexuality pattern alteration
- Social isolation
- Trauma, high risk for

Paget's disease
- Cardiac output, decreased
- Fatigue
- Injury, high risk for
- Mobility impairment
- Pain

Paralysis (hemiplegia, paraplegia, quadriplegia)
- Adjustment impairment
- Caregiver role strain
- Caregiver role strain, high risk for
- Coping, ineffective family
- Coping, ineffective individual
- Grieving, dysfunctional
- Health maintenance alteration
- Hopelessness
- Incontinence, bowel
- Incontinence, reflex
- Mobility impairment
- Powerlessness
- Role performance alteration
- Sexuality pattern alteration
- Skin integrity impairment
- Skin integrity impairment, high risk for

Prolapsed intervertebral disk
- Incontinence, reflex
- Mobility impairment
- Pain
- Urinary elimination pattern alteration

Neonatal disorders

Birth trauma
- Growth and development alteration
- Hypothermia
- Injury, high risk for

Fetal alcohol syndrome
- Growth and development alteration

Hyperbilirubinemia
- Breast-feeding, interrupted
- Fluid volume deficit, high risk for
- Injury, high risk for
- Nutrition alteration: Less than body requirements

Meconium aspiration syndrome
- Breathing pattern, ineffective
- Injury, high risk for

Neonatal anomaly
- Breast-feeding, ineffective
- Breast-feeding, interrupted
- Infant feeding pattern, ineffective

Neurologic impairment (neonatal)
- Infant feeding pattern, ineffective

Perinatal asphyxia
- Aspiration, high risk for
- Breathing pattern, ineffective
- Coping, ineffective family
- Growth and development alteration
- Hypothermia
- Injury, high risk for

Postmaturity
- Skin integrity impairment
- Thermoregulation, ineffective

Prematurity
- Aspiration, high risk for
- Breast-feeding, ineffective
- Breast-feeding, interrupted
- Breathing pattern, ineffective
- Coping, ineffective family
- Growth and development alteration

- Hypothermia
- Infant feeding pattern, ineffective
- Nutrition alteration: Less than body requirements
- Parental role conflict
- Parenting alteration
- Parenting alteration, high risk for
- Thermoregulation, ineffective
- Verbal communication impairment

Sepsis
- Growth and development alteration
- Hypothermia
- Thermoregulation, ineffective
- Ventilation, spontaneous: Inability to sustain
- Ventilatory weaning response, dysfunctional

Neoplasms

– Activity intolerance
– Adjustment impairment
– Airway clearance, ineffective
– Anxiety
– Body image disturbance
– Caregiver role strain
– Caregiver role strain, high risk for
– Constipation
– Coping, defensive
– Coping, ineffective family
– Coping, ineffective individual
– Decisional conflict
– Denial
– Disuse syndrome, high risk for
– Diversional activity deficit
– Family process alteration
– Fluid volume deficit, high risk for
– Grieving, anticipatory
– Growth and development alteration
– Home maintenance management impairment
– Hopelessness
– Incontinence, urge
– Infection, high risk for
– Knowledge deficit
– Oral mucous membrane alteration
– Pain, chronic
– Powerlessness
– Self-care deficit
– Self-esteem, situational low
– Sexuality pattern alteration
– Skin integrity impairment
– Skin integrity impairment, high risk for
– Social isolation
– Tissue integrity impairment
– Tissue perfusion alteration (cerebral)
– Ventilatory weaning response, dysfunctional
– Violence, high risk for: Self-directed

Abdominal tumor
- Anxiety
- Pain
- Tissue perfusion alteration (venous)

Acoustic tumor
- Sensory or perceptual alteration (auditory)

Bladder cancer
- Incontinence, urge
- Pain
- Urinary elimination pattern alteration
- Urinary retention

Breast cancer
- Body image disturbance
- Fluid volume deficit, high risk for
- Pain

Facial tumor
- Body image disturbance
- Oral mucous membrane alteration
- Pain
- Self-esteem disturbance

Gastrointestinal tumor
- Constipation
- Diarrhea
- Nutrition alteration: Less than body requirements
- Tissue perfusion alteration (gastrointestinal)

Head or neck cancer
- Body image disturbance
- Oral mucous membrane alteration
- Pain

- Sensory or perceptual alteration (gustatory)
- Verbal communication impairment

Leukemia
- Altered protection
- Body temperature alteration, high risk for
- Gas exchange impairment
- Grieving, anticipatory
- Hopelessness
- Infection, high risk for
- Oral mucous membrane alteration
- Tissue integrity impairment

Lung cancer
- Activity intolerance
- Breathing pattern, ineffective
- Gas exchange impairment
- Powerlessness
- Verbal communication impairment

Lymphomas
- Altered protection
- Hopelessness
- Infection, high risk for

Multiple myeloma
- Altered protection
- Hopelessness
- Infection, high risk for

Nasal or sinus neoplasms
- Sensory or perceptual alteration (olfactory)

Nasopharyngeal tumor
- Sensory or perceptual alteration (auditory)

Pelvic tumor
- Incontinence, stress
- Pain
- Sexual dysfunction
- Urinary elimination pattern alteration

Prostate cancer
- Sexual dysfunction
- Urinary elimination pattern alteration
- Urinary retention

Neurologic disorders

Alcoholic cerebellar degeneration
- Verbal communication impairment

Altered level of consciousness
- Aspiration, high risk for
- Fluid volume deficit, high risk for
- Incontinence, functional
- Self-care deficit
- Thought process alteration

Alzheimer's disease
- Caregiver role strain
- Caregiver role strain, high risk for
- Coping, ineffective family
- Coping, ineffective individual
- Health maintenance alteration
- Home maintenance management impairment
- Hopelessness
- Incontinence, bowel
- Incontinence, functional
- Incontinence, stress
- Incontinence, urge
- Injury, high risk for
- Knowledge deficit
- Nutrition alteration: Less than body requirements
- Poisoning, high risk for
- Role performance alteration
- Self-care deficit
- Self-esteem, chronic low
- Sexuality pattern alteration
- Social interaction impairment
- Social isolation
- Thought process alteration
- Tissue integrity impairment
- Trauma, high risk for
- Verbal communication impairment
- Violence, high risk for

Amyotrophic lateral sclerosis
- Airway clearance, ineffective
- Breathing pattern, ineffective
- Caregiver role strain
- Caregiver role strain, high risk for
- Coping, family: Potential for growth
- Coping, ineffective family

- Coping, ineffective individual
- Grieving, anticipatory
- Health maintenance alteration
- Hopelessness
- Incontinence, bowel
- Mobility impairment
- Nutrition alteration: Less than body requirements
- Powerlessness
- Self-care deficit
- Self-esteem, chronic low
- Sexuality pattern alteration
- Social isolation
- Tissue integrity impairment
- Urinary elimination pattern alteration
- Ventilation, spontaneous: Inability to sustain
- Ventilatory weaning response, dysfunctional
- Verbal communication impairment

Bell's palsy
- Body image disturbance
- Neglect, unilateral
- Self-esteem, chronic low
- Self-esteem, situational low
- Sensory or perceptual alteration (gustatory)
- Sexuality pattern alteration
- Swallowing impairment

Brain abscess
- Airway clearance, ineffective
- Body image disturbance
- Injury, high risk for
- Mobility impairment
- Pain
- Self-esteem, chronic low
- Sensory or perceptual alteration
- Sexuality pattern alteration
- Skin integrity impairment
- Tissue perfusion alteration

Brain stem lesions
- Sensory or perceptial alteration (gustatory, olfactory)

Brain tumor
- Airway clearance, ineffective
- Altered protection
- Breathing pattern, ineffective
- Fear
- Health maintenance alteration
- Incontinence, bowel
- Incontinence, total
- Incontinence, urge
- Injury, high risk for
- Knowledge deficit
- Mobility impairment
- Neglect, unilateral
- Poisoning, high risk for
- Powerlessness
- Self-care deficit
- Self-esteem, chronic low
- Self-esteem, situational low
- Sensory or perceptual alteration (tactile)
- Sexuality pattern alteration
- Social interaction impairment
- Thermoregulation, ineffective
- Thought process alteration
- Tissue integrity impairment
- Tissue perfusion alteration
- Trauma, high risk for
- Verbal communication impairment
- Violence, high risk for

Cerebral aneurysm (berry aneurysm)
- Anxiety
- Mobility impairment
- Thermoregulation, ineffective
- Tissue integrity impairment
- Tissue perfusion alteration (cerebral)
- Verbal communication impairment

Cerebral edema
- Fluid volume excess
- Thermoregulation, ineffective
- Thought pattern alteration
- Tissue integrity impairment
- Tissue perfusion alteration (cerebral)

Cerebral palsy
- Caregiver role strain
- Caregiver role strain, high risk for
- Growth and development alteration
- Health maintenance alteration
- Mobility impairment
- Self-care deficit
- Self-esteem, chronic low
- Sensory or perceptual alteration (kinesthetic)
- Tissue integrity impairment
- Verbal communication impairment

Cerebral vasospasm
- Tissue perfusion alteration (cerebral)

Cerebrovascular accident
- Activity intolerance
- Activity intolerance, high risk for
- Airway clearance, ineffective
- Aspiration, high risk for
- Body image disturbance
- Breathing pattern, ineffective
- Caregiver role strain
- Caregiver role strain, high risk for
- Constipation, colonic
- Coping, ineffective family
- Disuse syndrome, high risk for
- Family process alteration
- Fatigue
- Gas exchange impairment
- Growth and development alteration
- Health maintenance alteration
- Home maintenance management impairment
- Hopelessness
- Hypothermia
- Incontinence, bowel
- Incontinence, functional
- Incontinence, reflex
- Incontinence, stress
- Incontinence, total
- Incontinence, urge
- Injury, high risk for
- Knowledge deficit
- Mobility impairment
- Neglect, unilateral
- Nutrition alteration: Less than body requirements
- Nutrition alteration: More than body requirements
- Poisoning, high risk for
- Powerlessness
- Self-care deficit
- Self-esteem, chronic low
- Self-esteem, situational low
- Sensory or perceptual alteration (tactile)
- Sexuality pattern alteration
- Skin integrity impairment
- Skin integrity impairment, high risk for
- Social interaction impairment
- Social isolation
- Swallowing impairment
- Thermoregulation, ineffective
- Thought process alteration
- Tissue perfusion alteration (cerebral)
- Trauma, high risk for
- Urinary elimination pattern alteration
- Verbal communication impairment

Coma
- Altered protection
- Constipation
- Incontinence, bowel
- Tissue integrity impairment

Encephalitis
- Activity intolerance
- Anxiety
- Constipation
- Coping, ineffective family
- Coping, ineffective individual
- Diversional activity deficit
- Fear
- Growth and development alteration
- Hopelessness
- Self-esteem, chronic low
- Sexuality pattern alteration
- Thermoregulation, ineffective
- Thought process alteration
- Tissue integrity impairment

Encephalopathy
- Health maintenance alteration
- Parenting alteration
- Self-esteem, chronic low
- Thought process alteration
- Tissue integrity impairment
- Verbal communication impairment
- Violence, high risk for

Guillain-Barré syndrome
- Activity intolerance
- Activity intolerance, high risk for
- Airway clearance, ineffective
- Anxiety
- Breathing pattern ineffective
- Coping, ineffective individual
- Fatigue
- Gas exchange impairment
- Incontinence, bowel
- Mobility impairment
- Pain
- Self-care deficit
- Self-esteem, chronic low

- Sensory or perceptual alteration (tactile)
- Sexuality pattern alteration
- Tissue integrity impairment
- Ventilation, spontaneous: Inability to sustain

Headache
- Pain
- Pain, chronic
- Sensory or perceptual alteration (tactile)
- Sexuality pattern alteration

Huntington's disease
- Caregiver role strain
- Caregiver role strain, high risk for
- Health maintenance alteration
- Incontinence, bowel
- Mobility impairment
- Self-care deficit
- Self-esteem, chronic low
- Tissue integrity impairment
- Verbal communication impairment

Hydrocephalus
- Coping, ineffective family
- Thermoregulation, ineffective
- Tissue integrity impairment
- Verbal communication impairment

Increased intracranial pressure
- Growth and development alteration
- Thermoregulation, ineffective
- Tissue integrity impairment

Meningitis
- Activity intolerance
- Hypothermia
- Incontinence, bowel
- Self-esteem, chronic low
- Sexuality pattern alteration
- Tissue integrity impairment
- Tissue perfusion alteration (cerebral)
- Verbal communication impairment

Multiple sclerosis
- Activity intolerance
- Activity intolerance, high risk for
- Airway clearance, ineffective
- Altered protection
- Caregiver role strain
- Caregiver role strain, high risk for
- Coping, family: Potential for growth
- Fatigue
- Grieving, anticipatory
- Health maintenance alteration
- Hopelessness
- Incontinence, bowel
- Incontinence, reflex
- Incontinence, total
- Incontinence, urge
- Infection, high risk for
- Management of therapeutic regimen, ineffective
- Mobility impairment
- Nutrition alteration: Less than body requirements
- Pain
- Self-care deficit
- Self-esteem, chronic low
- Sensory or perceptual alteration (kinesthetic, tactile)
- Sexuality pattern alteration
- Tissue integrity impairment
- Trauma, high risk for
- Urinary elimination pattern alteration
- Ventilation, spontaneous: Inability to sustain

Myasthenia gravis
- Airway clearance, ineffective
- Fatigue
- Gas exchange impairment
- Incontinence, bowel
- Mobility impairment
- Self-care deficit
- Self-esteem, chronic low
- Tissue integrity impairment
- Ventilatory weaning response, dysfunctional
- Verbal communication impairment

Organic brain syndrome
- Fluid volume deficit, high risk for
- Health maintenance alteration
- Incontinence, bowel
- Injury, high risk for
- Knowledge deficit
- Poisoning, high risk for
- Self-care deficit
- Self-esteem, chronic low
- Sensory or perceptual alteration
- Social interaction impairment
- Social isolation
- Thought process alteration

- Tissue integrity impairment
- Trauma, high risk for
- Verbal communication impairment
- Violence, high risk for

Parkinson's disease
- Activity intolerance
- Body image disturbance
- Breathing pattern ineffective
- Caregiver role strain
- Caregiver role strain, high risk for
- Constipation
- Coping, ineffective family
- Coping, ineffective individual
- Home maintenance management impairment
- Hopelessness
- Incontinence, reflex
- Incontinence, urge
- Injury, high risk for
- Knowledge deficit
- Management of therapeutic regimen, ineffective
- Mobility impairment
- Nutrition alteration: Less than body requirements
- Powerlessness
- Self-care deficit
- Self-esteem, chronic low
- Sensory or perceptual alteration
- Sexuality pattern alteration
- Social isolation
- Tissue integrity impairment
- Trauma, high risk for
- Ventilation, spontaneous: Inability to sustain
- Ventilatory weaning response, dysfunctional
- Verbal communication impairment

Peripheral neuritis
- Mobility impairment
- Pain
- Peripheral neurovascular dysfunction, high risk for
- Sensory or perceptual alteration (tactile)
- Skin integrity impairment, high risk for
- Swallowing impairment

Reye's syndrome
- Fluid volume deficit
- Growth and development alteration
- Mobility impairment
- Thermoregulation, ineffective

Seizure disorders
- Airway clearance, ineffective
- Anxiety
- Breathing pattern ineffective
- Growth and development alteration
- Incontinence, functional
- Injury, high risk for
- Powerlessness
- Self-esteem, chronic low
- Sensory or perceptual alteration (tactile)
- Sexuality pattern alteration
- Social isolation
- Tissue integrity impairment
- Trauma, high risk for

Spinal cord defects (myelomeningocele, spina bifida)
- Coping, family: Potential for growth
- Growth and development alteration
- Incontinence, total
- Self-esteem, chronic low
- Tissue integrity impairment
- Urinary elimination pattern alteration

Spinal tumor
- Breathing pattern ineffective
- Dysreflexia
- Incontinence, bowel
- Incontinence, reflex
- Incontinence, total
- Injury, high risk for
- Mobility impairment
- Self-care deficit
- Self-esteem, chronic low
- Self-esteem, situational low
- Sensory or perceptual alteration (kinesthetic)
- Sexuality pattern alteration
- Skin integrity impairment, high risk for
- Tissue integrity impairment
- Urinary elimination pattern alteration

Transient ischemic attack
- Sensory or perceptual alteration (tactile)
- Tissue perfusion alteration (cerebral)

Obstetric and gynecologic disorders

Abnormal rupture of membranes (premature, prolonged)
- Fluid volume deficit
- Hyperthermia
- Infection, high risk for

Abortion
- Grieving, dysfunctional
- Injury, high risk for
- Self-esteem disturbance
- Tissue perfusion alteration

Abruptio placentae
- Anxiety
- Grieving, dysfunctional
- Pain
- Tissue perfusion alteration

Amniotic fluid embolism
- Anxiety
- Injury, high risk for

Atrophic senile vaginitis
- Body image disturbance
- Incontinence, stress

Breast engorgement
- Breast-feeding, ineffective
- Infection, high risk for
- Pain
- Skin integrity impairment

Cyanotic maternal cardiac disease
- Cardiac output, decreased
- Injury, high risk for
- Tissue perfusion alteration

Ectopic pregnancy
- Fluid volume deficit
- Pain
- Tissue perfusion alteration

Endometriosis
- Anxiety
- Infection, high risk for
- Knowledge deficit
- Sexual dysfunction

Gestational diabetes
- Infection, high risk for
- Nutrition alteration: Less than body requirements

Hydatidiform mole
- Fluid volume deficit
- Grieving, anticipatory
- Pain

Hyperemesis gravidarum
- Fluid volume deficit
- Nutrition alteration: Less than body requirements
- Pain

Infertility
- Coping, ineffective individual
- Grieving, dysfunctional
- Knowledge deficit
- Self-esteem, situational low
- Self-esteem disturbance

Labor
- Anxiety
- Breast-feeding, effective
- Coping, ineffective individual
- Incontinence, total
- Injury, high risk for
- Knowledge deficit
- Pain
- Parenting alteration
- Parenting alteration, high risk for
- Self-esteem disturbance
- Skin integrity impairment

Maternal nipple anomaly
- Breast-feeding, ineffective
- Breast-feeding, interrupted
- Pain

Menopause
- Self-esteem disturbance
- Sexuality pattern alteration

Multiple births
- Anxiety
- Coping, ineffective individual
- Incontinence, stress
- Injury, high risk for
- Knowledge deficit
- Parenting alteration
- Parenting alteration, high risk for

Pelvic inflammatory disease
- Fluid volume deficit, high risk for
- Pain
- Sexual dysfunction
- Skin integrity impairment

Placenta previa
- Anxiety
- Grieving, dysfunctional
- Tissue perfusion alteration

Postpartum hemorrhage
- Anxiety
- Fluid volume deficit
- Tissue perfusion alteration

Pregnancy
- Anxiety
- Coping, ineffective individual
- Family process alteration
- Knowledge deficit
- Parenting alteration
- Parenting alteration, high risk for
- Tissue integrity impairment
- Tissue perfusion alteration (venous)

Pregnancy-induced hypertension
- Anxiety
- Diversional activity deficit
- Fear
- Fluid volume deficit
- Gas exchange impairment
- Injury, high risk for
- Oral mucous membrane alteration
- Pain
- Self-esteem, situational low
- Tissue perfusion alteration
- Urinary elimination pattern alteration

Premature labor
- Anxiety
- Breast-feeding, effective
- Breathing pattern, ineffective
- Coping, ineffective individual
- Injury, high risk for
- Knowledge deficit
- Parenting alteration
- Parenting alteration, high risk for
- Self-esteem disturbance

Puerperal infection
- Infection, high risk for
- Pain

Uterine leiomyoma (fibroid)
- Constipation
- Incontinence, urge
- Pain
- Urinary retention

Uterine prolapse
- Body image disturbance
- Incontinence, stress

Uterine rupture
- Fluid volume deficit
- Pain
- Tissue perfusion alteration

Vaginal atrophy
- Sexuality pattern alteration

Renal and urologic disorders

Acute renal failure
- Cardiac output, decreased
- Family process alteration
- Fear
- Fluid volume deficit
- Fluid volume excess
- Infection, high risk for
- Mobility impairment
- Self-care deficit
- Self-esteem, situational low
- Sensory or perceptual alteration
- Sexual dysfunction
- Skin integrity impairment
- Sleep pattern disturbance
- Thought process alteration
- Tissue perfusion alteration (renal)

Chronic renal failure
- Coping, ineffective family
- Denial
- Family process alteration
- Fluid volume excess
- Management of therapeutic regimen, ineffective
- Powerlessness
- Sexual dysfunction
- Skin integrity impairment, high risk for
- Tissue perfusion alteration (renal)

Glomerulonephritis
- Coping, ineffective family
- Fluid volume excess
- Infection, high risk for
- Mobility impairment
- Nutrition alteration: Less than body requirements
- Self-care deficit
- Tissue perfusion alteration

Hydronephrosis
- Coping, ineffective family
- Infection, high risk for
- Urinary elimination pattern alteration

Interstitial nephritis
- Fluid volume deficit
- Fluid volume excess
- Infection, high risk for
- Mobility impairment
- Self-care deficit
- Sensory or perceptual alteration
- Thought process alteration
- Tissue perfusion alteration

Polycystic kidney disease
- Tissue perfusion alteration (renal)

Pyelonephritis
- Fluid volume excess
- Infection, high risk for
- Mobility impairment
- Pain
- Self-care deficit
- Tissue perfusion alteration

Renal calculi
- Denial
- Infection, high risk for
- Pain
- Tissue perfusion alteration (renal)
- Urinary elimination pattern alteration
- Urinary retention

Renal disease: End-stage
- Caregiver role strain
- Caregiver role strain, high risk for
- Coping, defensive
- Coping, ineffective individual
- Decisional conflict
- Denial
- Grieving, anticipatory
- Grieving, dysfunctional
- Hopelessness
- Poisoning, high risk for
- Self-esteem, chronic low
- Sexuality pattern alteration

Urethrocele
- Incontinence, stress

Respiratory disorders

Acute respiratory failure
- Activity intolerance
- Anxiety
- Aspiration, high risk for
- Cardiac output, decreased
- Fear
- Gas exchange impairment
- Infection, high risk for
- Powerlessness
- Suffocation, high risk for
- Thought process alteration
- Tissue perfusion alteration (cardiopulmonary)
- Verbal communication impairment

Adult respiratory distress syndrome
- Airway clearance, ineffective
- Anxiety
- Breathing pattern ineffective
- Coping, ineffective individual
- Fluid volume deficit
- Gas exchange impairment
- Mobility impairment
- Nutrition alteration: Less than body requirements
- Self-care deficit
- Tissue perfusion alteration (cardiopulmonary)
- Ventilation, spontaneous: Inability to sustain
- Ventilatory weaning response, dysfunctional
- Verbal communication impairment

Airway obstruction
- Aspiration, high risk for
- Gas exchange impairment
- Ventilation, spontaneous: Inability to sustain
- Verbal communication impairment

Asthma
- Activity intolerance
- Airway clearance, ineffective
- Breathing pattern ineffective
- Coping, ineffective family
- Coping, ineffective individual
- Gas exchange impairment
- Health maintenance alteration
- Management of therapeutic regimen, ineffective
- Oral mucous membrane alteration
- Self-care deficit
- Verbal communication impairment

Atelectasis
- Airway clearance, ineffective
- Breathing pattern ineffective
- Coping, ineffective individual
- Fear
- Gas exchange impairment
- Mobility impairment
- Self-care deficit
- Verbal communication impairment

Bronchiectasis
- Airway clearance, ineffective
- Breathing pattern ineffective
- Coping, ineffective family
- Gas exchange impairment
- Mobility impairment
- Nutrition alteration: Less than body requirements
- Self-care deficit

Bronchiolitis, croup, and epiglottitis
- Breathing pattern ineffective
- Coping, ineffective family
- Fluid volume deficit, high risk for
- Gas exchange impairment

Chronic bronchitis and emphysema
- Activity intolerance
- Airway clearance, ineffective
- Breathing pattern ineffective
- Coping, ineffective family
- Coping, ineffective individual
- Fear
- Fluid volume deficit, high risk for
- Gas exchange impairment
- Health maintenance alteration
- Infection, high risk for
- Mobility impairment
- Nutrition alteration: Less than body requirements
- Oral mucous membrane alteration
- Self-care deficit

Chronic obstructive pulmonary disease
- Activity intolerance
- Airway clearance, ineffective
- Breathing pattern ineffective
- Caregiver role strain
- Caregiver role strain, high risk for
- Coping, ineffective family
- Denial
- Gas exchange impairment
- Home maintenance management impairment
- Hopelessness
- Infection, high risk for
- Injury, high risk for
- Knowledge deficit
- Management of therapeutic regimen, ineffective
- Nutrition alteration: More than body requirements
- Poisoning, high risk for
- Powerlessness
- Role performance alteration
- Self-esteem, chronic low
- Sleep pattern disturbance
- Suffocation, high risk for
- Tissue perfusion alteration (cardiopulmonary)
- Ventilation, spontaneous: Inability to sustain
- Ventilatory weaning response, dysfunctional
- Verbal communication impairment

Cor pulmonale
- Activity intolerance
- Airway clearance, ineffective
- Anxiety
- Breathing pattern ineffective
- Cardiac output, decreased
- Coping, ineffective individual
- Fatigue
- Fluid volume excess
- Gas exchange impairment
- Grieving, anticipatory
- Hopelessness
- Infection, high risk for
- Verbal communication impairment

Hemothorax
- Breathing pattern ineffective
- Fluid volume deficit
- Pain
- Tissue perfusion alteration
- Ventilation, spontaneous: Inability to sustain
- Verbal communication impairment

Interstitial lung disease
- Activity intolerance
- Airway clearance, ineffective
- Breathing pattern ineffective
- Gas exchange impairment

Lung abscess
- Infection, high risk for
- Pain
- Tissue perfusion alteration (cardiopulmonary)

Pleural effusion
- Breathing pattern ineffective
- Hyperthermia
- Infection, high risk for
- Ventilatory weaning response, dysfunctional

Pleurisy
- Breathing pattern ineffective
- Coping, ineffective family
- Gas exchange impairment
- Pain

Pneumonia
- Airway clearance, ineffective
- Anxiety
- Aspiration, high risk for
- Breathing pattern ineffective
- Fluid volume deficit, high risk for
- Gas exchange impairment
- Grieving, anticipatory
- Health maintenance alteration
- Infection, high risk for
- Mobility impairment
- Nutrition alteration: Less than body requirements
- Poisoning, high risk for
- Self-care deficit
- Tissue perfusion alteration (cardiopulmonary)
- Ventilation, spontaneous: Inability to sustain
- Verbal communication impairment

Pneumothorax
- Cardiac output, decreased
- Gas exchange impairment
- Infection, high risk for
- Pain
- Ventilation, spontaneous: Inability to sustain

Pulmonary disease
- Body temperature alteration, high risk for
- Coping, ineffective family
- Hopelessness
- Oral mucous membrane alteration
- Denial
- Tissue integrity impairment
- Ventilatory weaning response, dysfunctional

Pulmonary disease: End-stage
- Caregiver role strain
- Caregiver role strain, high risk for
- Coping, defensive
- Coping, ineffective individual
- Denial
- Grieving, anticipatory
- Grieving, dysfunctional
- Hopelessness

Pulmonary edema
- Activity intolerance
- Breathing pattern, ineffective
- Cardiac output, decreased
- Fear
- Fluid volume excess
- Gas exchange impairment
- Mobility impairment
- Self-care deficit
- Tissue perfusion alteration
- Ventilatory weaning response, dysfunctional
- Verbal communication impairment

Pulmonary embolus
- Activity intolerance
- Anxiety
- Breathing pattern, ineffective
- Cardiac output, decreased
- Fluid volume deficit
- Fluid volume deficit, high risk for
- Gas exchange impairment
- Mobility impairment
- Pain

• Tissue perfusion alteration (cardiopulmonary, venous)
• Verbal communication impairment

Respiratory distress syndrome (neonatal)
• Aspiration, high risk for
• Breathing pattern, ineffective
• Diversional activity deficit
• Thermoregulation, ineffective

Tuberculosis
• Airway clearance, ineffective
• Breathing pattern, ineffective
• Gas exchange impairment
• Social isolation

Sexual disorders

Chlamydia
• Infection, high risk for
• Sexual dysfunction

Genital herpes
• Infection, high risk for
• Powerlessness
• Sexuality pattern alteration
• Social isolation

Gonorrhea
• Incontinence, urge
• Infection, high risk for
• Sexuality pattern alteration

Male erectile dysfunction (impotence)
• Body image disturbance
• Self-esteem, situational low
• Sexual dysfunction
• Urinary retention

Premature ejaculation
• Self-esteem disturbance
• Sexual dysfunction

Syphilis
• Infection, high risk for
• Injury, high risk for
• Knowledge deficit

Trauma

– Body image disturbance
– Sensory or perceptual alteration
– Violence, high risk for

Asphyxia
• Aspiration, high risk for
• Breathing pattern, ineffective
• Growth and development alteration
• Hypothermia

Burns
• Altered protection
• Body image disturbance
• Body temperature alteration, high risk for
• Breathing pattern, ineffective
• Diversional activity deficit
• Fluid volume deficit
• Fluid volume deficit, high risk for
• Fluid volume excess
• Grieving, dysfunctional
• Hopelessness
• Infection, high risk for
• Injury, high risk for
• Mobility impairment
• Pain
• Parenting alteration
• Parenting alteration, high risk for
• Powerlessness
• Self-esteem disturbance
• Skin integrity impairment
• Social isolation
• Thermoregulation, ineffective
• Tissue perfusion alteration
• Trauma, high risk for
• Ventilation, spontaneous: Inability to sustain
• Ventilatory weaning response, dysfunctional

Chest trauma
• Airway clearance, ineffective
• Aspiration, high risk for
• Breathing pattern, ineffective
• Ventilatory weaning response, dysfunctional

Child abuse (battered child syndrome, neglect, shaken baby syndrome)
- Parenting alteration
- Parenting alteration, high risk for

Dislocation
- Activity intolerance
- Activity intolerance, high risk for
- Anxiety
- Mobility impairment

Drug overdose or toxicity
- Coping, ineffective individual
- Gas exchange impairment
- Hyperthermia
- Hypothermia
- Incontinence, functional
- Poisoning, high risk for
- Suffocation, high risk for
- Thermoregulation, ineffective
- Thought process alteration
- Trauma, high risk for
- Verbal communication impairment
- Violence, high risk for

Fractures
- Activity intolerance
- Activity intolerance, high risk for
- Breathing pattern, ineffective
- Coping, ineffective family
- Denial
- Disuse syndrome, high risk for
- Diversional activity deficit
- Fluid volume deficit
- Hopelessness
- Incontinence, stress
- Injury, high risk for
- Mobility impairment
- Oral mucous membrane alteration
- Pain
- Parenting alteration
- Parenting alteration, high risk for
- Role performance alteration
- Self-care deficit
- Sensory or perceptual alteration (gustatory, olfactory)
- Skin integrity impairment
- Skin integrity impairment, high risk for
- Trauma, high risk for
- Verbal communication impairment

Frostbite
- Hypothermia
- Skin integrity impairment, high risk for
- Tissue perfusion alteration (peripheral)

Head injury (craniocerebral, facial)
- Activity intolerance
- Activity intolerance, high risk for
- Aspiration, high risk for
- Body image disturbance
- Body temperature alteration, high risk for
- Disuse syndrome, high risk for
- Fear
- Fluid volume deficit, high risk for
- Gas exchange impairment
- Growth and development alteration
- Health maintenance alteration
- Incontinence, bowel
- Incontinence, functional
- Incontinence, urge
- Injury, high risk for
- Knowledge deficit
- Mobility impairment
- Neglect, unilateral
- Nutrition alteration: Less than body requirements
- Parenting alteration
- Parenting alteration, high risk for
- Poisoning, high risk for
- Posttrauma response
- Powerlessness
- Self-care deficit
- Sensory or perceptual alteration (auditory, gustatory, olfactory, tactile)
- Social interation impairment
- Swallowing impairment
- Thermoregulation, ineffective
- Thought process alteration
- Tissue perfusion alteration (cerebral)
- Trauma, high risk for
- Violence, high risk for

Heat exhaustion or heatstroke
- Body temperature alteration, high risk for
- Hyperthermia
- Oral mucous membrane alteration
- Thermoregulation, ineffective

Hyperthermia or hypothermia
- Body temperature alteration, high risk for
- Hyperthermia
- Hypothermia
- Knowledge deficit
- Neglect, unilateral
- Oral mucous membrane alteration
- Thermoregulation, ineffective

Incest
- Coping, ineffective individual
- Family process alteration
- Personal identity disturbance
- Posttrauma response
- Rape-trauma syndrome

Inhalation injuries
- Injury, high risk for
- Suffocation, high risk for
- Thermoregulation, ineffective

Multisystemic trauma
- Anxiety
- Fluid volume deficit
- Infection, high risk for
- Powerlessness
- Self-care deficit
- Suffocation, high risk for
- Tissue perfusion alteration
- Trauma, high risk for
- Ventilatory weaning response, dysfunctional

Near-drowning episode
- Suffocation, high risk for
- Thermoregulation, ineffective

Neuromuscular trauma
- Aspiration, high risk for
- Disuse syndrome, high risk for
- Incontinence, total
- Skin integrity impairment
- Skin integrity impairment, high risk for

Orthopedic injuries
- Body image disturbance
- Growth and development alteration
- Hopelessness
- Mobility impairment
- Sexuality pattern alteration

Poisoning
- Aspiration, high risk for
- Coping, ineffective family
- Injury, high risk for
- Poisoning, high risk for
- Sensory or perceptual alteration (olfactory, tactile)
- Tissue perfusion alteration (renal)

Radiation exposure, accidental
- Diarrhea
- Fatigue
- Fluid volume deficit
- Infection, high risk for
- Skin integrity impairment
- Tissue integrity impairment

Rape
- Posttrauma response
- Rape-trauma syndrome
- Self-esteem disturbance

Soft-tissue injuries (infant)
- Parenting alteration
- Parenting alteration, high risk for

Spinal cord injury
- Activity intolerance
- Activity intolerance, high risk for
- Adjustment impairment
- Airway clearance, ineffective
- Body image disturbance
- Constipation
- Disuse syndrome, high risk for
- Diversional activity deficit
- Dysreflexia
- Fear
- Gas exchange impairment
- Grieving, dysfunctional
- Growth and development alteration
- Health maintenance alteration
- Hopelessness
- Incontinence, bowel
- Incontinence, reflex
- Incontinence, total
- Incontinence, urge
- Infection, high risk for
- Management of therapeutic regimen, ineffective
- Mobility impairment
- Posttrauma response
- Powerlessness

- Self-care deficit
- Sensory or perceptual alteration (kinesthetic, tactile)
- Sexual dysfunction
- Sexuality pattern alteration
- Skin integrity impairment, high risk for
- Social isolation
- Trauma, high risk for
- Urinary elimination pattern alteration
- Urinary retention

Sunburn
- Body temperature alteration, high risk for
- Skin integrity impairment, high risk for

Multisystemic disorders

Chronic pain
- Adjustment impairment
- Coping, defensive
- Pain, chronic
- Self-esteem, chronic low

Deformity or disfigurement
- Adjustment impairment
- Body image disturbance
- Coping, defensive
- Self-esteem, chronic low

Degenerative disease
- Body temperature alteration, high risk for
- Coping, family: Potential for growth
- Coping, ineffective family
- Family process alteration
- Violence, high risk for: Self-directed

Dehydration
- Constipation
- Hyperthermia
- Thermoregulation, ineffective
- Tissue perfusion alteration

Failure to thrive
- Fluid volume deficit
- Fluid volume deficit, high risk for
- Growth and development alteration
- Nutrition alteration: Less than body requirements
- Parenting alteration
- Parenting alteration, high risk for

Hemorrhage
- Aspiration, high risk for
- Fluid volume deficit
- Growth and development alteration
- Oral mucous membrane alteration
- Thermoregulation, ineffective
- Tissue perfusion alteration (renal)
- Urinary elimination pattern alteration

Intoxication
- Aspiration, high risk for
- Hypothermia
- Sensory or perceptual alteration
- Thought process alteration
- Verbal communication impairment

Long-term disability
- Coping, family: Potential for growth
- Coping, ineffective family
- Diversional activity deficit
- Family process alteration
- Home maintenance management impairment
- Role performance alteration
- Violence, high risk for: Self-directed

Prolonged hospitalization
- Diversional activity deficit
- Parental role conflict
- Parenting alteration
- Parenting alteration, high risk for
- Self-esteem, situational low
- Sexuality pattern alteration

GORDON'S FUNCTIONAL HEALTH PATTERNS

Gordon has described a functional health pattern system to help identify and formulate nursing diagnoses. Based on general categories, this system allows for easy organization of basic nursing information obtained during your initial assessment. Flexible and adaptable, these functional health patterns can be used for patients in various states of health and illness, in any age-group, and in any clinical specialty. Presented below is a brief outline of Gordon's functional health patterns.

Learning to incorporate Gordon's concepts into your assessment format may require time and practice; however, the rewards of understanding the patient and identifying specific areas where you can intervene are well worth the effort. When using the following health pattern categories, obtain the nursing history from the patient's perspective through a series of specific questions designed to elicit information in an organized manner.

1. Health perception and health management pattern
- General health
- Health practices
- Concerns about illness
- Responsibility for health restoration and maintenance

2. Nutritional and metabolic pattern
- Daily food and fluid intake
- Weight loss or gain
- Appetite
- Dietary restrictions
- Healing potential of skin wounds or lesions
- General body status or condition

3. Elimination pattern
- Bowel elimination pattern or problem
- Urinary elimination pattern or problem
- Perspiration pattern or problem

4. Activity and exercise pattern
- Energy level
- Exercise pattern
- Perceived ability for (use Functional level code* below):
  - _ Bathing
  - _ Bed mobility
  - _ Cooking
  - _ Dressing
  - _ Feeding
  - _ General mobility
  - _ Grooming
  - _ Home maintenance
  - _ Shopping
  - _ Toileting

5. Sleep and rest pattern
- Sleep problems
- Rested or not rested after sleep
- Use of sleep aids

6. Cognitive and perceptual pattern
- Sensory status: Visual, auditory, olfactory, tactile, gustatory
- Memory
- Intelligence
- Pain or discomfort

7. Self-perception and self-concept pattern
- Feelings about self
- Body image
- Self-esteem
- Emotional state

***Functional level code**
Level 0 = Independent
Level I = Requires use of equipment or device
Level II = Requires assistance or supervision from another person
Level III = Requires assistance or supervision from another person and equipment or device
Level IV = Is dependent and does not participate

8. Role and relationship pattern
- Living arrangement
- Family or significant others
- Communication
- Role and responsibilities in family
- Socialization
- Finances

9. Sexuality and reproductive pattern
- Sexual relations
- Sexual satisfaction or dissatisfaction
- Contraceptive use and problems
- Reproductive and menstrual history

10. Coping and stress-tolerance pattern
- Stressors
- Coping mechanisms
- Major life changes
- Problem management

11. Value and belief pattern
- Satisfaction with life
- Spirituality and religious beliefs
- Religious practices
- Conflicts

12. Other
- Concerns not already discussed

Nursing diagnoses and Gordon's functional health patterns

1. Health perception and health management pattern
- Altered protection
- Disuse syndrome, high risk for
- Dysreflexia
- Health maintenance alteration
- Health-seeking behaviors
- Infection, high risk for
- Injury, high risk for
- Management of therapeutic regimen, ineffective
- Noncompliance
- Poisoning, high risk for
- Suffocation, high risk for

2. Nutritional and metabolic pattern
- Body temperature alteration, high risk for
- Breast-feeding, effective
- Breast-feeding, ineffective
- Breast-feeding, interrupted
- Fluid volume deficit
- Fluid volume deficit, high risk for
- Fluid volume excess
- Hyperthermia
- Hypothermia
- Infant feeding pattern, ineffective
- Nutrition alteration: Less than body requirements
- Nutrition alteration: More than body requirements
- Nutrition alteration, high risk for: More than body requirements
- Oral mucous membrane alteration
- Skin integrity impairment
- Skin integrity impairment, high risk for
- Swallowing impairment
- Thermoregulation, ineffective
- Tissue integrity impairment

3. Elimination pattern
- Constipation
- Diarrhea
- Incontinence, bowel
- Incontinence, functional
- Incontinence, reflex
- Incontinence, stress
- Incontinence, total
- Incontinence, urge
- Urinary elimination pattern alteration
- Urinary retention

4. Activity and exercise pattern
- Activity intolerance
- Activity intolerance, high risk for
- Airway clearance, ineffective
- Aspiration, high risk for
- Breathing pattern, ineffective
- Cardiac output, decreased
- Diversional activity deficit
- Gas exchange impairment
- Home maintenance management impairment
- Mobility impairment
- Neglect, unilateral
- Peripheral neurovascular dysfunction, high risk for

- Self-care deficit
- Tissue perfusion alteration
- Ventilation, spontaneous: Inability to sustain
- Ventilatory weaning response, dysfunctional

5. Sleep and rest pattern
- Fatigue
- Sleep pattern disturbance

6. Cognitive and perceptual pattern
- Knowledge deficit
- Pain
- Pain, chronic
- Sensory or perceptual alteration
- Thought process alteration

7. Self-perception and self-concept pattern
- Adjustment impairment
- Anxiety
- Body image disturbance
- Fear
- Grieving, anticipatory
- Hopelessness
- Personal identity disturbance
- Powerlessness
- Self-esteem, chronic low
- Self-esteem, situational low
- Self-esteem disturbance
- Self-mutilation, high risk for
- Violence, high risk for

8. Role and relationship pattern
- Family process alteration
- Grieving, anticipatory
- Grieving, dysfunctional
- Parental role conflict
- Parenting alteration
- Parenting alteration, high risk for
- Social interaction impairment
- Social isolation
- Verbal communication impairment
- Violence, high risk for

9. Sexuality and reproductive pattern
- Rape-trauma syndrome
- Sexual dysfunction
- Sexual pattern alteration

10. Coping and stress-tolerance pattern
- Caregiver role strain
- Caregiver role strain, high risk for
- Coping, defensive
- Coping, family: Potential for growth
- Coping, ineffective family
- Coping, ineffective individual
- Decisional conflict
- Denial
- Grieving, dysfunctional
- Growth and development alteration
- Relocation stress syndrome

11. Value and belief pattern
- Spiritual distress

NURSING DIAGNOSES AND MASLOW'S HIERARCHY OF NEEDS

The diagram below depicts Maslow's hierarchy of needs. You can use this system when determining priorities for patient care. Shown at left is the ascending hierarchy of human needs; the definitions at right explain the five need categories.

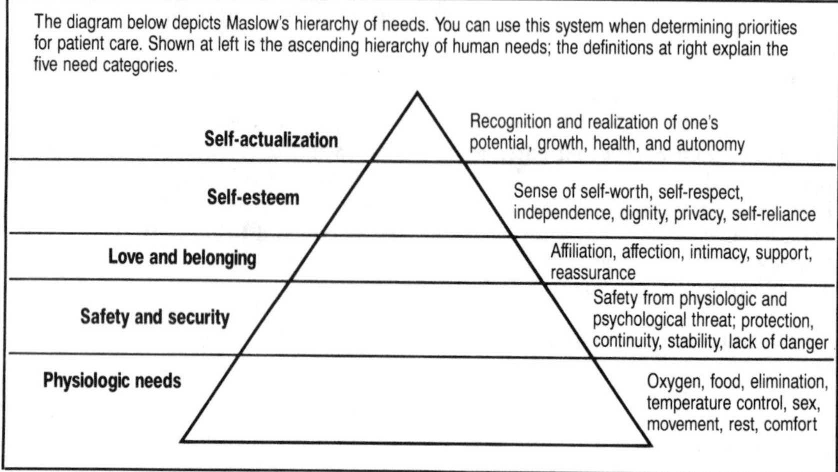

Maslow's hierarchy of needs is based on the idea that lower-level physiologic needs must be met before higher-level abstract needs can be met. Considering need categories as you identify patient problems will help you decide which nursing diagnoses to address first.

For example, a victim of physical abuse first needs his physical injuries treated (physiologic needs). Next, he may need protection from future episodes of abuse (safety and security). Moving up the hierarchy, you may then help the patient by providing support and reassurance (love and belonging). Long-term goals may include helping him build self-esteem. Keep in mind that a patient's need level may change throughout planning and intervention, so you'll have to continually reassess the patient and reevaluate his needs.

Read the descriptions of each category in the diagram; then see how you'd relate them to nursing diagnoses. Compare your evaluation with how the authors categorized the nursing diagnoses according to this hierarchy.

Self-actualization
- Growth and development alteration
- Health-seeking behaviors
- Knowledge deficit
- Spiritual distress

Self-esteem
- Adjustment impairment
- Body image disturbance
- Coping, defensive
- Coping, ineffective family
- Coping, ineffective individual
- Decisional conflict
- Denial
- Diversional activity deficit
- Hopelessness
- Noncompliance
- Personal identity disturbance
- Posttrauma response
- Powerlessness
- Rape-trauma syndrome
- Relocation stress syndrome
- Role performance alteration
- Self-esteem, chronic low
- Self-esteem, situational low
- Self-esteem disturbance
- Violence, high risk for

Love and belonging
- Caregiver role strain
- Caregiver role strain, high risk for
- Coping, family: Potential for growth
- Coping, ineffective family
- Family process alteration
- Parental role conflict
- Parenting alteration
- Social interaction impairment
- Social isolation

Safety and security
- Anxiety
- Disuse syndrome, high risk for
- Dysreflexia
- Fear
- Grieving, anticipatory
- Grieving, dysfunctional
- Health maintenance alteration
- Home maintenance management impairment
- Infection, high risk for
- Injury, high risk for
- Management of therapeutic regimen, ineffective
- Neglect, unilateral
- Poisoning, high risk for
- Self-mutilation, high risk for
- Suffocation, high risk for
- Trauma, high risk for
- Verbal communication impairment

Physiologic needs
- Activity intolerance
- Airway clearance, ineffective
- Altered protection
- Aspiration, high risk for
- Body temperature alteration, high risk for
- Breast-feeding, effective
- Breast-feeding, ineffective
- Breast-feeding, interrupted
- Breathing pattern, ineffective
- Cardiac output, decreased
- Constipation (colonic, perceived)
- Diarrhea
- Fatigue
- Fluid volume deficit
- Fluid volume excess
- Gas exchange impairment
- Hyperthermia
- Hypothermia
- Incontinence (bowel, functional, reflex, stress, total, urge)
- Infant feeding pattern, ineffective
- Mobility impairment
- Nutrition alteration
- Oral mucous membrane alteration
- Pain
- Pain, chronic
- Peripheral neurovascular dysfunction, high risk for
- Self-care deficit (specify)
- Sensory or perceptual alteration
- Sexual dysfunction
- Sexuality pattern alteration
- Skin integrity impairment
- Sleep pattern disturbance
- Swallowing impairment
- Thermoregulation, ineffective
- Thought process alteration
- Tissue integrity impairment
- Tissue perfusion alteration
- Urinary elimination pattern alteration
- Urinary retention
- Ventilation, spontaneous: Inability to sustain
- Ventilatory weaning response, dysfunctional

NURSING DIAGNOSES AND OREM'S UNIVERSAL SELF-CARE DEMANDS

Orem's concept of nursing focuses on self-care activities that individuals perform to maintain life, health, and well-being. In order to maintain integrated human functions, all individuals must meet *universal self-care demands.* If an individual is unable to satisfactorily meet these demands, the nurse intervenes by providing and managing care. According to Orem's theory, the goals of nursing include helping the patient to overcome circumstances that interfere with self-care and cause limitations and deficits. The list below uses Orem's universal self-care demands to group related nursing diagnoses.

Air
- Airway clearance, ineffective
- Aspiration, high risk for
- Breathing pattern, ineffective
- Gas exchange impairment
- Ventilation, spontaneous: Inability to sustain
- Ventilatory weaning response, dysfunctional

Water
- Cardiac output, decreased
- Fluid volume deficit
- Fluid volume deficit, high risk for
- Fluid volume excess
- Tissue perfusion alteration

Food
- Breast-feeding, effective
- Breast-feeding, ineffective
- Breast-feeding, interrupted
- Infant feeding pattern, ineffective
- Nutrition alteration: Less than body requirements
- Nutrition alteration: More than body requirements
- Nutrition alteration, high risk for: More than body requirements
- Oral mucous membrane alteration

Elimination
- Constipation
- Constipation, colonic
- Constipation, perceived
- Diarrhea
- Incontinence, bowel
- Incontinence, functional
- Incontinence, reflex
- Incontinence, stress
- Incontinence, total
- Incontinence, urge
- Skin integrity impairment
- Skin integrity impairment, high risk for
- Urinary elimination pattern alteration
- Urinary retention

Activity and rest
- Activity intolerance
- Activity intolerance, high risk for
- Disuse syndrome, high risk for
- Diversional activity deficit
- Fatigue
- Mobility impairment
- Neglect, unilateral
- Self-care deficit
- Sleep pattern disturbance

Solitude and social interaction
- Family process alteration
- Parental role conflict
- Parenting alteration
- Parenting alteration, high risk for
- Rape-trauma syndrome
- Role performance alteration
- Self-mutilation, high risk for
- Sexual dysfunction
- Sexuality pattern alteration
- Social interaction impairment
- Social isolation
- Verbal communication impairment
- Violence, high risk for

Prevention of hazards
- Altered protection
- Body temperature alteration, high risk for

- Dysreflexia
- Health maintenance alteration
- Health-seeking behaviors
- Home maintenance management impairment
- Hyperthermia
- Hypothermia
- Infection, high risk for
- Injury, high risk for
- Management of therapeutic regimen, ineffective
- Noncompliance
- Pain
- Pain, chronic
- Peripheral neurovascular dysfunction, high risk for
- Poisoning, high risk for
- Suffocation, high risk for
- Swallowing impairment
- Thermoregulation, ineffective
- Tissue integrity impairment
- Trauma, high risk for

Promotion of human functioning

- Adjustment impairment
- Anxiety
- Body image disturbance
- Caregiver role strain
- Caregiver role strain, high risk for
- Coping, defensive
- Coping, family: Potential for growth
- Coping, ineffective family
- Coping, ineffective individual
- Decisional conflict
- Denial
- Fear
- Grieving, anticipatory
- Grieving, dysfunctional
- Growth and development alteration
- Hopelessness
- Knowledge deficit
- Personal identity disturbance
- Posttrauma response
- Powerlessness
- Relocation stress syndrome
- Self-esteem, chronic low
- Self-esteem, situational low
- Self-esteem disturbance
- Sensory or perceptual alteration
- Spiritual distress
- Thought process alteration

HOME HEALTH CARE CLASSIFICATION

The Home Health Care Classification (HHCC) of nursing diagnoses and interventions developed by Virginia Saba at Georgetown University School of Nursing allows you to assess, classify, and code nursing care needs of home health care patients. This system revises, adapts, and expands upon the 104 currently approved North American Nursing Diagnosis Association (NANDA) nursing diagnoses.

In this system, 145 nursing diagnoses are used to describe patient needs. Each diagnosis has a five-character code: an initial letter code (A to T), representing one of the 20 identified *home health nursing components,* followed by a two-digit code corresponding to one of 50 *major diagnostic categories.* Two decimal place codes indicate the *diagnostic subcategory* (.1 to .9) and *expected outcome* (.01 to .03), respectively. For example, the classification system codes the diagnosis *Activity intolerance* as A01.1x:

- *A* identifies the nursing component *Activity*
- *01* identifies the diagnostic category *Activity alteration*
- *.1* identifies the diagnosis subcategory *Activity intolerance*
- *.0x* identifies the expected outcome: .01 for *improved, .02 for stabilized,* or .03 for *deteriorated.*

The list below contains the codes for the HHCC nursing diagnoses broken down by nursing component, diagnostic category, and diagnostic subcategory.

A: Activity component
Factors related to the body's use of energy.
01 Activity alteration
- 01.1 Activity intolerance
- 01.2 Activity intolerance risk
- 01.3 Diversional activity deficit
- 01.4 Fatigue
- 01.5 Physical mobility impairment
- 01.6 Sleep pattern disturbance

02 Musculoskeletal alteration

B: Bowel elimination component
Factors related to the GI system.
03 Bowel elimination alteration
- 03.1 Bowel incontinence
- 03.2 Colonic constipation
- 03.3 Diarrhea
- 03.4 Fecal impaction
- 03.5 Perceived constipation
- 03.6 Unspecified constipation

04 Gastrointestinal alteration

C: Cardiac component
Factors related to the heart and circulatory system.
05 Cardiac output alteration
06 Cardiovascular alteration
- 06.1 Blood pressure alteration

D: Cognitive component
Factors related to mental and cerebral processes.
07 Cerebral alteration
08 Knowledge deficit
- 08.1 Knowledge deficit of diagnostic test

• 08.2 Knowledge deficit of dietary regimen
• 08.3 Knowledge deficit of disease process
• 08.4 Knowledge deficit of fluid volume
• 08.5 Knowledge deficit of medication regimen
• 08.6 Knowledge deficit of safety precautions
• 08.7 Knowledge deficit of therapeutic regimen
09 Thought processes alteration

E: Coping component
Factors related to the ability to manage responsibilities, problems, or difficulties.
10 Dying process
11 Family coping impairment
• 11.1 Compromised family coping
• 11.2 Disabled family coping
12 Individual coping impairment
• 12.1 Adjustment impairment
• 12.2 Decisional conflict
• 12.3 Defensive coping
• 12.4 Denial
13 Posttrauma response
• 13.1 Rape trauma syndrome
14 Spiritual state alteration
• 14.1 Spiritual distress

F: Fluid volume component
Factors related to liquid consumption.
15 Fluid volume alteration
• 15.1 Fluid volume deficit
• 15.2 Fluid volume deficit risk
• 15.3 Fluid volume excess
• 15.4 Fluid volume excess risk

G: Health behavior component
Factors related to actions to sustain, maintain, or regain health.
16 Growth and development alteration
17 Health maintenance alteration
18 Health-seeking behavior alteration
19 Home maintenance alteration
20 Noncompliance
• 20.1 Noncompliance of diagnostic test
• 20.2 Noncompliance of dietary regimen
• 20.3 Noncompliance of fluid volume
• 20.4 Noncompliance of medication regimen
• 20.5 Noncompliance of safety precautions
• 20.6 Noncompliance of therapeutic regimen

H: Medication component
Factors related to drug therapy.
21 Medication risk
• 21.1 Polypharmacy

I: Metabolic component
Factors related to endocrine and immune processes.
22 Endocrine alteration
23 Immune alteration
• 23.1 Protection alteration

J: Nutritional component
Factors related to the intake of food and nutrients.
24 Nutrition alteration
• 24.1 Body nutrition deficit
• 24.2 Body nutrition deficit risk
• 24.3 Body nutrition excess
• 24.4 Body nutrition excess risk

K: Physical regulation component
Factors related to body processes.
25 Physical regulation alteration

• 25.1 Dysreflexia
• 25.2 Hyperthermia
• 25.3 Hypothermia
• 25.4 Thermoregulation impairment
• 25.5 Infection risk
• 25.6 Infection unspecified

L: Respiratory component
Factors related to breathing and the pulmonary system.
26 Respiration alteration
• 26.1 Airway clearance impairment
• 26.2 Breathing pattern impairment
• 26.3 Gas exchange impairment

M: Role relationship component
Factors related to interpersonal, work, social, and sexual interactions.
27 Role performance alteration
• 27.1 Parental role conflict
• 27.2 Parenting alteration
• 27.3 Sexual dysfunction
28 Communication impairment
• 28.1 Verbal impairment
29 Family processes alteration
30 Grieving
• 30.1 Anticipatory grieving
• 30.2 Dysfunctional grieving
31 Sexuality patterns alteration
32 Socialization alteration
• 32.1 Social interaction alteration
• 32.2 Social isolation

N: Safety component
Factors related to risk reduction and the prevention of injury or loss.
33 Injury risk
• 33.1 Aspiration risk
• 33.2 Disuse syndrome
• 33.3 Poisoning risk
• 33.4 Suffocation risk
• 33.5 Trauma risk
34 Violence risk

O: Self-care component
Factors related to the ability to perform self-maintenance activities.
35 Bathing or hygiene deficit
36 Dressing or grooming deficit
37 Feeding deficit
• 37.1 Breast-feeding impairment
• 37.2 Swallowing impairment
38 Self-care deficit
• 38.1 Activities of daily living (ADL) alteration
• 38.2 Instrumental activities of daily living (IADL) alteration
39 Toileting deficit

P: Self-concept component
Factors related to an individual's mental self-image.
40 Anxiety
41 Fear
42 Meaningfulness alteration
• 42.1 Hopelessness
• 42.2 Powerlessness
43 Self-concept alteration
• 43.1 Body image disturbance
• 43.2 Personal identity disturbance
• 43.3 Chronic low self-esteem disturbance
• 43.4 Situational self-esteem disturbance

Q: Sensory component
Factors related to the senses.
44 Sensory perceptual alteration
• 44.1 Auditory alteration
• 44.2 Gustatory alteration
• 44.3 Kinesthetic alteration
• 44.4 Olfactory alteration
• 44.5 Tactile alteration
• 44.6 Unilateral neglect
• 44.7 Visual alteration
45 Comfort alteration
• 45.1 Acute pain
• 45.2 Chronic pain
• 45.3 Unspecified pain

R: Skin integrity component
Factors related to the mucous membrane, corneal, integumentary, or subcutaneous structures of the body.
46 Skin integrity alteration
- 46.1 Oral mucous membranes impairment
- 46.2 Skin integrity impairment
- 46.3 Skin integrity impairment risk
- 46.4 Skin incision

47 Peripheral alteration

S: Tissue perfusion component
Factors related to oxygenation of tissues.
48 Tissue perfusion alteration

T: Urine elimination component
Factors related to the genitourinary system.
49 Urinary elimination alteration
- 49.1 Functional urinary incontinence
- 49.2 Reflex urinary incontinence
- 49.3 Stress urinary incontinence
- 49.4 Total urinary incontinence
- 49.5 Urge urinary incontinence
- 49.6 Urinary retention

50 Renal alteration

NURSING DIAGNOSIS CASE STUDIES

The following case studies show how to apply a nursing diagnosis to clinical practice.

ADULT HEALTH

Mike Bradley, age 28, comes from a Roman Catholic family of Irish and German descent. One month ago, Mike was diagnosed with acquired immunodeficiency syndrome (AIDS). Since then, he has experienced loss of appetite, weight loss of 10 lb (4.5 kg), hypersomnia, anergy, decreased concentration, and an overall sense of hopelessness.

Mike's despair at his diagnosis was exacerbated by a number of factors:

- a recent breakup with Jim, his companion of 5 years
- the death of a close friend from complications of AIDS 6 months ago
- fear of losing his job as a physical education teacher at a local high school
- fear of rejection by his family.

Two weeks ago, Mike began sleeping most of the day, missing work, and losing touch with family and friends. He expressed fleeting thoughts of suicide without a plan or intent. A week ago, though, he was admitted to the emergency department after an overdose of diazepam. Once he was stabilized, he was transferred to the psychiatric unit.

Developing a diagnosis

Jean Munson, RN, works in the psychiatric unit. Initially, she assessed Mike's overall status: blood pressure, 120/70 mm Hg; pulse rate, 72 beats/minute; respiratory rate, 18 breaths/minute; temperature, 98.6° F (37° C); height, 5′9″ (20.5 cm); and weight, 135 lb (61.25 kg) . Mike reported no allergies and stated that he occasionally takes diazepam to ease his anxiety.

Jean found Mike alert and oriented to time, place, and person. He was poorly groomed, spoke in a low monotone, and showed psychomotor retardation. He exhibited poor judgment and insight, limited immediate recall, a diminished attention span, an impoverished affect, and a despondent mood. Mike denied use of alcohol or recreational drugs, had no homicidal thoughts, and showed no psychotic behavior. He continued to speak of a wish to kill himself and seemed disappointed that this attempt was unsuccessful.

The medical record indicates that Mike has no history of depression or suicidal thoughts and no family history of mental illness. After taking Mike's history, Jean believes that he may attempt suicide again. Before addressing Mike's complicated emotional issues, her first priority is to ensure his safety. Therefore, she chooses as her top-priority diagnosis *high risk for self-directed violence, related to suicidal ideation and attempt.* Once Mike's safety is ensured, a number of nursing diagnoses, including *social isolation, hopelessness,* and *ineffective individual coping,* may help to address long-term needs.

Planning care

Jean realizes that during a short hospital stay, she realistically can't solve Mike's problems. Her goals must be achievable and to the point. She decides that her first goal is to prevent Mike from harming himself in the hospital. Once his safety is ensured, she hopes to help him express feelings of despair associated with his AIDS diagnosis. Ultimately, she hopes to help him realize that he needs support and take steps to contact appropriate sources of support. She documents the following outcomes in her plan of care:

- Patient does not harm himself while in hospital.
- He expresses feelings about AIDS and other life events.
- He admits that he needs ongoing help and support.
- He identifies and contacts appropriate sources of support.

Interventions

Although Jean is Mike's primary case manager, she seeks input from all members of the psychiatric patient care team on a daily basis. During team meetings, Jean incorporates the observations and recommendations of the team's psychiatrist, psychologist, social worker, therapists (art, music, occupational), and pharmacist into Mike's treatment plan and then discusses any modifications of the plan with him.

Immediately following Mike's admission to the unit, Jean initiates safety protocols and one-on-one observation until suicide precautions are discontinued. She informs Mike that she will help him control impulses to harm himself. She asks him to make a commitment not to harm himself and assures him that a staff member will check on him every hour for the first 24 hours, then every 2 hours. She explains that, while she is his case manager, other members of a team of professionals will be working to assist him.

Then Jean encourages Mike to express his feelings about his AIDS diagnosis. She tries to communicate to him that feelings like anger, despair, guilt, and hopelessness are not wrong and that he does not have to be ashamed of them. She encourages him to identify supportive persons to whom he can express feelings of depression. Jean advises him to seek out the company of others when he feels helpless and hopeless.

After 5 days of treatment, Mike meets with the team to voice his concerns and ask questions. This meeting also permits the team to evaluate Mike's progress and assess his readiness for discharge. Before he leaves the hospital, Jean refers him to agencies specializing in care and support of AIDS patients.

Evaluation

During Mike's 7-day hospitalization, Jean was able to get him to routinely practice safety measures, talk about his feelings, and ask for help. Most importantly, she helped him recognize his need for ongoing treatment and support. After discharge, he began outpatient psychotherapy and agreed to join a support group. Through careful planning, Jean was able to point this patient away from despair and toward making the most of his life.

ADOLESCENT HEALTH

Anne Gregory is a 14-year-old eighth grade student and the oldest of five children. Her father is a farmer; her mother takes care of the household and family. Anne has always been expected to help with the younger children. Quiet and studious, she is a straight-A student who demonstrates a strong desire to do everything perfectly. Anything falling short of perfection causes her to become visibly upset.

Less than a year ago, Anne weighed 120 lb (54.4 kg). Although heavier than most of her classmates, she wasn't obese. At the beginning of the school year, Anne's mother became pregnant with her fifth child. One of Anne's classmates told Anne that she, rather than her mother, looked pregnant. That was the moment Anne decided to diet.

Anne literally stopped eating. Within 1 month, she lost 10 lb (4.5 kg). After an additional 10-lb weight loss, Anne's parents began to worry. Dinner became a tense, unpleasant time as Mr. and Mrs. Gregory unsuccessfully attempted to get Anne to eat. They struggled with the problem until Anne's weight had dropped to 80 lb (36.3 kg).

Anne isolated herself from friends and family. She took long walks alone in the woods. Feeling frustrated and helpless, her parents sought medical assistance for Anne, who was hospitalized for a month.

Developing a diagnosis

Nora Aronson, RN, works in the eating disorders unit where Anne is a patient. She begins her assessment by evaluating Anne's vital signs, hydration status, weight, evidence of previous eating disorders, past dieting, and episodes of emesis. Nora considers Anne's physiologic status carefully to determine if she should suggest enteral feedings.

During the health history, she asks Anne questions about her attitudes and feelings toward food and toward her own appearance. She includes Mr. and Mrs. Gregory for part of the interview. She tries to understand Anne's role within her family and her relationship with her parents and younger siblings.

Nora notes that Anne still perceives herself as chubby. She seems to equate controlling her eating with maintaining self-discipline. She also expresses a desire to resemble the ultra-thin models who grace the pages of teenage fashion magazines.

Nora believes that real change for Anne means not only developing healthier eating habits, but also changing the way she feels about herself. Therefore, Nora chooses as her top-priority diagnosis *body image disturbance related to an eating disorder.*

Planning care

Nora's most important goal for Anne is helping her comply with the prescribed medical regimen to ensure her physiologic well-being. As a next step, she hopes to help Anne examine her perceptions and feelings about food, exercise, weight loss, and her appearance.

For change to be meaningful, Anne needs to realize for herself that her eating and exercise patterns are self-destructive. She also needs to understand how social values, such as society's emphasis on the ideal feminine shape, are influencing her behavior. In her plan of care, Nora documents the following outcome statements:

- Patient acknowledges that her eating habits are unhealthy.
- She requests help in controlling her eating patterns.
- She participates in decisions about her care and treatment.
- She attends a support group for people with eating disorders.
- She identifies new strategies for coping with stress.
- She expresses satisfaction with her appearance.

Interventions

First, Nora participates in implementing the medical regimen to ensure Anne's well-being. She also obtains a referral for psychiatric evaluation to help Anne deal with underlying emotional issues.

In working with Anne, Nora conveys a constructive, caring attitude. She takes steps to ensure continuity of care throughout her hospital stay and encourages Anne to express her feelings openly. Only if she is encouraged to deal with her feelings honestly will Anne be able to come to terms with the psychological issues behind her dangerous weight loss.

Nora consults with the dietician and arranges for her to visit Anne. Together, they make a list of foods that Anne likes most and plan meals and snacks for the next 3 days. The dietician's goal is to help plan high-calorie, nutritionally balanced meals that provide Anne with 2,500 kcal each day.

Nora and Anne make a contract in which Anne agrees to eat specific amounts of food to achieve her weight-gain goals. To promote adherence to the contract, Nora arranges to have Anne observed during meals and personally supervises all trips to the bathroom, to discourage purging.

Throughout Anne's stay, Nora remains in contact with her parents and reminds them of the importance of their emotional support. She urges them to attend family counseling sessions to explore their relationship with their daughter.

Nora uses behavior modification to reinforce healthful nutrition. Rewards include television and visitor privileges. To be effective, behavior modification must be consistent, allowing Anne to predict the consequences of her behavior. However, to set a good example, Nora avoids manipulating Anne or coercing her to participate in care or adhere to rules.

At discharge, Nora encourages Anne to participate in group discussions with peers who also have eating disorders. She has a final meeting with Anne's parents. At this meeting, she teaches the Gregorys how to detect signs that Anne may be relapsing into self-destructive eating patterns.

Evaluation

At the end of Anne's stay on the eating disorders unit, Nora is able to document significant progress. Anne has gained 10 lb (4.5 kg) and participates in a support group. The most important changes, however, involve Anne's insight about herself. She expresses an understanding that her radical weight loss is a sign that she needs help. She can state that her poor nutritional habits are endangering her health. Most importantly, she agrees that she must learn to develop self-esteem from within herself, not based on other people's perception of her appearance. Her parents also express a significantly improved understanding of their daughter's condition.

CHILD HEALTH

Tommy Garrett, age 4, was born with a bilateral cleft lip and palate. Tommy's lip was surgically closed when he was an infant, and the initial repair was recently revised. His palate was closed shortly before his third birthday. Aside from recurrent otitis media, he is well nourished and physically healthy. However, learning to speak has been a slow, tedious process.

Tommy has been in a speech rehabilitation program for the last 2 years. Speech therapy is especially important because Tommy can't articulate certain sounds and some of his words are unintelligible.

Tommy and his 6-year-old brother live with their 23-year-old mother. Mrs. Garrett is divorced, never completed high school, doesn't receive child support, and must survive on a low salary from her job in a fast-food restaurant. Many times, she has neglected to bring Tommy to therapy. Recently, he has missed six sessions in a row.

Developing a diagnosis

Katherine Lopez, RN, is a community health nurse who visits the Garretts in their home every other week. During her conversations with Mrs. Garrett, she has made the following observations:

- Mrs. Garrett expresses resentment of the interference from Katherine and other health care providers.
- She has little knowledge of normal child development.
- She frequently complains about the difficulty she has controlling her children.
- She hasn't established routines for such activities as mealtime or bedtime.
- She doesn't have time or resources to pay sufficient attention to developing Tommy's verbal communication.

- She has little social contact outside of work and her family.

Katherine realizes that before Tommy's speech impairment can be addressed, she needs to identify and address the problems within his family that are preventing him from receiving adequate help. Katherine selects the nursing diagnosis *ineffective family coping related to care of a child with special needs* as her first priority in developing a plan of care.

Planning care

Initially, Katherine hopes to get Mrs. Garrett to acknowledge Tommy's special needs and to discuss her feelings about them. The next step is to encourage her to accept outside help in caring for Tommy. To ensure effective change, she plans to work with Mrs. Garrett to help her better understand Tommy's physical, emotional, and developmental needs and to help her meet her own social and economic needs. Katherine documents the following outcomes in her plan of care:

- Parent acknowledges child's special needs.
- She accepts assistance from health care providers.
- She expresses increased confidence in her ability to meet child's needs.
- She takes appropriate steps to ensure her own economic and social well-being.

Interventions

Katherine listens to Mrs. Garrett without passing judgment and makes it clear that her goal is to help her and her family. Over time, she makes it clear that her offer of help is not intended to be a criticism of Mrs. Garrett's parenting skills. As their rapport improves, Katherine provides her with information on normal growth and development. She slowly explains specific ways in which Tommy deviates from the norm.

To help motivate Mrs. Garrett, Katherine involves her in the planning process. She works with Mrs. Garrett to develop realistic expectations for Tommy. Together, they establish simple, short-term goals to provide structure in the home and ensure that Tommy gets to his speech therapy session each week.

Katherine acts as a liaison between the family and other members of the multidisciplinary team, including Tommy's physician, psychologist, speech therapist, and occupational therapist. During team meetings, Katherine incorporates the observations and recommendations of other team members into Tommy's treatment plan. Then she discusses all alterations to the plan with Mrs. Garrett.

Prior to Tommy's discharge, Katherine provides Mrs. Garrett with information about educational programs, parent support groups, respite care agencies, health care providers, and religious organizations that provide support to struggling families. Katherine helps Mrs. Garrett understand that by taking steps to meet her own needs, such as increasing her social circle and arranging for respite periods away from her sons, she will be better prepared to care for her children.

Evaluation

After 3 months, Katherine can document significant improvement in family function. Mrs. Garrett demonstrates improvement in her communication skills. She can describe Tommy's developmental needs and is better able to express her own needs.

For his part, Tommy works to meet goals set by his mother, such as speaking slowly and enunciating words clearly, sitting at the table to eat meals, and playing with other children. Finally, the whole family demonstrates enhanced social functioning, with members interacting with extended family, peers, and new contacts from church and support groups.

MATERNAL-NEONATAL HEALTH

Mary Mason is a 28-year-old white primipara. At 39½ weeks' gestation, she went into labor. After determining that the child was a frank breech presentation, the doctor performed a cesarean section. Mrs. Mason gave birth to a 5-lb 3-oz (2,353-g) girl named Ashley. The Apgar score was 4/6; intermittent positive pressure was administered by face mask after the infant was suctioned. The infant received a preliminary diagnosis of Down's syndrome and was transferred immediately to the neonatal intensive care unit (NICU).

Before leaving the delivery room, Mary was told about the baby's condition and the tentative diagnosis. She was shocked. Her pregnancy had advanced normally, and she had received good prenatal care. At 17 weeks, her serum alpha-fetoprotein level was normal, so amniocentesis had not been performed.

Less than a week after birth, Ashley had surgery for a tracheoesophageal fistula. Again, Mary was not emotionally prepared to deal with her child's condition.

One week after giving birth, Mary was discharged. During the next week, she spent every day visiting Ashley in the NICU. Just when she was prepared for the baby's discharge, a barium swallow showed that the fistula had not fully healed. By this time, Mary was angry and afraid. After an additional week, healing was complete and the baby began feeding from a bottle.

Developing a diagnosis

Vera Washington, RN, works in the NICU of the hospital where Ashley is being treated. She has had frequent contact with the child's mother. During her visits, Mary exhibits intense emotional conflict over her child's condition. Her feelings range from rage to resignation. She talks about wanting the baby but doesn't know how she can cope. She seems to understand little about normal growth and development, let alone the care of a child with special needs.

While investigating the family history, Vera notes that Mary lives with the baby's father, Rob, but is not married to him. She has one sibling and a father, both of whom live in another area of the country. She questions whether Mary has adequate emotional support to cope with her current crisis.

After speaking with Mary and noting her history, Vera documents a diagnosis of *parenting alteration related to inadequate attachment to high-risk neonate.* She realizes that these early weeks will be crucial in determining the parents' relationship with their child and in building the confidence they need to face the challenges ahead.

Planning care

Vera realizes that the first step is to help Mary and her companion establish a bond with Ashley. She next needs to help them express their feelings and anxieties regarding Ashley's condition and their own parenting skills.

Vera's next task will be to get Mary and Rob to accept help in developing competent parenting skills. She hopes they will become involved in planning their baby's care. By the time the baby is ready for discharge, they must begin to demonstrate knowledge of her developmental needs and a willingness to use available support systems.

In her plan of care, Vera documents the following outcomes:

- Parents establish appropriate contact with neonate.
- They communicate feelings and anxieties regarding neonate's condition and their parenting skills.
- They demonstrate adequate knowledge of neonate's developmental needs.
- They become involved in planning and providing neonate's care.
- They use available support systems to assist with care of neonate.

Interventions

Vera encourages both parents to visit the NICU. Before the visit, Vera explains their baby's appearance along with the various supportive devices. She provides Mary with a picture of her baby to help her accept the reality of Ashley's birth and encourages both parents to express their anxieties. She tells them not to be ashamed of expressing such feelings as anger and guilt.

During their visits to the hospital, Vera assesses Mary and Rob's level of understanding of their baby's condition and their expectations for the future. She enlists the help of the hospital neonatologist to effectively educate them. Mary and Rob are encouraged to touch and talk to their baby, learning to care for her inside the secure hospital environment.

When the baby is discharged, Vera provides the parents with the NICU telephone number and encourages them to call at any time. She refers the family to social services for education, follow-up, and referrals as indicated.

Evaluation

In a follow-up visit, Vera can document satisfactory progress in the developing relationship between Ashley and her parents. Mary and Rob are comfortable in voicing their anxieties about their baby's condition and their ability to provide care. They display appropriate attachment behaviors and provide the baby with appropriate verbal, tactile, and auditory stimulation. Finally, they express an understanding of available sources of support and a willingness to contact them.

GERIATRIC HEALTH

John Marak is an 87-year-old Jewish male, born and raised in Hungary. He was admitted to the hospital from the nursing home where he has spent the past 5 years. His admitting medical diagnoses were aspiration pneumonia, end-stage cirrhosis of the liver, and esophageal varices. Two recent episodes of coffee-ground vomitus precipitated Mr. Marak's transfer to the hospital.

Mr. Marak has one son who brought him from his native Hungary 10 years ago. From the beginning, Mr. Marak's son has been insistent that everything possible be done to restore his father's health.

During the first week of Mr. Marak's hospitalization, the bleeding stopped and his lungs also improved. However, he was unable to swallow without serious danger of aspiration. Several attempts were made to insert a feeding tube but each time, Mr. Marak managed to pull it out. Total parenteral nutrition was initiated and continued for 3 weeks with intermittent attempts to restore a feeding tube. Each time the tube was inserted, Mr. Marak became agitated and combative until he succeeded in pulling it out.

Multidisciplinary group meetings with the son failed to convince him that his father's prognosis was extremely poor and that making Mr. Marak as comfortable as possible might be the best solution. Since Mr. Marak's competence was questionable, his pleas to the staff to "take me home" were given no consideration by his son.

Developing a diagnosis

Erica Donetti, RN, is a part of the multidisciplinary team caring for Mr. Marak. In her initial investigation of Mr. Marak's history, she noted that he had spent time in a concentration camp. As part of his religious tradition, Mr. Marak wears a hat at all times, keeps a prayer book at his bedside, and occasionally asks to be visited by a rabbi. His son is the only family member in close contact with him.

Mr. Marak is oriented to time, place, and person sporadically. He answers some questions in English, but often does not answer at all. Occasionally, he speaks Yiddish. When agitated, he speaks only Hungarian.

Erica realizes that because of his complex physiologic problems, a variety of nursing diagnoses, such as *nutrition alteration: less than body requirements, verbal communication impairment,* and *high risk for skin integrity impairment,* are appropriate for Mr. Marak. She also feels strongly that Mr. Marak needs help in dealing with the emotional and social consequences of aging, severe illness, and hospitalization. Therefore, she includes the nursing diagnosis *powerlessness related to loss of control over life situation* in her documentation.

Planning care

To help Mr. Marak cope with powerlessness, Erica plans to involve him in developing a schedule for his care. As much as possible, she will attempt to determine what his wishes are with regard to continued treatment. Erica eventually hopes to obtain Mr. Marak's expressed agreement with plans for his medical and nursing care. She also realizes that she needs to understand the reasons behind his son's insistence on continued medical treatment at all costs. In her plan of care, she documents the following outcomes:

- Patient participates in care-related decisions to the extent possible.
- He is given the opportunity to speak with a rabbi.
- He expresses his wishes with regard to continuation of life-sustaining treatment.
- His son expresses feelings related to his father's illness and treatment.
- Patient and son cooperate with multidisciplinary treatment team in determining appropriate course of action, with patient's expressed wishes being the most important consideration.

Interventions

First, Erica demonstrates to Mr. Marak her willingness to cooperate with aspects of care that are important to him. She posts a sign over his bed that reads: "Do Not Remove Hat Or Prayer Book," and "Keep Patient's Glasses On Him While He Is Awake."

Erica also helps Mr. Marak participate in decision making. She always asks his permission before providing care and refers to a list of questions in Hungarian that are posted over his bed. She explains each procedure before performing it.

To help determine Mr. Marak's wishes regarding treatment decisions, she consults with the hospital chaplaincy service about locating a rabbi whose opinion Mr. Marak will respect, possibly one who speaks Yiddish or Hungarian. She plans to arrange for a consultation regarding Jewish law on decisions related to terminating life-sustaining treatment.

Finally, Erica recognizes that she must help Mr. Marak's son come to terms with his father's illness. She has an opportunity to speak with him on a Sunday afternoon during a visit with his father. He expresses strong feelings of anger and guilt about his father's condition and relates the current crisis to his father's ordeal during the Holocaust. Erica asks him if he would agree to a meeting with the hospital's psychiatric nurse specialist. She also arranges a multidisciplinary conference to include staff members and Mr. Marak's son to determine the best course of action.

Evaluation

Despite his deteriorating condition, Mr. Marak gave clear indications that he was pleased with the staff's attention to his individual needs. He thanked Erica for arranging a visit with a rabbi. During this visit, he was able to clearly express his wish that his suffering not be artificially prolonged. Eventually, Mr. Marak returned to his nursing home, and his son accepted his right to die with dignity.

N.A.N.D.A. TAXONOMY I REVISED

The North American Nursing Diagnosis Association's *Taxonomy I Revised,* organized around nine human response patterns, is the currently accepted classification system for nursing diagnoses. The complete taxonomic structure is listed below.

Pattern 1. Exchanging: A human response pattern involving mutual giving and receiving

1.1.2.1	Altered nutrition: More than body requirements
1.1.2.2	Altered nutrition: Less than body requirements
1.1.2.3	Altered nutrition: Potential for more than body requirements
1.2.1.1	Risk for infection
1.2.2.1	Risk for altered body temperature
1.2.2.2	Hypothermia
1.2.2.3	Hyperthermia
1.2.2.4	Ineffective thermoregulation
1.2.3.1	Dysreflexia
1.3.1.1	Constipation
1.3.1.1.1	Perceived constipation
1.3.1.1.2	Colonic constipation
1.3.1.2	Diarrhea
1.3.1.3	Bowel incontinence
1.3.2	Altered urinary elimination
1.3.2.1.1	Stress incontinence
1.3.2.1.2	Reflex incontinence
1.3.2.1.3	Urge incontinence
1.3.2.1.4	Functional incontinence
1.3.2.1.5	Total incontinence
1.3.2.2	Urinary retention
1.4.1.1	Altered (specify type) tissue perfusion (renal, cerebral, cardiopulmonary, gastrointestinal, peripheral)
1.4.1.2.1	Fluid volume excess
1.4.1.2.2.1	Fluid volume deficit
1.4.1.2.2.2	Risk for fluid volume deficit
1.4.2.1	Decreased cardiac output
1.5.1.1	Impaired gas exchange
1.5.1.2	Ineffective airway clearance
1.5.1.3	Ineffective breathing pattern
1.5.1.3.1	Inability to sustain spontaneous ventilation
1.5.1.3.2	Dysfunctional ventilatory weaning response
1.6.1	Risk for injury
1.6.1.1	Risk for suffocation
1.6.1.2	Risk for poisoning
1.6.1.3	Risk for trauma
1.6.1.4	Risk for aspiration
1.6.1.5	Risk for disuse syndrome
1.6.2	Altered protection
1.6.2.1	Impaired tissue integrity
1.6.2.1.1	Altered oral mucous membrane
1.6.2.1.2.1	Impaired skin integrity
1.6.2.1.2.2	Risk for impaired skin integrity
1.7.1	Decreased adaptive capacity: Intracranial*
1.8	Energy field disturbance*

Pattern 2. Communicating: A human response pattern involving sending messages

2.1.1.1	Impaired verbal communication

Pattern 3. Relating: A human response pattern involving establishing bonds

3.1.1	Impaired social interaction
3.1.2	Social isolation
3.1.3	Risk for loneliness*
3.2.1	Altered role performance
3.2.1.1.1	Altered parenting
3.2.1.1.2	Risk for altered parenting
3.2.1.1.2.1	Risk for altered parent/infant/child attachment*
3.2.1.2.1	Sexual dysfunction
3.2.2	Altered family processes
3.2.2.1	Caregiver role strain
3.2.2.2	Risk for caregiver role strain
3.2.2.3.1	Altered family process: Alcoholism*
3.2.3.1	Parental role conflict
3.3	Altered sexuality patterns

*indicates 1 of the 19 diagnoses recently approved by NANDA

Pattern 4. Valuing: A human response pattern involving the assigning of relative worth

4.1.1 Spiritual distress (distress of the human spirit)
4.2 Potential for enhanced spiritual well-being*

Pattern 5. Choosing: A human response pattern involving the selection of alternatives

5.1.1.1 Ineffective individual coping
5.1.1.1.1 Impaired adjustment
5.1.1.1.2 Defensive coping
5.1.1.1.3 Ineffective denial
5.1.2.1.1 Ineffective family coping: Disabling
5.1.2.1.2 Ineffective family coping: Compromised
5.1.2.2 Family coping: Potential for growth
5.1.3.1 Potential for enhanced community coping*
5.1.3.2 Ineffective community coping*
5.2.1 Ineffective management of therapeutic regimen: Individual
5.2.1.1 Noncompliance (specify)
5.2.2 Ineffective management of therapeutic regimen: Families*
5.2.3 Ineffective management of therapeutic regimen: Community*
5.2.4 Effective management of therapeutic regimen: Individual*
5.3.1.1 Decisional conflict (specify)
5.4 Health-seeking behaviors

Pattern 6. Moving: A human response pattern involving activity

6.1.1.1 Impaired physical mobility
6.1.1.1.1 Risk for peripheral neurovascular dysfunction
6.1.1.1.2 Risk for perioperative postioning injury*
6.1.1.2 Activity intolerance
6.1.1.2.1 Fatigue
6.1.1.3 Risk for activity intolerance
6.2.1 Sleep pattern disturbance
6.3.1.1 Diversional activity deficit
6.4.1.1 Impaired home maintenance management
6.4.2 Altered health maintenance
6.5.1 Feeding self-care deficit
6.5.1.1 Impaired swallowing
6.5.1.2 Ineffective breast-feeding
6.5.1.2.1 Interrupted breast-feeding
6.5.1.3 Effective breast-feeding
6.5.1.4 Ineffective infant feeding pattern
6.5.2 Bathing or hygiene self-care deficit
6.5.3 Dressing or grooming self-care deficit
6.5.4 Toileting self-care deficit
6.6 Altered growth and development
6.7 Relocation stress syndrome
6.8.1 Risk for disorganized infant behavior*
6.8.2 Disorganized infant behavior*
6.8.3 Potential for enhanced organized infant behavior*

Pattern 7. Perceiving: A human response pattern involving the reception of information

7.1.1 Body image disturbance
7.1.2 Self-esteem disturbance
7.1.2.1 Chronic low self-esteem
7.1.2.2 Situational low self-esteem
7.1.3 Personal identity disturbance
7.2 Sensory or perceptual alterations (specify—visual, auditory, kinesthetic, gustatory, tactile, olfactory)
7.2.1.1 Unilateral neglect
7.3.1 Hopelessness
7.3.2 Powerlessness

Pattern 8. Knowing: A human response pattern involving the meaning associated with information

8.1.1 Knowledge deficit (specify)
8.2.1 Impaired environmental interpretation syndrome*
8.2.2 Acute confusion*
8.2.3 Chronic confusion*
8.3 Altered thought processes
8.3.1 Impaired memory*

*indicates 1 of the 19 diagnoses recently approved by NANDA

Pattern 9. Feeling: A human response pattern involving the subjective awareness of information

9.1.1	Pain
9.1.1.1	Chronic pain
9.2.1.1	Dysfunctional grieving
9.2.1.2	Anticipatory grieving
9.2.2	Risk for violence: Self-directed or directed at others
9.2.2.1	Risk for self-mutilation
9.2.3	Post-trauma response
9.2.3.1	Rape-trauma syndrome
9.2.3.1.1	Rape-trauma syndrome: Compound reaction
9.2.3.1.2	Rape-trauma syndrome: Silent reaction
9.3.1	Anxiety
9.3.2	Fear

*indicates 1 of the 19 diagnoses recently approved by NANDA

NEW NURSING DIAGNOSES

Confusion, acute

Definition

Abrupt onset of changes in attention span, cognition, psychomotor activity, level of consciousness, or sleep-wake cycle

Assessment

- Age, sex, level of education, occupation, recent immigration
- Health history, including use of medications, recent surgery, allergies, history of alcoholism, drug abuse, or depression
- Neurologic status, including level of consciousness (LOC), orientation, thought and speech, mood, affect, memory, visual and spatial ability, judgment and insight, psychomotor activity, perceptions; delusions, illusions, hallucinations; pain level; recent behavioral changes; history of transient ischemic attacks (TIAs), head injury, early dementia, acquired immunodeficiency syndrome, schizophrenia
- Cardiovascular status, including vital signs, skin color, posture, auscultation of carotid artery and heart sounds, history of coronary artery disease or hypertension
- Respiratory status, including rate, depth, and pattern of respirations; auscultation for breath sounds; smoking history; shortness of breath; history of chronic obstructive pulmonary disease, cancer, tuberculosis
- Sensory status, including results of vision and hearing examination,use of corrective lenses or hearing aid, history of eye or ear disorders
- Nutritional status, including typical daily food intake, weight loss
- Sleep status, including recent change in sleep pattern or environment (recent hospitalization)

Defining characteristics

- Altered attention span
- Altered sleep patterns
- Changes in recent, remote, and immediate memory
- Disorientation to time, place, person, circumstances, or situation
- Confabulation
- Fluctuations in psychomotor activity
- Inability to initiate and follow through with goal-directed behavior
- Impaired ability to reason, solve problems, make decisions, conceptualize, or interpret the environment
- Inappropriate affect
- Inappropriate social behavior

Associated disorders and conditions

Alcoholism, cerebrovascular accident, delirium, dementia, drug abuse, infection, TIAs, head trauma, hypoxemia or hypercapnia, sensory deprivation

Expected outcomes

- Patient does not experience injury.
- Patient's neurologic status does not deteriorate.
- Family members report an improved ability to cope with the patient's confused state.
- Patient starts to participate in activities of daily living (ADLs).
- Patient reports feeling increasingly calm.
- Patient and family members state the causes of acute confusion.
- Patient and family members express an understanding of the importance of informing other health care providers about episode of acute confusion.

Interventions and rationales

- Assess the patient's LOC and changes in behavior *to provide baseline for comparison with ongoing assessment findings.*

• Have a staff member stay at the patient's bedside, if necessary, *to protect the patient from harm.*
• Enlist the aid of a family member *to help calm the patient.*
• Limit noise and environmental stimulation *to prevent the patient from becoming more confused.*
• Review all medications *to find out if adverse effects of drug therapy may be the cause of confusion.*
• Monitor neurologic status on a regular basis *to detect any improvement or decline in the patient's neurologic function.*
• Use appropriate safety measures *to protect the patient from injury.* Avoid physical restraints *to avoid agitating the patient.*
• Address the patient by name and tell him your name *to foster his awareness of self and environment.*
• Give the patient short, simple explanations each time you perform a procedure or task *to decrease confusion.*
• Schedule nursing care to provide quiet times for the patient *to help avoid sensory overload.*
• Mention time, place, and date frequently throughout the day. Have a clock and a calendar where the patient can easily see them. Refer to these aids when orienting him *to foster awareness of self and environment.*
• Keep the patient's possessions in the same place as much as possible. *A consistent, stable environment reduces confusion and frustration and aids completion of ADLs.*
• Ask family members to bring labeled family photos and other favorite articles *to create a more secure environment for the patient.*
• Plan the patient's routine and be as consistent as possible in following it. *A consistent plan aids task completion and reduces confusion.*
• Speak slowly and clearly and allow the patient ample time to respond *to reduce his frustration and promote task completion.*
• Encourage the patient to perform ADLs, dividing tasks into small, critical units. Be patient and specific in providing instructions. Allow time for the patient to perform each task. *These measures enhance his self-esteem as well as help prevent complications related to inactivity.*
• Encourage family members to share stories and discuss familiar people and events with the patient. *Sharing stories and familiar subjects promotes a sense of continuity, aids memory, and creates a sense of security and comfort.* Note that if the patient's short-term memory is impaired, his remote memory still may be intact.
• Support family members' attempts to interact with the patient *to provide positive reinforcement.*
• Allow time before and after visits for family members to express feelings. *Listening to the family members in an open and nonjudgmental manner will help them cope with the patient's illness. Listening to their opinions may also help you assess and monitor the patient's condition.*
• Reassure the patient and family members that confusion will be temporary *to help relieve their anxiety.* Always include the patient in discussions.
• Confer with the doctor about diagnostic test results, patient's progress in behavior, and LOC. *A collaborative approach to treatment helps ensure high-quality care and continuity of care.*
• Discuss the episode of acute confusion with the patient and family. Make sure they understand the cause of confusion. Review measures family members can take at home to help the patient if he begins to exhibit signs of confusion:
  – Give the patient short explanations of activities.
  – Remind the patient of time, place, and date frequently.
  – Speak slowly and clearly to the patient and allow him time to respond.
  – Provide the patient with a consistent routine.

Teaching will empower the patient and

family members to take greater responsibility for their health care needs.
• Stress to the patient and family members that, in the future, they should inform health care providers about the episode of acute confusion *to help ensure continuity of care*.

Evaluation statements
Patient:
• does not experience injury during episode of acute confusion.
• receives an appropriate diagnostic workup to identify and treat the cause of confusion.
• performs ADLs to the extent possible.
• exhibits a mental status within the normal range.
• reports feelings of increased calm.
• expresses an understanding of the episode of acute confusion.

Family members:
• report an increased ability to cope with the patient's confused state.

Patient and family members:
• express understanding of measures to take should confusion recur
• express an understanding of the importance of telling future health care providers about episode of acute confusion.

Confusion, chronic

Definition
An irreversible, long-standing, or progressive deterioration of intellect and personality characterized by decreased ability to interpret environmental stimuli; decreased capacity for thought; and disturbances of memory, orientation, and behavior

Assessment
• Age, sex
• Neurologic status, including level of consciousness, orientation, thought and speech, mood, affect, memory, visual and spatial ability, judgment and insight, psychomotor activity, perceptions; recent behavior changes; lethargy, restlessness, short-term memory loss, sleep disturbance; history of multiple infarctions, transient ischemic attacks, Parkinson's disease, cerebral infarcts, seizures, alcohol or drug abuse
• Self-care status, including ability to perform instrumental or routine activities of daily living (ADLs)
• Family status, including marital status, economic status, living arrangements, presence of caregiver and relationship to patient, caregiver's perception of patient's abilities

Defining characteristics
• Altered attention span
• Altered sleep patterns
• Changes in recent, remote, and immediate memory
• Disorientation to time, place, person, or situation
• Confabulation
• Fluctuations in psychomotor activity
• Inability to initiate and follow through with goal-directed behavior
• Impaired ability to reason, abstract, and solve problems; make decisions; conceptualize; or interpret the environment
• Inappropriate affect
• Inappropriate social behavior

Associated disorders
Acquired immunodeficiency syndrome, Alzheimer's disease, cerebrovascular accident, dementia, head trauma, Korsakoff's psychosis, multi-infarct dementia

Expected outcomes
• Patient's cognitive abilities, behavior, and self-care status are carefully assessed.
• Patient is assessed for signs of depression.
• Patient's weight is measured and documented.
• Family members discuss their ability to provide care for the patient.
• Patient is provided with a structured environment to ensure maximum functioning.
• Family members or caregiver describe strategies to help the patient cope with chronic confusion.

• Patient participates in selected activities to the extent possible.
• Safety of the patient's home environment is assessed.
• If necessary, patient and family members prepare for relocation to long-term care facility.
• Patient receives adequate emotional support to help him cope with stress of moving to a new environment.
• Staff at the patient's new residence receive clear instructions regarding measures to help the patient cope with chronic confusion.

Interventions and rationales
• Assess the patient's cognitive abilities and changes in behavior *to provide baseline data for comparison with ongoing assessment findings.*
• Encourage family members to watch you perform mental status assessments *to give them a more accurate view of the patient's abilities.*
• Evaluate the patient's ability to care for himself, including his ability to function alone and drive a car. *Safety is a primary concern.*
• Assess the patient for depression *to determine the need for treatment.*
• Weigh the patient, document your findings, and include instructions for regular weighing as part of the care plan *to monitor the patient's nutritional status.*
• Ask family members about their ability to provide care for the patient *to assess their need for assistance.* Be sure to project an attentive and nonjudgmental attitude when listening to them *to help ensure that you receive accurate information.*
• Take steps to provide a stable physical environment and consistent daily routine for the patient. *Stability and consistent structure enhance functioning.*
• Teach family members or caregiver strategies to help the patient cope with his condition:
  – Place an identification bracelet on the patient *to promote safety.*
  – Touch the patient *to convey acceptance.*
  – Avoid unfamiliar situations when possible *to help ensure a consistent environment.*
  – Provide structured rest periods *to prevent fatigue and reduce stress.*
  – Avoid asking questions the patient can't answer – for example, questions that test his orientation to time, place, person, or situation – *to avoid frustrating him.*
  – Provide finger foods if the patient will not sit and eat *to ensure adequate nutrition.*
  – Select activities based on the patient's interests and abilities and praise him for participating in activities *to enhance his sense of self-worth.*
  – Use TV and radio carefully *to avoid sensory overload, which may exacerbate confusion.*
  – Limit choices the patient has to make *to provide structure and avoid confusion.*
  – Label familiar photos with names of individuals pictured *to provide a sense of security.*
  – Use symbols, rather than written signs, to identify the patient's room, the bathroom, and other facilities *to help the patient identify surroundings.*
  – Place the patient's name in large block letters on clothing and other belongings *to help the patient recognize his belongings and prevent them from becoming lost.*
• If possible, make a home visit *to assess the safety of the patient's living environment.*
• Assist family members in contacting appropriate community services. If necessary, act as an advocate for the patient within the health care system *to help secure services needed for ongoing care.*
• Provide family members with information concerning long-term health care facilities. If necessary, assist family members in moving the patient to a nursing home or other long-term care setting. *A patient with chronic confusion may require ongoing skilled nursing care.*

• If the patient is to be moved to a long-term care facility, explain to him the decision in as simple and gentle terms as possible *to facilitate comprehension.* Allow the patient to express his feelings regarding the move *to facilitate grieving over the loss of independence.* Provide psychological support to the patient and family members *to alleviate stress they will experience during the relocation.*
• Communicate all aspects of the discharge plan to the staff at the patient's new residence, including:
  – measures to ensure a stable environment and consistent routine
  – the need to monitor the patient's ongoing ability to perform ADLs
  – measures to ensure adequate nutrition
  – interventions to provide emotional support to patient and family members.

Documenting a discharge plan and communicating it to caregivers helps to ensure continuity of care. Interventions should seek to ensure the patient's dignity and rights.

Evaluation statements

Patient:
• experiences no injury because of chronic confusion.
• undergoes a complete diagnostic workup to rule out any reversible cause of confusion.
• participates in appropriate activities.
• functions to maximum ability in a stable and structured environment.
• receives adequate nutrition.
• receives adequate emotional support before, during, and after relocation to long-term care facility.
• expresses feelings regarding living arrangement in the nursing home.

Family members:
• discuss openly their ability to provide for the patient.
• describe strategies to help the patient cope with chronic confusion.
• receive adequate information regarding long-term care options to make informed decisions regarding the patient's future.

■ Coping, ineffective community

related to increased levels of teen pregnancy

Definition

Difficulty experienced by a community in confronting social, health, or economic problems; in this instance, problems experienced by a community in controlling an escalating teen-pregnancy rate

Assessment

• Community demographics, including age and sex distribution, ethnic groups, racial groups, religious groups, education and income levels
• Family status, including family composition (percentage of single-parent families in the community); ability of families to meet their physical, social, emotional, and economic needs; responsibilities assumed by teens in the care of siblings
• Community health status, including prevalence of health problems in the community; beliefs, values, and attitudes about health and illness; attitudes toward sex and sexuality; availability of health care services; community members' use of health care services
• Prevalence of teen pregnancies; attitudes toward teen mothers and their infants; incidence of sexually transmitted diseases, low-birth-weight neonates, and congenital abnormalities
• Education system, including availability of sex education in schools; willingness of parents to allow children to participate
• Teenagers' knowledge about sex and sexuality
• Political system, including government officials' support for or opposition to sex education
• Attitude of religious groups toward sex and sexuality; religious groups' influence on educators
• Transportation availability to clinics and other social services; recreation opportunities for adolescents

- Welfare and health care system; reliance of teen mothers on welfare for support

Defining characteristics
- Absence of education or support for sexually active teenagers
- Absence of programs for pregnancy testing, counseling, or teaching young women to care for infants
- Absence of sex education in the home, school, and community
- Excessive community conflicts over what to teach adolescents or preadolescent children about sex
- Failure of teenagers to perceive long-term effects of having babies
- High incidence of infants who are born prematurely or with health problems.
- High rate of teen pregnancy
- Lack of access to birth control devices for teenagers
- Lack of community support for preventive sex education
- Perception by teenagers that teachers and parents are uncaring, disapproving, or unavailable to help
- Poor prenatal care, which threatens the health of the adolescent mother and infant

Associated disorders and conditions
Mother: sexually transmitted diseases, drug and alcohol abuse
Child: developmental delays, hepatitis, lack of immunizations, malnutrition, human immunodeficiency virus infection, neglect and failure to thrive

Expected outcomes
- Community members express awareness of the seriousness of the high adolescent pregnancy rate in their community.
- Community members express the need for a plan to reduce the prevalence of teen pregnancies.
- Community members develop and implement plans to reduce teen pregnancy.
- Community members evaluate the success of the plan in meeting goals and objectives.
- Community members continue to revise the plan to prevent teen pregnancy as necessary.

Interventions and rationales
- Assess teenagers' knowledge about sex and sexuality *to determine their educational needs.*
- Work with schools to develop pregnancy prevention programs *to give the adolescent information about the risks, problems, and complications of early pregnancy.*
- Work closely with individual adolescents who are pregnant *to assess their needs and provide care.*
- Implement an outreach and health promotion program *to raise community members' awareness of the need to approach teen pregnancy as a community problem.* Consider taking the following steps:
  - Work with teachers, school psychologists, counselors, students, and the parent-teacher association to determine the extent of the teen pregnancy problem among the adolescent population.
  - Encourage local youth groups, churches, and social service organizations to feature guest speakers on pregnancy prevention at their meetings.
  - Contact representatives of local corporations to ask for funding for educational programs.
- Help community members (school nurses, counselors, teachers) recognize adolescent girls who need counseling regarding such issues as peer pressure to be sexually active and the long-term consequences of pregnancy. Remind community members of the importance of listening attentively and remaining nonjudgmental. *Alert adults who take a nonjudgmental approach will have more success in effectively communicating advice to adolescents.*
- Provide education on preventive birth-control measures (including abstinence from sex) and have this information available at school. *Access to information at school provides adolescents with*

a safe environment in which to seek help.
• Establish clubs for adolescent girls in the community. The goal of these clubs is to foster self-esteem. During club meetings, members should have the opportunity to openly discuss difficult questions such as:
– why girls consider a baby as a status symbol
– how to respond to peer pressure to be sexually active.
Improved self-esteem has been found the most effective way to reduce teen pregnancies.
• Encourage adolescents to participate in peer-support networks where they can openly discuss social and dating pressure and other issues related to teen pregnancy *to allow adolescents an opportunity to openly express their feelings and obtain support from peers.*
• Encourage community members to establish school-based clinics in which the teens can have access to reproductive-system models, pregnancy tests, and nonprescription birth-control measures *to support the teenagers who make the decision to protect themselves from unwanted pregnancies.*
• Develop a list of referrals for teenagers, such as hospitals with human sexuality courses, charities that provide prenatal care and childbirth services, women's clinics, and Planned Parenthood *to compensate for restricted access to information in the adolescent's home or school.*
• Encourage community members to implement an information campaign to educate adolescents, parents, and community members about the problems associated with teen pregnancy. *To be effective in reducing pregnancy rates, an education program must involve the entire community.*
• Work with community members to evaluate the effectiveness of the teen pregnancy prevention program and assist with modifying the program as needed *to ensure the program's effectiveness and promote use of the program as a model for preventive health.*
• Collect statistical data from the schools to analyze the teen pregnancy rates *to help evaluate the effectiveness of the prevention program.*

Evaluation statements
Community members:
• express the need for a plan to reduce teen pregnancy.
• develop a plan to reduce the incidence of teen pregnancies.
• establish an outreach and health promotion program.
• establish school-based sex-education and self-esteem programs.
• report a reduction in the rate of teen pregnancy.

■ Coping, potential for enhanced community

related to immunization

Definition
Potential for a community to improve its ability to meet the social, economic, or health-related needs of its residents. This example describes efforts to improve childhood immunization programs.

Assessment
• Community demographics, including age and sex distribution, ethnic groups, racial groups, religious groups, education and income levels
• Community health status, including residents' beliefs, values, and attitudes about health and illness; availability of health care services; residents' use of health care services; prevalence of childhood illnesses in the community
• Education system, including educational level of adult population; state law or school system's requirements for immunization before school attendance
• Religious institutions and their support for or objections to immunization
• Social services, including availability of clinics and other social services; access to health care; welfare system; parents' dependence on welfare for support

Defining characteristics

- Absence of education regarding childhood immunization in the community.
- Absence of an immunization requirement for school entrance
- Lack of community support for childhood immunization programs
- Potential for an outbreak of a communicable disease because of lack of proper immunization among transient groups (despite established community immunization programs and school requirements)

Expected outcomes

- Community members express understanding of problems associated with failure to immunize the population.
- Community members express understanding of the need for a plan to reduce the number of children who are not immunized.
- Community members establish a plan of action to increase the rate of immunizations and ensure adequate protection from communicable diseases.
- Community members work to reduce the spread of communicable diseases and increase the rate of immunization within the community.
- Community members evaluate established plans for ensuring that all children become immunized and make changes to plans as necessary.

Interventions and rationales

- Work with community members to pinpoint potential problems associated with inadequate immunization of the population *to ensure adequate protection against communicable disease.* Consider taking the following steps:
  - Identify new members of the community, such as immigrants and refugees, *to help reach parents who need information about immunization.*
  - Identify parents who do not follow through with the required series of immunizations *to protect children from incomplete immunization.*
- Encourage community members to implement a program to disseminate information about the problems associated with inadequate immunization *to educate residents and promote the community's established immunization program.*
- Provide extensive education about communicable disease and the importance of immunizations *to empower community residents and help decrease the risk of communicable disease.*
- Encourage health departments, clinics, and practitioners' offices to provide information on the recommended childhood immunization schedule to the public *to foster education about immunization.*
- Contact parents of children who are not immunized in person or by handwritten note. Make it clear that your purpose in promoting immunization is to protect their child from illness *to build parents' trust in immunization programs.*
- Provide immunization information in the parents' first language *to overcome lack of understanding caused by language barriers.*
- Develop a list of referrals for parents of children who are not immunized. Include information on low-cost health insurance, city health centers, and well-baby clinics *to encourage compliance.*
- Coordinate with local nursing schools, health department nurses, and other interested nursing groups to provide the necessary number of professionals to deliver adequate immunizations *to reduce the risk of communicable disease.*
- Conduct a follow-up survey on immunization rates *to measure the effectiveness of educational efforts.*
- Collect statistical data from community sources, such as the health department and schools, *to continue to identify children who have not been immunized.*

Evaluation statements

Community members:

- put forth a plan to meet the community's immunization needs.
- develop a plan that contains definite actions, yet allows for modifications.

• make changes to the plan that help solve problems and further the goal of meeting the community's immunization needs.
• implement a program to disseminate information about the problems associated with inadequate immunization.

Energy field disturbance

Definition
Disharmony in a person's inner sense of well-being that results in physical, emotional, or spiritual distress

Assessment
• Psychological status, including anxiety, fatigue, depression, somatic complaints, recent lifestyle changes (death of loved one, conflict in a relationship, or loss of job)
• Health status, including presence of disorder that is life-threatening or requires surgery
• Sensory status, including pain, disorders that may affect senses
• Spiritual status, including religious beliefs and affiliation; support system; helplessness, hopelessness, anger, withdrawal
• Caregiver's readiness to provide therapeutic healing, including education and training in therapeutic touch or similar treatment technique

Defining characteristics
• Agitation
• Altered self-esteem or self-concept
• Anger
• Anxiety
• Depression
• Fatigue
• Irritability
• Pain
• Poor wound healing
• Restlessness

Associated disorders
Amputation, cancer, infection, rheumatoid arthritis, trauma, any illness that is life-threatening or requires surgery

Expected outcomes
• Patient feels increasingly relaxed, as demonstrated by slower and deeper breathing, skin flushing in treated area, audible sighing, or reports of feeling more relaxed.
• Patient visualizes images that relax him.
• Patient reports feeling less tension or pain.
• Patient continues to receive treatments that help to relax him and promote inner well-being.
• Patient uses self-healing techniques, such as meditation, guided imagery, yoga, or prayer.
• Patient expresses increased sense of well-being.

Interventions and rationales
• Implement measures to promote therapeutic healing. Place your hands 4" to 6" (10 to 15 cm) above the patient's body. Pass your hands over the entire skin surface. *This technique helps you become attuned to the patient's energy field, the flow of energy that surrounds a person's being.* With experience and training in therapeutic touch or similar treatment, a practitioner can identify sensory cues to energy field disturbances, such as heat, cold, tingling, or an electric sensation.
• Try to gain the patient's cooperation as you perform healing techniques such as therapeutic touch *to enhance effectiveness of healing techniques and foster participation in spiritual aspects of care.*
• Continue to treat the patient using therapeutic healing techniques. *One treatment rarely restores a full sense of inner well-being.*
• Suggest that the patient use self-healing techniques, such as meditation, guided imagery, yoga, or prayer, *to encourage the patient to participate in his care.*

Evaluation statements
Patient:
• reports an improvement in symptoms or shows signs of increased comfort.

- expresses an understanding of actions that can be performed to promote relaxation and inner well-being.
- uses self-healing techniques, such as meditation, guided imagery, yoga, or exercise.
- reports an increased sense of well-being.

Environmental interpretation syndrome, impaired

Definition

Consistent lack of orientation to person, place, time, or circumstances that lasts for more than 6 months and necessitates placement in a protective environment

Assessment

- Cultural status, including age, sex, level of education, occupation, living arrangements, nationality, race, ethnic group, religion, personal habits
- Family status, including marital status, family composition, family members' ability to meet patient's needs
- Cardiovascular status, including vital signs, skin color (especially lips and nails); chest pain, fatigue on exertion, dyspnea, dizziness; electrocardiography or echocardiography results
- Neurologic status, including level of consciousness (LOC), motor activity, thought and speech, mood and affect, memory, attention span, judgment, orientation, comprehension, perception; cerebellar function, cranial nerve function, sensation, reflexes, pupillary response; medications
- Psychological status, including changes in appearance, appetite, energy level, motivation, personal hygiene, self-image, self-esteem, sleep patterns, LOC; alcohol and drug use, life changes (recent divorce, separation, job loss, loss of a loved one, relocation)
- Psychiatric history, including age at onset of illness; severity of symptoms; impact on functioning; type of treatment and response
- Self-care status, including functional ability (muscle tone, size, and strength; range of motion, coordination); daily activities (dressing, grooming, bathing, toileting, hygiene); use of adaptive equipment
- Social status, including interaction with others, ability to function in social or occupational roles
- Sensory status, including presence of visual or hearing deficits, use of hearing aid or eyeglasses

Defining characteristics

- Consistent disorientation to environment
- Chronic confusion
- Inability to reason, concentrate, or follow simple directions
- Loss of occupation or social function resulting from memory decline
- Slow response to questions

Associated disorders

Acquired immunodeficiency syndrome, Alzheimer's disease, angina, atherosclerosis, brain tumor, cerebral aneurysm, cerebrovascular accident, dementia, epilepsy, head trauma, human immunodeficiency virus infection, hypertension, multiple sclerosis, organic brain disorders, substance abuse, transient ischemic attacks

Expected outcomes

- Clear, concise goals for coping with disorientation are communicated to the patient and caregiver.
- Patient acknowledges and responds to efforts by others to establish communication.
- Patient remains oriented to environment to the fullest extent possible.
- Family members participate in efforts to help patient cope with disorientation.
- Patient and caregiver express feelings associated with disorientation.
- Patient remains free from injury.
- Caregiver describes measures for helping patient cope with disorientation.
- Family members demonstrate reorientation techniques.
- Family members describe ways to ensure that home is made safe for patient.

• Caregiver describes plans to continue to help patient cope with disorientation in the least restrictive way possible.
• Caregiver, in cooperation with patient, identifies and contacts appropriate support services.

Interventions and rationales

• Spend time with the patient and caregiver *to establish a trusting relationship.*
• Be clear, concise, and direct in establishing goals and skills for coping with disorientation *so the patient and caregiver can understand them.*
• Consider performing the following interventions:
  – Assess the patient's sight and hearing, and assist him with glasses or a hearing aid as necessary.
  – Minimize distractions by turning off radios or television.
  – When speaking to the patient, face him, maintain eye contact, and smile.
  – Speak slowly in clear, low tones, using simple direct language. Repeat your remarks as needed.
  – Be aware that the patient may be sensitive to your unspoken feelings about him.

These measures will help foster communication with the patient. Successful communication is necessary to implement interventions.
• Orient the patient to reality as needed *to improve his awareness of himself and his environment:*
  – Call him by name.
  – Tell him your name.
  – Provide background information (place, time, date) frequently throughout the day. Reinforce this information verbally and by using a reality orientation board.
  – Orient him to his environment.
• Place the patient's photograph or name on the room door *to aid memory and help him find his room.*
• Keep items in the same places. *A consistent, stable environment reduces confusion, decreases frustration, and aids successful completion of activities of daily living.*
• Ask family members to provide the patient with photographs (labeled with the name and relationship on the back) and favorite belongings. *Belongings may spark his memory and promote a sense of security.*
• Don't discourage the patient from wandering. *Wandering stimulates circulation, decreases contracture formation, reduces stress, and provides a feeling of freedom.* Place the patient in a room close to the nursing station, clear the area of as many hazards as possible, make sure he wears an identification bracelet, and provide hospital security with a recent photograph of him *to prevent the patient from getting lost or being injured.*
• Encourage the patient to interact with others *to increase social activity and ease the isolation that may result from disorientation.*
• Provide reassurance and praise the patient for completing simple tasks *to increase the patient's self-esteem.*
• Help the patient and caregiver identify feelings associated with disorientation *to help improve their ability to cope.*
• Work with the patient and caregiver to establish goals for coping with disorientation in the least restrictive way *to maximize independence and reduce feelings of loneliness.*
• Demonstrate reorientation techniques to family members and provide time for supervised return demonstrations *to prepare them to cope with the patient when he returns home.*
• Instruct family members on how to maintain a safe home environment for the patient. *The patient may be unable to consider his own safety needs.*
• Refer the patient and caregiver to appropriate social service and mental health care agencies *to ensure continued care.*

Evaluation statements

Staff members:
• communicate clear, concise goals for coping with disorientation to the patient and caregiver.

Patient:
- acknowledges and responds to efforts by others to establish communication.
- remains oriented to environment to the fullest extent possible.
- expresses feelings associated with disorientation.
- remains free from injury.

Caregiver:
- describes measures for helping patient cope with disorientation.
- describes plans to help patient cope with disorientation in the least restrictive way possible.
- identifies and contacts appropriate support services.

Family members:
- participate in efforts to help patient cope with disorientation.
- demonstrate reorientation techniques.
- describe measures to improve safety of home for patient.

Family process alteration: Alcoholism

Definition
Ineffective family functioning related to alcohol abuse in one or more members, often leading to conflict, denial of problems, resistance to change, ineffective problem solving, and a series of self-perpetuating crises

Assessment
- Family status, including alcoholic family member's ability to function in occupational and family roles, ability of other family members to function in their roles, family conflicts, financial status, rituals during holidays and family celebrations
- Coping patterns, including type and number of changes family has experienced recently, usual response to stress, ability to adapt to change, use of support systems for assistance
- Family health history, including medication use, mental illness, stress-related illnesses, history of alcohol or drug abuse, evidence of emotional, physical, or sexual abuse of spouse or children
- Parental status, including age, marital status, number and ages of dependent children, knowledge of normal child behavior
- Drinking pattern, including continuous or binge drinking, periods of abstinence and relapse, use of other substances, symptoms of withdrawal, past drinking patterns and treatment
- Psychological status, including self-image and self-esteem, functional ability, independence level, problem-solving skills, decision-making skills
- Spiritual status, including affiliation with a religious group; religious practices

Defining characteristics
- Altered role functioning, including inability of alcoholic family member to function in occupational and family roles, attempt by other family members to compensate for alcoholic member's inability to fulfill roles, assumption of adult roles by older children
- Anger, anxiety, and depression
- Conflict between parents and between children and parents
- Deterioration in family relationships
- Distancing behaviors
- Feelings of rejection, guilt, hopelessness, and mistrust
- Inability of family to meet physical and emotional needs of its members
- Isolation of family from outside support systems
- Poor academic performance in children
- Poor self-esteem in family members
- Stress-related physical problems

Associated disorders
Alcohol abuse, amnesic disorders, anxiety disorders, cardiovascular disease, conduct disorder, delirium, dementia, depression, drug abuse, encephalopathy, esophageal varices, liver disease, nutritional deficiencies, peripheral neuropathy, personality disorders, sexual disorders, ulcers

Expected outcomes

- Family members acknowledge there is a problem with alcoholism within the family.
- Alcoholic family member signs a contract stating that he agrees to abstain from alcohol.
- Family members sign contracts stating that they will not engage in abusive behavior.
- Family members communicate their needs using "I" statements.
- Parents take steps to reassert appropriate boundaries with children and to resume parental responsibilities.
- Family members discuss problems in an open, safe environment.
- Family members acknowledge their strengths and progress they have made in resolving problems.
- The number and intensity of family crises diminish.
- Family members state their plans to continue to seek counseling and attend appropriate support groups.

Interventions and rationales

- Encourage family members to acknowledge that there is a problem with alcoholism within the family *to break through family denial*. Encourage individual family members to take responsibility for their problems. *Problems cannot be addressed until family members take responsibility for them.*
- Inform the alcoholic family member that he will have to address his alcoholism before progress can be made in rebuilding the family. Tell him that abstinence with the help of a support group like Alcoholics Anonymous (AA) is the only proven effective treatment for alcoholism *to establish abstinence as the basis for treatment.*
- Ask the alcoholic family member to sign a contract stating that he will abstain from alcohol *to help him take responsibility for his behavior.*
- Help family members evaluate the consequences of abusive and violent behavior. Inform them that any suspected abuse will be reported. Ask family members to sign contracts stating that they will not be abusive to each other *to help ensure safety of family members.*
- Teach family members to communicate their needs assertively. Encourage family members to use "I" statements to express feelings—for example, "I'm mad because you didn't show up for the school play like you promised." *Using "I" statements may help family members get in touch with and talk about feelings.*
- Discuss with parents their ideas and beliefs regarding parental authority. Ask them if they feel they have abdicated authority. Work with parents to develop steps to reassert parental authority *to reestablish appropriate boundaries and relieve children of the need to assume parental roles.*
- Provide an opportunity for family members to discuss conflicts in an open, safe atmosphere *to decrease anxiety and help family members develop confidence in their ability to resolve problems.*
- Assist family members in identifying their strengths and the progress they have made in addressing problems *to build self-esteem.*
- Encourage family members to continue to seek counseling *to enhance interpersonal skills and strengthen the family unit.*
- Encourage family members to participate in AA, Alanon, or Alateen to *foster recovery.*

Evaluation statements

Alcoholic family member:

- signs a contract stating that he agrees to abstain from alcohol.

Parents:

- take steps to reassert appropriate boundaries with children and to resume parental responsibilities.

Family members:

- acknowledge that there is a problem with alcoholism.
- sign contracts stating that they will not engage in abusive behavior.
- communicate their needs using "I" statements.

• discuss problems in an open, safe environment.
• acknowledge their strengths and the progress they have made in resolving problems.
• state their plans to continue to seek counseling and attend appropriate support groups.

Infant behavior, disorganized

related to pain, prematurity, oral problems, motor problems, feeding intolerance, environmental overstimulation, or lack of stimulation

Definition
A disturbance in infant behavior, such as inappropriate responses to stimuli, problems regulating physiologic function, or apparent inability to interact with the environment. "Disorganized infant behavior" is a term used to describe difficulty in infant behavioral or neurologic development which may lead to problems with the infant's ability to relate to the environment and interfere with parent-infant attachment.

Assessment
• Cardiovascular status, including pulse, respirations
• Gastrointestinal status, including feeding pattern, food tolerance, defecation pattern, ability to maintain adequate weight, abdominal bloating, abdominal distention
• Neurologic status, including muscle tone, newborn reflexes, excessive crying, lethargy, irritability, seizures, tremors; Brazelton Neonatal Behavioral Assessment, Dubowitz Gestational Age Assessment
• Sensory status, including responsiveness to visual, tactile, or auditory stimuli; experience with pain
• Parental status, including knowledge of normal growth and development
• Sleep status, including sleep patterns, usual hours of sleep
• Parents' psychological status, including energy level, motivation, self-image, competence, recent life changes, experience with children, eye contact and interaction with infant

Defining characteristics
• Evidence of problems in behavioral and neurologic development, such as:
 – deficient response to visual and auditory stimuli
 – excessive crying
 – hyperextension of arms and legs
 – irregular sleep pattern or difficulty obtaining adequate sleep
 – tremors, startles, twitches
 – excessive yawning, apnea

Associated disorders
Colic, prematurity, failure to thrive

Expected outcomes
• Parents learn to identify the infant's behavioral cues.
• Parents express understanding of appropriate responses to their infant's behavioral cues.
• Parents are able to identify their own emotional responses to their infant's behavior.
• Parents identify means to help the infant overcome his behavioral disturbance by recognizing the infant's needs and responding appropriately.
• Parents report improved ability to cope with stress of caring for the infant.
• Infant begins to show appropriate signs of maturation, such as longer periods of sleep, shorter periods of crying, longer periods of being awake and alert, smoother transitions between behavioral states, and responding positively to parents' interventions.
• Parents express positive feelings about their ability to care for the infant.

Interventions and rationales
• Explain to the parents that infant maturation is a developmental process and that their participation is crucial *to help them understand the importance of nurturing the infant.*
• Explain to the parents that their actions can help modify some of their in-

fant's behavior. However, make it clear that infant maturation is not completely within their control. *This explanation may help decrease the parents' feelings of incompetence.*

• Explain to the parents that infants give behavioral cues that indicate their needs. Discuss appropriate ways to respond to these behavioral cues, for example,:
  – providing stimulation that does not overwhelm the infant
  – stopping stimulation when the infant gives behavioral cues, such as yawning, looking away, or becoming agitated
  – finding methods to calm the infant if he becomes agitated (swaddling, gentle rocking, quiet vocalizations)

• Assist the parents in identifying and coping with their responses to their infant's behavioral disturbance *to help them recognize and adjust their response patterns. When the infant doesn't respond positively to them, the parents may feel inadequate or become frustrated. They need to understand that these reactions are normal.*

• Demonstrate appropriate ways of interacting with the infant *to show parents how to identify and interpret the infant's behavioral cues and how to respond appropriately. For example, if the infant becomes agitated, it may be because of overstimulation. At this point, the parents should stop stimulating the infant and allow him to rest.*

• Explore with parents ways to cope with the stress imposed by the infant's behavior *to help them develop better coping skills.*

• Praise the parents when they demonstrate appropriate methods of interacting with the infant *to provide positive reinforcement.*

• Provide the parents with information on sources of support and special infant services *to help them cope with the infant's long-term needs.*

Evaluation statements

Parents:

• exhibit less frustration with the infant.

• state their understanding of their infant's behavioral cues.

• discuss appropriate ways of responding to their infant's behavior.

• identify ways to help their infant overcome his behavioral disturbance.

• identify ways to improve their ability to cope with the infant's responses.

• identify resources for help with their infant.

■ Infant behavior, potential for enhanced organization

Definition

State in which an infant's behavioral development is satisfactory but can be improved

Assessment

• Cardiovascular status, including infant's pulse, respirations

• Gastrointestinal status, including feeding pattern, food tolerance, defecation pattern, ability to maintain adequate weight, abdominal distention, abdominal bloating

• Neurologic status, including excessive crying, poor sleep patterns, lethargy, irritability, seizures, tremors, muscle tone, newborn reflexes; Brazelton Neonatal Behavioral Assessment, Dubowitz Gestational Age Assessment

• Sensory status, including infant's responsiveness to visual, tactile, or auditory stimuli; experience with pain

• Sleep status, including usual hours of sleep

• Parental status, including knowledge of normal growth and development

• Parents' psychological status, including energy level, motivation, experience with children, eye contact and interaction with infant, Home Observation Measurement of the Environment

Defining characteristics

• Evidence of behavioral development in an infant, such as:
  – definite sleep-wake states

– the ability to be consoled and calmed down and to respond positively to parents
– responsiveness to visual and auditory stimuli
– stable physiologic measures

Associated disorders
This plan of care may apply to any infant.

Expected outcomes
• Parents express understanding of their role in their infant's behavioral development.
• Parents express confidence in their ability to interpret behavioral cues from their infant.
• Parents identify means to promote the infant's behavioral development.
• Parents express positive feelings about their ability to care for their infant.

Interventions and rationales
• Explain to the parents that infant maturation is a developmental process. Further explain that infants exhibit three behavioral states: sleeping, crying, and being awake and alert. Also explain that infants provide behavioral cues that indicate their needs. *Education will help parents understand the importance of nurturing the infant and prepare them to respond to the infant's behavioral cues.*
• Explain to the parents that their actions can help promote infant development. Make it clear, however, that infant maturation is not completely within their control. *This explanation may decrease feelings of anxiety and incompetence and help to prevent unrealistic expectations.*
• Demonstrate appropriate ways of interacting with the infant, such as moderate stimulation, gentle rocking, and quiet vocalizations, *to assist parents in identifying the most effective methods of interacting with their child.*
• Help the parents interpret behavioral cues from their infant *to foster healthy parent-child interaction.* For example, help them recognize when the infant is awake and alert and point out to them that this is a good time to provide stimulation.
• Assist the parents in identifying ways they can promote their infant's development, such as providing stimulation by shaking a rattle in front of the infant, talking to the infant in a gentle voice, and looking at the infant when feeding him *to encourage practices that promote the infant's development. Sensory experiences promote cognitive development.*
• Explore with the parents ways to cope with the stress caused by the infant's behavior *to increase their coping skills.*
• Praise the parents for their attempts to enhance their interaction with the infant to provide positive reinforcement.
• Provide the parents with information on sources of support and special infant services *to encourage them to continue to foster their infant's development.*

Evaluation statements
Parents:
• express an understanding of their infant's behavioral development.
• express confidence in their ability to recognize behavioral cues from their infant.
• identify activities that foster positive responses from their infant.
• provide appropriate sensory and tactile stimulation for their infant.
• identify resources for help with their infant.

Infant behavior, risk for disorganization

related to pain, prematurity, oral problems, motor problems, feeding intolerance, environmental overstimulation, or lack of stimulation

Definition
Risk for behavioral disturbance in an infant. "Disorganized infant behavior" is a term used to describe difficulty in infant behavioral or neurologic development which may lead to problems with

the infant's ability to relate to the environment and interfere with parent-infant attachment.

Assessment

- Cardiovascular status, including infant's pulse, respirations
- Gastrointestinal status, including infant's feeding pattern, defecation pattern, food tolerance, ability to maintain adequate weight, abdominal bloating, abdominal distention
- Neurologic status, including muscle tone, newborn reflexes, excessive crying, lethargy, irritability, seizures, tremors; Brazelton Neonatal Behavioral Assessment, Dubowitz Gestational Age Assessment
- Sensory status, including infant's responsiveness to visual, tactile, or auditory stimuli; experience with pain
- Sleep status, including sleep pattern, usual hours of sleep
- Parental status, including knowledge of normal growth and development
- Parents' psychological status, including energy level, motivation, experience with children, eye contact and interaction with infant

Risk factors

- Factors that may disturb an infant's behavioral development, such as:
  - environmental overstimulation
  - invasive or painful procedures
  - oral or motor problems
  - pain
  - prematurity
  - lack of stimulation or physical contact

Associated disorders

Colic, prematurity, failure to thrive

Expected outcomes

- Parents identify factors that place their infant at risk for a behavioral disturbance.
- Parents identify potential signs of behavioral disturbance in their infant.
- Parents describe appropriate ways to interact with their infant.
- Parents identify their reactions to their infant (including ways of coping with occasional frustration and anger).
- Parents express positive feelings about their ability to care for their infant.

Interventions and rationales

- Explain to the parents that infant maturation is a developmental process and that their participation is crucial *to help them understand the importance of nurturing the infant.*
- Explain to the parents that their actions can help modify some of their infant's behavior. However, make it clear that infant maturation is not completely within their control. *This explanation will decrease parents' feelings of incompetence.*
- Explain to the parents that certain risk factors may interfere with the infant's ability to achieve optimal development. These risk factors include overstimulation, lack of stimulation, lack of physical contact, or painful medical procedures. *Educating the parents will help them understand their role in interpreting the infant's behavioral cues and providing appropriate stimulation.*
- Describe for the parents the potential signs of a behavioral disturbance in an infant:
  - inappropriate responses to stimuli, such as failure to respond to human contact or a tendency to become agitated with human contact
  - physiologic regulatory problems, such as a breathing disturbance in a premature infant
  - apparent inability to interact with the environment.

Education will help the parents recognize if their infant has a problem in behavioral development.

- Demonstrate appropriate ways of interacting with the infant *to assist parents in identifying and interpreting the infant's behavioral cues and in responding appropriately.* For example, help them recognize when the baby is awake and alert, and help them understand when the baby needs more stimulation, such as being spoken to or being held.

• Explore with parents ways to cope with the stress imposed by the infant's behavior *to increase their coping skills.* Help them identify their emotional responses to the infant's behavior *to help them recognize and adjust their response patterns.* Explain that it's normal for parents to experience feelings of inadequacy, frustration, or anger if their infant doesn't respond positively to them.
• Praise the parents when they demonstrate appropriate methods of interacting with the infant *to provide positive reinforcement.*
• Provide the parents with information on sources of support and special infant services *to help them cope with the infant's long-term needs.*

Evaluation statements

Parents:
• identify risk factors for behavioral disturbance.
• identify potential signs of a behavioral disturbance in their infant.
• identify actions that promote their infant's development.
• report improvement in their ability to cope with the stress of raising an infant.
• identify resources for help with their infant.

Intracranial adaptive capacity, decreased

Definition

A state in which physiologic mechanisms that normally compensate for increased intracranial volumes are compromised, resulting in disproportionate increases in intracranial pressure (ICP) in response to stimuli

Assessment

• Cardiovascular status, including vital signs; skin color and temperature; carotid and apical pulses, heart sounds; jugular vein distention; electrocardiography; history of hypertension
• Gastrointestinal status, including bowel patterns; dietary intake; abdominal inspection, palpation, and auscultation
• Musculoskeletal status, including range of motion (ROM); joint and muscle symmetry; muscle size, strength, and tone; functional mobility; contractures, subluxation, dislocation, atrophy; previous trauma, degenerative joint diseases
• Neurologic status, including mental status; cranial nerve function; cerebellar function; reflexes (deep tendon, superficial, and pathological [Babinski's reflex]); peripheral sensory system (pain, position, and vibration); pupillary size and reactivity; use of anticonvulsant, neuroleptic, antidepressant, antimanic, analgesic, or illicit drugs; history of head injury; alcohol abuse; lethargy, restlessness, stupor, headaches, seizures, tremors, paresthesia, paresis, incoordination, ticks, fasciculation, pain, abnormal posturing (decorticate or decerebrate); computed tomography scan, magnetic resonance imaging, cerebral arteriography, electroencephalography, evoked potential studies, Glasgow Coma Scale
• Respiratory status, including chest expansion; rate, depth, and pattern of respirations; tracheal position; fremitus; auscultation of lung fields; arterial blood gas (ABG) analysis, pulse oximetry, mixed venous oxygen saturation; history of lung disease; tobacco use; use of bronchodilators, antibiotics, diuretics
• Sensory status, including visual acuity, auditory acuity, use of hearing aid or glasses, tactile sensitivity eye disorders, hearing loss, psychiatric disorders

Defining characteristics

• ICP monitoring that reveals:
  – baseline ICP equal to or greater than 10 mm Hg; wide amplitude ICP waveform
  – disproportionate increase in ICP following single nursing maneuver
  – elevated P2 ICP waveform
  – volume pressure response test variation (volume-pressure ratio greater

than 2, pressure-volume index less than 10)
– repeated increases in ICP exceeding 10 mm Hg for more than 5 minutes following external stimuli

Associated disorders
Arteriovenous malformation, brain injuries, brain tumors, cerebral abscesses and aneurysms, cerebral hypoxia, cerebral ischemia, cerebrovascular accident, cranial surgery, hydrocephalus, intracranial hemorrhage, Reye's syndrome

Expected outcomes
• Patient maintains a patent airway.
• Patient maintains effective breathing patterns.
• Patient maintains normal ABG levels.
• Patient shows no evidence of fever.
• Patient's position facilitates venous drainage from the brain.
• Patient does not experience a sustained rise in ICP in response to stimulation.
• Patient's environment is modified to reduce noxious stimuli.
• Patient maintains regular bowel function.
• Patient maintains skin integrity.
• Patient remains free of signs and symptoms of infection.
• Patient shows no evidence of neurologic compromise.
• Patient and family members express feelings about treatment and recovery.

Interventions and rationales
• Perform a thorough nursing history and head-to-toe assessment and document *to establish a baseline of the patient's condition for future comparison and to ensure continuity and consistency of care among nursing staff.*
• Monitor neurologic status, including level of consciousness, pupillary size and reactivity, eye movement, selected reflexes, and motor and sensory function *to identify changes indicative of increased ICP.*
• Monitor vital signs and hemodynamic parameters (mean arterial blood pressure, pulmonary artery pressure) *to assess hemodynamic stability and to note trends.*
• Maintain ICP monitoring systems, if used. Use aseptic technique for dressing changes. Maintain a closed system. *Aseptic technique prevents contamination of equipment and subsequent infections.*
• Monitor ICP waveforms for trends over time (A waves, B waves, C waves). Assess intracranial pulse waves (P1 percussion waves, P2 tidal waves, P3 dicrotic waves). Monitor for damped waveforms, absent waveforms, or abnormally high or low readings. *Waveforms provide information about cerebral compliance. Cerebral compliance is the body's attempt to cope with changes in intracranial content (brain tissue, blood volume, and cerebral spinal fluid). Compliance is expressed as a mathematical ratio between volume and pressure changes within the skull.*
• Assess cerebral perfusion pressure. *Adequate cerebral perfusion pressure is critical to prevent cerebral ischemia. Cerebral perfusion pressure is calculated by taking the mean arterial pressure and subtracting the ICP.*
• Assess temperature every 2 hours. *Fever increases cerebral metabolic demands, cerebral blood flow, and ICP.*
• Maintain a patent airway. Assess rate, depth, and rhythm of respirations *to monitor lung expansion and presence of abnormal sounds.*
• Suction the patient only if needed. Limit suctioning to 10 to 15 seconds per pass of the catheter. *Suctioning stimulates coughing and Valsalva's maneuver; Valsalva's maneuvers increase intrathoracic pressure, decrease cerebral venous drainage, and increase cerebral blood volume, resulting in increased ICP.*
• Hyperoxygenate the lungs with 100% oxygen for 1 minute before and after suctioning. *Hypercapnia results in cerebral vasodilation, increased cerebral blood volume, and increased ICP. Preoxygenation helps avoid hypoxemia and tissue ischemia.*

- Administer lidocaine, if prescribed, I.V. or into the endotracheal (ET) tube before suctioning. *Lidocaine suppresses the cough reflex, thereby preventing increases in ICP.*
- Monitor ABG levels. Observe for signs and symptoms of respiratory distress. *Hypercapnia results in vasodilation, increased cerebral blood volume, and increased ICP. Hypoxia may contribute to tissue ischemia.*
- Elevate the head of the bed 15 to 30 degrees or as ordered. Keep the patient's head and neck straight. Use sandbags, rolled towels, or small pillows to keep the head in a neutral position. Avoid hip flexion of 90 degrees or more. *Neutral head position promotes venous drainage from the head. Some positions cause increased intra-abdominal and intrathoracic pressure that can interfere with venous drainage from the head.*
- When performing neurologic assessment, use the minimal amount of stimuli required to obtain a response. *Unpleasant or painful stimuli increase ICP.*
- Limit environmental noise as much as possible. Auditory stimuli can contribute *to increased ICP.*
- Monitor for seizure activity. Maintain seizure precautions. Administer anticonvulsant drugs as prescribed. *Tonic-clonic seizures increase intrathoracic pressure, decrease cerebral venous outflow, and increase cerebral blood volume, thereby raising ICP.*
- Maintain intake and output. Maintain fluid restriction, if ordered. *Fluid restriction assists in decreasing extracellular fluid from the body, thereby decreasing ICP.*
- Administer osmotic diuretics, if prescribed. Monitor for signs and symptoms of dehydration (increased sodium, serum osmolality, decreased urine output). *Osmotic diuretics are given to pull fluid from nonedematous areas of the brain, thereby decreasing ICP.*
- Administer loop diuretics, if prescribed, *to decrease water in injured brain tissue and to decrease overall body water, thereby reducing cerebral edema and lowering ICP.* Monitor for signs of dehydration and hypokalemia—*adverse effects of diuretics.*
- Turn and reposition the patient every 2 hours and as needed *to prevent pressure ulcer formation.*
- While turning, keep the patient's head in a neutral position *to promote venous drainage from the head.*
- Use a draw sheet for repositioning the patient. Instruct the patient to exhale, if conscious, when turning or moving in bed, *to avoid Valsalva maneuvers, which can increase ICP by increasing intrathoracic and intra-abdominal pressures.*
- Monitor and record bowel movements. Administer stool softeners, as prescribed. Instruct the patient not to hold his breath or strain on defecation. *Straining associated with constipation can cause a Valsalva's maneuver and resultant increases in ICP.*
- Instruct the patient, if he is able to follow simple commands, to avoid pushing against a footboard or digging heels into the mattress when moving up in bed. Remove footboards if possible, especially if the patient has decerebrate or abnormal posturing. *Isometric muscle contraction can increase ICP.*
- Perform passive ROM exercises *to maintain muscle tone and prevent atrophy and contractures.*
- Maintain normothermia. Administer antipyretics if ordered. Apply a hypothermia blanket. Assess rectal temperature every 30 minutes while on the blanket. Control shivering. Administer chlorpromazine if prescribed. *Shivering causes isometric muscle contraction, which can increase ICP.*
- Continue frequent neurologic assessment. Compare results with previous findings. *Frequent assessment allows for the detection of subtle changes in neurologic signs that indicate improvement or deterioration in the patient's status.*
- Try to limit painful procedures, if possible. Avoid unnecessary tension or pulling on tubes (ET tube, indwelling

urinary catheter). *Unpleasant or painful stimuli increase ICP.*
• Involve family members in gentle stroking of the patient's face, hand, or arm. *Recent studies have shown touch provided by family members may lower ICP in some patients.*
• Speak in a low, soft voice. Provide nursing care in a calm, reassuring manner. Explain all procedures before touching the patient. *Explanations can help prevent emotional upsets that may increase ICP.*
• Avoid discussion of upsetting topics near the patient's bedside. The patient may be upset by discussion of his prognosis, treatment procedures, or his level of pain. Instruct the patient's family members not to discuss upsetting topics within the patient's hearing range. *Emotional upsets may increase ICP.*
• Ask family members to bring in audiotapes of familiar voices and the patient's favorite music. Play audiotapes through earphones, if appropriate. *Family members' voices and preferred music have been shown to decrease ICP in some patients.*
• Provide uninterrupted rest periods as much as possible. Avoid awakening the patient during rapid eye movement (REM) sleep. *Cerebral blood flow increases during REM sleep.* Do not carry out nursing activities known to increase ICP during that time. *Nursing procedures performed during REM sleep may cause additional elevations in the patient's ICP.*
• Schedule sufficient time, at least 10 minutes, between nursing care activities (bathing, turning, suctioning) *to allow the patient to rest and to avoid cumulative effects of continuous activity on ICP. Close spacing of activities has been known to cause sustained increases of ICP.*
• Encourage the patient and family to ventilate feelings associated with diagnosis, treatment, and recovery. *Expression of feelings helps the patient and family cope with treatment.*
• Refer the patient and family to appropriate support groups *to assist them in dealing with the injury, diagnosis, or recovery.*

Evaluation statements

Patient:
• maintains effective breathing patterns, a patent airway, and normal ABG levels.
• shows no signs or symptoms of infection.
• maintains proper positioning to facilitate venous drainage from the brain.
• avoids Valsalva's maneuver.
• is free of constipation.
• has intact skin.
• shows no evidence of neurologic compromise or sustained increases in ICP.

Patient's environment:
• contains fewer noxious stimuli as a result of modifications.

Patient and family members:
• openly express fear, anxiety, anger, and other feelings associated with treatment and recovery.

Loneliness, risk for

Definition

A subjective state in which an individual is at risk for experiencing vague dysphoria associated with feelings of isolation from others

Assessment

• Family status, including family composition, presence of a spouse, ability of family to meet patient's physical and emotional needs; conflicts between patient's needs and the family's ability to meet them; feelings of self-worth of family members
• Psychological status, including changes in appetite, behavior, energy level, mood, motivation, self-image, self-esteem, or sleep patterns; alcohol and drug consumption; recent death, job loss, loss of loved one, or relocation; psychiatric history
• Social status, including interpersonal skills, size of social network, quality of relationships, degree of trust in others, level of self-esteem, ability to function

in social and occupational roles
• Health history, including medical illness, mental illness, disabilities, deformities
• Spiritual status, including religious or church affiliation; description of faith and religious practices; support network (family, clergy, friends)

Risk factors
• Deformity or disfigurement
• Difficulty in marriage or long-term relationship
• Geographic separation from family and friends
• Impaired mobility
• Lack of affiliation with social institutions
• Lack of participation in social activities
• Medical or psychiatric diagnosis that carries social stigma (for example, acquired immunodeficiency syndrome [AIDS], cancer, or schizophrenia)
• Physical isolation
• Poor health
• Poor interpersonal skills
• Poverty
• Recent divorce or death of loved one
• Recent relocation
• Troubled family relationships
• Unemployment

Associated disorders and treatments
AIDS, antisocial disorder, anxiety disorder, arthritis, attention-deficit hyperactivity disorder, cancer, cerebrovascular accident, communication disorder, conduct disorder, depression, eating disorder, head or neck surgery, herpes simplex type II, human immunodeficiency virus infection, incontinence, learning disorder, mental retardation, mood disorders, obsessive-compulsive disorder, oppositional defiant disorder, organic mental disorder, panic disorder, parent-child relational problem, Parkinson's disease, personality disorders, pervasive developmental disorder, *Pneumocystis carinii* pneumonia, posttraumatic stress disorder, relational problems, schizoaffective disorder, separation anxiety disorder, sexual dysfunction, spinal cord injuries, tuberculosis, vision loss

Expected outcomes
• Patient identifies feelings of loneliness and the desire to socialize more.
• Patient identifies behaviors that lead to loneliness.
• Patient identifies persons who are likely to be supportive and accepting of him.
• Patient spends times with others.
• Patient is comfortable in social settings, interacting with peers, and receives support from others.
• Patient makes specific plans to continue involvement with others, such as through recreational activities or social interaction groups.

Interventions and rationales
• Spend sufficient time with the patient to allow him to express his feelings of loneliness *to establish a trusting relationship.*
• Inform the patient that you will help him express feelings of loneliness and identify ways to increase social activity *to bring the issue into the open and help the patient understand that your goal is to help him.*
• Work with the patient in identifying factors and behaviors that have contributed to loneliness *to begin changing behaviors that may alienate others.*
• Help the patient identify feelings associated with loneliness *to lessen their impact and mobilize energy to counteract them.*
• Help the patient curb feelings of loneliness by encouraging one-on-one interaction with others who are likely to accept him – for example, church members or patients with similar health problems – *to promote feelings of acceptance and support.*
• Encourage the patient to address needs assertively. *By being assertive, the patient assumes responsibility for getting his needs met, without anger or guilt.*
• As the patient's comfort level improves, encourage him to attend group

activities and social functions *to promote use of social skills.*
- Help the patient identify social activities he can initiate, such as becoming active in a support group or volunteer organization, *to foster feelings of control and increase social contacts.*
- Help the patient accept the fact that other people may view him differently because of his illness and explore ways of coping with their reactions. *The stigma associated with illness is a reality and the patient must learn to cope with it.*
- Work with the patient in establishing goals for reducing feelings of loneliness once he leaves the health care setting *to focus energy on specific objectives.*
- Refer the patient and family to social service agencies, mental health center, and appropriate support groups *to ensure continued care and maintain social involvement.*

Evaluation statements

Patient:
- identifies problems associated with loneliness.
- attends and participates in group activities.
- initiates conversations with peers.
- describes coping mechanisms that can reduce feelings of loneliness.

Management of therapeutic regimen, effective individual

Definition

An effective pattern of regulating and integrating into daily life a program for treating illness and its sequelae

Assessment

- Family status, including marital status, family composition
- Psychological status, including changes in appetite, behavior, energy level, mood, motivation, self-image, sleep; alcohol and drug use; life changes; psychiatric history; blood and urine toxicology
- Self-care status, including ability to carry out voluntary activities; use of adaptive devices; neurologic, sensory, or psychological impairment
- Social status, including communication skills, size of social network, quality of relationships, degree of trust in others, ability to function in social and occupational roles
- Spiritual status, including religious or church affiliation, religious practices, support network (family, clergy, friends)

Defining characteristics

- Expressed desire to manage treatment and to reduce risk factors for progression of illness
- Appropriate choices made with regard to daily activities for meeting the goals of treatment or prevention program
- Symptoms within normal range

Expected outcomes

- Patient recognizes potential problems and can identify needs.
- Patient works toward establishing objectives to meet needs.
- Patient makes plans to ensure meeting future needs.

Interventions and rationales

- Help the patient identify needs, potential problems, and sources of stress *to maintain the highest level of well-being.*
- Help the patient identify the resources necessary to meet needs and develop strategies for using these resources *to solve problems.*
- Assist the patient in identifying major stressors in his life and which of his needs demand immediate attention. Help to establish priorities for addressing problems *to focus energy on important issues.*
- Once the patient has established priorities for addressing problems, help him to clarify those problems he seeks to have addressed first *to expedite resolving them.*
- Encourage the patient to contact appropriate agencies *so that they can give*

preventive care, reduce stress, and enhance the patient's well-being.
- Continue to monitor the patient's progress in identifying needs, problems, and stressors *to reinforce the patient's efforts to obtain maximum well-being.*
- Support the patient's plans for meeting future needs *to foster independence.*

Evaluation statements

Patient:
- establishes a plan to meet therapeutic needs.
- includes specific actions in the plan.
- makes changes to the plan that are beneficial in meeting needs and solving problems.

■ Management of therapeutic regimen, ineffective community

related to drug and alcohol abuse among teenagers

Definition

An unsatisfactory pattern of integrating programs for preventing and treating health problems into the community

Assessment
- Community demographics, including age and sex distribution, ethnic groups, education and income levels
- Prevalence of health problems in the community; availability of health care services; community use of health care services
- Drug and alcohol use among teenagers in high school, including reports of episodes of blackouts, injuries, accidents, mental health problems; reports from teachers (changes in student behaviors and attitudes, failing grades); increased incidence of school absenteeism, dropouts, encounters with the police and legal system; reports from school psychologist and counselors
- Problems that may be associated with drug and alcohol abuse, such as automobile accidents, homicides, suicides, domestic violence, burglaries, increased teenage pregnancy, sexually transmitted diseases, low-birth-weight neonates, and congenital abnormalities

Defining characteristics
- Absence of a drug or alcohol abuse clinic in the community
- Absence of programs for screening, counseling, treatment, and rehabilitation of drug and alcohol abuse
- Higher-than-normal incidence of health problems in the community
- High incidence of dysfunctional or single-parent families
- High incidence of family drug or alcohol abuse
- Lack of knowledge about the effects of drugs and alcohol
- Lack of recreational facilities
- Maladaptive behaviors, such as antisocial behavior and social isolation
- Perception on the part of teenagers that their use of alcohol and drugs does not constitute abuse
- Reports from teenagers that teachers and parents are uncaring, disapproving, or unavailable to help
- Unexpected acceleration of drug and alcohol abuse

Associated disorders

Adolescent antisocial behavior, alcoholism, mood disorders, oppositional defiant disorder, parent-child relational problem, substance-related disorders (intoxication, withdrawal, dependence, psychoses)

Expected outcomes
- Community members express the need for a plan to reduce the prevalence of drug and alcohol abuse.
- Community members develop a plan to reduce the prevalence of drug and alcohol abuse.
- Community members demonstrate an ongoing commitment to maintaining drug education and outreach programs for the benefit of local teenagers.
- Teenagers report an understanding of the negative effects of drug and alcohol abuse on their health, their families, and the community.

Interventions and rationales

- Implement an outreach and health promotion program *to raise community members' awareness of the need to approach drug and alcohol abuse as a community problem.* Consider taking the following steps:
  - working with teachers, school psychologists, counselors, students, and the parent-teacher association to educate parents and teenagers about the risk factors and signs and symptoms of drug abuse
  - placing anti-drug posters in local teenage hangouts
  - encouraging local youth groups, churches, and social service organizations to feature guest speakers on drug and alcohol abuse at their meetings
  - contacting representatives of local corporations and asking for funding for educational and recreational programs.
- Encourage community members to establish a drug and alcohol counseling program *to provide early identification of teenagers at high risk for drug and alcohol abuse.* Educate people who will be working with teenagers about the importance of remaining nonjudgmental and open-minded and of maintaining confidentiality *to foster trust.*
- Counsel teenagers to participate in outreach and health promotion programs *to allow for early identification, intervention, treatment, and anticipatory guidance.*
- Establish a school-based drug and alcohol education program *to provide knowledge regarding the risks of drug and alcohol abuse.* The drug and alcohol education program should include teaching about self-esteem issues, assertiveness skills, stress management, coping with peer pressure, and factual information about drugs and alcohol. Participation in recreational activities should also be part of the program. *To be effective, a drug and alcohol education program should use a holistic approach that confronts teenagers' emotional needs and encourages them to make informed choices.*
- Develop a learning packet for community residents *to increase the community's understanding of drug and alcohol abuse.* With this knowledge, parents and others can act as advocates for teenagers.
- Conduct a follow-up survey on drug and alcohol use *to measure the effectiveness of the screening, education, and treatment programs.*

Evaluation statements

Community members:

- express the need for a plan to reduce drug and alcohol abuse.
- develop a plan to reduce the incidence (new cases) and prevalence (current number of people with problem) of drug and alcohol abuse.
- establish an outreach and health promotion program.
- establish school-based drug and alcohol abuse programs.
- report an increased understanding of drug and alcohol abuse.

Teenagers:

- attend programs on self-esteem, assertiveness skills, and stress management.
- identify risk factors and signs and symptoms of drug and alcohol abuse.
- discuss ways of coping with peer pressure and other stressors.
- discuss the dangers of drug and alcohol abuse.
- participate in newly established school recreational activities.
- report an increased understanding of the negative effects of drug and alcohol use on their health, their families, and the community.

■ Management of therapeutic regimen, ineffective family

related to family conflict, complex therapy, economic difficulties, or difficulty coping with the health care system

Definition

Difficulty integrating measures to cope with illness into a family's daily routine

Assessment

- Family status, including marital status, family composition, communication patterns, coping skills, drug or alcohol abuse, psychiatric history, beliefs and attitudes about health and illness
- Health status, including chronic or terminal illness, severely disabling physical conditions
- Socioeconomic factors, including family's financial status, insurance, accessibility of health care, availability of health care providers, transportation system
- Social status, including communication skills, size of social network, degree of trust in others, level of self-esteem, ability to function in social and occupational roles
- Spiritual status, including religious or church affiliation, description of faith and religious practices

Defining characteristics

- Accelerated illness of family member
- Desire to manage treatment
- Difficulty with regulating or integrating treatment
- Family activities that are not conducive to meeting the goals of treatment or prevention
- Inattention to illness or its sequelae
- Presence of risk factors for progression of illness

Associated disorders

Adolescent adjustment disorder, acquired immunodeficiency syndrome, arthritis, attention-deficit hyperactivity disorder, cancer, chronic obstructive pulmonary disease, coronary artery disease, eating disorders, Parkinson's disease, posttraumatic stress disorder, renal failure, spinal cord injury, substance abuse

Expected outcomes

- Family members participate in family therapy sessions.
- Family members openly express feelings regarding illness of relative.
- Family members express desire to have assistance in resolving conflicts.
- Family members identify behaviors that lead to conflict.
- Family members demonstrate an increased ability to assert their needs in an appropriate manner.
- Family members cooperate in finding ways to incorporate therapeutic regimen into their lifestyle.
- Family members establish goals and strategies for coping with future conflict.
- Family members plan for future course of illness.

Interventions and rationales

- Spend time with the family, get to know each family member individually, and establish a trusting relationship with each family member *to help identify measures that will increase family cohesiveness.*
- Encourage family members to attend and participate in family therapy sessions *to strengthen the family unit and promote resolution of conflict.*
- Help the family members describe feelings associated with the illness of their relative *to bring family conflict into the open. Unresolved family conflicts may prevent family members from fully implementing the therapeutic regimen.*
- Elicit family members' personal beliefs about illness and review relevant information *to establish their support for improving management of therapeutic regimen.*
- Educate family members about pathophysiology of illness and explain relationship between pathophysiology and therapeutic regimen. *If family members know the reasons for specific behaviors, they may be more willing to adjust their lifestyle.*
- Work with family members to identify behaviors that have contributed to family conflict and to help them identify alternative behaviors *to promote resolution of the conflict.*
- Encourage family members to address individual needs in an assertive manner to *promote healthy interactions within their family.*

• Help family members clarify values associated with their lifestyle *to enhance understanding of conflicts between their lifestyle and the demands of the therapeutic regimen.*
• Work with family members to develop a daily routine for managing the therapeutic regimen that fits with their lifestyle. *Collaboration with family members makes it possible to incorporate lifestyle factors, such as culture, family dynamics, and finances, into the plan for managing illness.*
• Assist family members in modifying factors (such as lack of supportive behaviors among family members) that interfere with treatment management *to enhance the level of care.*
• Work with the family in establishing goals for coping with conflicts *to focus their energy on achievable objectives and foster hope.*
• Refer the family members to appropriate agencies, if needed. *This can ensure continued family support and help reduce conflicts.*
• Help family members plan for the future course of the illness. *Planning enhances the family members' abilities to develop an appropriate strategy to manage the therapeutic regimen.*

Evaluation statements

Family members:
• identify unresolved conflicts.
• attend and participate in family therapy sessions.
• express a desire to resolve conflicts.
• describe coping mechanisms that can reduce conflicts.
• successfully incorporate components of the therapeutic regimen into daily activities.
• carry out the therapeutic regimen.
• establish a plan for coping with the future course of illness.

Memory impairment

Definition

Inability to remember or recall bits of information or behavioral skills

Assessment

• Age, sex, level of education, occupation, living arrangements
• Cardiovascular status, including vital signs, apical pulse, pulse rate and rhythm, heart sounds; color of skin, lips, and nails; fatigue on exertion, dyspnea, dizziness; history of hypertension, chest pain, anoxia; complete blood count and differential, thyroid studies, electrocardiography, echocardiography
• Family status, including marital status, household composition; presence of a spouse; length of marriage, divorce, or widowhood
• Neurologic status, including mental status (abstract thinking, insight regarding present situation, judgment, long- and short-term memory, cognition, orientation to person, place, and time), level of consciousness, sensory ability, fine and gross motor functioning; history of neurologic disorder, head injury, or psychiatric illness; medication use; computed tomography scan, magnetic resonance imaging, cerebral angiography, electroencephalography, toxicology studies, thyroid function, serotonin levels
• Psychological status, including changes in appetite, behavior, energy level, mood, motivation, self-image, self-esteem, sleep patterns; alcohol and drug consumption; recent divorce, separation, death, job loss, loss of loved one, relocation, or physical or emotional trauma; psychiatric history
• Self-care status, including ability to carry out voluntary activities, use of adaptive equipment

Associated disorders

Alzheimer's disease, atherosclerosis, cerebral aneurysm, cerebrovascular accident, concussion, epilepsy, head injury, human immunodeficiency virus infection, multi-infarct dementia, multiple sclerosis, organic brain disorders, substance abuse, transient ischemic attacks

Defining characteristics
- Confabulation
- Confusion
- Decreased social skills
- Denial of memory loss
- Disorientation
- Distortions
- Labile affect
- Loss of intellectual ability
- Poor memory and judgment

Expected outcomes
- Patient expresses feelings about memory impairment.
- Patient acknowledges the need to take measures to cope with memory impairment.
- Patient identifies coping skills to deal with memory impairment.
- Patient and family members state specific plans to modify lifestyle.
- Patient and family members establish realistic goals to deal with further loss of memory.

Interventions and rationales
- Observe the patient's thought processes during every shift. Document and report any changes. *Changes may indicate progressive improvement or a decline in the patient's underlying condition.*
- Implement appropriate safety measures to protect the patient from injury. *He may be unable to provide for his own safety needs.*
- Call the patient by name and tell him your name. Provide background information (place, time, date) frequently throughout the day *to provide reality orientation.* Use a reality orientation board *to visually reinforce reality orientation.*
- Spend sufficient time with the patient to allow him to become comfortable discussing memory loss *to establish a trusting relationship.*
- Inform the patient that you are aware of his memory loss and that you will help him cope with his condition *to bring the issue into the open and help the patient understand that your goal is to help him.*
- Be clear, concise, and direct in establishing goals *so that the patient can maximize use of his remaining cognitive skills.*
- Offer short, simple explanations to the patient each time you carry out any medical or nursing procedure *to avoid confusion.*
- Label the patient's personal possessions and photos, keeping them in the same place as much as possible, *to reduce confusion and create a secure environment.*
- Encourage the patient to develop a consistent routine for performing activities of daily living *to enhance his self-esteem and increase his self-awareness and awareness of environment.*
- Teach the patient ways to cope with memory loss—for example, using a beeper to remind him when to eat or take medications, using a pillbox organized by days of the week, keeping lists in notebooks or a pocket calendar, or having family members or friends remind him of important tasks. *Reminders help to limit the amount of information the patient must maintain in his memory.*
- Encourage the patient to interact with others *to increase social involvement, which may decline with memory loss.*
- Encourage the patient to express feelings associated with impaired memory *to reduce the impact of memory impairment on the patient's self-image and to lessen anxiety.*
- Help the patient and family members establish goals for coping with memory loss. Discuss with family members the need to maintain the least restrictive environment possible. Instruct them on how to maintain a safe home environment for the patient. *This helps ensure that the patient's needs are met and promotes his independence.*
- Demonstrate reorientation techniques to family members and provide time for supervised return demonstrations *to prepare them to cope with the patient with memory impairment.*
- Help family members identify appropriate community support groups, men-

tal health services, and social service agencies *to assist in coping with the effects of the patient's illness or injury.*

Evaluation statements

Patient:
- identifies problems associated with memory loss.
- attends and participates in group activities.
- describes mechanisms for coping with memory loss.
- adapts skills that help strengthen memory.

Parent-infant or parent-child attachment, risk for altered

Definition

Disrupted interaction between parents and an infant or child that interferes with the development of a protective, nurturing relationship

Assessment

- Family status, including marital status, composition of family, ages of family members, ability of family to meet physical and emotional needs of its members, evidence of abuse, health history
- Parental status, including level of education, knowledge of normal growth and development, stability of relationship, available support systems
- Parents' psychological status, including energy level, motivation, recent life changes, psychiatric history, maternal history of drug abuse, alcohol or antidepressant use by either partner
- Infant's neurologic status, including muscle tone, reflexes; infant lethargy, irritability, seizures, tremors; Brazelton Neonatal Behavioral Assessment, Dubowitz Gestational Age Assessment; Bayley Scales of Infant Development
- Infant's sensory status, including vision or hearing loss; visual and auditory-evoked potentials, audiometric tests
- Sleep pattern, including infant's usual hours of sleep

Risk factors

- Anxiety over parental role
- Illness in the infant or child that doesn't allow initiation of contact with parents
- Inability of parents to meet their personal needs
- Lack of privacy
- Physical barriers
- Prematurity of infant
- Separation
- Substance abuse

Associated disorders and conditions

Blindness, child abuse, hearing loss, persistent pervasive developmental disorder, prematurity

Expected outcomes

- Parents initiate positive interaction with infant, as evidenced by mutual responsiveness and eye contact.
- Parents touch the infant appropriately, call him by name, and speak to him.
- Infant responds by becoming calmer when touched and soothed by parents.
- Parents express confidence in their ability to respond to the infant's needs.
- Parents respond appropriately to the infant and express positive feelings about him.
- Parents express confidence in their ability to care for the infant at home.
- Parents recognize when assistance is needed.
- Infant responds positively to the parents.

Interventions and rationales

- Perform an ongoing assessment of parent and infant interaction *to evaluate whether parent-infant attachment is proceeding normally.*
- Speak positively about the infant in the parents' presence *to encourage the parents to develop a positive view of the infant.*
- Maintain eye contact with the infant when caring for him, talk to him, and touch him appropriately *to demonstrate for the parents healthy interactions with the infant.*
- Assist the parents in learning to understand behavioral cues from the in-

fant. For example, the infant may become fussy when he is ready for a nap or may pull his ear if he has an earache. *Developing a better understanding of their infant's behavior will decrease the parents' frustration and help them to care more effectively for their infant.*
• Provide the parents and the infant with privacy *to facilitate attachment.*
• Assess the parents' knowledge of infant care and development *to develop an appropriate teaching plan.*
• Assist and teach the parents to provide physical care for the infant *to increase their sense of competence and self-confidence.*
• Encourage the parents to make eye contact with the infant, caress and talk to him in a soothing tone, call him by name, and make positive remarks about him *to foster a healthy parent-child attachment and to help ensure the child's well-being.*
• Observe the parents; note whether their responses to the infant are appropriate. Complement them when they exhibit successful parenting skills *to increase their confidence.*
• Discuss life changes precipitated by the birth of an infant *to help the parents express their frustrations and feelings about role changes.* Topics may include altered finances, changes in living space, caretaking arrangements, and new roles and responsibilities for the parents and siblings.
• Provide the parents with sources of ongoing support and care *to ensure adequate follow-up.*
• Assess the home environment. Discuss adaptations that need to be made at home *to increase the parents' confidence about caring for the infant.*

Evaluation statements

Parents:
• exhibit positive responses to the infant, making eye contact with him, caressing and talking to him, calling him by name, and making positive remarks about him.
• respond to the infant's behavioral cues, provide stimulation when he is alert and ready, do not overstimulate him, and recognize when he needs to nap.
• provide usual infant care with confidence.
• talk to each other about the infant.
• express concerns and worries about the infant.
• state available resources for assistance.
• express their understanding of role changes and possible responses.

Infant:
• responds positively to the parents, shows interest in their faces, and becomes calm when soothed by them.
• feeds and sleeps well.

Spiritual well-being, potential for enhanced

Definition

Process of developing the inner self by interconnecting physical, psychological, and spiritual strengths

Assessment

• Spiritual status, including personal religious habits; religious or church affiliation; embarrassment at practicing religious rituals; beliefs opposed by family, peers, health care providers
• Health history, including medical conditions that change body image, chronic or terminal illness, debilitating disease
• Psychological status, including reactions to illness and disability, change in appetite, energy level, motivation, personal hygiene, self-image, sleep, sex drive; alcohol or drug abuse; moodiness; recent divorce, job loss, losses through separation or death; personality traits, relationships with peers
• Self-care status, including neurologic, musculoskeletal, sensory or psychological impairment; ability to carry out activities and adapt

- Family status, including marital status; communication patterns
- Nutritional status, including malabsorption or nutritional deficiencies, obesity, anorexia, bulimia, weight loss or gain, nausea, vomiting, fainting, constipation, diarrhea, pallor, irritability, cravings, food hoarding, alteration in personal habits such as exercise, drug and alcohol use, and use of laxatives
- Sleep pattern status, including hours of sleep, energy level before and after sleep, difficulty falling asleep, nocturnal awakening, early morning awakening, hypersomnia, insomnia, sleep pattern reversal

Defining characteristics
- Disturbance in belief system
- Inability to carry out religious practices due to medical illness or hospitalization
- Ineffective coping skills
- Loss of appetite, disturbed sleep pattern, changes in exercise and eating patterns
- Poor family communication and support regarding religious beliefs and expectations
- Statements indicating doubts about belief system and spiritual emptiness

Associated disorders and conditions
Alcoholism, anorexia, bipolar disorder, bulimia, chronic or terminal illness, depression, dyssomnia, malabsorption, obesity, parasomnia, sleep apnea, suicidal tendencies, any condition requiring surgery

Expected outcomes
- Patient discusses spiritual conflicts.
- Patient is provided with opportunity to meet with chosen religious authority.
- Patient is supported in his efforts to pursue enhanced spiritual well-being.
- Patient pursues religious or spiritual practices to the extent that he feels comfortable.
- Patient openly discusses effects of illness on his beliefs and other spiritual issues.
- Patient describes plan to continue to enhance spiritual well-being.
- Patient receives referrals for continued support.

Interventions and rationales
- Monitor for potential signs of spiritual distress that might harm the patient's well-being (altered self-care, sleep pattern disturbance, and change in exercise and eating habits) *to plan appropriate interventions.*
- Assess the significance of spirituality in the patient's life and in coping with illness. Note whether the patient participates in religious rituals, observes religious practices (such as prayer, meditation, or dietary restrictions), or wishes to discuss spiritual beliefs. Keep an open view of what constitutes spirituality. *Before the nurse can intervene in spiritual matters, she must determine if spirituality is significant for the patient.*
- Ask the patient if his illness has affected his spiritual outlook and tell him you are willing to help him address spiritual issues if he so wishes *to reduce isolation and help bring issues related to spiritual distress out into the open.*
- Ask the patient if he wishes to discuss spiritual concerns with a chosen religious authority *to allow access to expert spiritual care resources.*
- Encourage the patient to pursue spiritual questions. Reassure him that spiritual concerns are valid and that by strengthening his spirituality he can enhance his own overall well-being *to demonstrate acceptance.*
- Provide the patient with resources for coping with spiritual distress (such as referrals to religious or spiritual organizations or books on prayer and meditation) *to enhance his opportunity to attend to spiritual needs.* Make sure those selected are appropriate with regard to the patient's religious affiliation and spiritual beliefs *to demonstrate respect for his beliefs and values.* If you lack knowledge about the patient's be-

liefs and practices, consult his chosen religious authority *to best meet the patient's needs.*
- Help the patient arrange travel to a place selected for prayer, reflection, or contemplation. Use such resources as church-affiliated vans or volunteer escorts *to enhance the patient's contact with outside sources of support.*
- Demonstrate to the patient that you are willing to discuss issues related to spirituality, such as the patient's view of God, how illness has affected his religious beliefs, or how hospital stays affect his spiritual practices *to bring spiritual issues into the open.* Keep an open mind when listening. Keep the conversation focused on the patient's spiritual values and the role they play in recovering from illness and coping with changes in body image *to ensure that interaction between the nurse and patient remains therapeutic.*
- Discuss with the patient the importance of maintaining a healthy diet, getting regular exercise and sleep, and maintaining healthy interaction with family and friends. *A patient in spiritual distress may neglect his day-to-day well-being.*
- Praise the patient for taking time to attend to his spiritual needs and encourage him to continue to develop his spirituality once he leaves the health care setting *to provide continued encouragement.*
- Provide the patient with referrals to appropriate religious groups, spiritually-centered organizations, and social service organizations. Consider such resources as parish nurses, home-visiting services, and computer networks *to help provide continued opportunity for spiritual development and to ensure continuity of care.*

Evaluation statements

Patient:
- discusses spiritual conflicts.
- is provided with opportunity to meet with chosen religious authority.
- recognizes and verbalizes the support he's been given in his efforts to pursue enhanced spiritual well-being.
- pursues religious or spiritual practices to the extent he feels comfortable.
- discusses effects of illness on his beliefs and other spiritual issues openly.
- identifies the religious resources offered outside the hospital or agency.
- expresses increased confidence in his ability to cope with changes in body image and maintain spiritual values in the face of long-term or chronic illness
- maintains healthy eating pattern, exercise schedule, and sleep pattern.
- describes plan to continue to enhance spiritual well-being.

SELECTED REFERENCES

Behrman, R.E., and Kliegman, R., eds. *Nelson Textbook of Pediatrics,* 14th ed. Philadelphia: W.B. Saunders Co., 1992.

Better Documentation. Clinical Skillbuilders Series. Springhouse, Pa.: Springhouse Corp., 1992.

Betz, C.L., et al. *Family-Centered Nursing Care of Children,* 2nd ed. Philadelphia: W.B. Saunders Co., 1994.

Carroll-Johnson, R.M., ed. *Classification of Nursing Diagnoses: Proceedings of the Tenth Conference.* Philadelphia: J.B. Lippincott Co., 1994.

Carroll-Johnson, R.M., ed. *Classification of Nursing Diagnoses: Proceedings of the Ninth Conference.* Philadelphia: J.B. Lippincott Co., 1991.

Chenitz, W.C., et al., eds. *Clinical Gerontological Nursing.* Philadelphia: W.B. Saunders Co., 1991.

Cochran, I., et al. "Stroke Care: Piecing Together the Long-Term Picture," *Nursing94* 24(6):34-41, June 1994.

Cohen, S.M., et al. *Maternal, Neonatal, and Women's Health Nursing.* Springhouse, Pa.: Springhouse Corp., 1991.

Compton, P. "Drug Abuse: A Self-Care Deficit," *Journal of Psychosocial Nursing and Mental Health Services* 27(3):22-26, March 1989.

Craven, R.F., and Hirnle, C.J. *Fundamentals of Nursing: Human Health and Function.* Philadelphia: J.B. Lippincott Co., 1992.

Diagnostic and Statistical Manual of Mental Disorders, 4th ed. Washington, D.C.: American Psychiatric Association, 1994.

Diseases. Springhouse Pa.: Springhouse Corp., 1993.

Dolan, M.B. *Community and Home Health Care Plans.* Springhouse, Pa.: Springhouse Corp., 1990.

Dyer, J.G., et al. *Psychiatric Nursing Diagnoses.* Springhouse, Pa.: Springhouse Corp., 1995.

Eliopoulous, C. *Caring for the Elderly in Diverse Care Settings.* Philadelphia: J.B. Lippincott Co., 1990.

Fuller, J., and Schaller-Ayers, J. *Health Assessment: A Nursing Approach,* 2nd ed. Philadelphia: J.B. Lippincott Co., 1994.

Gilliss, C.L. "The Family Dimension of Cardiovascular Care," *Canadian Journal of Cardiovascular Nursing* 2(1):3-8, April 1991.

Gleeson, B. "After Myocardial Infarction: How to Teach a Patient in Denial," *Nursing91* 21(5):48-56, May 1991.

Gordon, M. *Nursing Diagnosis: Process and Application,* 3rd ed. St. Louis: Mosby-Year Book, 1994.

Grant, A.B. *The Professional Nurse: Issues and Actions.* Springhouse, Pa.: Springhouse Corp., 1994.

Handbook of Medical-Surgical Nursing. Springhouse, Pa.: Springhouse Corp., 1994.

Holzemer, W.L., et al. "Nursing Care Plans for Patients with HIV/AIDS: Confusion or Consensus?" *Journal of Advanced Nursing* 16(3):257-61, March 1991.

Ignatavicius, D.D., and Bayne, M.V. *Medical-Surgical Nursing: A Nursing Process Approach.* Philadelphia: W.B. Saunders Co., 1991.

Iyer, P.W., "Thirteen Charting Rules to Keep You Legally Safe, Part 1," *Nursing91* 21(6):40-45, June 1991.

Iyer, P.W., et al. *Nursing Process and Nursing Diagnosis,* 2nd ed. Philadelphia: W.B. Saunders Co., 1991.

Illustrated Manual of Nursing Practice, 2nd ed. Springhouse, Pa.: Springhouse Corp., 1994.

Jaffe, M.S., and Melson, K.A. *Maternal-Infant Health Care Planning,* 2nd ed. Springhouse, Pa.: Springhouse Corp., 1995.

Kenner, C.A. *Nurse's Clinical Guide to Neonatal Care.* Springhouse Pa.: Springhouse Corp., 1992.

Kerfoot, S.J. "An Adolescent 'Problem' Patient: Child or Adult?" *Rehabilitation Nursing* 18(6):400-401, November-December, 1993.

Kidd, P.S., et al., "Driving Practices, Risk-Taking Motivations, and Alcohol Use Among Adolescent Drivers: A Pilot Study," *Journal of Emergency Nursing* 19(4):292-96, August 1993.

Kirsch, E. "Treating Nursing's Response to Nursing Diagnosis," *Journal of Emergency Nursing* 17(3):125-26, June 1991.

Krupnick, S., and Wade, A. *Psychiatric Care Planning.* Springhouse, Pa.: Springhouse Corp., 1993.

Lubkin, I.M. *Chronic Illness: Impact and Interventions,* 2nd ed. Boston: Jones & Bartlett, 1990.

Maas, M., et al. *Nursing Diagnoses and Interventions for the Elderly.* Redwood City, Calif.: Addison-Wesley Nursing, 1991.

MacLaren, A. *Nurse's Clinical Guide to Maternity Care.* Springhouse, Pa.: Springhouse Corp., 1992.

Mastering Documentation. Springhouse, Pa.: Springhouse Corp., 1995.

McFarland, G.K., and Thomas, M.D. *Psychiatric Mental Health Nursing.* Philadelphia: J.B. Lippincott Co., 1991.

Meeker, M.H., and Rothrock, J.C., eds. *Alexander's Care of the Patient in Surgery,* 9th ed. St. Louis: Mosby-Year Book, Inc., 1991.

Musolf, J.M. "Easing the Impact of the Family Caregiver's Role," *Rehabilitation Nursing* 16(2):82-84, March-April 1991.

NANDA Nursing Diagnoses: Definitions and Classification. Philadelphia: North American Nursing Diagnosis Association, 1992.

Newman, D.K., and Smith, D.A.J. *Geriatric Care Plans.* Springhouse, Pa.: Springhouse Corp., 1991.

Nursing Procedures. Springhouse, Pa.: Springhouse Corp., 1992.

Nursing Process in Clinical Practice. Springhouse, Pa.: Springhouse Corp., 1993.

Phipps, W.J., et al. *Medical-Surgical Nursing: Concepts and Clinical Practice,* 4th ed. St. Louis: Mosby-Year Book, Inc., 1991.

Rothrock, J.C. *Perioperative Nursing Care Planning.* St. Louis: Mosby-Year Book, Inc., 1990.

Saba, V.K., and Zuckerman, A.E., "A New Home Health Classification Method," *Caring* 11(10):27-34, October 1992.

Seifert, P.C., and Grandusky, R.J. "Nursing Diagnoses: Their Use in Developing Care Plans," *AORN Journal* 51(4):1008-21, 1023-26, April 1990.

Standards and Recommended Practices for Perioperative Nursing. Denver: Association of Operating Room Nurses, 1991.

Standards of Clinical Nursing Practice. Kansas City, Mo.: American Nurses' Association, 1991.

Tackenberg, J. "Teaching Caregivers about Alzheimer's Disease," *Nursing92* 22(5):75-82, May 1992.

Taylor, C.M., and Sparks, S.M. *Nursing Diagnosis Cards,* 7th ed. Springhouse, Pa.: Springhouse Corp., 1993.

Tirk, J.E. "Determining Discharge Priorities," *Nursing92* 22(7):55, July 1992.

Ufema, J. "Helping Loved Ones Say Goodbye," *Nursing91* 21(10):42-43, October 1991.

INDEX

Nursing diagnoses and related etiologies appear in italicized type.

Nursing diagnoses and related etiologies appear in italicized type.

D

E

F

Nursing diagnoses and related etiologies appear in italicized type.

Nursing diagnoses and related etiologies appear in italicized type.

T

Nursing diagnoses and related etiologies appear in italicized type.